Prostate Cancer Imaging
An Engineering and Clinical Perspective

Edited by
Ayman El-Baz
Gyan Pareek
Jasjit S. Suri

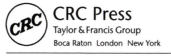

CRC Press
Taylor & Francis Group
Boca Raton London New York

CRC Press is an imprint of the
Taylor & Francis Group, an **informa** business

CRC Press
Taylor & Francis Group
6000 Broken Sound Parkway NW, Suite 300
Boca Raton, FL 33487-2742

© 2019 by Taylor & Francis Group, LLC
CRC Press is an imprint of Taylor & Francis Group, an Informa business

No claim to original U.S. Government works

Printed in Canada on acid-free paper

International Standard Book Number-13: 978-1-4987-8623-2 (Hardback)

Visit the Taylor & Francis Web site at
http://www.taylorandfrancis.com

and the CRC Press Web site at
http://www.crcpress.com

Dedication

This book is dedicated with love and affection to my mother and father, whose loving spirit sustains me still.

Ayman El-Baz

This book is dedicated to my late parents, whose love will always be in my heart.

Jasjit S. Suri

This book is dedicated to Natwar Kumar Pareek—a great urologist, father and mentor, and to my loving wife Gina and two children Niki and Sonya.

Gyan Pareek

Contents

Preface

This book covers novel strategies of the state-of-the-art approaches for automated noninvasive systems for early prostate cancer diagnostics. Prostate cancer is the most frequently diagnosed malignancy after skin cancer and the second leading cause of male cancer-related deaths in the United States after lung cancer. However, early detection of prostate cancer increases chances of patients' survival. Generally, CAD systems analyze the prostate images in three steps: (i) prostate segmentation; (ii) prostate description or feature extraction, and (iii) classification of the prostate status.

Current diagnosing of prostate carcinoma combines digital rectal examination (DRE), prostate-specific antigen (PSA) blood test, and needle biopsy. Each of these techniques have their own shortcomings. The biopsy is the most precise, but is a highly invasive, expensive, and painful method for detecting prostate cancer and determining its aggressiveness. Therefore accurate, highly sensitive and specific, but noninvasive diagnostic techniques are in significant demand. Today's CAD systems analyze images from various modalities, such as ultrasound, computed tomography (CT), and MRI, to detect and localize prostate cancer, as well as evaluate its size and extent.

The main aim of this book is to help advance scientific research within the broad field of early detection of prostate cancer. This book focuses on major trends and challenges in this area, and it presents work aimed at identifying new techniques and their use in biomedical image analysis.

Ayman El-Baz
Gyan Pareek
Jasjit S. Suri

Acknowledgements

The completion of this book could not have been possible without the participation and assistance of so many people whose names may not all be enumerated. Their contributions are sincerely appreciated and gratefully acknowledged. However, the editors would like to express their deep appreciation and indebtedness particularly to Dr. Ali H. Mahmoud and Dr. Ahmed M. Shalaby for their endless support. We would like to further thank all the collaborators, which include engineers, scientists, and physicians from industries and academics all around the globe for their friendship and support. Lastly, we would like to thank our families for their constant love, support and understanding.

Ayman El-Baz
Gyan Pareek
Jasjit S. Suri

Editors

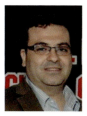

Ayman El-Baz is a Professor, University Scholar, and Chair of the Bioengineering Department at the University of Louisville, Kentucky. Dr. El-Baz earned his bachelor's and master's degrees in Electrical Engineering in 1997 and 2001, respectively. He earned his doctoral degree in electrical engineering from the University of Louisville in 2006. In 2009, Dr. El-Baz was named a Coulter Fellow for his contributions to the field of biomedical translational research. Dr. El-Baz has 15 years of hands-on experience in the fields of bio-imaging modeling and noninvasive computer-assisted diagnosis systems. He has authored or coauthored more than 450 technical articles (105 journals, 15 books, 50 book chapters, 175 refereed-conference papers, 100 abstracts, and 15 US patents).

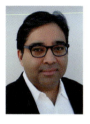

Gyan Pareek is the Director of Minimally Invasive Urologic Surgery, and Assistant Professor of Surgery (Urology) at the Alpert Medical School of Brown University. Dr. Pareek has been a full-time faculty member since completing his Minimally Invasive and Endourology fellowship at the University of Wisconsin in 2005. Dr. Pareek is the director of the Brown medical student urology course (URO-415). He is particularly passionate about resident teaching and is actively involved with the residents as a clinical and research mentor through the Brown Medical Student Mentoring Program. Dr. Pareek is a member of the urology staff at Rhode Island Hospital, Miriam Hospital, Providence VA Medical Center, and Memorial Hospital of Rhode Island.

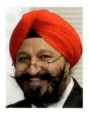

Jasjit S. Suri is an innovator, scientist, visionary, industrialist, and internationally known leader in biomedical engineering. Dr. Suri has spent over 24 years in the field of biomedical engineering/devices and its management. He received his doctorate from the University of Washington, Seattle, and his MBA from Weatherhead, Case Western Reserve University, Cleveland, Ohio. Dr. Suri was awarded the President's Gold medal in 1980 and the Fellow of American Institute of Medical and Biological Engineering for his outstanding contributions.

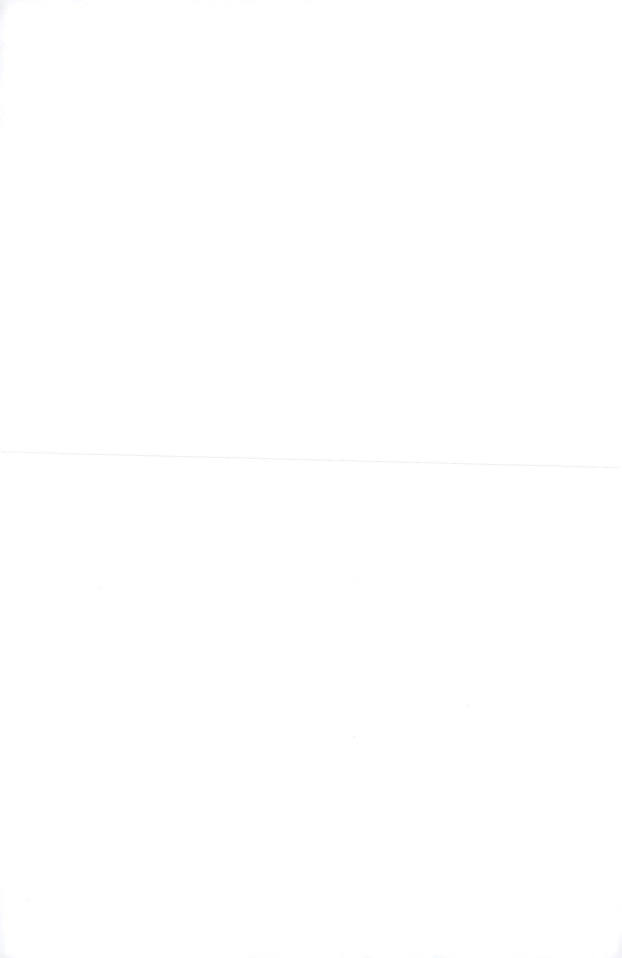

Contributors

Ahmed Aboulfotouh
Faculty of Computers and Information
Mansoura University
Mansoura, Egypt

Ruba Alkadi
Khalifa University of Science and Technology
Abu Dhabi, United Arab Emirates

Murali K. Ankem
Department of Urology
University of Louisville School of Medicine
Louisville, Kentucky

Winston Barzell
Urology Treatment Center
Sarasota, Florida

Jonathan B. Bloom
Urologic Oncology Branch
Center for Cancer Research
National Cancer Institute
National Institutes of Health
Bethesda, Maryland

Joseph Brito
Division of Urology
Rhode Island Hospital and The Miriam
    Hospital
Providence, Rhode Island

H. Abraham Chiang
Department of Urology
Brigham and Women's Hospital
Harvard Medical School
Boston, Massachusetts

Adnan Dervishi
Department of Urology
University of Louisville School of Medicine
Louisville, Kentucky

A. El-Baz
Electronics and Communication Engineering
    Department
Mansoura University
Mansoura, Egypt

Ayman El-Baz
BioImaging Laboratory
Bioengineering Department
University of Louisville
Louisville, Kentucky

Mohamed Abou El-Ghar
Radiology Department
Urology and Nephrology Center
Mansoura University
Mansoura, Egypt

Adel Elmagharaby
Department of Computer Engineering and
    Computer Science
University of Louisville
Louisville, Kentucky

Moumen El-Melegy
Department of Computer Engineering
Assiut University
Asyut, Egypt

Mohammed Elmogy
Faculty of Computers and Information
Mansoura University
Mansoura, Egypt

and

BioImaging Laboratory
Bioengineering Department
University of Louisville
Louisville, Kentucky

Sammy Elsamra
Department of Urology
Robert Wood Johnson Medical School
New Brunswick, New Jersey

Jennifer Fantasia
Warren Alpert Medical School of Brown
    University
and
Division of Urology
Rhode Island Hospital and The Miriam
    Hospital
Providence, Rhode Island

Baowei Fei
Department of Radiology and Imaging
    Sciences
Emory University School of Medicine
Atlanta, Georgia

Dagan Feng
Biomedical & Multimedia Information
    Technology (BMIT) Research Group
School of Information Technologies
The University of Sydney
New South Wales, Australia

Boris Gershman
Warren Alpert Medical School of Brown
    University
and
Division of Urology
Rhode Island Hospital and The Miriam
    Hospital
and
Minimally Invasive Urology Institute
The Miriam Hospital
Providence, Rhode Island

Valentina Giannini
Candiolo Cancer Institute (FPO-IRCCS)
Candiolo, Italy

and

Department of Surgical Sciences
University of Turin
Turin, Italy

Samuel A. Gold
Urologic Oncology Branch
Center for Cancer Research
National Cancer Institute
National Institutes of Health
Bethesda, Maryland

Dragan Golijanin
Warren Alpert Medical School of Brown
    University
and
Division of Urology
Rhode Island Hospital and The Miriam
    Hospital
and
Minimally Invasive Urology Institute
The Miriam Hospital
Providence, Rhode Island

D. Grand
Department of Radiology
Brown Medical School
Providence, Rhode Island

Scott Greenberg
Department of Urology
University of Massachusetts Medical School
University of Massachusetts Memorial Health
    Care
Worcester, Massachusetts

Graham R. Hale
Urologic Oncology Branch
Center for Cancer Research
National Cancer Institute
National Institutes of Health
Bethesda, Maryland

George E. Haleblian
Department of Urology
Brigham and Women's Hospital
Harvard Medical School
Boston, Massachusetts

Daniel Kaplon
Urology Treatment Center
Sarasota, Florida

Mohamed Khadra
Department of Urology at the Nepean Hospital
and
Sydney Medical School Nepean
The University of Sydney
New South Wales, Australia

F. Khalifa
Electronics and Communication Engineering
    Department
Mansoura University
Mansoura, Egypt

and

Bioengineering Department
University of Louisville
Louisville, Kentucky

Jinman Kim
Biomedical & Multimedia Information
    Technology (BMIT) Research Group
School of Information Technologies
The University of Sydney
New South Wales, Australia

Guillaume Lemaître
CDS Paris-Saclay, Parietal team, Inria, CEA
Université Paris-Saclay
Palaiseau, France

Changyang Li
Biomedical & Multimedia Information
    Technology (BMIT) Research Group
School of Information Technologies
The University of Sydney
New South Wales, Australia

Daniel Margolis
Weill Cornell Medicine
Weill Cornell Imaging
New York-Presbyterian
New York City, New York

Robert Martí
Computer Vision and Robotics Group
    (ViCOROB)
Universitat de Girona
Girona, Spain

Simone Mazzetti
Candiolo Cancer Institute (FPO-IRCCS)
Candiolo, Italy

and

Department of Surgical Sciences
University of Turin
Turin, Italy

Patrick McClure
BioImaging Laboratory
Bioengineering Department
University of Louisville
Louisville, Kentucky

Timothy D. McClure
Weill Cornell Medicine
Lefrak Center for Robotic Surgery
New York City, New York

Fabrice Meriaudeau
CISIR, Electrical & Electronic Engineering
    Department
Universiti Teknologi Petronas
Seri Iskandar, Malaysia

Gyan Pareek
Department of Urology
Brown Medical School
Providence, Rhode Island

Rutveej Patel
Department of Urology
Robert Wood Johnson Medical School
New Brunswick, New Jersey

Sutchin R. Patel
Department of Urology
University of Wisconsin School of Medicine
    and Public Health
Madison, Wisconsin

J. Pereira
Department of Urology
Brown Medical School
Providence, Rhode Island

Peter A. Pinto
Urologic Oncology Branch
Center for Cancer Research
National Cancer Institute
National Institutes of Health
Bethesda, Maryland

Kareem N. Rayn
Urologic Oncology Branch
Center for Cancer Research
National Cancer Institute
National Institutes of Health
Bethesda, Maryland

Islam Reda
Faculty of Computers and Information
Mansoura University
Mansoura, Egypt

and

BioImaging Laboratory
Bioengineering Department
University of Louisville
Louisville, Kentucky

Daniele Regge
Candiolo Cancer Institute (FPO-IRCCS)
Candiolo, Italy

and

Department of Surgical Sciences
University of Turin
Turin, Italy

Joseph Renzulli, II
Warren Alpert Medical School of Brown
    University
and
Division of Urology
Rhode Island Hospital and The Miriam
    Hospital
and
Minimally Invasive Urology Institute
The Miriam Hospital
Providence, Rhode Island

Filippo Russo
Candiolo Cancer Institute (FPO-IRCCS)
Candiolo, Italy

Peter N. Schlegel
Weill Cornell Medicine
Urologist-in-Chief
New York Presbyterian/Weill Cornell
New York City, New York

A. Shalaby
Electronics and Communication Engineering
    Department
Mansoura University
Mansoura, Egypt

Ahmed Shalaby
BioImaging Laboratory
Bioengineering Department
University of Louisville
Louisville, Kentucky

Jasjit S. Suri
Global Biomedical Technologies, Inc.
and
AtheroPoint LLC
Roseville, California

Fatma Taher
College of Technological Innovation
Zayed University
Dubai, United Arab Emirates

Vladimir Valera
Urologic Oncology Branch
Center for Cancer Research
National Cancer Institute
National Institutes of Health
Bethesda, Maryland

Danielle Velez
Division of Urology
Rhode Island Hospital and The Miriam
    Hospital
Providence, Rhode Island

Xiuying Wang
Biomedical & Multimedia Information
    Technology (BMIT) Research Group
School of Information Technologies
The University of Sydney
New South Wales, Australia

Naoufel Werghi
Department of Electrical and Computer
    Engineering
Khalifa University
Abu-Dhabi, United Arab Emirates

Ke Yan
Biomedical & Multimedia Information
    Technology (BMIT) Research Group
School of Information Technologies
The University of Sydney
New South Wales, Australia

Jennifer Yates
Department of Urology
University of Massachusetts Medical School
University of Massachusetts Memorial Health
    Care
Worcester, Massachusetts

1 History of Imaging for Prostate Cancer

Sutchin R. Patel

CONTENTS

The detection of prostate cancer has primarily been based on the use of serum prostate-specific antigen (PSA) along with a digital rectal exam (DRE). Prior to the introduction of transrectal ultrasound, digital guidance was used for the performance of prostate biopsies. The improvements in medical imaging have allowed for the ability to detect clinically significant lesions as well as the extent of disease (1).

THE HISTORY OF ULTRASONOGRAPHY

Studies during the nineteenth century into the measurement of the speed of sound in water paved the way for the development of SONAR (SOund Navigation And Ranging) (2). Jean-Daniel Colladon, a Swiss physicist, in 1826 performed an experiment where he struck an underwater bell in Lake Geneva and simultaneously ignited gunpowder. The flash of the gunpowder was observed by Colladon 10 miles away and he heard the sound of the bell with an underwater trumpet. By measuring the time interval between these two events, Colladon was able to calculate the speed of sound in a body of water (Lake Geneva) (3). This experiment has been seen as the birth of underwater acoustics. John William Strutt (also known as Lord Rayleigh) was a physicist, who won the Nobel Prize in Physics in 1904 for discovering the element Argon. He predicted the existence of surface acoustic waves that travel on the surface of solids (called Rayleigh waves) and, in 1877, published *The Theory of Sound*, which became the foundation for the science of ultrasound (4) (Figure 1.1).

In 1880, Pierre and Jacques Curie made an important discovery that eventually led to the development of the modern-day ultrasound transducer. The Curie brothers observed that when pressure was applied to crystals of quartz an electric charge was generated (3). The charge was directly proportional to the force applied to it and the phenomenon was called "piezoelectricity" from the Greek word meaning "to press." Current ultrasound transducers contain piezoelectric crystals.

On April 15, 1912, the Titanic sank in the North Atlantic after striking an iceberg, and the ensuing public outcry led to significant interest in the development of a device to detect underwater objects (2). Constantin Chilowsky, a Russian expatriate living in Switzerland, was an electrical engineer who became interested in echo ranging because of the sinking of the Titanic. German U-boat attacks on

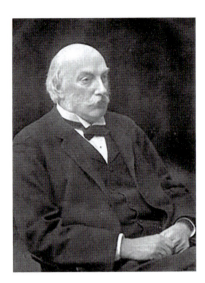

FIGURE 1.1   John William Strutt, 3rd Baron Rayleigh (1842–1919).

Allied shipping heightened his interest in developing SONAR (5). In 1915, Chilowsky developed a working hydrophone in conjunction with Paul Langevin, an eminent French physicist. Their work contributed much to the knowledge of generating and receiving ultrasound waves, which was an important part of the pulse echo principle of SONAR. Funding for research was exhausted at the end of World War I and the efforts shifted toward measuring the depth of the ocean floor. The quest for naval superiority and the submarine versus antisubmarine battles of World War II renewed interest in SONAR development (2).

An understanding of the historical milestones of ultrasound require knowledge of transmission and pulse reflection methods, as well as A, B, and M modes of ultrasound. Early ultrasound used the transmission method where ultrasound measured the ultrasonic waves that passed through a specimen (6). The amount of sound waves not absorbed from the intervening tissue was recorded. The pulse reflection method placed the receiver and transmitter on the same side of the specimen and the amount of sound reflected was then recorded. Amplitude or A-mode was a one-dimensional image that displayed the amplitude or strength of a wave along the vertical axis and time on the horizontal axis (2). Brightness or B-mode, which is commonly used today, is a two-dimensional characterization of tissue where each dot or pixel on the screen represents an individual amplitude spike. In currently used models, amplitudes of varying intensity are assigned shades from black to white. M-motion or motion mode ultrasound relates the amplitude of the ultrasound wave to the imaging of moving structures (such as cardiac muscle).

DEVELOPMENT OF MEDICAL ULTRASONOGRAPHY

George Ludwig and Francis Struthers, working at the Naval Medical Research Institute in Bethesda, Maryland, were among the first to use echo technique in biologic tissue. Because they were employed by the military their work was considered restricted information and was not published in medical journals (2).

John Julian Wild was an English-trained surgeon who immigrated to the United States after World War II (Figure 1.2). Working in Owen Wangensteen's laboratory at the University of Minnesota, using A-mode imaging and a 15 MHz transducer, Wild measured the thickness of the bowel wall in a large water tank (7). Ahead of his time, Wild felt that "it should be possible to detect tumors of the accessible portions of the gastroenterological tract both by density changes and also in all probability of the tumor tissue to fail to contract" (2). Wild managed to develop a scanning device that was

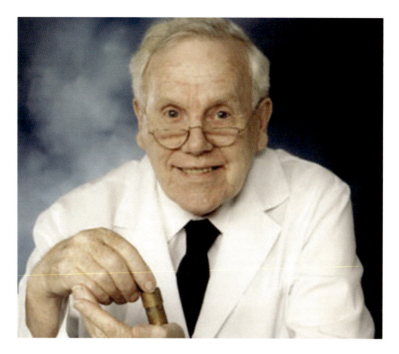

FIGURE 1.2   John Julian Wild (1914–2009).

used to screen patients for breast cancer and also developed transrectal and transvaginal transducers (2,8). With this instrument he imaged a brain tumor in a pathology specimen and localized a brain tumor in a patient after a craniotomy (2).

Douglass Howry played an important role in the development of ultrasound and ultrasonic devices in the 1940s. Unlike Wild, Howry worked more on the development of the equipment and the applied theory of ultrasound rather than on its clinical application. Howry's goal was to produce an instrument that was "in a manner comparable to the actual gross sectioning of structures in the pathological laboratory" (9). Working with W. Roderic Bliss, an electrical engineer, Howry built the first B-mode scanner in 1949. In the late 1950s, Howry and colleagues developed an ultrasound scanner with a semicircular pan containing a plastic window that was later developed into a direct-contact scanner. In 1961, Ralph Meyerdirk and William Wright produced the prototype for the first handheld contact scanner in the United States (10). Ian Donald at the University of Glasgow used an A-mode ultrasound machine to differentiate various types of tissues in recently excised fibroids and ovarian cysts. Donald and his colleagues in Glasgow contributed significant research in regard to ultrasonography in the field of obstetrics and gynecology. He incidentally discovered that a full urinary bladder provided a natural acoustic window for the transmission of ultrasound waves through the pelvis, thus allowing pelvic structures to be imaged more clearly (2,11).

TRANSRECTAL ULTRASONOGRAPHY

Anatomic ultrasound imaging is the oldest and most widely used technique to image the prostate. Watanabe et al. were the first to describe the use of transrectal ultrasound (TRUS) imaging of the prostate with a 3.5 MHz transducer in 1974 (12,13). Prostate cancer lesions have been classically described as hypoechoic lesions on TRUS imaging (14,15). However, the low specificity and positive predictive value (PPV) of TRUS imaging was a clear limitation as other conditions such as prostatitis or focal infarcts could also show hypoechoic characteristics. Lee et al. showed that the positive predictive value of TRUS by itself was 41%, the PPV dropped to 24% if the DRE was normal, 12% if the PSA was normal, and only 5% if both the DRE and PSA levels were normal (16).

In 1989, Hodge et al. explored the utility of adding lesion-directed biopsies to specific hypoechoic areas found on ultrasound compared to the standard non-targeted TRUS-guided systematic prostate biopsy. In 136 men with abnormal prostates on DRE, they found that directed biopsies toward hypoechoic areas within the prostate added very little yield since in 80/83 patients, prostate cancer was detected by the non-targeted systematic biopsies. The addition of TRUS-guided cores to hypoechoic lesions increased the yield by only 5% (17). Thus TRUS imaging by itself has been inadequate for the diagnosis, characterization, and targeting of prostate cancer due to poor resolution, low specificity, and its negative predictive value. The main concerns of the technique include failure to detect prostate cancer (due to poor spatial resolution of lesions), inaccurate risk stratification (from under sampling in cases of small volume disease, transition zone or anteriorly located tumors) and high detection rate of small clinically insignificant prostate cancer (18–20). Most prostate cancer tissue is known to be harder or stiffer than normal prostate tissue (the digital rectal exam is predicated on the physician detecting harder or abnormal lumps of cancer tissue). With real-time elastography imaging tissue, the physician induces a mechanical excitation in the prostate tissue and then images the response using real-time ultrasound (21). Techniques include strain elastography, acoustic radiation force impulse imaging, and shear wave elastography. Despite some promising results, an absolute quantitative threshold to distinguish benign from malignant tissue still remains to be determined. Thus transrectal ultrasound guidance continues to be used principally to guide systematic 12-core biopsies of the prostate.

HISTORY OF MAGNETIC RESONANCE IMAGING

Nikola Tesla discovered the rotating magnetic field in 1882. In 1937, Columbia University Professor Isidor Rabi, working at the Pupin Physics Laboratory in New York City, recognized that the atomic nuclei show their presence by absorbing or emitting radio waves when exposed to a magnetic field and this quantum effect was then called nuclear magnetic resonance (NMR) (Figure 1.3). Rabi won the 1944 Nobel Prize in Physics for his "resonance method for recording the magnetic properties of atomic nuclei" (22).

Felix Bloch and Edward Purcell, in 1946, independently discovered the magnetic resonance phenomena when they studied the magnetic resonance properties of atoms and molecules in solids and liquids (compared to the study of individual atoms or molecules by Rabi using a molecular beam method). They were both awarded the Nobel Prize in 1952 for their work (23). The famous physicist Niels Bohr described the principles of NMR when he stated, "You know, what these people do is really clever. They put little spies into the molecules and send radio signals to them and they have to radio back what they are seeing" (24).

It was not until the 1970s that NMR went beyond application as a research tool in chemical and physical analysis and was applied to medicine. In 1971, Raymond Damadian, a physician working at Brooklyn's Downstate Medical Center, showed that nuclear magnetic relaxation of times of healthy tissues and cancerous tissue differed due to water content (25). Damadian would apply for a patent for an "apparatus and method for detecting cancer in tissue" in 1972 and his patent would be approved in 1974 (26). In 1973, Paul C. Lauterbur, a chemist at the State University of New York, Stony Brook, produced the first NMR image of a test tube filled with water. Raymond Damadian would then, in 1977, build the first MRI scanner assisted by his two postdoctoral students Michael Goldsmith and Larry Minkoff at the Downstate Medical Center. Dr. Damadian initially volunteered his own body for the first MRI scan but it was unsuccessful. His associates told him he was too obese and thus Dr. Minkoff's skinnier torso was used to create the first human MRI scan on July 3, 1977 (24,26).

Sir Peter Mansfield improved the mathematics behind MRI when he suggested gradients as a way to spatially localize NMR signals, and developed the echo-planar technique that allowed images to be produced in seconds and later become the basis for fast magnetic resonance imaging (24). He shared the 2003 Nobel Prize in Physiology or Medicine with Paul Lauterbur "for their discoveries concerning magnetic resonance imaging."

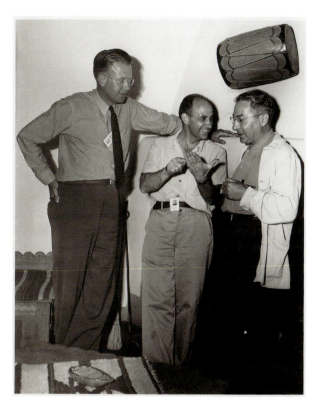

FIGURE 1.3   Isidor Rabi (1898–1988; right) with fellow Nobel Prize winners Ernest O. Lawrence (left) and Enrico Fermi (center).

In 1956, the "Tesla" unit (T) was introduced as a derived unit of the strength of a magnetic field by the International Electrotechnical Commission Committee of Action in Munich, Germany. MRI machines are calibrated in Tesla units. The stronger the magnetic field, the stronger the amount of radio signals that can be elicited of the body's atoms and therefore the higher quality of the MRI image.

CONVENTIONAL MRI

Conventional magnetic resonance imaging is composed of a T1-weighted (T1W) and T2-weighted (T2W) spin echo imaging. T1W imaging offers little benefit to prostate cancer tumor detection and characterization but it does have value in detecting post-biopsy hemorrhage, which appears hyperintense on T1W imaging. T2W imaging is the main sequence used for prostate MR imaging. It has high spatial resolution and allows for clear visualization of prostatic zonal anatomy and the capsule. T2W imaging for prostate cancer detection is non-specific as a region of low signal intensity can also be seen by prostatitis, atrophy, scar tissue, and hemorrhage (27). T2W MRI, which was generally performed with lower magnet field strengths, was limited due to poor specificity and high inter- and intraobserver variability, partially due to the lack of standardization in reporting of prostate MRI (28).

MULTIPARAMETRIC MRI

Multiparametric MRI (mpMRI) has been promising when used for localization and targeting of suspicious prostate lesions. Using a 1.5 Tesla (T) or 3.0T MR scanner with a pelvic phased-array surface coil in combination with an endorectal coil (ERC). A higher magnet strength (3T) can increase signal-to-noise ratio to provide increased resolution so that an ERC may not be needed (29,30). The use of an ERC along with a pelvic phased-array coil has been shown to enhance visualization of surrounding pelvic tissue, which can help identify the presence of extraprostatic extension and seminal vesicle invasion as well as an increase in the sensitivity for detecting prostate cancer (31).

MR spectroscopy that quantified relative levels of metabolites, such as choline, citrate, creatine, and polyamines, was utilized for enhanced prostate cancer detection but has been phased out as a sequence in mpMRI (32). A combination of functional and anatomical sequences (such as T1W, T2W, diffusion-weighted imaging, and dynamic contrast-enhanced MRI) allow for localization and characterization (prostate imaging-reporting and data system, PI-RADS) of prostate lesions. Increasing suspicion (PI-RADS ≥4) has been shown to correlate with a higher risk of prostate cancer on fusion biopsy (33). MRI fusion biopsies have seen an increase in use with reproducible results outside of academic centers (34). Prostate fusion biopsy combines the strength of MRI imaging with the easy applicability of the TRUS imaging/biopsy platform that is very familiar to urologists using office-based platforms (Artemis [Eigen], UroNav [Invivo/Philips], Urostation [Koelis], etc.) to allow the onlay of pre-procedure MRI to guide prostate biopsy in real time. Software-based platforms (Artemis, UroNav, Koelis, etc.) incorporate complex algorithms to register and co-display MR and TRUS images for guidance during biopsy (35). The benefit of prostate fusion biopsy has been documented in men with prior negative prostate biopsy, men with cancer located outside of the standard 12-core biopsy pattern, and in men diagnosed with low-risk prostate cancer (36,37).

IMAGING FOR PROSTATE CANCER STAGING

Computed tomography and MRI in conjunction with whole-body bone scintigraphy have formed the basis for accurate staging for prostate cancer and the detection of metastatic lesions. Prostate cancer staging involves assessment of extraprostatic extension, seminal vesicle involvement, and lymph node and bone involvement. MpMRI has been studied as a tool to predict organ-confined prostate cancer on final pathology but has shown poor sensitivity (47%) for pathological extraprostatic extension (38,39).

The current standard imaging test for bone metastasis is whole-body bone scintigraphy. A bone scan is indicated per NCCN (National Comprehensive Cancer Network) guidelines in patients who initially present with high-risk prostate cancer (T1 disease with a PSA ≥ 20 ng/mL, T2 disease with a PSA ≥ 10 ng/mL, Gleason score ≥8 or T3/T4 disease), any stage of disease with symptoms of bone metastasis, biochemical recurrence post radical prostatectomy, or increasing PSA or abnormal DRE after radiotherapy (40).

Single-photon scintigraphic imaging is performed using a bone-seeking radiopharmaceutical ^{99m}Tc-methylene disphosphonate (^{99m}Tc-MDP). This radiotracer mimics high metabolic states of fast-growing cancer cells align the nuclear camera to quantify these areas using a bone scan index. Bone scintigraphy, however, has relatively poor specificity (42%) for osteoblastic bone metastasis (41). False positive findings attributed to the poor specificity for bone scan can occur with Paget's disease, prior trauma, infections, or metabolic disorders such as hyperparathyroidism.

Prostacint (Cytogen, Princeton NJ), In-111 capromab pendetide, is a radiolabeled antibody targeted to the prostate-specific membrane antigen (PSMA), which is a glycoprotein expressed in both benign and neoplastic prostatic epithelial cells applied clinically in 1996 following FDA approval. It is upregulated in hormone-resistant states and in metastatic disease (42,43). Unfortunately, Prostacint has limited predictive value in imaging the prostate fossa, particularly following radiation therapy, has low sensitivity for detecting osseous metastasis, and is technically demanding, thus it was not widely adopted (44,45). Novel small molecule imaging PSMA ligands have been developed to attempt to address these limitations. Molecular imaging strategies for evaluating prostate cancer try to capitalize on the increased metabolic needs of cancer cells, tumor-specific expression of androgen receptor membrane proteins, or the osteoblastic reaction adjacent to bone marrow metastasis.

PET involves imaging of radiolabeled tracers inside the prostate after IV administration using gamma rays (28). It tends to be used for cancer staging, assessing biochemical failure after radiotherapy, or metastatic involvement. PET imaging highlights the metabolic molecular of cellular activity of prostate cells and is used in conjunction with anatomical imaging in the form of PET/MRI or PET/CT. The different PET methods are characterized by the choice of tracer used and the targeted biological process: metabolism (18 F-fluodeoxyglucose is the most common radiotracter used to monitor glucose metabolism in tumor cell), cellular proliferation (1-amino-3-fluurine-18-fluorcylobutane-1-carboxylic acid [18-FACBC], 11C-choline, and 18 F-flurocholine), and receptor binding (PMSA-based radiotracers: 64 Cu-labeled aptomers and 11C-, 18F-, 68Ga-, and 86Y-labeled low molecular weight inhibitors of PSMA) (46).

CONCLUSIONS

Despite newer imaging technology, advances in prostate cancer imaging have historically been slow to develop. The history of the development of ultrasonography as well as advances in MRI illustrate how we have reached our current methods to image the prostate. The recent software and imaging platforms developed for prostate fusion biopsies have begun to move us from an essentially blind biopsy process to a more targeted approach. Thus the history of prostate imaging has shown us that the continued advances in the field of radiology have benefited our ability to better image and biopsy the prostate.

REFERENCES

1. Taneja SS. Imaging in the diagnosis and management of prostate cancer. *Rev Urol* 2004;6:101–113.
2. Newman PG, Rozycki GS. The history of ultrasound. *Surg Clin North Am* 1998;78:179–195.
3. Hackmann W. Introduction. *Seek and Strike*, London, UK, Crown, 1984, pp. xxiv–xxv.
4. Hackmann W. Underwater acoustics before the first world war. In *Seek and Strike*, London, UK, Crown, 1984, pp. 1–10.
5. Hackmann W. Underwater acoustics before the first world war. In *Seek and Strike*, London, UK, Crown, 1984, pp. 73–95.
6. Wild JJ, Reid JM. Diagnostic use of ultrasound. *Br J Phys Med* 1956;19:248–257.
7. Wild JJ. The use of ultrasonic pulses for the measurement of biologic tissues and the detection of tissue density changes. *Surgery* 1950;27:183–187.
8. Wild JJ, Reid JM. Further pilot echographic studies of the histologic structures of tumors of the living intact human breast. *Am J Pathol* 1952;28:839–861.
9. Koch EB. In the image of science? Negotiating the development of diagnostic ultrasound in the cultures of surgery and radiology. *Technol Cult* 1993;34:858–893.
10. Goldberg BB, Gramiak R, Freimanis AK. Early history of diagnostic ultrasound: The role of American radiologists. *AJR* 1993;160:189–194.
11. Donald I. Sonar: The story of an experiment. *Ultrasound Med Biol* 1974;1:109–117.
12. Watanabe H, Kaiho H, Shima M et al. Development and application of new equipment for transrectal ultrasonography. *J Clin Ultrasound* 1974;2:91–98.
13. Watanabe H, Igari D, Tanahashi Y et al. Transrectal ultrasonography of the prostate. *J Urol* 1975;114:734–739.
14. Lee F, Gray JM, McLeary RD et al. Transrectal ultrasound in the diagnosis of prostate cancer: Location, echogenicity, histopathology, and staging. *Prostate* 1985;7:117–129.
15. Griffiths GJ, Clements R, Jones DR et al. The ultrasound appearances of prostatic cancer with histological correlation. *Clin Radiol* 1987;38:219–227.
16. Lee F, Torp-Pedersen S, Littrup PJ et al. Hypoechoic lesions of the prostate: Clinical relevance to tumor size, digital rectal examination, and prostate specific antigen. *Radiology* 1989;170:29–32.
17. Hodge KK, McNeal JE, Terris MK et al. Random systematic versus directed ultrasound guided transrectal core biopsies of the prostate. *J Urol* 1989;142:71–74.
18. Serefoglu EC, Altinova S, Ugras NS et al. How reliable is 12-core prostate biopsy procedure in the detection of prostate cancer? *Can Urol Assoc J* 2013;7:E293–E298.

19. Volkin D, Turkbey B, Hoang AN et al. Multiparametric magnetic resonance imaging (MRI) and subsequent MRI/ultrasonography fusion guided biopsy increase the detection of anteriorly located prostate cancers. *BJU Int* 2014;114:E43–E49.
20. Nevoux P, Ouzzare A, Ahmed HU et al. Quantitative tissue analyses of prostate cancer foci in an unselected cystoprostatectomy series. *BJU Int* 2012;110:517–523.
21. Good DW, Stewart GD, Hammer S et al. Elasticity as a biomarker for prostate cancer: A systematic review. *BJU Int* 2014;113:523–534.
22. Shampo MA, Kyle RA, Steensma DP. Isidor Rabi-1944 Nobel laureate in physics. *Mayo Clin Proc* 2012;87:e11.
23. Shampo MA, Kyle RA. Felix Bloch—developer of magnetic resonance imaging. *Mayo Clin Proc* 1995;70:889.
24. MRI's Inside Story. *The Economist*, The Economist Group Limited, London, UK, December 4, 2003.
25. Damadian R. Tumor detection by nuclear magnetic resonance. *Science* 1971;171:1151–1153.
26. Macchia RJ, Termine JE, Buchen CD et al. Magnetic resonance imaging and the controversy of the 2003 Nobel Prize in Physiology or Medicine. *J Urol* 2007;178:783–785.
27. Kirkham AP, Emberton M, Allen C. How good is MRI at detecting and characterizing cancer within the prostate. *Eur Urol* 2006;50:1163–1174.
28. George AK, Turkbey B, Valayil SG et al. A urologist's perspective on prostate cancer imaging: Past, present, and future. *Abdom Radiol* 2016;41:805–816.
29. Turkbey B, Merino MJ, Gallardo EC et al. Comparison of endorectal coil and nonendorectal coil T2W and diffusion-weighted MRI at 3 Tesla for localizing prostate cancer: Correlation with whole-mount histopathology. *J Magn Reson Imaging* 2014;39:1443–1448.
30. Lourneco AP, Donegan L, Khalil H et al. Improving outcomes of screening breast MRI with practice evolution: Initial clinical experience with 3T compared to 1.5T. *J Magn Reson Imaging* 2014;39:535–539.
31. Costa DN, Yuan Q, Xi Y et al. Comparison of prostate cancer detection at 3-T MRI with and without an endorectal coil: A prospective, paired-patient study. *Urol Oncol* 2016;34:225.e7–225.e13.
32. Weinreb JC, Blume JD, Coakley FV et al. Prostate cancer: Sextant localization at MR imaging and MR spectroscopic imaging before prostatectomy-results of ACRIN prospective multi-institutional clinic-pathologic study. *Radiology* 2009;251:122–133.
33. Weinreb JC, Barentsz JO, Choyke PL et al. PI-RADS prostate imaging: Reporting and data system: 2015, Version 2. *Eur Urol* 2016;69:16–40.
34. Rastinehad AR, Abboud SF, George AK et al. Reproducibility of multiparametric MRI and fusion-guided prostate biopsy: Multi-institutional external validation by a propensity score matched cohort. *J Urol* 2016;195:1737–1743.
35. Kongnyuy M, George AK, Rastinehad AR et al. Magnetic resonance imaging-ultrasound fusion-guided prostate biopsy: Review of technology, techniques, and outcomes. *Curr Urol Rep* 2016;17:32.
36. Sankineni S, George AK, Brown AM et al. Posterior subcapsular prostate cancer: Identification with mp MRI and MRI/TRUS fusion-guided biopsy. *Abdom Imaging* 2015;40:2557–2565.
37. Delongchamps NB, Peyromaure M, Schull A et al. Prebiopsy magnetic resonance imaging and prostate cancer detection: Comparison of random and targeted biopsies. *J Urol* 2013;189:493–499.
38. Gupta RT, Faridi KF, Singh AA et al. Comparing 3-T multiparametric MRI and partin tables to predict organ-confined prostate cancer after radical prostatectomy. *Urol Oncol* 2014;32:1292–1299.
39. Raskolnikov D, George AK, Rais-Bahrami S et al. The role of magnetic resonance image guided prostate biopsy in stratifying men for risk of extracapsular extension in radical prostatectomy. *J Urol* 2015;194:105–111.
40. *NCCN Guidelines 2.2016 Prostate Cancer.* 2016. www. NCCN.org.
41. Damle NA, Bal C, Bandopadhyaga GP et al. The role of 18F-fluoride PET-CT in the detection of bone metastasis in patients with breast, lung and prostate carcinoma: A comparison with FDG PET/CT and 99mTc-MDP bone scan. *Jpn J Radiol* 2013;31:262–269.
42. Fair WR, Israeli RS, Heston WD. Prostate-specific membrane antigen. *Prostate* 1997;32:140–148.
43. Elgamal AA, Holmes EH, Su SL et al. Prostate-specific membrane antigen (PMSA): Current benefits and future value. *Semin Surg Oncol* 2000;18:10–16.
44. Haseman MK, Reed NL, Rosenthal SA. Monoclonal antibody imaging of occult prostate cancer in patients with elevated prostate-specific antigen. Positron emission tomography and biopsy correlation. *Clin Nucl Med* 1996;21:131–140.
45. Dotan ZA. Bone imaging in prostate cancer. *Nat Clin Prac Urol* 2008;5:434–444.
46. Wibner AG, Burger IA, Sala E et al. Molecular imaging of prostate cancer. *RadioGraphics* 2016;36:142–161.

2 Transrectal Ultrasound (TRUS)-Guided Prostate Biopsy
Historical Perspective and Contemporary Clinical Application

Jennifer Fantasia, Dragan Golijanin, and Boris Gershman

CONTENTS

INTRODUCTION

Prostate cancer is the most common cancer in men and the second leading cause of cancer mortality (Siegel et al. 2017). In 2017, there were an estimated 161,360 new cases and 26,730 deaths attributed to prostate cancer (Siegel et al. 2017). Despite substantial changes in screening for prostate cancer over the last 40 years, transrectal ultrasound (TRUS)-guided prostate biopsy remains the diagnostic standard and is utilized to establish tissue diagnosis in the overwhelming majority of prostate cancer cases (Carter et al. 2013). It is estimated that more than 1 million TRUS-guided prostate biopsies are performed annually in the United States, with important implications for both cost and potential morbidity (Aubry et al. 2013). Accordingly, clinicians must understand the underlying principles behind this imaging modality to safely perform biopsies and accurately interpret imaging findings relevant to the clinical management of their patients.

HISTORICAL PERSPECTIVE

As an internal male reproductive organ, physical examination of the prostate requires digital rectal examination (DRE). Historically, a DRE suspicious for malignancy would constitute the indication for performing a prostate biopsy. Initially, prostate biopsy was performed via a transperineal approach as first described by Barringer in 1922 (Barringer 1922). In 1937 Astraldi described performance of prostate biopsy by transrectal digital guidance (Astraldi 1937). Digitally guided biopsies remained common practice until the development of ultrasonography and its clinical application to prostate imaging. The advent of ultrasonography allowed for imaging of the prostate, first reported in 1952 by Wild and Reid, followed by Takahashi in 1963 (Wild and Reid 1952; Takahashi and Ouchi 1963). The quality of such imaging was technically limited until the late 1960s, when Watanabe performed the first successful TRUS-guided biopsy (Watanabe et al. 1968). Subsequent advances in ultrasound imaging have since made it the primary imaging modality to evaluate the prostate for both benign and malignant processes. To accurately perform and interpret a TRUS of the prostate, it is critical for the practicing urologist to have a strong understanding of both the underlying prostatic anatomy as well as an understanding of the physical properties of ultrasound for optimal image acquisition and interpretation (Figure 2.1).

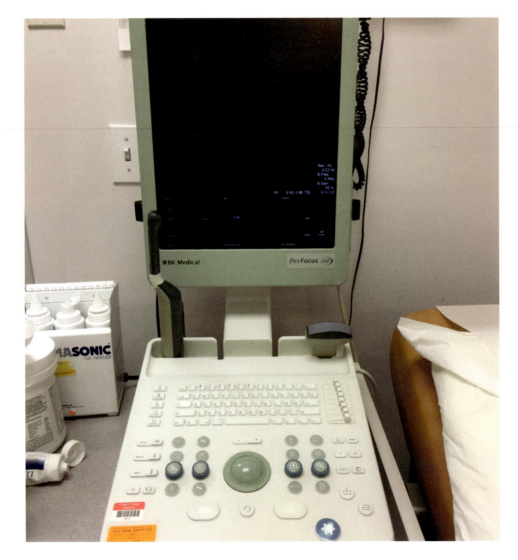

FIGURE 2.1 Ultrasound platform.

PROSTATE ANATOMY AND HISTOLOGICAL ARCHITECTURE

The prostate is a glandular organ positioned above the urogenital diaphragm and below the bladder neck superiorly; it rests behind the pubic symphysis anteriorly, with the rectum posteriorly. The urethra courses through the entire length of the prostate, from the base of the prostate to its apex. Additional structures that may be visualized during ultrasound of the prostate include the seminal vesicles and vasa deferentia.

Histologically, the prostate has traditionally been divided into different zones based on location and tissue types (McNeal 1981). These zones have important clinical implications based on observed patterns of pathology, both benign and malignant. Traditional zones of the prostate include the anterior fibromuscular stroma (AFS), the transitional zone (TZ), peri-urethral zone, central zone (CZ), and peripheral zone (PZ). The majority of prostatic malignancies arise from the peripheral and central zones of the prostate, both located posteriorly in the gland. This pattern was reported by Stamey (1995) based on observations from gross and histological findings obtained from radical prostatectomy specimens. In contrast, the transitional zone is more likely to harbor adenomas from benign prostatic hyperplasia. While there is no distinct delineation of these zones on ultrasound, the transitional zone—which may be particularly enlarged in cases of benign prostatic hyperplasia—demonstrates a more heterogeneous echogenicity as compared with the central and peripheral zones (Halpern 2002).

TECHNICAL ASPECTS OF PROSTATE ULTRASONOGRAPHY

Ultrasonography involves the passage of sound waves through tissues, allowing the interface between the sound wave and tissue to be communicated back to the transducer to reveal information about tissue structure, composition, and density (Kossoff 2000). The transducer uses alternating electrical current pulses to stimulate mechanical energy from the internal transducer crystals; as these crystals expand and contract, the mechanical energy is converted into sound waves which pass from the transducer, through a coupling agent (gel), and into the tissue. As the longitudinal sound waves travel through tissue, a portion of the sound wave energy is reflected back to the transducer to be converted to mechanical, then electrical, energy, which is then reconstructed to create the visual ultrasound image (Kossoff 2000).

Certain parameters of the ultrasound can be manipulated by the provider to optimize image acquisition. Ultrasound frequency is an important parameter, as manipulation of the frequency will alter the tissue penetration of the sound waves (Kossoff 2002). A high frequency results in a higher-resolution image, with greater discrimination between various tissues and possible lesions, but comes at the expense of decreased tissue penetration. The majority of prostate TRUS are performed at a frequency of 6–10 Hz, although recent studies have described high-resolution ultrasound using high frequencies up to 29 MHz (Ghai et al. 2016). A working knowledge of the technical aspects of the imaging modality will allow the practitioner to set optimal parameters for various clinical indications. For example, the posterior central and peripheral zones are optimally imaged with a higher-frequency setting, whereas the anterior prostate may require a lower-frequency for improved tissue penetration.

The most common form of ultrasound performed for prostate TRUS is a gray-scale modality. The amplitude of the sound wave determines the brightness of the pixelation on the image, and the image should be calibrated so that the peripheral zone reflects a medium gray color (Kossoff 2002). Terminology describing the echogenicity, or brightness, of the imaging ranges from hyperechoic (bright) to hypoechoic (dark), with the peripheral zone set as the reference. *Anechoic* is the term used to describe complete absence of echogenicity as is seen with the passage of sound waves through fluid. The echogenicity of tissue is due to the reverberation of the sound wave against the particles of the tissue (Kossoff 2002). Thus, a denser tissue will result in a more echogenic image.

Historically, the echogenicity of lesions within the prostate was felt to correlate with malignant lesions. In 1989, Hodge reported that TRUS prostate biopsy of hypoechoic lesions correlated with a palpable abnormality on DRE in 90% of cases, with histological diagnosis of prostate cancer confirmed in 66% of biopsies obtained from correlating lesions (Hodge 1989). Still, prostate cancers may be hypoechoic, hyperechoic, or anechoic (Shinohara et al. 1989). Indeed, 39% of lesions are isoechoic on ultrasound (Shinohara et al. 1989). Nonetheless, although hypoechoic lesions are not pathognomonic of prostate cancer, such abnormalities still provide visual targets for areas of concern at the time of biopsy.

TECHNICAL ASPECTS OF PERFORMING TRUS-GUIDED PROSTATE BIOPSY

Prior to biopsy, the patient is instructed to perform a cleansing enema to evacuate the rectum of stool to allow for enhanced visualization of the prostate as well as to potentially decrease the risk for infectious complications. Most commonly, the patient is positioned in the left lateral decubitus position, with knees drawn to the chest. Alternatively, some facilities utilize a prone position for performing biopsy. A DRE should be performed prior to insertion of the probe to evaluate for associated pathology that may prevent successful TRUS (e.g., rectal mass, stricture, patient intolerance) as well as to confirm any palpable abnormalities. The ultrasound probe is lubricated with a gel that serves as a coupling agent and placed into a sterile sleeve (Figures 2.2 and 2.3).

The mapping, or initial survey, of the prostate begins with scanning the gland in both axial and sagittal planes to obtain an accurate volume estimate. The width and the length of the gland are obtained in the axial plane, while the length is measured in the sagittal plane. Prostate volume is then estimated by the ultrasound platform, typically by calculating the geometric volume of the prostate as an ellipsoid. The prostate is then inspected from base to apex for characteristics such as overall gland contour, echogenicity, and appearance of the seminal vesicles and vasa deferentia. The echogenicity of the prostate should be symmetrical between lobes with a clear sonographic capsule differentiating between the prostate gland and peri-prostatic tissues (Figures 2.4 and 2.5).

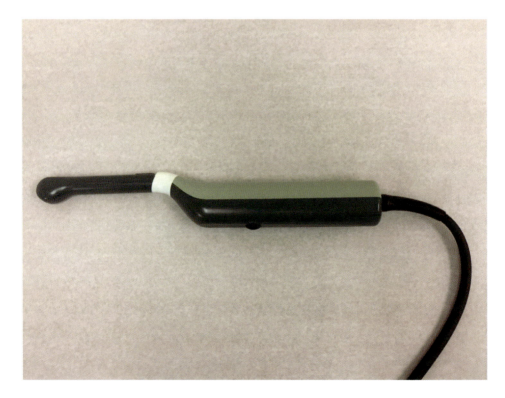

FIGURE 2.2   End-fire ultrasound probe/transducer.

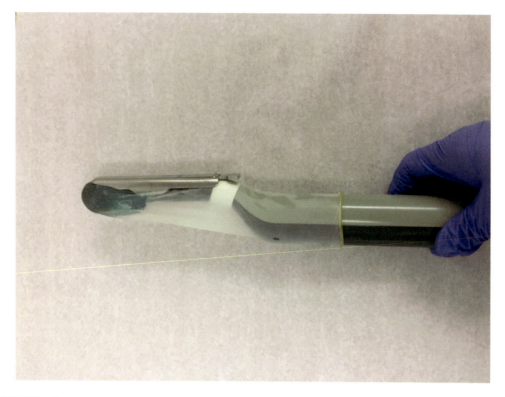

FIGURE 2.3 Ultrasound probe with coupling gel and needle guide.

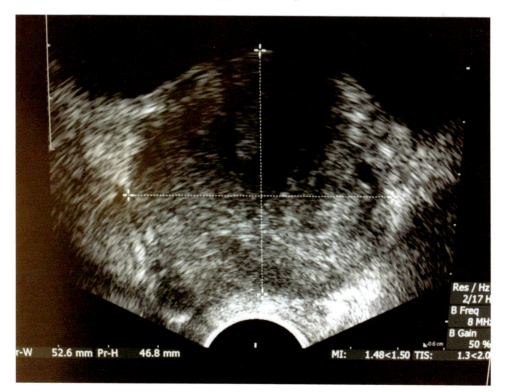

FIGURE 2.4 Axial view of prostate with measurements.

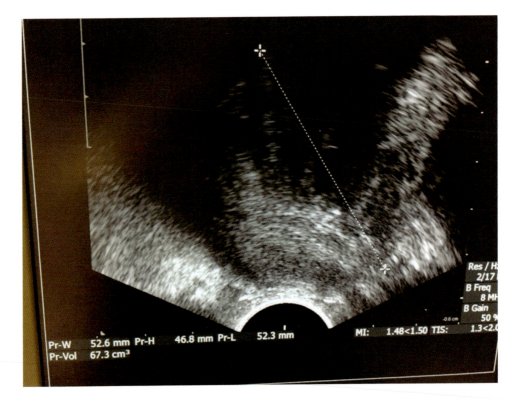

Pr-W 52.6 mm Pr-H 46.8 mm Pr-L 52.3 mm   MI: 1.48<1.50 TIS: 1.3<2.0
Pr-Vol 67.3 cm³

Res / H:
2/17
B Freq
8 MH
B Gain
50 %

FIGURE 2.5   Sagittal view of the prostate with measurement.

There are two types of ultrasound probes used for prostate biopsy that provide imaging in different orientations. This has important implications regarding how the probe is manipulated to view different aspects of the prostate. The end-fire probe relays an image from either directly in front of the probe or at a very slight angle. Thus, to obtain lateral views of the prostate—important for both administration of local anesthetic as well as obtaining sample cores from the most lateral lobes of the prostate—the probe handle must be angled laterally away from the target of interest. This requires that the patient be positioned such that the handle can be moved up and down with the anus as a fulcrum to successfully visualize the right and left lobes. In contrast, the side-fire probe relays an image laterally from the probe and thus rotation of the probe allows for complete imaging of the prostate, including right and left lateral lobes.

CLINICAL ASPECTS OF TRUS PROSTATE BIOPSY

INDICATIONS

Indications for performance of prostate biopsy include elevated prostate-specific antigen (PSA), abnormal PSA kinetics, or abnormal DRE suspicious for malignancy (Carter et al. 2014). Contemporary clinical guidelines advocate shared decision making—a discussion between patients and providers of the risks and benefits of PSA screening—to prevent overdiagnosis and overtreatment of clinically insignificant prostate cancer (Carter et al. 2014). While prostate TRUS without biopsy may be performed for a variety benign indications—including obtaining accurate prostate size measurements as part of evaluation for voiding dysfunction, evaluation of azoospermia, and suspected prostatic infection—this chapter will focus on TRUS-guided prostate biopsy.

TRUS-guided prostate biopsy is the standard of care diagnostic test for elevated PSA in the biopsy-naïve setting, and in recent years it has been increasingly applied for monitoring of active surveillance. However, the diagnosis of prostate cancer by systematic sampling of the prostate is a relatively unique paradigm in oncology as it represents a random sampling of the gland rather than targeted biopsy of a radiographically apparent lesion. Accordingly, there is a risk of sampling error whereby clinically significant disease may not be captured. This limitation has presented a challenge to both the diagnosis and management of prostate cancer, resulting the introduction of prostate MRI and MRI-U/S fusion biopsy. This technology is increasingly utilized for patients on active surveillance and for patients with elevated PSA undergoing repeat biopsy (AUA 2016). Still, TRUS-guided biopsy is an integral component even when MRI fusion is applied.

CONTRAINDICATIONS

Contraindications to TRUS-guided prostate biopsy including active urinary infection, coagulopathy, and rectal anomalies that preclude the procedure (e.g., rectal stricture, which may result in inability to tolerate rectal introduction of the TRUS probe; or absence of rectum, as in patients with total proctocolectomy). Active urinary infection is associated with high risk of serious infectious complications. Similarly, coagulopathy can result in severe bleeding complications. Some patients may require sedation to successfully undergo the procedure, either due to concomitant ano-rectal pathology or anxiety.

PREPARATION

The procedure is reviewed in detail including post-procedural recovery. Informed consent is obtained after discussion of the indication(s), risks, benefits, and alternatives to the procedure, including potential complications and possible implications based on biopsy results.

Management of antiplatelet or anticoagulation therapy prior to prostate biopsy has important considerations for risk of post-biopsy bleeding complications and has been studied extensively. Current American Urological Association (AUA) guidelines recommend that patients may continue use of low-dose aspirin as this has not been associated with increased risk of significant bleeding complications (Culkin et al. 2014). Other antiplatelet agents (e.g., clopidogrel) or anticoagulation therapy should be discontinued based on the half-life of the medication so that coagulopathy is fully reversed at the time of the procedure. Clopidogrel should be discontinued 5–7 days prior to biopsy. Novel oral anticoagulants should be held for 2–5 days prior to the procedure, depending on the agent. For patients on warfarin, a normalized INR should be documented prior to biopsy. For patients at high risk of a venous thromboembolic event, if antiplatelet or anticoagulation therapy is held (e.g., recent cardiac stent, mechanical prosthetic valve), the clinician should consider bridging with heparin or low-molecular-weight heparin prior to biopsy.

Infectious complications have received growing attention in recent years given increasing risk of serious infectious complications following prostate biopsy (Loeb et al. 2011). Peri-procedural antibiotic prophylaxis mitigates this risk. Identified risk factors include healthcare workers, prior antibiotic exposure within 6 months, and recent international travel to areas with high rates of resistance (Anderson et al. 2015). AUA guidelines recommend that all patients undergoing prostate biopsy receive antibiotic prophylaxis against coliform, or intestinal, bacteria including E. coli, klebsiella, proteus, enterobacter, serrattia, enterococcus, and anaerobes (Wolf et al. 2008). However, since the clinical introduction of prostate biopsy, antimicrobial resistance patterns have significantly increased, correlating with a 4% increase in the risk of hospitalization, largely due to the infectious complications of TRUS prostate biopsy in the setting of antibiotic-resistant bacteria

(Nam et al. 2010). Currently, the AUA guidelines published in 2014 still recommend either fluo-roquinolone-based or first-, second-, or third-generation cephalosporin antibiotic prophylaxis as a first-line therapy, for a duration of <24 hours. Alternative prophylactic regimens include Bactrim and aminoglycosides or aztreonam.

Increased recognition of antimicrobial resistance profiles has also stimulated extensive research to establish best practices with emphasis on safety, antibiotic stewardship, and cost-effectiveness. Recent data suggests that rectal swabs may identify patients with fluoroquinolone resistance for tailored antimicrobial therapy (Taylor et al. 2012). Others recommend use of local and up-to-date antibiograms to assess for current patterns of resistance and to inform choice of prophylactic agent (Liss et al. 2017). Another approach is to include the addition of a second antimicrobial agent (e.g., gentamicin) at the time of biopsy for "augmented" antimicrobial pro-phylaxis (Womble et al. 2015).

BIOPSY TECHNIQUE AND PATTERNS

After the initial survey of the prostate, local anesthesia is administered. Acknowledging the potential for patient discomfort and peri-procedural anxiety, several studies have evaluated dif-ferent methods of analgesia. While abroad it is more common to utilize intravenous sedation or systemic pain medication in the form of opioids, peri-prostatic nerve block remains the gold standard and is the most frequently used in the United States (Bjurlin et al. 2014). This block is performed by targeting the neurovascular bundles that lie laterally at the junction of the prostate and the seminal vesicles. This area can be identified as a hyperechoic region due to the presence of peri-prostatic fat. Most commonly, 5 mL of local anesthetic (1%–2% lidocaine or bupivacaine) can be used to infiltrate the plane containing the neurovascular bundles bilaterally. The anesthetic agent can be administered either as one single injection per side or via multiple injections per side (Cantiello et al. 2012).

The biopsy cores are obtained using a spring-loaded core needle biopsy gun, usually 18-gauge. The ultrasound probe is designed with a trough for the biopsy needle and the needle itself is etched to enhance its visualization on ultrasound; many ultrasound devices also include a marker ruler in the parasagittal plane to facilitate accurate placement of the needle to obtain samples. Historically, lesions were targeted either by palpation or by correlating hypoechoic findings on ultrasound. However, many malignant lesions cannot be distinguished by ultrasound or palpation. Accordingly, a systematic sampling of the prostate using a sextant model was purposed by Hodge et al. (1989). Biopsies were obtained from the base, mid, and apex bilaterally. However, this sampling scheme failed to adequately sample areas of the prostate, particularly at the lateral peripheral zone. This was confirmed by correlating pathological findings from radical prostatectomy specimens (McNeal et al. 1988). Current guidelines recommended performing a 12-core biopsy pattern, including the original sextant biopsy template plus additional samples at the lateral base, mid, and apex, as well as the targeted biopsy of any palpable abnormalities or suspicious lesions on imaging (Bjurlin et al. 2013) (Figures 2.6 through 2.10).

COMPLICATIONS

Although a commonly performed procedure, TRUS-guided prostate biopsy may be associated with potential morbidity which can have substantial impact on both the patient and the health-care system. Physical complications are often classified into noninfectious (i.e., pain; bleeding complications including hematuria, hematospremia, and rectal bleeding; urinary retention) and infectious complications (i.e., bacteriuria, urinary tract infection, bacteremia, sepsis). Reported

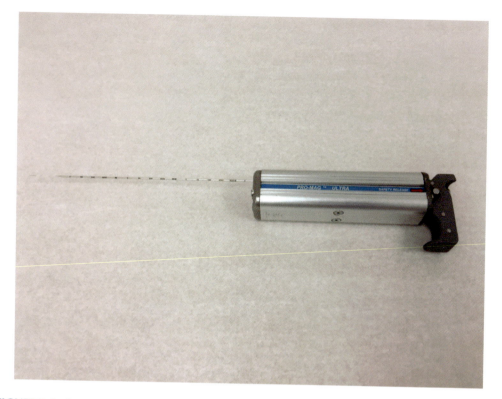

FIGURE 2.6 Prostate biopsy gun.

rates of complications vary widely in the literature depending on patient cohort, biopsy technique, and definitions of endpoints.

Most complications as usually self-limited and resolve over days to weeks. Bleeding complications can be mitigated by appropriate peri-procedural management of antiplatelet or anticoagulation medications. The most common complication experienced is hematospermia, which affects over 30% of patients and resolves spontaneously in most instances (Heidenreich et al. 2014). Similarly, nearly 15% of patients experience mild hematuria with spontaneous resolution (Heidenreich et al. 2014). Approximately 2% of patients experience rectal bleeding lasting longer than 2 days, and <1% develop urinary retention (Heidenreich et al. 2014).

Infectious complications range in severity, from the symptomatic urinary tract infection that can be safely managed with oral antibiotics to sepsis requiring hospitalization. Indeed, the vast majority of prostate biopsy complications requiring hospitalization are infectious in nature (Loeb et al. 2013). Associated risk factors for patients who ultimately require hospitalization following TRUS prostate biopsy include diabetes and enlarged prostate (Loeb et al. 2013). Rates of urinary tract infections following TRUS prostate biopsy vary between 2% and 6%, while the rate of hospitalization after TRUS prostate biopsy for febrile illness ranges between 0.6% and 4.1% (Heidenreich et al. 2014; Nam et al. 2014). Recent studies suggest an increase in the rates of infectious complications requiring hospitalization compared to historical trends (Loeb et al. 2013). Consistently, these infectious complications are associated with antimicrobial-resistant bacteria (Loeb et al. 2013). These trends continue to fuel the research to optimize antimicrobial prophylaxis.

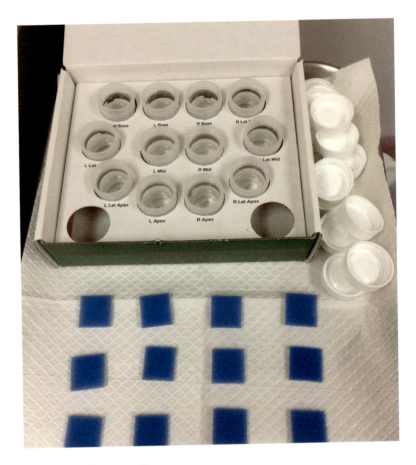

FIGURE 2.7   Prostate specimen samples.

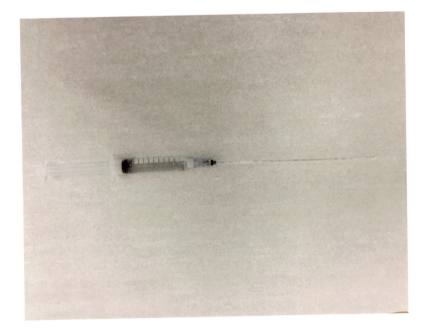

FIGURE 2.8   Spinal needle used to inject local anesthetic.

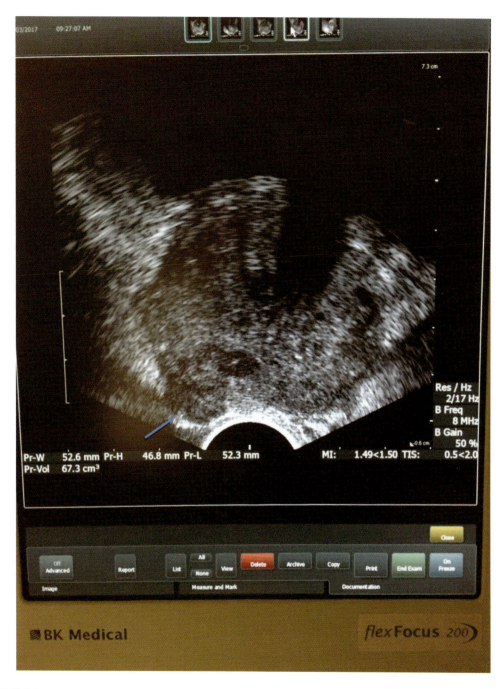

FIGURE 2.9 Axial view of prostate with hypoechoic lesion at the right lateral posterior prostate (arrow).

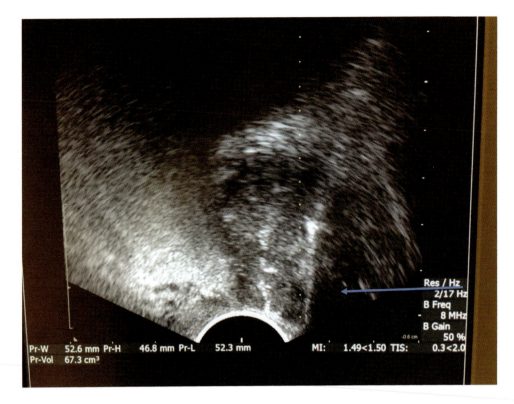

Res / Hz
2/17 Hz
B Freq
8 MHz
B Gain
50 %
-0.6 cm

Pr-W   52.6 mm Pr-H   46.8 mm Pr-L   52.3 mm   MI: 1.49<1.50 TIS: 0.3<2.0
Pr-Vol 67.3 cm³

FIGURE 2.10   Sagittal view with needle guide and needle tract after biopsy.

FUTURE DIRECTIONS

Recent technical advancements in the field of ultrasonography are currently being evaluated in hopes of refining the diagnostic ability for TRUS prostate biopsy. Color Doppler ultrasound is now being used to assess areas of increased vascularity within the prostate, which may correlate with malignant change, to allow for targeted biopsies. In one study, this imaging technique was shown to increase cancer detection rates and provide more accurate diagnosis. However, the sensitivity remains low, with as many as 45% of malignant lesions failing to demonstrate any sonographic findings (Halpern et al. 2000). To further improve the diagnostic accuracy, intravenous microbubble contrast agents have been utilized to better delineate the microvasculature associated with malignant lesions. In early studies, the use of contrast-enhanced ultrasound has improved the sensitivity for the detection of prostate cancers (Halpern et al. 2000). With improved sonographic demonstration of lesions, the use of the 3D ultrasound has also been investigated to improve the accuracy of biopsy (Bjurlin et al. 2014). Finally, the fusion of real-time ultrasound imaging with a detailed MRI-based mapping of the prostate, MRI-U/S fusion biopsy, has emerged as a novel contemporary paradigm in prostate biopsy. MRI-fusion biopsy will be addressed in detail in Chapter 5.

REFERENCES

Anderson E, Leahy O, Cheng AC, Grummet J. Risk factors for infection following prostate biopsy: A case control study. *BMC Infect Dis* 2015;15:580.

Astraldi A. Diagnosis of cancer of the prostate: Biopsy by rectal route. *Urol Cutan Rev* 1937;41:421–427.

Aubry W, Lieberthal R, Willis A et al. Budget impact model: Epigenetic assay can help avoid unnecessary repeated prostate biopsies and reduce healthcare spending. *Am Health Drug Benefits* 2013;6:15–24.

Barringer BS. Carcinoma of the prostate. *Surg Gynecol Obstet* 1922;34:168–176.

Bjurlin MA, Carter HB, Schellhammer P et al. Optimization of initial prostate biopsy in clinical practice: Sampling, labeling and specimen processing. *J Urol* 2013;189:2039–2046.

Cantiello F, Cicione A, Autorino R et al. Pelvic plexus block is more effective than periprostatic nerve block for pain control during office transrectal ultrasound guided prostate biopsy: A single center, prospective, randomized, double arm study. *J Urol* 2012;188(2):417–421. doi:10.1016/j.juro.2012.04.003.

Carter HB, Albertsen PC, Barry MJ et al. Early detection of prostate cancer: AUA Guideline. *J Urol* 2013;190(2):419–426. doi:10.1016/j.juro.2013.04.119.

Culkin DJ, Exaire EJ, Green D et al. Anticoagulation and antiplatelet therapy in urological practice: ICUD/AUA review paper. *J Urol* 2014;192(4):1026–1034. doi:10.1016/j.juro.2014.04.103.

Ghai S, Eure G, Fradet V et al. Assessing cancer risk on novel 29 MHz micro-ultrasound images of the prostate: Creation of the micro-ultrasound protocol for prostate risk identification. *J Urol* 2016;196(2):562–569.

Halpern EJ. Anatomy of the prostate gland. In Halpern EJ, Cochlin DL, Goldberg BB (Eds.), *Imaging of the Prostate*. London, UK: Martin Dunitz, 2002. pp. 3–15.

Halpern EJ, Verkh L, Forsberg F et al. Initial experience with contrast-enhanced sonography of the prostate. *AJR Am J Roentgenol* 2000;174:1575–1580.

Heidenreich A, Bastian PJ, Bellmunt J et al. EAU guidelines on prostate cancer. I. Screening, diagnosis, and local treatment with curative intent: Update 2013. *Eur Urol* 2014;65:124–137.

Hodge KK, McNeal JE, Terris M et al. Random systematic versus directed ultrasound guided transrectal core biopsies of the prostate. *J Urol* 1989;142:71–74.

Joint Consensus Panel of the American Urological Association and Society of Abdominal Radiology. Prostate MRI and MRI-targeted biopsy in patients with prior negative biopsy-Collaborative Initiative of the American Urological Association and the Society of Abdominal Radiology's prostate cancer disease-focused panel. April 2016. Available at: https://www.auanet.org/common/pdf/education/clinical-guidance/Consensus-Statement-Prostate-MRI-and-MRI-Targeted-Biopsy.pdf.

Kossoff G. Basic physics and imaging characteristics of ultrasound. *World J Surg* 2000;24:134–142.

Liss MA, Ehdaie B, Loeb S et al. An update of the American Urological Association white paper on the prevention and treatment of the more common complications related to prostate biopsy. *J Urol* 2017;198(2):329–334.

Loeb S. Antimicrobial prophylaxis for transrectal ultrasound biopsy. *American Urology Association Update Series*, Lesson 1, 2013;32:1–8.

Loeb S, Carter HB, Berndt SI et al. Complications after prostate biopsy: Data from SEER-Medicare. *J Urol* 2011;186(5):1830–1834. doi:10.1016/j.juro.2011.06.057.

Loeb S, Vellekoop A, Ahmed HU et al. Systematic review of complications of prostate biopsy. *Eur Urol* 2013;64:876–892.

McNeal JE. The zonal anatomy of the prostate. *Prostate* 1981;2:35–49.

McNeal JE, Redwine EA, Freiha FS et al. Zonal distribution of prostatic adenocarcinoma: Correlation with histologic pattern and direction of spread. *Am J Surg Pathol* 1988;12:897–906.

Nam RK, Saskin R, Lee Y et al. Increasing hospital admission rates for urological complications after transrectal ultrasound guided prostate biopsy. *J Urol* 2010;189:S12–S17.

Shinohara K, Wheeler TM, Scardino PT. The appearance of prostate cancer on transrectal ultrasonography: Correlation of imaging and pathological examinations. *J Urol* 1989;142:76–82.

Siegel RL, Miller KD, Jemal A. Cancer statistics, 2017. *CA Cancer J Clin* 67:7–30. doi:10.3322/caac.21387.

Stamey TA. Making the most out of six systematic sextant biopsies. *Urology* 1995;45(1):2–12.

Takahashi H, Ouchi T. The ultrasonic diagnosis in the field of urology. *Proc Jpn Soc Ultrasonic Med* 1963;3:7.

Taylor AK, Zembower TR, Nadler RB et al. Targeted antimicrobial prophylaxis using rectal swab cultures in men undergoing transrectal ultrasound guided prostate biopsy is associated with reduced incidence of postoperative infectious complications and cost of care. *J Urol* 2012;187(4):1275–1279. doi:10.1016/j.juro.2011.11.115.

Watanabe H, Kato H, Kato T et al. [Diagnostic application of ultrasonotomography to the prostate]. *Nippon Hinyokika Gakkai Zasshi* 1968;59:273–279.

Wild JJ, Reid JM. Application of echo-ranging techniques to the determination of structure of biological tissues. *Science* 1952;115:226–230.

Wolf JS Jr., Bennett CJ, Dmochowski RR et al. Urologic Surgery Antimicrobial Prophylaxis Best Practice Policy Panel. Best practice policy statement on urologic surgery antimicrobial prophylaxis. *J Urol* 2008;179(4):1379–1390. doi:10.1016/j.juro.2008.01.068. Erratum in: *J Urol*. 2008;180(5):2262–2263.

Womble PR, Linsell SM, Gao Y et al. Michigan Urological Surgery Improvement Collaborative. A statewide intervention to reduce hospitalizations after prostate biopsy. *J Urol* 2015;194(2):403–409. doi:10.1016/j.juro.2015.03.126.

3 Current Active Surveillance Protocol for Prostate Cancer

Scott Greenberg and Jennifer Yates

CONTENTS

INTRODUCTION

The landscape of prostate cancer screening, diagnosis, and treatment is changing rapidly. The most active areas of research and development are arguably occurring in the treatment of advanced and metastatic prostate cancer. With the introduction of abiraterone and enzalutamide, the paradigm for advanced prostate cancer management has significantly changed. On the other end of the prostate cancer spectrum, screening for prostate cancer has become a controversial topic. The changes introduced by the United States Preventive Services Task Force's (USPSTF) prostate cancer screening recommendations has had a major impact on attitudes toward screening and actual screening practices. Once recent review of studies assessing the impact of the USPSTF grade "D" recommendation found that prevalence of low-risk prostate cancer has decreased since 2012 (Lee et al. 2017). Additional studies of prostate cancer epidemiology over the next decade may continue to reveal a shift in the stage at diagnosis, a concern to urologists who will be tasked with treating more advanced prostate cancer.

The concept of active surveillance (AS) arose from the desire to minimize overtreatment of prostate cancer, coupled with the realization that many men have indolent cancers that may never be troublesome in their lifetimes. Active surveillance must be distinguished from watchful waiting (WW), as they have dramatically different goals of care. Active surveillance is utilized for men presumed to have a more indolent cancer that poses no immediate threat to their health. The goal of AS is to intervene if necessary while the disease is localized and treatable. In contrast, WW is best suited for older or more co-morbid patients with limited life expectancies. There is no intent to "cure," but rather minimize the risk of morbidity related to advanced prostate cancer.

Over the past 10 years, several randomized controlled trials supported the growing belief that many patients with prostate cancer are overtreated with modalities such as radiation (RT) and radical prostatectomy (RP). In 2014, the results of a long-term Scandinavian study, SPCG-4, were published (Bill-Axelson et al. 2014). The authors assigned patients to either watchful waiting or RP, and followed them for a mean of 23.2 years. The patients included in the study displayed higher-risk characteristics than the other two randomized trials reported below. The mean prostate-specific antigen (PSA) was 13 ng/dL and the majority had palpable disease. The authors found that RP decreased the overall risk of death from any cause by 12.7 percentage points, and the risk of death from prostate cancer decreased by 17.7 percentage points. The long-term mortality benefits of RP were greatest in patients younger than 65 years of age.

In contrast, the Prostate Cancer Intervention versus Observation Trial (PIVOT) (Wilt et al. 2012) included patients with lower-risk characteristics, who were randomized to either observation or RP. During a median follow-up period of 10 years, all-cause mortality was reduced only by 2.9 percentage points, and prostate cancer specific mortality was reduced by 2.6 percentage points. However, the cohort that appeared to benefit the most from RP included men with a PSA greater than 10 ng/mL, and possibly those patients with intermediate- or high-risk disease. The results of the study were criticized due to low statistical power, thus this should be taken into consideration when comparing observation and RP.

Finally, the United Kingdom Prostate Testing for Cancer and Treatment (ProtecT) trial randomized patients to AS, RP, or RT (Hamdy et al. 2016). Patients included in the study displayed predominantly low-risk characteristics, with 77% of patients diagnosed with Gleason 3+3 disease, and 76% had clinical stage T1c disease. Cancer-specific and all-cause mortality were similar at 10 years, regardless of the assigned treatment group. The rate of clinical progression and metastatic disease were lower in the treatment groups, but this could not be extrapolated to conclude that treatment leads to significant differences in disease-specific or overall survival.

Acknowledging that a certain cohort of men with prostate cancer are at risk for overtreatment, the challenge becomes identifying those patients with indolent cancer who can be safely enrolled in an AS program. A number of AS protocols have published series with robust follow-up, demonstrating the safety of AS in the well-selected cohort of patients. Table 3.1 lists the inclusion criteria for several of the larger prospective AS series. In general, most AS programs utilize well-established criteria for low-risk disease. The Epstein criteria, first described in 1994, risk-stratify patients based on tumor volume (low risk, <0.2 cm^3), the presence of Gleason 4 or 5 disease (low risk, no Gleason 4 or 5), and clinically localized disease (Epstein et al. 1994). The criteria were revised to include PSA density less than 0.15 ng/mL, fewer than 3 positive biopsy cores, and less than 50% of core involvement with cancer. Another widely used risk calculator was described by D'Amico and colleagues (1999), and utilizes PSA, clinical stage, and Gleason score when determining risk. The National Comprehensive Cancer Network (NCCN) expanded the calculation of risk to include both low-risk and very low-risk patients. The variables considered when risk-stratifying patients include clinical stage, PSA, number of positive cores, percentage positive of involved cores, and PSA density (PSAD) (NCCN.org).

TABLE 3.1

Inclusion Criteria for Large Prospective AS Programs

AS Protocol	PSA	Clinical Stage	Percent Cores Involved (%)	Gleason Grade	Number of Positive Cores
Toronto[*]	≤10[a]	—	—	≤3+3; 3+4[c]	—
JHU[†]	(PSAD <0.15 ng/mL)	≤T2[a]	≤50	≤6	≤2
PRIAS[b,‡]	≤10 and PSAD <0.2 ng/mL	≤T2[c]	—	≤6	≤2
UCSF[§]	≤10	≤T2[a]	≤50	≤6	≤33%

[a] Age less than 70.

[b] Prior to 2012 (i.e., original protocol).

[c] Gleason 3+4 included if shorter life expectancy/comorbidities.

[*] Klotz, L. et al., *J. Clin. Oncol.*, 33, 272–277, 2015.

[†] Tosoian, J.J. et al., *J. Clin. Oncol.*, 29, 2185–2190, 2011.

[‡] Bokhorst, L.P. et al., *Eur. Urol.*, 70, 954–960, 2016.

[§] Welty, C.J. et al., *J. Urol.*, 193, 807–811, 2015.

Recognizing that many patients with prostate cancer harbor indolent disease, the International Society of Urological Pathology (ISUP) introduced a change in the categorization of prostate cancer. The new grading system was validated in a large cohort of patients (Epstein et al. 2016), and is being introduced into clinical guidelines. The new system includes five groups: Group 1 (Gleason grade 6 or less); Group 2 (Gleason grade 3+4); Group 3 (Gleason grade 4+3); Group 4 (Gleason grade 8); Group 5 (Gleason grade 9 and 10). Placement of patients into risk categories such as these may facilitate selection of patients for AS. Patients in Group 1 can also be reassured that their disease is unlikely to lead to long-term morbidity and mortality, understandably a concern in any patient diagnosed with cancer.

This chapter introduces imaging modalities and biomarkers that are useful adjuncts to standard clinical variables in selecting patients for and monitoring patients on AS. Historically, repeat biopsy has remained a mainstay of AS protocols, important for both confirmation of low-risk disease, and for monitoring for progression of disease. Despite confirmatory biopsy being a well-accepted foundation of AS, many patients either decline or are not offered repeat biopsies. One series reviewing the SEER database, including 5,192 patients on an AS protocol, found that only 13% of patients underwent prostate biopsies more than 2 years into the protocol (Loeb et al. 2016). Older age and higher rates of comorbidities were associated with a lower rate of biopsy, while recent diagnosis and higher income were associated with a higher rate of biopsy. The importance of repeat biopsy was highlighted in a study of patients identified as appropriate candidates for AS (King et al. 2013). Repeat biopsy disqualified 17% of patients based on increase in cancer volume of grade.

The outcomes of selected patients on AS protocols are defined in several prospective studies, listed in Table 3.2. Despite favorable outcomes for most patients enrolled in AS, there has not been a rapid adoption of this treatment modality. A recent review of the United States National Cancer Database revealed that only 12.1% of men eligible for AS were enrolled (Maurice et al. 2015). The authors also found that the clinical application of AS was not based only on risk stratification, but other factors such as practice setting (academic) and region within the country also influenced enrollment in AS. With the inclusion of AS in widely accepted guidelines, AS may be offered to more patients across wider demographic and geographic patient populations.

Guidelines for prostate cancer treatment from major oncologic organizations now reflect the incorporation of AS into urologists' treatment paradigms. Notably, the NCCN, the European Association of Urology (EAU), and the American Urological Association (AUA) guidelines now address AS for lower-risk patients.

TABLE 3.2

Outcomes of Large Prospective AS Programs

AS Protocol	Median Follow-Up	Overall Survival	CSS	Metastases Free Survival	Treatment Rate
Toronto[*]	6.4		98.1% at 10 years 94.3% at 15 years		5 years 24.3% 10 years 36.5% 15 years 45%
JHU[†]	5	93% at 10 years	99.9% at 10 years	99.4% at 10 years	50% curative intervention at 10 years
PRIAS[‡]	10	—	—	—	52% at 5 years 73% at 10 years
UCSF[§]	5	98%	100%	100%	40% at 5 years

[*] Klotz, L. et al., *J. Clin. Oncol.*, 33, 272–277, 2015.
[†] Tosoian, J.J. et al., *J. Clin. Oncol.*, 29, 2185–2190, 2011.
[‡] Bokhorst, L.P. et al., *Eur. Urol.*, 70, 954–960, 2016.
[§] Welty, C.J. et al., *J. Urol.*, 193, 807–811, 2015.

CURRENT ACTIVE SURVEILLANCE PROTOCOL FOR PROSTATE CANCER

IMAGING

Multiparametric magnetic resonance imaging (mpMRI) is becoming the modality of choice for prostate cancer imaging due to its superior ability to diagnose and risk-stratify disease (Scarpato and Barocas 2016). Multiparametric MRI imaging combines anatomic imaging with functional and molecular imaging to produce a PI-RADS (Prostate Imaging-Reporting and Data System) score to quantify the overall probability of clinically significant prostate cancer (Hassanzadeh et al. 2017). Initially, mpMRI was scored using PI-RADS v1 which consisted of T2-weighted imaging, MR spectroscopy (metabolic imaging), diffusion-weighted imaging (DWI), and dynamic contrast-enhanced (DCE) MRI. In 2015, PI-RADS v2 was adopted and removed MR spectroscopy from the scoring equation as it is believed that this study added little value to the mpMRI interpretation. PI-RADS v2 has since been validated, but has been shown to have moderate interobserver variability (Hassanzadeh et al. 2017).

One of mpMRI's greatest strengths is its ability to accurately detect and discriminate clinically significant disease (i.e., higher-volume and higher-grade disease) from more indolent forms of disease in patients with suspected and known prostate cancer. Several studies have demonstrated the high negative predictive value (NPV) of mpMRI for intermediate- and high-risk prostate cancers. A recent study by Lu et al. (2017) evaluated men with negative prostate mpMRI by subsequently performing 12-core systematic mapping biopsy. In subgroup analysis, biopsy revealed prostate cancer in 44.8% (13/29) of men already on AS, but only 2 of those 29 men had Gleason ≥ 7 disease. They concluded that while the NPV for any prostate cancer on mpMRI in the AS cohort was only 55.2%, the NPV for clinically significant (Gleason ≥ 7 disease) was 93.1%. Studies that evaluate both patients without a diagnosis of prostate cancer and patients already on an AS protocol have demonstrated a NPV of up to 98% for mpMRI (Siddiqui et al. 2015). Given that the prostate cancer treatment paradigm is shifting to only treat clinically significant cancers that are likely to have detrimental effects on quality of life and longevity—mpMRI shows great promise for reducing the overdetection and overtreatment of prostate cancer.

In addition to mpMRI's strong NPV, other studies have demonstrated the high sensitivity of mpMRI for detecting clinically significant cancers by allowing improved targeting of suspicious areas on biopsy. Siddiqui et al. (2015) compared detection rates of intermediate- and high-risk prostate cancer in men who received targeted MR/ultrasound fusion prostate biopsies, standard 12-core extended-sextant biopsies, and combined modalities (i.e., MR/US fusion and extended-sextant biopsies). The group found that targeted biopsies diagnosed 30% more high-risk cancers and 17% fewer low-risk cancers versus standard biopsy methods. Interestingly, when combining targeted fusion biopsy with standard 12-core biopsy, 22% more cancers were detected than with targeted fusion biopsy alone—however, 83% of these tumors were low risk. Despite most tumors being low risk, the knowledge that some high-grade tumors may be missed with MR/US fusion alone has led to recommendations to undergo the combined method rather than MR/US fusion guided biopsy or standard sextant biopsy alone (Hansen et al. 2016). Hansen et al. found that in 343 men with PI-RADs 3–5 lesions, systematic (templated 24-core) biopsies missed 13 of 138 clinically significant lesions, defined as Gleason score 7–10. Likewise, targeted biopsies missed 12 of 138 clinically significant lesions—thus leading the authors to conclude that combining targeted and systematic biopsy is superior to either method alone (Hansen et al. 2016).

Given mpMRI's strong negative predictive value and high sensitivity for detecting clinically significant disease, it stands to reason that mpMRI has the potential to serve as a useful tool in monitoring disease in patients diagnosed with low-grade, localized prostate cancer who elect to undergo active surveillance. A 2017 anonymous survey by the National Cancer Institute that polled over 300 urologists found that 72.5% of respondents used mpMRI to monitor patients on active surveillance (Muthigi et al. 2017). Two important benefits mpMRI confers to patients undergoing AS are its ability to accurately detect disease progression and upgrading lesions. A recent study found that of 259 men with Gleason 3+3 or 3+4 disease detected by MRI/US fusion and subsequently enrolled in AS, 32 of 33 (97%) of upgraded lesions (to at least 4+3) occurred at sites visible on MRI or at three-dimensional digitally tracked sites of previously biopsied tumor (Nassiri et al. 2017). The authors concluded that during AS, tracking and targeting tumor foci with MRI/US fusion biopsy allows for improved detection of clinically significant cancers. Additionally, Almeida et al. (2016) demonstrated the utility of mpMRI in accurately grading and staging patients eligible for AS. The authors prospectively analyzed 73 patients with low-risk disease who elected prostatectomy rather than AS. Prior to prostatectomy, all men underwent mpMRI. They found that 92% of patients who were upstaged and 76% with upgraded based on prostatectomy pathology had a PI-RADS 4–5 lesion seen on mpMRI. The authors did not report whether these mpMRI lesions mapped to the same location in the prostatectomy specimen. The authors concluded that PI-RADS 4–5 lesions are strong predictors for clinically significant cancer in AS candidates (Almeida et al. 2016).

Another application of mpMRI in active surveillance is the use of apparent diffusion coefficient (ADC) to assess the need for re-biopsy. ADC is derived from diffusion weighted imaging (DWI) and used with T2-weighted MRI to identify tumor nodules on diagnostic imaging (Morgan et al. 2017). In poorly differentiated tumors—including those in prostate cancer—ADC values are lower (Morgan et al. 2017). A strong inverse correlation has been documented between ADC and Gleason grade and this relationship can help risk-stratify men undergoing AS for need to repeat biopsy of suspicious prostate lesions (Tosoian et al. 2016). Men with low-grade prostate cancer on biopsy but a discordant finding on mpMRI ADC may be good candidates for re-biopsy as the lesion may contain undiscovered clinically significant tumor. However, it should be noted that the benefit of ADC may not be applicable to all men—specifically those on 5-alpha-reductase inhibitors (5-ARIs). A prospective, randomized, placebo-controlled trial analyzing 37 men on AS found that men taking dutasteride for 6 months had less conspicuous lesions (defined as peripheral zone divided by tumor ADC) than their counterparts taking a placebo (Giganit et al. 2017). This difference was largely due to a significant increase in tumor ADC in men on dutasteride. Thus, men on 5-ARIs undergoing AS protocols utilizing mpMRI/ADC may require a lower threshold for re-biopsy compared to their non-5-ARIs counterparts.

In addition to ADC's utility in risk stratification of clinically significant tumors for men undergoing AS, it may also be clinically useful in monitoring the growth kinetics of these lesions. A recent study measured longitudinal change in dominant prostatic lesions volume compared to changes in ADC on mpMRI in patients on AS for prostate cancer. They discovered that ADC and tumor volume are negatively correlated, and variability of volume measurement by a single expert observer at a single center is >60%. However, the measured ADC variability was only ~5% (Morgan et al. 2017). Thus, calculating the change in ADC may be a more reliable tool for measuring tumor growth than measuring change in volume on mpMRI in prostate cancer surveillance.

Despite the advantages that mpMRI offers to patients undergoing prostate cancer AS, there is still no consensus regarding the use of mpMRI in this cohort. Multiparametric MRI and fusion biopsy are still in their relative infancy compared to imaging modalities and biopsy techniques used in other fields. Much of the research performed on the use of mpMRI in AS have taken place in high-volume academic centers. The application of this data to the community setting has not been evaluated and warrants additional study. In addition, the optimal application and appropriate sequencing of mpMRI in AS has not yet been fully defined (Schulmann et al. 2017). As more data is obtained from long-term studies measuring outcomes from prostate cancer patients on AS, current guidelines and consensus statements will likely be revised to reflect the application of mpMRI in AS.

MOLECULAR MARKERS

There has been increasing interest in the application of tissue-based molecular profiling tests to provide more data points for patients considering AS for low-grade prostate cancer. Three commonly utilized genomic assays include Decipher™, Oncotype DX®, and Prolaris®.

Decipher™ analyzes 1.4 million genomic markers, which represents 46,000 RNA sequences, by utilizing transcriptome-wide microarrays (Syed et al. 2017). The test focuses on 22 genes that are highly associated with prostate cancer (cell proliferation, androgen signaling, motility, differentiation, and immune modulation) and assigns the patient a value on the continuum from 0 to 1 to categorize the risk for metastatic disease at 5 years following radical prostatectomy—higher values are associated with worse outcomes (Knudsen et al. 2016, Syed et al. 2017). Several studies have validated Decipher™ in high-risk patients after radical prostatectomy; specifically, as a predictor for metastatic disease, biochemical recurrence, and prostate cancer mortality (Syed et al. 2017). While Decipher™ is not currently used as a tool for AS, further investigation may find clinical utility for men undergoing prostate cancer monitoring. A recent study found that RNA obtained from biopsy specimen and the subsequent radical prostatectomy specimen demonstrated correlation of $r = 0.70$ on Decipher™ testing (Knudsen et al. 2016). This correlation of biopsy and prostatectomy RNA supports use of Decipher™ on prostate biopsy tissue, but further research is necessary to evaluate any incremental benefit it may bestow to men on AS.

Oncotype DX® utilizes small-volume tissue samples (1mm) to generate a Genomic Prostate Score (GPS) by using reverse transcription polymerase chain reaction (RT-PCR) to measure the expression of a 17-gene panel (Tosoian et al. 2016, Syed et al. 2017). Of these genes, 12 are involved with carcinogenesis (not prostate-specific) and the other 5 are reference genes (Tosoian et al. 2016). Like Decipher™, Oncotype DX® was originally used for predicting the risk of metastasis after radical prostatectomy. However, in 2014, Klein et al. demonstrated that in biopsy tissues, this 17-gene assay improves prediction of the presence of clinically significant disease (high Gleason grade or non-organ-confined). The authors concluded that Oncotype DX® may have an application in selecting patients for AS (Klein et al. 2014). While this tissue-based test has potential to benefit patients considering AS, there is a paucity of literature assessing outcomes in the AS cohort.

Prolaris®, like Oncotype DX®, also uses RT-PCR to measure expression of genes associated with prostate cancer to create a score that is used to predict the likelihood of cancer progression, prostate cancer specific mortality, and aggressive pathologic features after prostatectomy (Syed et al. 2017). Prolaris® uses 1 mm of continuous tumor tissue to measure tumor cell proliferation. A 46-gene panel consisting of 31 cell cycle genes and 15 housekeeping genes is utilized to produce a cell cycle progression (CCP) score. The CCP score has been associated with likelihood of biochemical recurrence after prostatectomy. However, it has not been shown to be an independent predictor of mortality in men with Gleason 3+3 disease (Tosoian et al. 2016, Syed et al. 2017). Its potential application to patients on AS is unclear, as many of these patients are diagnosed with Gleason 6 prostate cancer.

Although there is a paucity of long-term prospective data for these molecular tests in the AS population, the NCCN does acknowledge that men with clinically localized prostate cancer undergoing AS may consider these genetic assays in deciding whether to enter an AS protocol (Syed et al. 2017). These tests have the potential to serve as a useful tool to alert patients and physicians to the presence of previously unidentified clinically significant cancer and thus prompt repeat biopsy or imaging with mpMRI.

SERUM TESTS

In addition to the widely used PSA serum test for prostate cancer detection and active surveillance, several other serum-based tests are also under clinical investigation for use in the AS population. These tests utilize PSA (Human Kallikrein 3; hK3), other Human Tissue Kallikreins, and their derivatives to risk stratify men and may help with decisions regarding their cancer management.

The PHI (Prostate Health Index) test uses total PSA (tPSA) and two derivatives to calculate a score that is then used to stratify men into risk categories. The PHI is calculated using the proPSA, a PSA isoform that has been shown to outperform PSA and free PSA in prostate cancer detection, and free PSA (Boegemann et al. 2016). This score was initially used to predict extracapsular spread, Gleason score, and upgrading at radical prostatectomy, but evidence from a 2012 paper by Tosoian et al. found -2proPSA and PHI score to have improved predictive accuracy over tPSA and %fPSA for reclassifying men on AS to higher-grade prostate cancer on follow-up (Tosoian et al. 2012, Syed et al. 2017).

The 4K score uses PSA (hK3), hK2, free PSA, and intact PSA (iPSA) along with age, digital rectal exam (DRE), and biopsy history to stratify patients into low-, intermediate-, and high-risk groups for the presence of clinically significant prostate cancer (Syed et al. 2017). This risk stratification has been successful in predicting development of metastatic prostate cancer within 20 years (Stattin et al. 2015). Further studies have suggested that 4K score predicts the presence of more aggressive cancer on prostate biopsy in men with initially diagnosed low-grade prostate cancer, which has the potential to make the 4K score a valuable tool for men deciding on AS versus immediate intervention (Syed et al. 2017).

While both PHI and the 4K scores show much promise, currently, there is a lack of long-term prospective data for these serum markers in the AS setting. Although the preliminary evidence supports the use of PHI and 4K scores in the AS population, further longitudinal studies are needed before they are widely incorporated into AS protocols.

URINE TESTS

Currently, two urine biomarkers show promise for men interested in pursuing AS—Prostate Cancer Antigen 3 Gene (PCA3) and TMPRSS2::ERG ("T2ERG").

PCA3 is a non-coding mRNA that is overexpressed 10- to 100-fold in prostate cancers compared to non-neoplastic prostate tissue. Expression is even higher in more poorly differentiated tumors (Filella et al. 2013). To obtain PCA3 for measurement in the urine, an examiner performs prostate massage through DRE. The first-catch urine (20–30 mL) is then collected and analyzed for PCA3 mRNA level and, as a control, PSA mRNA level. In 2012, the FDA approved PCA3 testing to risk-stratify patients with a prior negative biopsy to determine need for repeat biopsy (Syed et al. 2017). In 2017, a study from Johns Hopkins evaluating the PCA3 results from the men on their AS program found that the 11% of men who underwent Gleason grade reclassification (Gleason score >6) had higher first PCA3 score ($p = 0.007$) and subsequent PCA3 scores ($p = 0.002$) (Tosoian et al. 2017). Interestingly, longitudinal changes (increase or decrease PCA3 score in the same patient) did not affect a patient's risk of Gleason reclassification. In their multivariable model, the initial PCA3 score remained significantly associated with Gleason grade reclassification leading the authors to conclude that PCA3 provides additional prognostic information in patients undergoing or interested in AS (Tosoian et al. 2017).

As with PCA3, the transcription products of T2ERG can be collected in the urine after prostate massage. T2ERG is a fusion protein of the TMPRSS2 gene (21q22.3) and the ERG gene (21q22.2) that is present in ~40% to 80% of prostate cancers (Yu et al. 2010). TMPRSS2 is an androgen-sensitive gene and ERG is an ETS family transcription factor that is considered a key prostate cancer oncogene (Squire 2009). Like the BCR:ABL gene translocation in chronic myeloid leukemia (CML), a deletion in the long arm of chromosome 21 places the ERG gene immediately downstream of the androgen responsive TMPRSS2 gene. ERG will then drive the overexpression of TMPRSS2. This overexpression with loss of PTEN leads to unregulated cellular proliferation, anti-apoptotic activity, and additional cell cycle events that lead to malignant cells (Squire 2009). A study of 265 patients on AS with median follow-up of 4.1 years found ERG-positive tumors had a 58.6% risk of disease progression versus 21.7% in the ERG-negative cohort (hazard ratio 2.45) (Berg 2016). There is limited literature on the long-term outcomes of urinary T2ERG's predictive value in AS and further research is warranted.

CONCLUSION

Within the last decade, a shift in the treatment of lower stage and grade prostate cancer has made active surveillance an increasingly popular management option. The challenge lies in selecting the appropriate patient, the patient with indolent disease who does not harbor more aggressive cancer that could pose a threat to their longevity. The refinement of mpMRI has offered clinicians a tool both for selecting patients for AS and for monitoring patients on AS. In combination with currently utilized clinical parameters, mpMRI and molecular markers may offer patients and clinicians a nomogram to risk-stratify prostate cancer and select those patients who will benefit the most from AS.

REFERENCES

Almeida GL, Petralia G, Ferro M et al. Role of multi-parametric magnetic resonance image and PIRADS score in patients with prostate cancer eligible for active surveillance according PRIAS criteria. *Urol Int* 2016;96:459–469.

Berg KD. The prognostic and predictive value of TMPRSS2-ERG gene fusion and ERG protein expression in prostate cancer biopsies. *Dan Med J* 2016;63:B5319.

Bill-Axelson A, Holmberg L, Garmo H et al. Radical prostatectomy or watchful waiting in early prostate cancer. *N Engl J Med* 2014;370(10):932–942.

Boegemann M, Stephan C, Cammann H et al. The percentage of prostate-specific antigen (PSA) isoform [-2] proPSA and the Prostate Health Index improve the diagnostic accuracy for clinically relevant prostate cancer at initial and repeat biopsy compared with total PSA and percentage free PSA in men aged ≤65 years. *BJU Int* 2016;117:72–79.

Bokhorst LP, Valdagni R, Rannikko A et al. A decade of active surveillance in the PRIAS study: An update and evaluation of the criteria used to recommend a switch to active treatment. *Eur Urol* 2016;70:954–960.

D'Amico AV, Whittington R, Malkowicz SB et al. Pretreatment nomogram for prostate-specific antigen recurrence after radical prostatectomy or external-beam radiation therapy for clinically localized prostate cancer. *J Clin Oncol* 1999;17:168–172.

Epstein JI, Walsh PC, Carmichael M et al. Pathologic and clinical findings to predict tumor extend of nonpalpable (Stage T1c) prostate cancer. *JAMA* 1994;271(5):368–374.

Epstein JI, Zelefsky MJ, Sjoberg DD et al. A contemporary prostate cancer grading system: A validated alternative to the Gleason score. *Eur Urol* 2016;69(3):428–443.

Filella X, Foj L, Mila M et al. PCA3 in the detection and management of early prostate cancer. *Tumour Biol* 2013;34:1337–1347.

Giganit F, Moore CM, Robertson NL. MRI findings in men on active surveillance for prostate cancer: Does dutasteride make MRI visible lesions less conspicuous? Results from a placebo-controlled, randomised clinical trial. *Eur Radiol* 2017;27(11):4767–4774.

Hamdy FC, Donovan JL, Lane JA et al. 10-year outcomes after monitoring, surgery, or radiotherapy for localized prostate cancer. *N Engl J Med* 2016;375:1415–1424.

Hansen NL, Kesch C, Barrett T et al. Multicentre evaluation of targeted and systematic biopsies using magnetic resonance and ultrasound image-fusion guided transperineal prostate biopsy in patients with a previous negative biopsy. *BJU Int* 2016;120(5):631–638.

Hassanzadeh E, Glazer DI, Dunne RM et al. Prostate imaging reporting and data system version 2 (PI-RADS v2): A pictorial review. *Abdom Radiol* 2017;42:278–289.

King AC, Livermore A, Laurila TA et al. Impact of immediate TRUS rebiopsy in a patient cohort considering active surveillance for favorable risk prostate cancer. *Urol Oncol* 2013;31(6):739–743.

Klein EA, Cooperberg MR, Magi-Galluzzi C et al. A 17-gene assay to predict prostate cancer aggressiveness in the context of Gleason grade heterogeneity, tumor multifocality, and biopsy undersampling. *Eur Urol* 2014;66:550–560.

Klotz L, Vesprini D, Sethukavalan P et al. Long-term follow-up of a large active surveillance cohort of patients with prostate cancer. *J Clin Oncol* 2015;33:272–277.

Knudsen BS, Kim HL, Erho N et al. Application of a clinical whole-transcriptome assay for staging and prognosis of prostate cancer diagnosed in needle core biopsy specimens. *J Mol Diagn* 2016;18:295–406.

Lee DJ Mallin K, Graves AJ et al. Recent changes in prostate cancer screening practices and prostate cancer epidemiology. *J Urol* 2017;198(6):1230–1240.

Loeb S, Walter D, Curnyn C et al. How active is active surveillance? Intensity of follow-up during active surveillance for prostate cancer in the United States. *J Urol* 2016;196(3):721–726.

Lu AJ, Syed JS, Nguyen KA et al. Negative multiparametric magnetic resonance imaging of the prostate predicts absence of clinically significant prostate cancer on 12-core template prostate biopsy. *Urology* 2017;105:118–122.

Maurice MJ, Abouassaly R, Kim SP, Zhu H. Contemporary nationwide patterns of active surveillance use for prostate cancer. *JAMA Intern Med* 2015;175(9):1569–1571.

Morgan VA, Parker C, MacDonald A et al. Monitoring tumor volume in patients with prostate cancer undergoing active surveillance: Is MRI apparent diffusion coefficient indicative of tumor growth? *AJR AM J Roentgenol* 2017;209:620–628.

Muthigi A, Sidana A, George AK et al. Current beliefs and practice patterns among urologists regarding prostate magnetic resonance imaging and magnetic resonance-targeted biopsy. *Urol Oncol* 2017;35:32.e1–32.e7.

Nassiri N, Margolis DJ, Natarajan S et al. Targeted biopsy to detect Gleason score upgrading during active surveillance for men with low versus intermediate risk prostate cancer. *J Urol* 2017;197:632–639.

NCCN Guidelines. https://www.nccn.org/professionals/physician_gls/pdf/prostate.pdf.

Scarpato KR, Barocas DA. Use of mpMRI in active surveillance for localized prostate cancer. *Urol Oncol* 2016;34:320–325.

Schulmann AA, Sze C, Tsivian E et al. The contemporary role of multiparametric magnetic resonance imaging in active surveillance for prostate cancer. *Curr Urol Rep* 2017;18:52.

Siddiqui MM, Rais-Bahrami S, Turkbey B et al. Comparison of MR/ultrasound fusion-guided biopsy with ultrasound-guided biopsy for the diagnosis of prostate cancer. *JAMA* 2015;313:390–397.

Squire JA. TMPRSS2-ERG and PTEN loss in prostate cancer. *Nat Genet* 2009;41:509–510.

Stattin P, Vickers AJ, Sjoberg DD et al. Improving the specificity of screening for lethal prostate cancer using prostate-specific antigen and a panel of kallikrein markers: A nested case-control study. *Eur Urol* 2015;68:207–213.

Syed JS, Javier-Desloges J, Tatzel S et al. Current management strategy for active surveillance in prostate cancer. *Curr Oncol Rep* 2017;19:11.

Tosoian JJ, Loeb S, Epstein JI et al. Active surveillance of prostate cancer: Use, outcomes, imaging, and diagnostic tools. *Am Soc Clin Oncol Educ Book* 2016;35:e235–e245.

Tosoian JJ, Loeb S, Feng Z et al. Association of [-2]proPSA with biopsy reclassification during active surveillance for prostate cancer. *J Urol* 2012;188:1131–1136.

Tosoian JJ, Patel HD, Mamawala M et al. Longitudinal assessment of urinary PCA3 for predicting prostate cancer grade reclassification in favorable-risk men during active surveillance. *Prostate Cancer Prostatic Dis* 2017;20:339–342.

Tosoian JJ, Trock BJ, Landis P et al. Active surveillance program for prostate cancer: An update of the Johns Hopkins experience. *J Clin Oncol* 2011;29(16):2185–2190.

Welty CJ, Cowan JE, Nguyen H et al. Extended follow-up and risk factors for disease reclassification in a large active surveillance cohort for localized prostate cancer. *J Urol* 2015;193(3):807–811.

Wilt TJ, Brawer MK, Jones KM et al. Radical prostatectomy versus observation for localized prostate cancer. *N Engl J Med* 2012;367:203–213.

Yu J, Yu J, Ram-Shankar M et al. An integrated network of androgen receptor, polycomb, and TMPRSS2-ERG gene fusions in prostate cancer progression. *Cancer Cell* 2010;17:443–454.

4 Prostate MRI

J. Pereira, Gyan Pareek, and D. Grand

CONTENTS

INTRODUCTION

Prostate cancer (PCa) is the most prevalent cancer among men in the United States, with an estimated incidence of 180,890 cases in 2016.[1] Screening for prostate cancer has traditionally consisted of a digital rectal exam and prostate-specific antigen testing. Following a positive screening evaluation, transrectal ultrasound-guided prostate biopsy is the gold standard for pathologic diagnosis prior to treatment. However, while ultrasound is used to target regions of the prostate, it is unable to reliably identify focal, high-risk nodules.[2] Essentially, the prostate remains the last organ that is routinely biopsied "blind." As such, the incorporation of precise prostate imaging in the evaluation for PCa has become a topic of great interest. First described as a tool for prostate imaging in the 1980s, MRI has been shown to reliably detect and exclude high-risk prostate cancer and can provide targeting of these lesions for transrectal biopsy.[3–5] As the use of prostate MRI grew, the Prostate Imaging-Reporting and Data System (PI-RADS) was introduced, which outlines standards for MRI technique, interpretation, and reporting.[6,7]

MULTIPARAMETRIC MRI OF THE PROSTATE

The key benefit of MRI for prostate imaging is its exquisite soft-tissue contrast, which allows for differentiation of benign and malignant nodules. Multiparametric MRI (mpMRI) refers to the combination of both anatomic and physiologic imaging sequences, including diffusion-weighted imaging (DWI) and dynamic contrast-enhanced imaging (DCE).[7,8] Together, anatomic and physiologic data are assessed to arrive at an overall impression of the risk of clinically significant prostate cancer in any given prostate lesion.

ANATOMIC SEQUENCES

T1- and T2-weighted images serve as the anatomic sequences on which MRI imaging is based. Each imaging sequence is acquired using specific parameters that take advantage of the tissues intrinsic properties. This allows the sequences to highlight the tissues differently and provide complimentary information. On T1WI, water will have low intensity signal and appear dark, while fat displays high intensity signal and appears bright. In comparison water and fat will both appear bright, displaying high signal intensity on T2WI.[9] (Of note, fat can be made to appear dark on either T1- or T2-weighted sequences using fat suppression techniques.)

The soft-tissue contrast of T1WI in the prostate is quite poor. The primary use of T1WI is to identify areas of prostatic hemorrhage (commonly present when MRI is performed following biopsy) to prevent mistaking blood products for suspicious lesions (both of which may be dark on T2WI).[10] Rapid T1WI is performed following intravenous administration of gadolinium to assess perfusion of focal prostatic lesions.

The excellent soft-tissue contrast of T2WI provides detailed information on the anatomic zones of the prostate: the peripheral zone (PZ), transitional zone (TZ), central zone, and anterior fibromuscular zone.[10,11] The PZ is largest anatomic zone in young men, accounting for approximately 75% of total prostate volume, and is the location of over 70% of carcinomas. The PZ forms the subcapsular portion of the prostate surrounding the distal urethra and consists of a large posterior portion, as well as smaller anterior area often referred to as the anterior horn of the PZ. On T2WI, the normal PZ is noted to have intermediate to high signal intensity (Figure 4.1). PCa in the PZ, however, will appear as an area of low signal intensity amongst the higher signal intense background of normal PZ tissue. Unfortunately, low T2 signal in the peripheral zone is not pathognomonic for PCa. Prostatitis and hemorrhage (often post-biopsy) may have a similar appearance. As such, additional imaging sequences are used to differentiate between benign and malignant causes of these findings on T2WI of the PZ.[8,10,12]

The TZ surrounds the proximal urethra and is the site of benign prostatic hyperplasia (BPH) growth. Due to the growth of the TZ with age, the appearance of the PZ on T2WI is variable. BPH nodules in the TZ appear as round well-defined areas of inhomogeneous material with variable signal intensity that are circumscribed by a low signal intensity rim.[13] While BPH lesions may be difficult to discern from areas of PCa with similar signal intensity, other radiologic features help differentiate a malignant lesion. These include homogeneity of the lesion, a lenticular shape, ill-defined or irregular edges of the lesion, and invasion of the urethra or anterior fibromuscular zone.[10] As is true with the TZ, the central zone is also found to be of variable signal intensity and when compressed by an enlarged TZ the two zones are indiscernible from one another on T2WI. The anterior fibromuscular zone is identified as a dense area of low signal intensity posterior to the retropubic fat pad.[7,11]

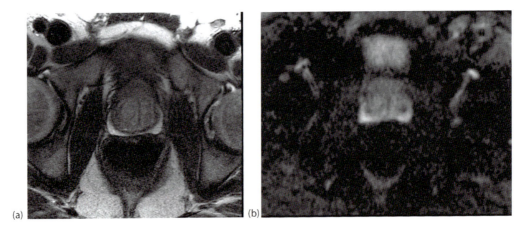

(a)   (b)

FIGURE 4.1   Axial T2-weighted image (a) and apparent diffusion coefficient mapping (b) demonstrating a normal peripheral zone.

DIFFUSION-WEIGHTED IMAGING

As mentioned previously, malignant lesions of the prostate appear as an area of low signal intensity on T2WI. However, these lesions may be difficult to distinguish from other benign pathologies with similar signal intensity. DWI helps to further differentiate benign and malignant lesions using structural differences in the tissue types.[7,8,11]

DWI is based on the diffusion of free water protons in cells. The level of diffusion weighting used during a study is referred to as the *b value*. When multiple *b* values are acquired, an apparent diffusion coefficient (ADC) can be calculated for the tissues being studied. The ADC is a measurement of the ability of water molecules to move freely within tissues. The ADC map is a graphical representation of the diffusion coefficient in each voxel of the image.[8,10,11]

Normal tissues are predominantly composed of extra-cellular space, through which water molecules can easily diffuse (picture walking from end to end of an empty subway car at 10:00 pm). In contrast, cancerous tissues have a much higher cellular density, replacing this large, open extra-cellular space with impenetrable cell membranes (now picture trying to walk from end to end of the same subway car at rush hour). Higher cellular density results in restricted diffusion, which corresponds to a low ADC.

That malignant lesions have been shown to have significantly lower ADCs than benign lesions is especially useful to distinguish BPH nodules of the TZ from PCa. The use of DWI in combination with T2WI has been shown to dramatically improve the sensitivity and specificity of PCa detection on MRI, when compared to T2WI alone. Additionally, the ADC directly correlates with the Gleason score of a lesion. That is, the lower the ADC, the higher the Gleason score.[11]

Unfortunately, there is overlap of the ADC values of benign and malignant prostatic lesions. Therefore, there is no concrete threshold ADC indicative of malignancy. More recently, investigators have shown that additional information can be gathered using high *b* value imaging (HBVI), using a *b* value greater than 1400 sec/mm^2. On these images, signal is preserved in areas of restricted diffusion on standard DWI and thus malignant lesions will appear hyperintense. This may be especially helpful in identifying malignant lesions near the anterior fibromuscular zone and in subcapsular or apical regions.[11]

DYNAMIC CONTRAST ENHANCEMENT

Dynamic contrast enhancement (DCE) is another method used to differentiate between benign and malignant tissues. This technique uses T1-weighted images obtained at multiple time points following IV contrast administration.[8] The prostate is commonly imaged 4–6 times/minute for approximately 5 minutes, after which the uptake and washout of the gadolinium is measured.

Compared to normal prostate tissue, PCa tissues are hypervascular due to increased angiogenesis. This results in earlier uptake and more rapid washout of contrast in malignant tissues. Enhancement can be evaluated qualitatively, semi-quantitatively, or quantitatively. Qualitative analysis is performed by visual inspection of the obtained images for signal intensity. Semi-quantitative techniques introduce uptake washout parameters such as integral area under the gadolinium concentration time curves, wash-in gradient, maximum signal intensity, time-to-peak enhancement, and start of enhancement. Quantitative evaluation uses complex pharmacokinetic models to further evaluate contrast uptake and washout.[8,10,14]

Despite early excitement, DCE has more recently been shown to be of only marginal benefit in the diagnosis of prostate cancer. Prostatitis in the peripheral zone and BPH in the central zone can both be hypervascular and mimic the appearance of PCa. The second version of PI-RADS includes an updated scoring system that relegates the role of DCE to helping sway borderline lesions toward suspicious categories if hypervacular.[7]

SIGNAL-TO-NOISE RATIO IN MRI OF THE PROSTATE

In order to acquire the best possible images of the prostate, MRI protocols seek to optimize the signal-to-noise ratio (SNR), as a higher SNR translates into higher spatial resolution and thus higher-quality images. SNR is affected by many factors but the two most important to the discussion of prostate MRI is the field strength of the magnet and the distance between the prostate and the "antennae" (receiving coil).[9]

MRI is commonly performed using magnetic field strengths of 1.5 Tesla (T) or 3T. SNR increases linearly with the strength of the magnetic field. Thus, MRI acquired at 3T will have nearly twice the SNR of a 1.5T scan. However, the SNR increases exponentially as the receiving coil (antennae) is moved closer to the organ of interest. Surface coils placed on the pelvis should always be used and may be combined with an endorectal coil (ERC) to exploit this benefit of proximity.[9] ERCs may be especially useful when obtaining sequences with inherently low SNR such as DWI.[11] In MRI, though, there is no free lunch. The ERC may compress the prostate and distort its anatomy on imaging. Also, ERCs are often quite uncomfortable, which leads to patient motion and image degradation.[14] The use of external coils alone can achieve high-quality images with adequate SNR, particularly when paired with a high magnetic field strength. Adequate images can be obtained with or without an ERC, using a 1.5T or 3T machine, though data comparing techniques is limited. Currently, PI-RADS version 2 (v2) recommends that radiologists strive to achieve the best possible images with the equipment available.[7]

REPORTING WITH PI-RADS

Prior to the introduction of the PI-RADS v1 in 2012, the protocols used for imaging and the systems used to report imaging findings were not standardized, which greatly hindered the acceptance of mpMRI of the prostate. Earlier reporting systems had largely been developed and used by individual institutions without external validation or consensus. Using the Breast Imaging-Reporting and Data System (BI-RADS) as a model, the European Society of Urogenital Radiologists (ESUR) sought to introduce guidelines for the performance, interpretation, and reporting of mpMRI of the prostate.[6,15] After its introduction, PI-RADS v1 was validated in several clinical and research settings. The systems' success lead to its joint revision by the ESUR, the American College of Radiology, and the AdMeTech Foundation in 2015. PI-RADS v2 focuses on the identification of clinically significant PCa, defined as disease with a Gleason score of 7 or higher, total volume of 0.5 cm^3 or larger, or with extra prostatic extension (EPE).[7]

As in the original version, PI-RADS v2 assigns a score of 1–5 to prostatic lesions based on their probability of containing clinically significant disease. A score of 1 indicates that clinically significant disease is highly unlikely to be present, while a score of 5 indicates that clinically significant disease is highly likely to be present. Biopsy is typically recommended for lesions with a PI-RADS scores of 4 or 5, though other clinical factors may play a role in the decision to biopsy lesions of lower scores.[7]

In PI-RADS v2, the primary and secondary MR sequence used for scoring is determined by the location of the lesion. A lesion that is evaluated as having a score of 1, 2, 4, or 5 using the primary sequence will maintain that number as the overall PI-RADS score. Scores of 3 on the primary sequence, however, are reevaluated using the secondary sequence to determine if the overall PI-RADS score will remain at 3 or be upgraded to 4. The primary and secondary sequences for a lesion in the PZ are the DWI and DCE sequences, while the primary and secondary sequences for a lesion in the TZ are the T2WI and DWI, respectively. MR spectroscopy, which had been recommended in PI-RADS v1, is no longer included in PI-RADS v2.[7]

Evaluation of a Lesion in the Peripheral Zone

The primary sequence for the evaluation of a PZ lesion is DWI (Table 4.1). When evaluation of a PZ lesion on DWI is performed, the signal intensity of the lesion should be compared to that of normal tissue in the same anatomic zone. If a lesion appears normal on DWI and HBVI, it is assigned a PI-RADS score of 1, while a lesion displaying indistinct hypointensity on ADC is scored as a 2. Lesions that appear mild to moderately hypointense on ADC and are isointense or mildly hyperintense on HBVI are assigned a PI-RADS score of 3. If a lesion is noted to have a focal area of obvious hypointensity on ADC (Figure 4.2) with definite hyperintensity on HBVI and a size less than 1.5 cm in its greatest dimension, it is given a score of 4. If a lesion has the appearance of a lesion with a score of 4 but is measured to be greater than 1.5 cm on greatest dimension or has any evidence of extra-capsular extension, it is assigned a score of 5.[7]

The secondary sequence used for evaluation of a PZ tumor is DCE (Table 4.1). Unlike the other sequences, a numeric scale is not used to describe DCE images. Lesions are only evaluated for the presence or absence of enhancement during this sequence. A lesion is considered to enhance if a focal area enhances earlier than or at the same time (but more profoundly) than the surrounding tissues. If the area of enhancement does not correspond to a lesion identified on T2WI or DCE, it is not considered true enhancement. Similarly, if the area of enhancement corresponds to a lesion that is clearly identified as BPH on T2WI, it is not considered to be true

TABLE 4.1

Peripheral Zone Lesion Evaluation and Scoring with PI-RADS Version 2

Sequence	Score	Description
Primary sequence: DWI[a]	1	Lesion appears normal on DWI and HBVI[b]
	2	Lesion displays indistinct hypo intensity on ADC[c] mapping
	3	Lesion appears mild to moderately hypointense on ADC mapping and isointense or mildly hyperintense on HBVI
		Note: Positive DCE[d] upgrades PI-RADS score to 4
	4	Lesion noted to have a focal area of obvious hypointensity on ADC mapping with definite hyperintensity on HBVI and a size <1.5 cm in its greatest dimension
	5	Lesion noted to have a focal area of obvious hypointensity on ADC mapping with definite hyperintensity on HBVI and a size ≥1.5 cm in its greatest dimension
Secondary sequence: DCE[d]	Positive	Lesion demonstrates a focal area that enhances earlier or more profoundly than the surrounding tissues
	Negative	Lesion shows no difference in enhancement compared to surrounding tissues OR
		Area of enhancement does not correspond to the lesion identified on T2WI[e] OR
		Area of enhancement corresponds to a lesion which is clearly identified as BPH[f] on T2WI, it is not considered to be true enhancement

[a] Diffusion-weighted imaging.
[b] High *b* value imaging.
[c] Apparent diffusion coefficient.
[d] Dynamic contrast enhancement.
[e] T2-weighted imaging.
[f] Benign prostatic hyperplasia.

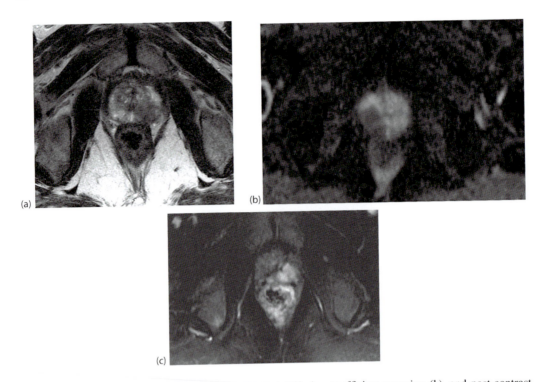

FIGURE 4.2 Axial T2-weighted image (a), apparent diffusion coefficient mapping (b), and post-contrast T1-weighted image demonstrating a large peripheral zone mass (c).

enhancement. When a PZ lesion is scored as a 3 on DWI, the overall PI-RADS score should be upgrade to a 4 if enhancement is noted on DCE.[7]

In the case of PZ lesions, T2WI is only used for PI-RADS scoring if DWI is unavailable. As mentioned previously, malignant lesions of the PZ observed on T2WI will appear as hypointense focal lesions. If the lesion does not appear hypointense on T2WI it is given a score of 1. If an area of hypointensity is noted to have a linear or wedge-shaped appearance, or if a diffuse hypointense area with no distinct margin is noted, the lesion is scored a 2. If a lesion is noted to have heterogeneous signal intensity or if it is a non-circumscribed area of moderate hypointensity, it is scored a 3. A well-circumscribed lesion with homogenous hypointensity of less than 1.5 cm in its largest dimension is considered a 4. If a lesion is larger than 1.5 cm or displays EPE, it is scored a 5.[7]

EVALUATION OF A LESION IN THE TRANSITIONAL ZONE

In the evaluation of a lesion in the TZ, the T2WI serves as the primary sequence for PI-RADS scoring (Table 4.2). In the TZ, malignant lesions will appear as poorly circumscribed areas of hypointensity. If no change in signal is noted in the lesion compared to surrounding tissues, it is given a score of 1. When a well-circumscribed hypointense lesion, or a well-encapsulated heterogeneously intense lesion (consistent with BPH) is seen, it is given a score of 2 (Figure 4.3). A lesion with unclear margins and heterogeneous signal intensity should be scored as a 3. Any lenticular or non-circumscribed lesion with moderate hypointensity that is less than 1.5 cm in its greatest dimension should be scored as a 4. If a lesion with a similar appearance to that of a 4 is larger than 1.5 cm or displays EPE, it is given a score of 5.[7]

The secondary sequence used to score a lesion in the TZ is DWI. Evaluation for a TZ lesion on DWI is performed in the same manner described previously for PZ lesions (Table 4.2). When a TZ

TABLE 4.2

Transition Zone Lesion Evaluation and Scoring with PI-RADS Version 2

Sequence	Score	Description
Primary sequence: T2WI[a]	1	Lesion demonstrates no change in signal compared to surrounding tissues
	2	Lesion is hypointense and well circumscribed hypointense OR Lesion is well encapsulated and heterogeneously intense (consistent with BPH[b])
	3	Lesion with unclear margins, and heterogeneous signal intensity Note: Score ≥4 on DWI[c] upgrades PI-RADS score to 4
	4	Lesion is lenticular or non-circumscribed with moderate hypointensity and a size <1.5 cm in its greatest dimension
	5	Lesion is lenticular or non-circumscribed with moderate hypointensity and a size ≥1.5 cm in its greatest dimension
Secondary sequence: DWI[c]	1	Lesion appears normal on DWI[c] and HBVI[d]
	2	Lesion displays indistinct hypointensity on ADC[e] mapping
	3	Lesion appears mild to moderately hypointense on ADC mapping and isointense or mildly hyperintense on HBVI
	4	Lesion noted to have a focal area of obvious hypointensity on ADC mapping with definite hyperintensity on HBVI and a size <1.5 cm in its greatest dimension
	5	Lesion noted to have a focal area of obvious hypointensity on ADC mapping with definite hyperintensity on HBVI and a size ≥1.5 cm in its greatest dimension

[a] T2-weighted imaging.
[b] Benign prostatic hyperplasia.
[c] Diffusion-weighted imaging.

[d] High *b* value imaging.
[e] Apparent diffusion coefficient.

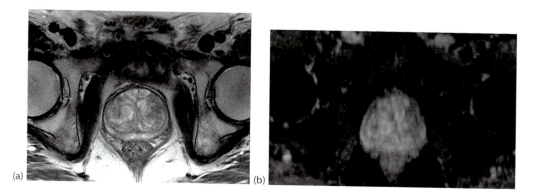

FIGURE 4.3 Axial T2-weighted image (a) and apparent diffusion coefficient mapping (b) demonstrating a lesion with diffuse low T2 signal without restricted diffusion likely due to chronic prostatitis; PI-RADS score: 2.

lesion is given a score of 3 on T2WI, DWI should be evaluated to determine if that lesion will receive a final PI-RADS score of 3 or be upgraded to a 4. If the lesion is evaluated to have a score of 5, the overall score is upgraded to 4. If the DWI score is valuated to be 4 or lower, the overall PI-RADS score will remain a 3. Of note, DCE does not play a role in the scoring of TZ lesions.[7]

As part of PI-RADS, a standardized method of reporting findings on mpMRI of the prostate was outlined. In addition to the scoring of lesions, radiologists should also describe lesion size and location. PI-RADS utilizes a standardized mapping system which describes 39 distinct sectors of the prostate that should be used to describe the location of lesions or other notable findings. According to PI-RADS v2, up to four lesions should be described and from these a dominant lesion should be identified. The dominant lesion is the lesion with the highest PI-RADS score. If multiple lesions have the same PI-RADS score, a lesion with EPE is considered dominant. If no lesions demonstrate EPE, the largest lesion is dominant. If more than four lesions are present, the four lesions with the highest likelihood of representing clinically significant cancer should be reported.[7,8]

CLINICAL APPLICATIONS OF PROSTATE MRI

The clinical applications of prostatic MRI include the staging, diagnosis, and surveillance of PCa.[5,8,10,16,17] A growing body of evidence continues to support the use of MRI for several of these indications. Current guidelines focus on the use of MRI of the prostate for the detection of clinically significant PCa in men with a prior negative biopsy and for the staging of clinically proven intermediate or high-risk disease.[18]

Transrectal ultrasound-guided prostate biopsy remains the standard procedure for initial prostate biopsy but false negative results are common.[19] As such, the use of MRI guidance to perform targeted prostate biopsies has been an area of interest. Studies have demonstrated that the use of mpMRI for targeted prostate biopsy increases the detection rates of clinically significant PCa,[10,18] while decreasing the detection rates of clinically insignificant disease. Use of target biopsies alone, however, may fail to detect some clinically significant disease when compared to the use of targeted biopsy in conjunction with standard prostate biopsy.[18] The clinical significance of the use of mpMRI for targeted biopsy in the biopsy-naïve man remains controversial, especially in light of the cost associated with the procedure.[17]

MRI has proven to be most useful in the diagnosis of significant cancers when clinical suspicion for PCa remains high despite negative biopsies.[19] Recently, the American College of Radiology and the American Urological Association released a joint consensus statement on the use of MRI targeted prostate biopsy in men with a prior negative biopsy. Use of targeted biopsies in this setting results in the detection of clinically significant disease in 11%–54% of cases. It is recommended that at least two biopsy cores are obtained from each suspicious lesion identified on MRI and that these be performed in conjunction with a standard biopsy.[18]

Active surveillance (AS) has become a mainstay in the treatment of low- and some intermediate-grade PCa. An AS protocol monitors for disease progression via the use of prostate-specific antigen (PSA) testing, digital rectal exam (DRE), and prostate biopsy. AS protocols vary by institution, but typically PSA testing and DRE are performed every 3–6 months and prostate biopsy is performed every 12–18 months. Prostate MRI is not yet considered a standard part of AS, but it has been studied as an adjunct. During AS, an unchanged mpMRI has been shown to have a negative predictive value of 80% for upstaging of disease on subsequent prostate biopsy.[17] Currently, mpMRI of the prostate is not sufficient to serve as the primary modality of surveillance, but further research and technological improvements may change this.

Finally, prostate MRI is a valuable tool in the staging of prostate cancer. MRI has been shown to be equivalent to CT or PET scan for the identification of metastatic disease in regional lymph nodes.[5] MRI has also been shown to be highly specific for the identification of EPE and SVI (Figure 4.4), with specificity rates of 91% and 97% respectively.[5] Obtaining MRI prior to treatment can influence the choice of treatment modality and help to inform surgical planning.

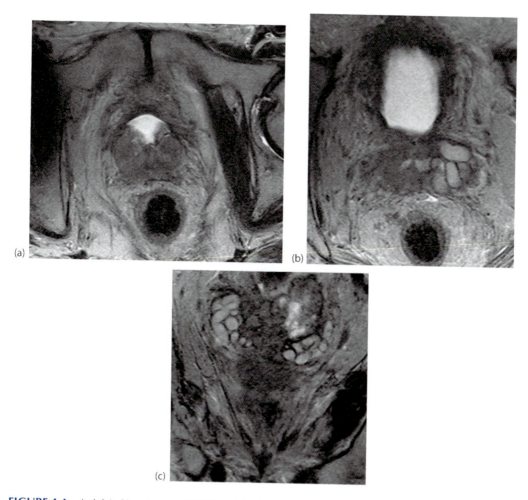

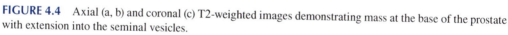

FIGURE 4.4 Axial (a, b) and coronal (c) T2-weighted images demonstrating mass at the base of the prostate with extension into the seminal vesicles.

CONCLUSIONS

Utilization of MRI to aid in the diagnosis and management of PCa has increased exponentially in recent years and will likely continue to expand in the near future. MRI confidently identifies clinically significant cancer, supplanting "overdiagnosis" with accurate and actionable diagnosis. MRI is also particularly useful to identify and target occult malignancy when clinical suspicion remains high despite negative prior biopsies. Finally, as increasing numbers of patients choose active surveillance over immediate, definitive treatment, MRI will likely play a large role in disease monitoring. PI-RADS provides a template for standardized communication between radiologists and urologists, which should improve clarity of reporting and interobserver variability.

REFERENCES

1. *SEER Cancer Statistics Factsheets: Prostate Cancer.* Bethesda, MD: National Cancer Institute, vol. 2016, 2016.
2. Loeb, S., Eastham, J. A. Diagnosis and staging of prostate cancer. In: *Campbell-Walsh Urology*, 11th ed. Edited by A. J. Wein, L. R. Kavoussi, A. W. Partin et al. Philadelphia, PA: Elsevier, pp. 2601–2608, 2016.

3. Steyn, J. H., Smith, F. W. Nuclear magnetic resonance imaging of the prostate. *Br J Urol*, **54:** 726, 1982.

4. Hricak, H., Williams, R. D., Spring, D. B. et al. Anatomy and pathology of the male pelvis by magnetic resonance imaging. *AJR Am J Roentgenol*, **141:** 1101, 1983.

5. Coakley, F. V., Oto, A., Alexander, L. F. et al. ACR appropriateness criteria(R) prostate cancer-pretreatment detection, surveillance, and staging. *J Am Coll Radiol*, **14:** S245, 2017.

6. Barentsz, J. O., Richenberg, J., Clements, R. et al. ESUR prostate MR guidelines 2012. *Eur Radiol*, **22:** 746, 2012.

7. Weinreb, J. C., Barentsz, J. O., Choyke, P. L. et al. PI-RADS prostate imaging - Reporting and data system: 2015, version 2. *Eur Urol*, **69:** 16, 2016.

8. Kiechle, J., Pahwa, S., Gulani, V. et al. Magnetic resonance imaging for prostate cancer: What the urologist needs to know. *Minerva Urol Nefrol*, **67:** 201, 2015.

9. Moser, E., Stadlbauer, A., Windischberger, C. et al. Magnetic resonance imaging methodology. *Eur J Nucl Med Mol Imaging*, **36 Suppl 1:** S30, 2009.

10. Shaish, H., Taneja, S. S., Rosenkrantz, A. B. Prostate MR imaging: An update. *Radiol Clin North Am*, **55:** 303, 2017.

11. Riches, S. F., deSouza, N. M. *Extra-cranial Applications of Diffusion-Weighted MRI.* Edited by B. Taouli. Cambridge, UK: Cambridge University Press, pp. 72–85, 2011.

12. Guneyli, S., Erdem, C. Z., Erdem, L. O. Magnetic resonance imaging of prostate cancer. *Clin Imaging*, **40:** 601, 2016.

13. Guneyli, S., Ward, E., Thomas, S. et al. Magnetic resonance imaging of benign prostatic hyperplasia. *Diagn Interv Radiol*, **22:** 215, 2016.

14. Barrett, T., Turkbey, B., Choyke, P. L. PI-RADS version 2: What you need to know. *Clin Radiol*, **70:** 1165, 2015.

15. Dickinson, L., Ahmed, H. U., Allen, C. et al. Scoring systems used for the interpretation and reporting of multiparametric MRI for prostate cancer detection, localization, and characterization: Could standardization lead to improved utilization of imaging within the diagnostic pathway? *J Magn Reson Imaging*, **37:** 48, 2013.

16. De Visschere, P. J., Briganti, A., Futterer, J. J. et al. Role of multiparametric magnetic resonance imaging in early detection of prostate cancer. *Insights Imaging*, **7:** 205, 2016.

17. Fulgham, P. F., Rukstalis, D. B., Turkbey, I. B. et al. AUA policy statement on the use of multiparametric magnetic resonance imaging in the diagnosis, staging and management of prostate cancer. *J Urol*, **198:** 832, 2017.

18. Rosenkrantz, A. B., Verma, S., Choyke, P. et al. Prostate magnetic resonance imaging and magnetic resonance imaging targeted biopsy in patients with a prior negative biopsy: A consensus statement by AUA and SAR. *J Urol*, **196:** 1613, 2016.

19. Gomella, L. G., Halpern, E. J., Trabulsi, E. J. Prostate biopsy: Techniques and imaging. In: *Campbell-Walsh Urology*, 11th ed. Edited by A. J. Wein, L. R. Kavoussi, A. W. Partin et al. Philadelphia, PA: Elsevier, pp. 2579–2592, 2016.

5 Current Role and Evolution of MRI Fusion Biopsy for Prostate Cancer

Danielle Velez, Joseph Brito, and Joseph Renzulli II

CONTENTS

The American Urology Association (AUA) recommends screening for prostate cancer (PCa) in men aged 55–70 who are without risk factors or family history.[1] Screening involves a digital rectal exam (DRE) and serum prostate-specific antigen (PSA), the combination of which helps to provide a level of risk of prostate cancer to the patient. The gold standard for the actual diagnosis of prostate cancer remains the transrectal ultrasound-guided biopsy (TRUS biopsy), which relies on a standard sextant template, randomly sampling the prostate at the base, mid, and apex levels, with two samples taken from each level from the right and left lobes, resulting in 12 cores. While it has proven to be a useful tool, ultrasound (US) alone is inadequate for visualizing suspicious prostatic lesions. Although cores are obtained in a systematic fashion, there is a risk of the biopsy needle missing a focus of intermediate- or high-risk prostate cancer.[2] Prostate biopsy itself is not without morbidity, as it is uncomfortable and invasive, can lead to transient hematuria and hematochezia, and carries a rate of post-biopsy sepsis from 0.6% to 5.7%.[3]

MRI-guided prostate biopsy has gained popularity in the last decade, with the promise of improving the detection rate of clinically significant prostate cancer in patients undergoing biopsy. Here we present a brief history of the utilization of MRI in the realm of prostate cancer, as well as indications for its utility in the diagnosis and treatment of this disease.

MRI HISTORY

Magnetic resonance imaging (MRI) was first utilized in 1977. Since its inception, the ability for MRI to detect and stage malignancy has been further refined and explored. In 1983, Hricak performed 25 pelvic MRIs using a 0.35T magnet, noting that in the prostate cancer patients, malignant tissue had a characteristically higher intensity signal than the surrounding benign gland.[4]

Modern MRI generally employs the more powerful 3T magnet. Paralleling the increase in imaging quality, the use of MRI in the diagnosis and staging of prostate cancer has become an increasingly common implement in the urologist's arsenal. As discussed previously, inherent sampling error in the standard sextant TRUS biopsy risks understaging of patient disease. Alternatively, random biopsies may uncover only clinically indolent disease with little or no risk of progression, creating a situation where the risks of a radical prostatectomy or radiation therapy outweigh its benefits. The United States Preventative Services Task Force (USPSTF) recommended against screening for prostate cancer in their 2008 guidelines. The task force concluded that treatment for prostate cancer diagnosed by screening exposes patients to the risks of treatment, including erectile dysfunction, urinary incontinence, bowel dysfunction, or even death, without proof that this population would have ever experienced cancer-related symptoms in their lifetime.[5] MRI allows the urologist to image the prostate in great detail, offering the opportunity to identify regions of interest for subsequent biopsy. Using this image as a map in real time to ensure tissue acquisition of the suspicious areas can further increase the biopsy yield for clinically significant (Gleason 7 or greater) disease.[6]

MULTIPARAMETRIC MRI

With increasing utilization of prostate MRI, select phases (or parameters) have become favored for detection of disease. Today, the industry consensus is for the multiparametric MRI (mpMRI) to include high-resolution T2-weighted images, and at least two functional techniques, diffusion-weighted imaging (DWI) and dynamic contrast enhancement (DCE), with or without MR spectroscopy. The combination of these images allows mpMRI to detect higher-grade disease, thus reducing the diagnosis and subsequent treatment of clinically indolent cancers.

Radiologists use the Prostate Imaging-Reporting and Data System (PI-RADS) to categorize lesions seen under mpMRI. Created under the International Prostate MRI Working Group in 2007, and then revised by the American College of Radiology and the European Society of Urogenital Radiology in 2015, the PI-RADS v2 system standardized the classification and reporting of prostate MRI lesions, which greatly facilitated in multicenter clinical evaluation and implementation.[7]

PI-RADS v2 uses a 5-point scale to assign a likelihood that the combination of mpMRI findings on T2WI, DWI, DCE correlates to a clinically significant focus of cancer within the gland:

- PI-RADS 1—Very low (clinically significant cancer is highly unlikely to be present)
- PI-RADS 2—Low (clinically significant cancer is unlikely to be present)
- PI-RADS 3—Intermediate (the presence of clinically significant cancer is equivocal)
- PI-RADS 4—High (clinically significant cancer is likely to be present)
- PI-RADS 5—Very high (clinically significant cancer is highly likely to be present)

Even with standardized reporting, there is still substantial variability in mpMRI interpretation. Garcia-Reyes et al.[8] showed that dedicated mpMRI education programs, and ultimately radiology experience, are required for diagnostic accuracy. Five blinded radiology fellows evaluated 31 mpMRIs, which had already been evaluated by board-certified radiologists with at least 5 years of prostate mpMRI experience. The radiology reads were then compared to final histopathology findings after radical prostatectomy. The fellows then underwent a dedicated mpMRI education program, and reevalauted the images. Cancer detection increased from 74.2% to 87.7% ($p = 0.003$), with Gleason score accuracy increasing from 54.8% to 73.5% ($p = 0.0005$) after education.

T2-weighted images reflect the tissue water content, and are used to establish prostatic anatomy. Cancerous lesions appear as poorly defined, low-signal intensity foci. Alone, T2WI carries a specificity and sensitivity of only 88% and 74%, respectively, as the lesions appear similar to benign prostatic hyperplasia in the peripheral zone, or even biopsy-related hemorrhage.[9] To prevent confusion during MRI fusion biopsy, the American College of Radiology recommends waiting at least 6 weeks between initial prostate biopsy and MRI fusion biopsy to allow for bleeding resolution.[7]

For this reason, T2WI is combined with functional imaging to improve mpMRI sensitivity and specificity. Diffusion-weighted imaging measures the random Brownian motion of water molecules

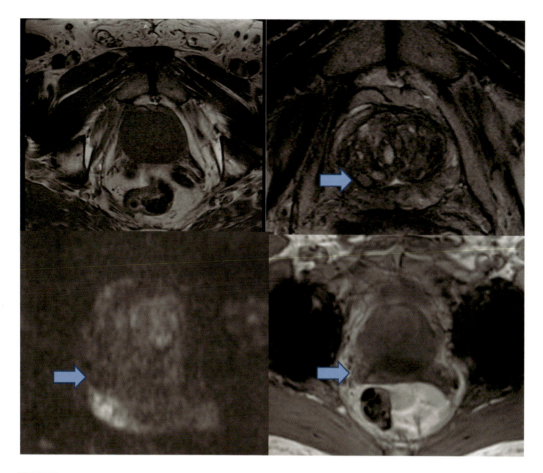

FIGURE 5.1 3T prostate MRI of a 71-year-old male with on active surveillance for low-risk T1 Gleason 6 prostate cancer. PSA 2.8. Arrows point to a PI-RADS 4 lesion in the right mid-gland, peripheral zone, as seen on different MRI sequences. Top left: unable to visualize lesion on T1 sequence. Top right: hypointense lesion on T2 sequence. Bottom left: DWI, notable for decreased ADC. Bottom right: VIBE imaging.

within tissues. Denser tissues have less movement, and therefore lower diffusion coefficients. The change in the tissue density is measured as the apparent diffusion coefficient (ADC). On DWI, cancerous lesions are defined by a high diffusion coefficient and low ADC. Diffusion-weighted imaging is particularly important, as the lesions identified on this phase have been shown to have a higher likelihood of being clinically significant (i.e., Gleason grade $\geq$7).[10]

Dynamic contrast-enhanced MRI evaluates tumor vascularity by imaging the prostate pre- and post-gadolinium administration. Magnetic resonance spectroscopic imaging (MRSI) relies on elevated choline and lower citrate in cancerous as opposed to benign tissue. It is useful in predicting the presence or absence of cancer and can provide information on the aggressiveness of the disease, further improving the specificity and sensitivity of mpMRI over T2WI alone (Figure 5.1).

INDICATIONS FOR mpMRI AND MRI FUSION BIOPSY

As more mpMRIs and MRI fusion biopsies are performed, the clinical scenarios where the technology has a benefit over traditional TRUS biopsies are also evolving and expanding. TRUS biopsy remains the gold standard for prostate cancer diagnosis. However, there is a rapidly growing body of literature to support a role for MRI fusion biopsy, as detailed in the 2016 guidelines released by the

AUA and the Society of Abdominal Radiology. Overall, the literature recommends consideration of mpMRI and MRI fusion biopsy in:[2,11]

- Patients considering active surveillance, or those currently on active surveillance, to ensure that this is the most appropriate management strategy
- Patients with history of prior negative prostate biopsy but continued suspicion of prostate cancer, usually due to rising PSA and/or abnormal DRE

In 2012, the European Society of Urogenital Radiologists (ESUR)[10] also released clinical guidelines, including a decision-making flowchart (Figure 5.2) focused on further prostate imaging after a patient's first TRUS biopsy. For low-risk patients deciding between treatment versus active surveillance, mpMRI may detect the presence of intermediate- to high-risk disease. Targeted biopsy of these "hot" lesions minimizes the sampling error of the standard TRUS biopsy, potentially removing active surveillance as an appropriate option if that lesion proves to be clinically significant.

Intermediate-risk patients may benefit more from information on disease location, such as the presence or absence of extraprostatic extension, to aid decision making on nerve-sparing and surgical approach. The ESUR concluded that Detection Protocols are most appropriate in the low-risk population, limiting the MRI to a 30-minute protocol, without an endorectal coil, covering the entire prostate with T2WI, DCE, and DWI phases. This differs slightly from the Staging Protocol, where a longer-MRI scan is required (45 minutes), due to the addition of magnetic resonance spectroscopic imaging (MRSI).

MRI provides the clinician with information regarding tumor volume, aggressiveness, and location. Particularly for anterior lesions, which may be missed on standard template biopsy, or for small lesions—mpMRI has enough sensitivity to detect tumors at least 0.5 mL in volume.[10]

But in the era of joint decision making between provider and patient, it is not the volume of information but the quality that counts. Multiparametric MRI favors the detection of high-risk disease. By identifying these lesions, mpMRI helps the provider to establish the population that would truly benefit from intervention. Simultaneously, by ignoring low-risk lesions, patients avoid the morbidity

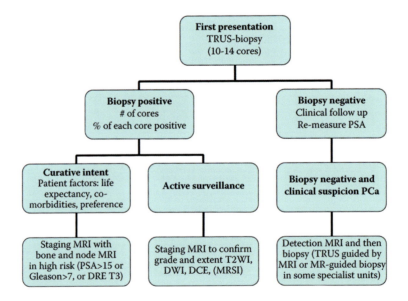

FIGURE 5.2 ESUR prostate imaging algorithm. Detection MRI: <30 minute protocol consisting of the T2WI, DWI, and DCE images. Staging MRI: 45-minute protocol to evaluate for extraprostatic extension, using the above images ± MRSI. (From Barentsz, J. et al., *Eur. Radiol.*, 22, 746–757, 2012.)

of low-yield biopsies and ultimately the overtreatment of disease that is unlikely to change their quality of life or life expectancy.

Vargas et al.[12] sought to assess the value of mpMRI and MRI fusion biopsy in men with clinically low-risk prostate cancer prior to placement on active surveillance. In this retrospective review, 388 men underwent mpMRI, followed by confirmatory biopsy, which included 12 cores plus a sampling of suspicious areas by US, MRI, or DRE. Seventy-nine men were upgraded to Gleason $\geq$3+4 on confirmatory biopsy. They also noted the high negative predictive value of a PI-RADS 2 lesion for disease upgrading (0.96–1.0), compared to the high sensitivity of a PI-RADS 5 lesion (0.87–0.98) for upgrading on confirmatory biopsy.

Active surveillance protocols often require repeat prostate biopsy. Alberts et al.[13] examined 210 men on AS with Gleason 6 disease who underwent a mpMRI at 3 months from diagnosis, at confirmatory biopsy 1 year from diagnosis, or after one or more repeat TRUS biopsies. The authors found that 64% of the men had a "positive" MRI, defined as detection of a PI-RADS $\geq$3 lesion, with 24% upgraded to Gleason $\geq$3+4 disease after re-biopsy. This finding was similar across the three groups (23%, 23%, and 27%, respectively). Although this was not directly compared to a control group of TRUS biopsy patients, the study was important in that it established that whether the mpMRI is performed early or later in the active surveillance course, its detection of higher-grade disease allows the patient to make better informed decisions about their selected management strategy. When performed earlier, MRI fusion biopsy may help to prevent unnecessary additional biopsies, which may not detect advancement of disease. Timely targeted biopsy may also lead to earlier treatment for clinically significant disease, which may help to improve cancer-specific survival.

The second indication for mpMRI and MRI-fusion biopsy is patients with negative biopsy but continued concern for undetected prostate cancer. Lee et al.[14] evaluated the efficacy of targeted biopsy using MRI in men with a previously negative prostate biopsy and rising PSA. Eighty seven men underwent mpMRI prior to biopsy, which was performed in a cognitive fusion technique (see below), obtaining the standard 12-core biopsy as well as targeted biopsies of suspicious lesions identified on MRI. Suspicious MRI lesions were seen in 94.2% of the men, with 56% of those patients having prostate cancer in at least one core biopsy (targeted or template). Of the prostate cores, 28.8% of the targeted cores, versus 3.6% of the template cores, ($p = 0.012$) contained prostate cancer. Only two patients had a negative MRI but finding of cancer within 1 of the 12 standard template cores. Furthermore, only five patients were found to have insignificant prostate cancer by Epstein criteria on MRI-targeted biopsy.

Taken together, these studies demonstrate the ability of mpMRI to visualize higher Gleason grade disease and to identify targetable lesions during re-biopsy. This technique helps to more accurately grade and stage a patient's disease, thereby decreasing the number of unnecessary biopsies a patient may have to undergo. MRI may also aid in patient selection for enrollment in or continuation of active surveillance protocols.

METHODS FOR MRI FUSION BIOPSY

Multiple methods for performing MRI-guided prostate biopsy have been described. In-bore, magnetic resonance-guided biopsy (MRG-biopsy) was the first method developed to sample MRI-visualized prostatic lesions. It requires the use of MRI-safe needles, which are placed into the lesions identified on MRI, and the location of the needle prior to its withdrawal is confirmed via MRI. Drawbacks to this method are that it is time-consuming, and therefore more uncomfortable to the patient, who must lay in the prone or decubitus position with a rectal probe in place. It is also more financially taxing, requiring access to the MRI scanner, the software, and MRI-safe needles. However, this method is very precise, and may be most helpful in patients with an altered anatomy (i.e., post abdominal-perineal resection).[2]

The so-called cognitive fusion or visual registration approach relies mostly on operative ability to use anatomic landmarks on ultrasound and MRI to manually guide the needle into the

MRI-identified lesions.[2] "Anatomic fiducials" include cysts, bony landmarks, and calcifications. Although this technique does not require as much equipment and time as the MRG biopsy, it is heavily dependent on operator experience and technique. Smaller lesions, anterior masses, and those at the lateral edge or apex can be particularly difficult to sample with cognitive fusion biopsy.[11]

Finally, software-based registration platforms overlay the mpMRI onto the real-time US images, giving the provider a map of the prostate and its lesions, in addition to real-time ultrasound feedback on needle location. Alignment is achieved in a rigid or elastic fashion. First, a prostatic sweep is performed with the ultrasound probe, creating a 3D reconstruction of the prostate. Rigid registration projects the mpMRI over the 3D ultrasound image and aligns the contour of the prostate and its landmarks under MRI to the US in an unchanging fashion. This does not correct for changes in prostate anatomy that may occur with patient repositioning or probe movement. Elastic registration attempts to compensate for the prostate deformation during the course of the biopsy, although in the process can cause some anatomic distortion by sacrificing internal architecture for continuously aligned contours.[2,15] In both rigid and elastic registration, the software tracks the movement of the ultrasound probe so that the fused US/MRI image remains accurate. Today, most software-based registration platforms have evolved to allow for a combination of elastic and rigid registration to maximize accuracy (Figure 5.3).

A literature review by Wegelin et al.[15] found no statistically significant benefit to any of the techniques described above in the detection of clinically significant prostate cancer. Any of the MRI fusion biopsies, regardless of the technique, were superior to routine TRUS in detecting clinically

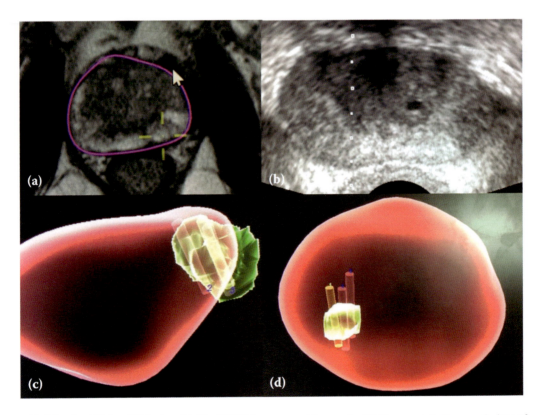

FIGURE 5.3 MRI to US fusion. (a) The T2WI is contoured in purple. (b) Transrectal ultrasound view of the same prostate (c) and (d). The TRUS and MRI prostatic images are combined, to create a 3D mapping of the prostate, including the location of previously detected suspicious lesions on MRI. In a rigid system, the surgeon would manually overlap prostate contour taken from the MRI to the prostate viewed under TRUS. In an elastic system, the software automatically compensates for differences in prostate shape/contour.

significant prostate cancer (OR 1.16, range 1.02–1.32). Pooled sensitivities for prostate cancer diagnosis were 0.72 (95% CI 0.62–0.81), 0.81 (95% CI 0.75–0.85), and 0.89 (95% CI 0.78–0.95) for cognitive-fusion biopsy, software-based biopsy, and in-bore MRI-guided biopsy, respectively.

MRI fusion biopsy programs also rely on tracking software to visualize the TRUS probe position and needle advancement in three dimensions, helping the provider to accurately target the lesion of interest.[2] The tracking software is also able to store the needle's location for each of its biopsy cores, allowing providers to re-sample the same areas on subsequent biopsies.

There are several ways to track the biopsy needle, and even more software systems to fine-tune these methods within clinical practice. One is electromagnetic tracking, which relies on a solenoid sensor on the TRUS biopsy probe, which generates a constantly changing magnetic field and subsequent electric current, which is then relayed to the computer to create a 3D image. The UroNav® system (Invivo Corporation), reports a registration and tracking error of 2–3 mm when the biopsy probe is positioned just proximal to the lesion of interest prior to deployment of the biopsy needle.[16]

Robotic arms affixed to the biopsy table and fitted with position-encoded sensors have also been used to track the 3D position of the biopsy probe. In this technique, as movement of the probe is controlled by the robotic arm, its motion is restricted to rotation along a fixed axis. One example of position-encoded sensors is the Artemis (Eigen), pictured below (Figure 5.4).

Finally, image-based tracking uses elastic registration and the 3D image of the prostate to track the ultrasound probe. A second 3D TRUS image is obtained after firing the prostate biopsy, to confirm the needle's position. The Urostation (Koelis) is an image-based software tracking system.

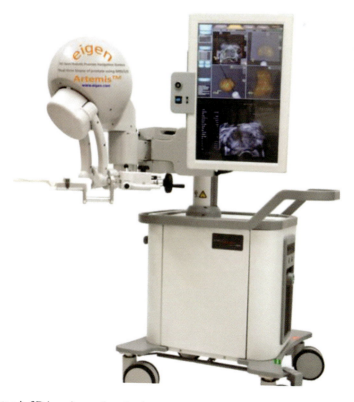

FIGURE 5.4 Artemis 3D imaging and navigation for prostate biopsy (Eigen). (From http://www.eigen.com/products/artemis.shtml.[17])

MRI FUSION BIOPSY VERSUS THE GOLD STANDARD

As more institutions adopt mpMRI and MRI fusion biopsy into practice, more data has been generated to compare the MRI fusion biopsy performance to that of the traditional template TRUS biopsy.

Costs associated with MRI/TRUS fusion technologies include the upfront financial investment in equipment and software, a heavy time commitment for training and traversing the learning curve of the technology, as well as the more long-term cost of maintenance and upgrading. However, the challenges that a practice faces in initiating an MRI fusion biopsy program are supported by a wealth of research supporting the use of MRI fusion biopsy over TRUS.

As previously mentioned, Lee et al.[14] noted that of their 87 patients with a previously negative biopsy and rising PSA, only 8 of the 46 newly identified prostate cancers (17.4%) would have been biopsied if only a traditional TRUS biopsy had been performed without mpMRI and MRI fusion biopsy.

Pokorny et al.[6] reported on the cancer detection rate for 226 biopsy-naïve men, with rising PSA and/or abnormal DRE after undergoing an mpMRI. Men with PI-RADS ≥3 lesions first underwent MRI fusion biopsy, and then 30 minutes later a standard sextant TRUS biopsy. Men with PI-RADS 1–2 lesions underwent TRUS biopsy alone. MRI-guided biopsy was performed in 142 men, versus 223 TRUS biopsies. Prostate cancer was diagnosed in 69.7% of the MRI-guided biopsy patients, versus 56.5% of the TRUS biopsy patients; in addition, MRI-guided biopsy detected more intermediate- to high-risk disease: 93.9% versus 62.7% ($p < 0.01$). MRI-guided biopsy also did not detect as much low-risk disease (6.1% vs. 62.7%, $p < 0.001$) as the standard TRUS biopsy. If the patients had only undergone MRI-guided biopsy for the PI-RADS 3 or greater lesions, fewer would have been exposed to the risks of biopsy, only to be diagnosed with a low-risk disease that does not warrant intervention.

Other studies have failed to establish a statistically significant difference in prostate cancer detection rate between TRUS and MRI-guided biopsy. Mendhiratta et al.[18] performed MRI fusion biopsy and TRUS biopsy in 161 men with a history of at least one negative prostate biopsy. Prostate cancer detection rates were similar, with MRI detecting 21.7% of cancers, and TRUS biopsy 18.6% ($p = 0.36$). However, looking at cancer detection rates per Gleason grade, MRI-guided biopsies detected more of the Gleason ≥7 cancers than TRUS biopsy (14.9% vs. 9.3%, $p = 0.02$). This is consistent with the basic intention of mpMRI, in that it is geared to the diagnosis of high-risk lesions, rather than clinically insignificant disease.

CONCLUSIONS

As a clinician's responsibility is to weigh the risks and benefits of every test and intervention, choosing the diagnostic test with the greatest yield for actionable diagnoses is in the best interest of the patient. In its current state, MRI fusion biopsy has been shown to outperform standard TRUS biopsy in the detection of intermediate- to high-risk disease. But as the techniques for performing mpMRI become more refined, and US/MRI fusion software improves, indications for the utilization of mpMRI in the management of both newly diagnosed and monitored prostate cancer are expected to evolve and expand.

REFERENCES

1. Carter, H.B. et al. Early detection of prostate cancer: AUA guidelines. *Journal of Urology* 2013;190(2):419–426.
2. Kongnyuy, M. et al. Magnetic resonance imaging-ultrasound fusion-guided prostate biopsy: Review of technology, techniques, and outcomes. *Current Urology Reports* 2016;17(4):32.
3. Anderson, E. et al. Risk factors for infection following prostate biopsy: A case control study. *BMC Infectious Disease* 2015;15:580.

4. Hricak, H. et al. Anatomy and pathology of the male pelvis by magnetic resonance imaging. *American Journal of Roentgenology* 1983;141:1101–1110.
5. USPSTF. Screening for prostate cancer: U.S. Preventive Services Task Force Recommendation Statement. *Annals of Internal Medicine* 2008;149:185–191.
6. Pokorny, M. et al. Prospective study of diagnostic accuracy comparing prostate cancer detection by transrectal ultrasound–guided biopsy versus magnetic resonance (MR) imaging with subsequent MR-guided biopsy in men without previous prostate biopsies. *European Urology* 2014;66:22–29.
7. *Prostate Imaging-Reporting and Data System (PIRADS), 2015 Version 2.* American College of Radiology.
8. Garcia-Reyes, K. et al. Detection of prostate cancer with multiparametric MRI (mpMRI): Effect of dedicated reader education on accuracy and confidence of index and anterior cancer diagnosis. *Abdominal Imaging* 2015;40:134–142.
9. Tyson, M. et al. Magnetic resonance-ultrasound fusion prostate biopsy in the diagnosis of prostate cancer. *Urologic Oncology* 2016;34:326–332.
10. Barentsz, J. et al. ESUR prostate MR guidelines 2012. *European Radiology* 2012;22:746–757.
11. Rosenkrantz, B. et al. Prostate magnetic resonance imaging and magnetic resonance imaging targeted biopsy in patients with a prior negative biopsy: A consensus statement by AUA and SAR. *Journal of Urology* 2016;196:1613–1618.
12. Vargas, H. et al. Magnetic resonance imaging for predicting prostate biopsy findings in patients considered for active surveillance of clinically low risk prostate cancer. *Journal of Urology* 2012;188:1732–1738.
13. Alberts, A.R. et al. Risk-stratification based on magnetic resonance imaging and prostate-specific antigen density may reduce unnecessary follow-up biopsy procedures in men on active surveillance for low-risk prostate cancer. *BJU International* 2017;120:511–519.
14. Lee, S.H. et al. Magnetic resonance imaging targeted biopsy in men with previously negative prostate biopsy results. *Journal of Endourology* 2012;26:787–791.
15. Wegelin, O. et al. Comparing three different techniques for magnetic resonance imaging-targeted prostate biopsies: A systematic review of in-bore versus magnetic resonance imaging-transrectal ultrasound fusion versus cognitive registration. Is there a preferred technique? *European Urology* 2017;71:517–531.
16. Invivocorp.com/solutions/prostate-solutions/uronav/
17. http://www.eigen.com/products/artemis.shtml
18. Mendhiratta, N. et al. Prebiopsy MRI and MRI-ultrasound fusion targeted prostate biopsy in men with previous negative biopsies: Impact on repeat biopsy strategies. *Oncology* 2015;86:1192–1200.

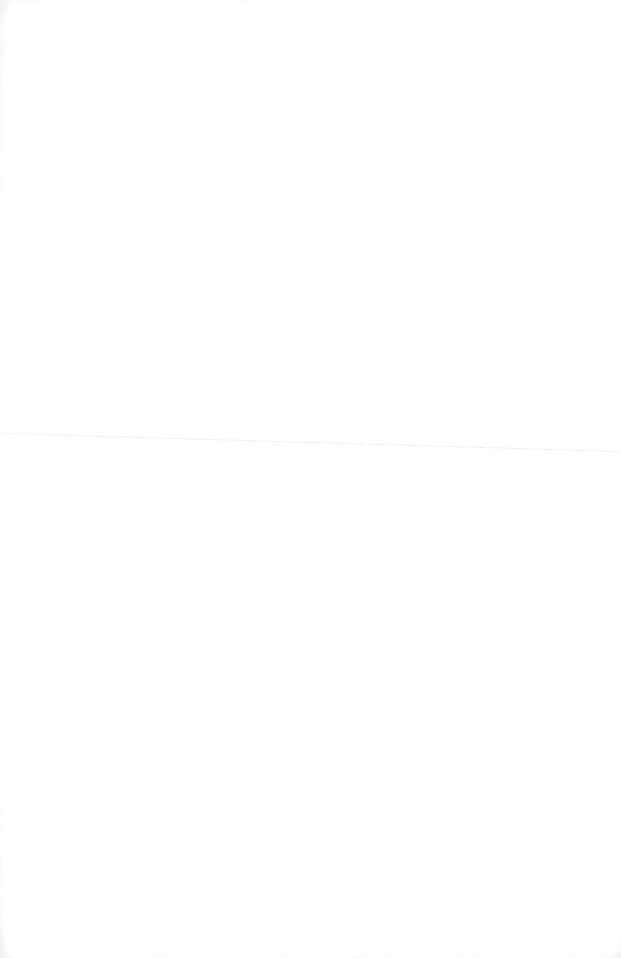

6 Current Role of Focal Therapy for Prostate Cancer

H. Abraham Chiang and George E. Haleblian

CONTENTS

INTRODUCTION

BACKGROUND

Prostate cancer is a prevalent malignancy, but the natural progression of disease is heterogeneous. Hence, current management of clinically localized prostate cancer depends on disease risk stratification. Standard of care management options include active surveillance, radical prostatectomy, and radiation with or without androgen deprivation therapy. Of note, it is estimated that up to 20%–55% of patients on active surveillance transition to definitive treatment (Wilt et al. 2012; Hamdy et al. 2016). With advancements in early prostate cancer detection and treatment, the 10-year prostate cancer–specific survival rate for patients with clinically localized prostate cancer is excellent at approximately 99%. The morbidities associated with radical prostatectomy and radiation are significant and can gravely impact a patient's quality of life. Rates of erectile dysfunction (ED) and urinary incontinence after definitive treatment are estimated to be 60%–80% and 20%–40%, respectively (Resnick et al. 2013; Wilt et al. 2017).

In recent years, multiple groups have published results of randomized controlled trials comparing definitive therapy to active surveillance for clinically localized prostate cancer. One such trial is the ProtecT trial, which compared radical prostatectomy, radiation therapy, and active surveillance in men with predominantly low-risk prostate cancer. After 10 years of follow-up, this trial demonstrated no overall or prostate cancer–specific survival with definitive treatment when compared to active surveillance (although rates of disease progression and metastasis were higher with active surveillance) (Hamdy et al. 2016).

Altogether, the unclear survival benefit of definitive treatment for men with low- to intermediate-risk prostate cancer combined with morbidities associated with treatment have fueled debate regarding overtreatment of clinically localized prostate cancer. In this setting, there has been increasing interest in developing less radical, less morbid therapies for the management of clinically localized prostate cancer.

The adoption of less radical therapies has already occurred for the management most other solid organ malignancies. Within the field of urology, this transition can be appreciated in the management of small renal masses. Classically, small renal masses suspicious for malignancy were managed with radical nephrectomy. While this was associated with favorable oncologic outcomes, the consequences of being left with a solitary kidney can be significant, and patients with impaired baseline renal function may not be operative candidates for radical nephrectomy. With development of less radical treatment options, such as partial nephrectomy and percutaneous ablation therapies, patients now have less morbid yet oncologically sound options.

Interestingly, prostate cancer has remained an exception to this trend toward partial or focal organ therapy. One reason for this is the belief that prostate cancer is inherently a multifocal disease and hence not amenable for focal treatment. However, there is increasing appreciation that not all prostate cancer is clinically significant, raising the possibility that (1) indolent prostate cancer lesions may not require treatment and (2) ablation of clinically significant index lesions may be sufficient in providing desired oncologic outcomes while decreasing morbidities associated with more radical, whole-gland treatment. Furthermore, advancements in diagnostic imaging modalities, such as prostate MRI, continue to improve our ability to discern clinically significant lesions from indolent ones with increasing accuracy. The significance of these developments is reflected in the renewed interest in investigation of focal therapy for prostate cancer.

The goal of this chapter is to review the technical aspects, oncologic outcomes, and functional outcomes with regard to various focal therapy modalities in the treatment of prostate cancer. The modalities reviewed include high-frequency focused ultrasound (HIFU), cryoablation, photodynamic therapy (PDT), laser interstitial thermotherapy (LITT), brachytherapy, irreversible electroporation (IRE), and radiofrequency ablation (RFA) (Table 6.1). Where applicable, the role of

TABLE 6.1

Technical Aspects of Various Focal Therapy Modalities

Modality	Energy Delivery	Ablation Mechanism	Route	Imaging Guidance
High-intensity focused ultrasound (HIFU)	Parabolic-focused ultrasound waves	Thermal: coagulative necrosis Mechanical: cavitation bubbles	Transurethral or transrectal	In-bore MRI (transurethral) MR-TRUS fusion (transrectal)
Cryoablation	Cryo-needles	Hypothermia	Transperineal	MRI Color doppler U/S
Photodynamic therapy (PDT)	Laser + photosensitizer + tissue oxygen	Formation of reactive oxygen species, vascular occlusion and tumor necrosis	Transperineal (intravenous photosensitizer)	MRI
Laser interstitial thermotherapy (LITT)	Laser	Thermal	Transperineal or transrectal	MRI
Brachytherapy	Radioactive seeds	DNA damage, cell death	Transperineal	MR-TRUS fusion
Irreversible electroporation (IRE)	Electric field	Cell membrane disruption, apoptosis	Transperineal	TRUS
Radiofrequency ablation (RFA)	Alternating current	Thermal	Transperineal	TRUS

imaging guidance modalities will also be discussed. It is important to note that focal therapy for prostate cancer remains in various stages of clinical trials and is not currently standard of care for the management of prostate cancer.

WHO SHOULD BE OFFERED FOCAL THERAPY?

Focal therapy for prostate cancer has been proposed for various clinical scenarios, including primary treatment of clinically localized prostate cancer, secondary treatment for recurrence, cytoreduction in more advanced or metastatic disease, as well as for palliation. Focal therapy indicated for primary treatment of clinically localized prostate cancer has the most robust body of evidence and hence will be the focus of this chapter.

From a technical standpoint, it seems reasonable that a patient with a unifocal clinically significant lesion (or at least disease restricted to one lobe) is better suited for focal therapy compared to those with multifocal or bilateral disease. Furthermore, the target lesion should be readily identifiable and spatially localizable using the radiographic modality guiding focal therapy delivery (i.e., ultrasound, CT, or MRI). Beyond this, the optimal selection criteria with respect to patient and disease characteristics remain poorly defined in literature. Thus far, the vast majority of patients included in clinical trials are in the low- to intermediate-risk categories, with some studies including high-risk patients as well (Table 6.2). Given that low- and intermediate-risk patients are at greater risk of "overtreatment" and exposure to morbidities associated with radical therapy, it stands to reason that these patients may gain the most from alternatives such as focal therapy.

IMAGING MODALITIES

Imaging serves two critical roles in focal therapy: (1) optimal patient selection based on disease/lesion characterization and (2) treatment planning and delivery.

Historically, ultrasound has been the most commonly used imaging modality of choice for evaluating the prostate. However, malignant prostatic lesions are not reliably visualized on ultrasound. Recent advancements in prostate MRI is having a profound effect in the detection and surveillance of prostate cancer. One study found that when compared to transrectal ultrasound (TRUS)-guided prostate biopsy, prostate MRI has higher sensitivity (93% vs. 48%) and negative predictive value (89% vs. 74%) in the detection of clinically significant prostate cancer (Ahmed et al. 2017). Furthermore, MRI provides good enumeration and spatial localization of suspicious lesions, qualities that are critical to effective focal therapy delivery. With accurate spatial localization, the margin of ablation can be decreased with decreased risk of injury to surrounding structures, such as the urethra, neurovascular bundle, and rectum. Furthermore, the overall volume of ablated tissue can be decreased, reducing procedure time.

MRI offers yet another benefit over alternative imaging modality in the form of thermometry. The majority of focal therapy modalities rely on some form of thermal ablation. Traditionally, this required the use of invasive temperature probes to monitor adequate ablation, as well as sparing of nearby critical structures from thermal spillover. It has now been demonstrated that MRI is capable of accurate real-time temperature monitoring, potentially obviating the need for additional invasive temperature monitoring probes (Ishihara et al. 1995). It is no surprise, then, that MRI is quickly being adopted as the imaging modality of choice for prostate focal therapy.

TABLE 6.2
Published Studies on Focal Therapy Organized by Ablation Modalities

Modality	Study	Follow-Up Length	# Patients Included	Risk Stratification	Prostate Cancer–Specific Survival	Clinically Significant Prostate Cancer on Post-treatment Biopsy	Erectile Dysfunction	Urinary Incontinence
HIFU	Golan (2017) Meta-analysis	6 months to 10 years	364	Low, intermediate, high	100%	8%	0%–48%	0%–10%
Cryoablation	Valerio (2017) Meta-analysis	26 months[a]	1950	Low, intermediate, high	100%	5.4%	18.5%	2%
PDT	Azzouzi (2017) Randomized controlled trial	24 months[a]	413	Low	100%	NR (51% any prostate cancer)	1%	1%
LITT	Valerio (2017) Meta-analysis	4.5 months[a]	50	Low, intermediate	100%	4.8%	0%	0%
Brachytherapy	Cosset (2013) Retrospective case series	28 months[a]	21	Low, intermediate	100%	0%	NR	4.8%
IRE	Ting (2015) Retrospective case series	7 months[a]	25	Low, intermediate	100%	25%	No change compared to pre-treatment	No change compared to pre-treatment
	Valerio (2017) Prospective case series	12 months[a]	19	Low, intermediate	100%	33.3%	8.3%	0%
RFA	Zlotta (1998) Proof-of-concept	NR	15	NR	NR	NR	NR	NR

[a] Median.
Abbreviation: NR = not reported.

FOCAL THERAPY MODALITIES

HIGH-INTENSITY FOCUSED ULTRASOUND (HIFU)

HIFU utilizes parabolic-focused ultrasound waves to ablate target tissue via two mechanisms. First, focused ultrasound wave energy is converted into thermal energy at the target tissue, triggering cell death by coagulative necrosis. During this process, target tissue can be heated up to 70°C–100°C within seconds of energy application. The second effect is mechanical: ultrasound waves interact with tissue water and generate negative pressure, thereby forming cavitation bubbles. The collapse of these cavitation bubbles transmits mechanical force, destroying adjacent tissue (Chaussy and Thüroff 2017). HIFU-mediated tissue ablation was first described in 1944 by Lynn and Putnam, and subsequently explored for ablation of prostatic adenomas in treatment of benign prostatic hyperplasia (BPH) in the 1990s. Ironically, HIFU was found to cause high rates of post-treatment urinary retention due to tissue edema and urethral sloughing and abandoned as a treatment for BPH. Nonetheless, HIFU did demonstrate considerable gland shrinkage after treatment, confirming its efficacy in prostatic tissue ablation.

HIFU energy is delivered using a transurethral or transrectal probe. Targeting of focused ultrasound is achieved by one of two mechanisms: (1) movement of the transducer or (2) electronic manipulation of the focal point (Chaussy and Thüroff 2017). An endorectal cooling device can be used to protect adjacent tissue from thermal injury (Ramsay et al. 2017). Although HIFU can be performed with ultrasound guidance, contemporary case series have increasingly leveraged MRI guidance. As previously discussed, MRI not only allows accurate spatial localization of the target lesion, but also provides real-time thermometry data. In a pilot study of five patients who underwent focal HIFU therapy just prior to radical prostatectomy, Ramsay et al. (2017) demonstrated that prostatic tissue ablation can be achieved with both spatial and thermal accuracy using MRI guidance. On surgical pathology, all index lesions were fully contained within the outer limit of thermal ablation.

Technical limitations of HIFU include limited tissue penetrance (24–40 mm depending on device model) that may preclude treatment of particularly large volume glands. Prostatic calcifications can also dissipate or deflect energy delivery. Furthermore, as in the case for all thermal ablative procedures, large vessels can act as heat sinks and limit adequate thermal ablation to nearby tissue.

In the United States, HIFU was approved for "prostatic tissue ablation" by the FDA in 2015. Europe, in contrast, has been using HIFU for many years, and as a result there is a large body of literature detailing its oncologic and functional outcomes. Golan et al. performed a meta-analysis of HIFU for focal ablation of prostate cancer, reviewing 13 studies (10 prospective, 2 comparative, 1 retrospective) for a total of 543 patients who received partial gland HIFU therapy. Nearly all patients undergoing primary treatment of prostate cancer had low- or intermediate-risk disease. Median follow-up ranged from 6 months to 10 years. Prostate cancer–specific survival was 100%. Of the 364 patients who underwent primary HIFU therapy followed by post-treatment prostate biopsy, 103 (28%) patients had a positive repeat biopsy, of whom 30 (8%) had clinically significant prostate cancer; 10% of patients went on to receive secondary therapy. Post-HIFU rates of ED and urinary incontinence ranged from 0% to 48% and 0% to 10%, respectively (Golan et al. 2017).

As is the case for all focal therapy modalities, interpretation of the above findings is limited by several issues. The type of pre- and post-treatment prostate biopsies were not standardized and included standard TRUS, targeted, and template biopsies. Furthermore, at least one study did not mandate post-treatment biopsies (i.e., post-treatment biopsy was performed for clinical suspicion of biochemical recurrence only). With regard to the functional outcomes, the definition of ED and urinary incontinence varied widely from study to study. Despite these limitations, the published literature suggests that HIFU is a relatively safe procedure with favorable functional outcomes when compared to standard of care radical therapies. Oncologic outcomes with respect to prostate cancer–specific survival appear no worse than standard of care, which is not surprising given that studies primarily focused on low- to intermediate-risk patients. However, the implications of residual clinically significant prostate cancer remain uncertain in the absence of longer follow-up and secondary outcome data regarding disease progression and development of metastatic disease. Randomized controlled trials comparing HIFU to standard of care therapies are lacking and needed to better evaluate the role of HIFU in the treatment of prostate cancer.

CRYOABLATION

Cryoablation is an FDA-approved treatment for prostate cancer, and as its name implies, achieves tissue ablation by exposing target lesions to extreme hypothermia. Early descriptions of prostate cryoablation date back to 1966 and were initially performed surgically (Gonder et al. 1966). With further refinement of cryoablation devices, percutaneous ablation became feasible in the 1990s by inserting cryo-needles transperineally under ultrasound guidance (Onik et al. 1993). Adjunct devices, such as urethra-warming catheters, can be used to protect nearby critical structures.

In recent years, MRI-guided cryoablation has been increasingly explored given its superior spatial localization compared to ultrasound, noninvasive thermal monitoring, and ability to clearly delineate frozen tissue post-treatment (Josan et al. 2009). A prospective feasibility study of software-assisted MRI-guided cryoablation enrolled 18 patients with intermediate- to high-risk disease. Early and late post-treatment MRI showed no radiographic evidence of residual disease within the ablated fields. Unfortunately, post-treatment biopsies were not obtained. Patients reported stable erectile and urinary symptoms compared to baseline at 12 month follow-up (Valerio et al. 2017c).

Valerio et al. performed a meta-analysis including 11 case series (9 retrospective and 2 prospective) evaluating the use of cryotherapy for treatment of prostate cancer. Ablation technique was most commonly hemi-gland ablation followed by focal ablation. Of the 1,950 patients included in this meta-analysis, the majority of patients were in the low- to intermediate-risk categories with a median PSA of 6.3. At a median follow-up of 26 months, prostate cancer–specific survival was 100%. Rate of clinically significant prostate cancer on post-treatment biopsy was 5.4%; 7.6% of patients underwent secondary treatment. Rates of ED and leak-free continence were 18.5% and 2%, respectively (Valerio et al. 2017a).

Overall, cryoablation appears to be a well-tolerated procedure with a relatively low sexual and genitourinary adverse side effect profile when compared to radical therapies. However, randomized controlled trials comparing cryoablation to standard of care therapies are needed to better assess oncologic and functional outcomes.

LASER-MEDIATED ABLATION: PHOTODYNAMIC THERAPY (PDT) AND LASER INTERSTITIAL THERMOTHERAPY (LITT)

Tissue ablation using lasers can be achieved by two different methods: PDT and LITT. PDT requires three components: a laser light source, photosensitizer, and target tissue oxygen. For prostate PDT, the photosensitizer is administered intravenously and the laser fibers are inserted into the target region transperineally. When the laser excites the photosensitizer at the target tissue, free radicals are generated, which in turn react with local tissue oxygen to create reactive oxygen species. Reactive oxygen species are highly cytotoxic and induce vascular occlusion and ultimately tumor necrosis (Lebdai et al. 2017). Given systemic circulation of the photosensitizing agent, patients are generally advised to avoid exposure to direct sunlight for a period of time.

Unique among focal therapy modalities, PDT has been compared to a standard of care therapy (active surveillance) in a randomized controlled trial. Azzouzi et al. recruited 413 patients with low-risk prostate cancer and randomized 206 to undergo PDT and 206 to active surveillance. After 24 months of follow-up, prostate cancer–specific survival in both groups was 100%. However, the rate of prostate cancer progression (from low-risk to intermediate- or high-risk disease) was lower for the PDT group compared to the active surveillance group (28% vs. 58%, HR 0.34, 95% CI 0.24–0.46; $p < 0.0001$). Patients in the PDT group were also more likely to have a negative prostate biopsy at 24 months compared to the active surveillance group (49% vs. 14%, HR 3.67, 95% CI 2.53–5.33; $p < 0.0001$). Finally, patients in the PDT group were less likely to undergo subsequent radical therapy when compared to those in the active surveillance group (6% vs. 29%, $p < 0.0001$). Clinically significant adverse side effects (National Cancer Institute grades 3–4) were rare, with ED and urinary incontinence occurring in 1% of patients for both PDT and active surveillance groups (Azzouzi et al. 2017).

Hence, Azzouzi et al. concluded that PDT may decrease risk of prostate cancer progression and increase likelihood of subsequent negative prostate biopsies when compared to active surveillance for patients with low-risk disease. Sexual and genitourinary toxicity profile associated with PDT treatment was comparable to active surveillance. Interestingly, patients who were randomized to PDT were less likely to undergo subsequent radical therapy. While this may be explained in part by higher rates of disease progression and positive post-treatment biopsies, it also raises the possibility that patient anxiety classically associated with active surveillance may be mitigated with focal therapy. Limitations of the study include the absence of intermediate-risk patients as well as comparison to other standard of care therapies, such as radical prostatectomy or radiation. Undoubtedly, recruitment for such randomized controlled trials would be more challenging. This study employed standard TRUS-guided biopsies, and hence another limitation is the inherent sampling error rate of prostate biopsies. Short of radical prostatectomy pathology specimens, template biopsies offer the most thorough sampling of the prostate followed by the standard TRUS-guided biopsy as a distant third. Nevertheless, this study provides valuable insight as the unique randomized controlled trial in the field of focal therapy for prostate cancer.

A second method of laser tissue ablation is LITT. LITT is distinct from PDT in that the laser light directly heats target tissue to achieve thermal ablation. Hence, a photosensitizer is not needed. A shortcoming of all thermal ablation modalities, including LITT, is thermal spillover and potential injury to adjacent tissue.

A meta-analysis of four prospective series evaluating LITT included 50 patients with low- to intermediate-risk prostate cancer. At a median follow-up of 4.5 months, the prostate cancer–specific survival rate was 100%. The rate of clinically significant prostate cancer on post-treatment biopsy was 4.8%. ED and urinary incontinence rates were 0% and 0%, respectively (Valerio et al. 2017a). Further studies are needed to better evaluate the safety and efficacy profile of LITT in the treatment of prostate cancer.

BRACHYTHERAPY

Whole-gland brachytherapy has long been used as a standard of care treatment for clinically localized prostate cancer. Pre-treatment mapping of the prostate is performed with ultrasound, CT or MRI. Once the prostate contour is determined, tissue ablation is achieved by placing radioactive seeds transperineally, typically under TRUS guidance with template. When compared to other standard of care treatments, brachytherapy offers several benefits. It is less invasive than prostatectomy and may be a viable option for patients who are not operative candidates. Furthermore, because the radioactive seeds can be "placed-and-forgotten," fewer hospital visits are required during treatment compared to external beam radiation. On the other hand, a major shortcoming of brachytherapy is a more pronounced genitourinary side effect profile when compared to radical prostatectomy or external beam radiation. It seems reasonable to deduce, then, that adapting brachytherapy from a whole-gland to focal ablation technique may reduce genitourinary side effects. As a demonstration of technical feasibility, a study has shown that hemi-gland brachytherapy, when compared to whole-gland brachytherapy, resulted in significant reduction in radiation dose to the contralateral gland, as well as to the urethra, neurovascular bundle, and rectum (Laing et al. 2016).

The largest published series of sub-total gland brachytherapy by Nguyen et al. includes 318 patients with low- to intermediate-risk disease. Notably, in this series sub-total gland ablation was performed by radiating the entire peripheral zone of the prostate, instead of hemi-gland or focal ablation. Hence, this technique does not fully conform to the idea of "focal therapy." Nonetheless, as the largest series in sub-total prostate brachytherapy, the study provides valuable insight with regards to oncologic outcomes. After a median follow-up of 61 months, prostate cancer-free survival was 99.7% and 3.5% of patients were found to have clinically significant prostate cancer post-treatment (Nguyen et al. 2012). Functional outcomes were not investigated.

Cosset et al. published preliminary data on a smaller series of 21 patients with low- to intermediate-risk disease who did undergo truly focal, lesion-directed brachytherapy. Of note, patient selection was narrowed to those with limited and localized tumors on two separate biopsies and MRI. Mean treatment volume was 34% of the total prostate volume. Follow-up and data collection is still underway, but of the five patients who have been biopsied post-treatment, none had clinically significant prostate cancer. ED and urinary toxicities at 1-year follow-up was found to be comparable to whole-gland brachytherapy (Cosset et al. 2013). Data from longer follow-up will provide further information regarding oncologic and functional outcomes of LITT.

IRREVERSIBLE ELECTROPORATION (IRE)

IRE achieves ablation by exerting a strong electric field to the target tissue, disrupting cell membranes and inducing apoptosis. This is in stark contrast to most other focal therapy modalities that involves thermal ablation and necrosis. As a direct consequence of its unique mechanism of action, IRE lacks thermal spillover to adjacent tissue and achieves a very sharp ablation boundary that is measured in cell layers (Lee et al. 2010). Technical feasibility of IRE has been demonstrated in non-curative intent trials where patients underwent IRE followed by radical prostatectomy. Surgical specimen pathology confirmed adequate target tissue ablation without skip lesions (Van den Bos et al. 2016).

A retrospective case series by Ting et al. included 25 patients with low- to intermediate-risk prostate cancer showed 100% prostate cancer–specific survival at 7 months of follow-up. On post-treatment biopsy, 25% of patients were found to have clinically significant prostate cancer, although none of these samples were from the treated field. Patient-reported erectile function and incontinence rates remained stable when compared to pre-treatment (Ting et al. 2016).

A more recent prospective case series by Valerio et al. included 19 patients with low- to intermediate-risk prostate cancer, and after follow-up of 12 months, prostate cancer–specific survival was 100%. Some 33.3% of patients were found to have clinically significant prostate cancer on post-treatment biopsy, but laterality/location of these positive samples were not specified, making it unclear whether these represented recurrences, inadequate ablation, or separate nontargeted lesions. One patient reported new onset ED and no patients had new urinary incontinence (Valerio et al. 2017b). All in all, data regarding IRE for treatment of prostate cancer remains scarce, and further trials are needed to assess its safety and efficacy profiles.

RADIOFREQUENCY

RFA uses alternating current to heat target tissue and induce coagulative necrosis. Although commonly used for cardiac ablation or treatment of small renal masses, very little data is available regarding the use of RFA for treatment of prostate cancer.

The only published case series for focal RFA of prostate cancer is a proof-of-concept study dating back to 1998. In this series, 15 patients received RFA with no intention to treat prior to radical prostatectomy. Both monopolar and bipolar energy were used and target lesions identified when visible on TRUS. Even if no suspicious lesions were visible, one or two ablative lesions were made in the gland. Surgical pathology demonstrated coagulative necrosis lesions in line with predicted lesion size. No oncologic or functional outcomes were measured (Zlotta et al. 1998).

CONCLUSION

Early detection and treatment of prostate cancer in the era of PSA screening has led to excellent disease-specific survival for patients. Unfortunately, this outcome has been achieved at the cost of overtreatment and significant morbidities associated with standard of care radical therapies. These shortcomings in the management of prostate cancer, combined with the ever-growing concerns of rising healthcare costs, have fueled interest in focal therapy as an alternative treatment modalities in select patients.

A multitude of focal ablation techniques including HIFU, cryoablation, PDT, LITT, brachytherapy, IRE, and RFA are actively being investigated. Of these, HIFU and cryoablation have been most thoroughly studied, particularly in patients with low- to intermediate-risk disease. In this patient population, studies have shown that radical therapy is comparable to active surveillance with regard to overall and disease-specific survival. Early results suggest that focal therapy may be associated with disease-specific survival comparable to these standard of care treatments.

However, a number of limitations must be addressed before focal therapy is recommended as a treatment option for patients with prostate cancer. For one, nearly all studies conducted thus far have been case series. Randomized controlled trials that compare focal therapy against standard of care treatments have been lacking and are only starting to be published. In the absence of such comparative efficacy trials, it is yet unfeasible to comment on the oncologic efficacy of focal therapy in the treatment of prostate cancer. Furthermore, as follow-up data for focal therapy matures, it will be interesting to see if differences in clinically meaningful secondary outcome measures, such as rates of disease progression or metastasis, become apparent.

From a functional standpoint, a goal of focal therapy is to spare nearby critical structures, such as the urethra, neurovascular bundle, and rectum. By ablating a small lesion, or even with hemigland ablation and sparing of contralateral structures, the expectation is that improved functional outcomes can be achieved. Data thus far suggest that functional outcomes with regard to ED and urinary incontinence are favorable when compared to standard of care radical therapies. However, interpretation of this data is limited by relatively short follow-up periods, large methodology variations in measuring of functional status, and small sample sizes for most modalities.

Above all, randomized controlled trials comparing focal therapy to standard of care therapies are needed to better assess both oncologic and functional outcomes. Thus far, one randomized controlled trial comparing PDT to active surveillance has been published by Azzouzi et al. and discussed this in chapter. Another randomized controlled trial currently underway is the partial prostate ablation versus radical prostatectomy (PART) trial, which recently completed recruitment. The first phase of the PART trial will randomize 80 patients with intermediate-risk prostate cancer to radical prostatectomy or HIFU. The goal of the first phase is to assess the feasibility of recruiting and randomizing an adequate number of participants. If successful, additional recruitment will be performed to assess oncologic and functional outcomes. Long-term data from randomized controlled trials such as this are needed before focal therapy will be accepted as standard of care treatment option for prostate cancer.

Finally, although not discussed in detail in this chapter, the role of focal therapy for recurrent and metastatic prostate cancer as well as for palliation is also being explored. Overall, the role of focal therapy for prostate cancer remains unclear and is not recommended as standard of care at this time. Nevertheless, if the evolution in management of other solid organ malignancies are a sign of things to come, we can expect focal therapy to play an increasing role as optimal patient selection and disease characterization become better defined, and as ablative technology continues to improve.

REFERENCES

Ahmed, H.U. et al., 2017. Diagnostic accuracy of multi-parametric MRI and TRUS biopsy in prostate cancer (PROMIS): A paired validating confirmatory study. *Lancet (London, England)*, 389(10071), 815–822.

Azzouzi, A.-R. et al., 2017. Padeliporfin vascular-targeted photodynamic therapy versus active surveillance in men with low-risk prostate cancer (CLIN1001 PCM301): An open-label, phase 3, randomised controlled trial. *The Lancet Oncology*, 18(2), 181–191.

Chaussy, C.G. and Thüroff, S., 2017. High-intensity focused ultrasound for the treatment of prostate cancer: A review. *Journal of Endourology*, 31(S1), S30–S37.

Cosset, J.-M. et al., 2013. Focal brachytherapy for selected low-risk prostate cancers: A pilot study. *Brachytherapy*, 12(4), 331–337.

Golan, R. et al., 2017. Partial gland treatment of prostate cancer utilizing high-intensity focused ultrasound in the primary and salvage setting: A systematic review. *The Journal of Urology*, 198(5), 1000–1009.

Gonder, M.J., Soanes, W.A. and Shulman, S., 1966. Cryosurgical treatment of the prostate. *Investigative Urology*, 3(4), 372–378.

Hamdy, F.C. et al., 2016. 10-year outcomes after monitoring, surgery, or radiotherapy for localized prostate cancer. *The New England Journal of Medicine*, 375(15), 1415–1424.

Ishihara, Y. et al., 1995. A precise and fast temperature mapping using water proton chemical shift. *Magnetic Resonance in Medicine*, 34(6), 814–823.

Josan, S. et al., 2009. MRI-guided cryoablation: In vivo assessment of focal canine prostate cryolesions. *Journal of Magnetic Resonance Imaging: JMRI*, 30(1), 169–176.

Laing, R. et al., 2016. Hemi-gland focal low dose rate prostate brachytherapy: An analysis of dosimetric outcomes. *Radiotherapy and Oncology: Journal of the European Society for Therapeutic Radiology and Oncology*, 121(2), 310–315.

Lebdai, S. et al., 2017. Vascular targeted photodynamic therapy with padeliporfin for low risk prostate cancer treatment: Midterm oncologic outcomes. *The Journal of Urology*, 198(2), 335–344.

Lee, E.W. et al., 2010. Advanced hepatic ablation technique for creating complete cell death: Irreversible electroporation. *Radiology*, 255(2), 426–433.

Nguyen, P.L. et al., 2012. Updated results of magnetic resonance imaging guided partial prostate brachytherapy for favorable risk prostate cancer: Implications for focal therapy. *The Journal of Urology*, 188(4), 1151–1156.

Onik, G.M. et al., 1993. Transrectal ultrasound-guided percutaneous radical cryosurgical ablation of the prostate. *Cancer*, 72(4), 1291–1299.

Ramsay, E. et al., 2017. Evaluation of focal ablation of magnetic resonance imaging defined prostate cancer using magnetic resonance imaging controlled transurethral ultrasound therapy with prostatectomy as the reference standard. *The Journal of Urology*, 197(1), 255–261.

Resnick, M.J. et al., 2013. Long-term functional outcomes after treatment for localized prostate cancer. *The New England Journal of Medicine*, 368(5), 436–445.

Ting, F. et al., 2016. Focal irreversible electroporation for prostate cancer: Functional outcomes and short-term oncological control. *Prostate Cancer and Prostatic Diseases*, 19(1), 46–52.

Valerio, M. et al., 2017a. New and established technology in focal ablation of the prostate: A systematic review. *European Urology*, 71(1), 17–34.

Valerio, M. et al., 2017b. Nanoknife electroporation ablation trial: A prospective development study investigating focal irreversible electroporation for localized prostate cancer. *The Journal of Urology*, 197(3 Pt 1), 647–654.

Valerio, M. et al., 2017c. Magnetic resonance imaging-transrectal ultrasound fusion focal cryotherapy of the prostate: A prospective development study. *Urologic Oncology*, 35(4), 150.e1–150.e7.

Van den Bos, W. et al., 2016. Histopathological outcomes after irreversible electroporation for prostate cancer: Results of an ablate and resect study. *The Journal of Urology*, 196(2), 552–559.

Wilt, T.J. et al., 2012. Radical prostatectomy versus observation for localized prostate cancer. *The New England Journal of Medicine*, 367(3), 203–213.

Wilt, T.J. et al., 2017. Follow-up of prostatectomy versus observation for early prostate cancer. *The New England Journal of Medicine*, 377(2), 132–142.

Zlotta, A.R. et al., 1998. Percutaneous transperineal radiofrequency ablation of prostate tumour: Safety, feasibility and pathological effects on human prostate cancer. *British Journal of Urology*, 81(2), 265–275.

7 High-Intensity Focused Ultrasound (HIFU)

Rutveej Patel and Sammy Elsamra

CONTENTS

INTRODUCTION

Ultrasound refers to sound waves that contain frequencies higher than the upper audible limit in human hearing, and is defined by the American National Standards Institute as sound at frequencies greater than approximately 20 kilohertz (20,000 hertz). Ultrasound devices operate in multiple levels of frequencies and have been used in the medical field as an imaging modality since the 1940s. Current ultrasound instruments typically operate at 1–18 megahertz. Ultrasonic images are created as a result of sending ultrasound pulses into tissue. This produces echoes off the tissue of varying degrees that can be recorded by the sensor and displayed as an image.

Ultrasound has an ability to interact with tissues and can propagate through them. This propagation creates cycles of increased and decreased pressure, which can manipulate tissue. While imaging ultrasound operates at higher frequencies, HIFU typically uses frequencies from 0.8 to 3.5 MHz. This results in a delivery of energy to the tissues much higher than the levels seen with diagnostic ultrasound. HIFU is in the category of therapeutic ultrasound, which is broadly divided into two subtypes: low-intensity and high-intensity. Other applications in this field include lithotripsy, targeted drug delivery, and ultrasound-mediated hemostasis or thrombolysis. High-intensity applications can also selectively destroy tissue.

HISTORY OF HIFU

The development of the modern ultrasound relies on the piezoelectric effect, which was first discovered in 1880 by Jacques and Pierre Curie. The piezoelectric effect is the ability of certain materials to generate an electric charge when mechanical stress is applied to them. This effect is also reversible—if a material generates electricity when external stress is applied, then it also has an ability to generate stress when an external electric field is applied. The piezoelectric effect was not incorporated into practical applications from its discovery until the initiation of World War I, when it was employed in the form of SONAR devices. As technology has advanced, new materials that can utilize the piezoelectric effect have been created and this phenomenon has been applied in many different industries.

Modern ultrasound transducers utilize the piezoelectric effect to produce and receive sound waves. Applying an electric field to a piezoelectric crystal will cause a realignment of the internal dipole structure, resulting in crystal lengthening or shortening. The size of the mechanical adjustment will depend on the voltage that is applied to the crystal. Running an alternating current through the crystal will cause vibrations at high speeds and this will produce an ultrasound. The wave will then bounce back off the tissue under investigation and will have a reverse effect on the crystal—the mechanical energy from the sound wave will cause the crystal to vibrate and this vibration will be converted into electric energy.

The history of HIFU can be traced back to the 1950s with the discovery, by Frank and William Fry, that high-frequency sound waves can generate localized tissue damage. Their initial interest into the study of the central nervous system led to the invention of instruments that generated, detected, and measured ultrasound. Their investigations and inventions led to understanding how ultrasound is scattered and attenuated, the degree to which different tissues can tolerate ultrasound, and further understanding of ultrasound parameters such as the speed of propagation. The equipment for these experiments was built from scratch and current modern-day devices are iterations of these initial devices.

The treatment of prostate cancer with HIFU was first reported in 1995 and 1996.[1,2] Transrectal HIFU continues to be a popular treatment alternative due to it being a minimally invasive treatment for localized disease. There is no requirement for an incision, and it can be performed with little to no bleeding. Patients do not require any hospitalization, and if they do develop a recurrence, the treatment can be repeated. Previous treatment with radiation or other local therapy also does not preclude patients from receiving HIFU for recurrences.[3] In late 2015, the United States Food and Drug Administration (FDA) approved HIFU for the ablation of prostate tissue. HIFU had been already approved for use in prostate tissue for ablation outside the United States by this point.

MECHANISM OF ACTION OF HIFU

HIFU can be delivered as a pulsed or continuous beam, and is applied as a pulse in medical devices and extracorporeal shock wave lithotripsy. Thermal ablation is the predominant mechanism of tissue destruction for the current HIFU devices, but mechanical effects also play a role. High-frequency vibration of a piezoelectric or piezoceramic transducer generates ultrasound waves that are focused into a focal point by an energy source. The probe uses an acoustic lens and converges multiple traversing beams of ultrasound onto the target. The individual beams pass through the tissue without any effect. However, at the focal point where the beams are concentrated, the energy is deposited for ablative effects. The temperature of the tissue at the focus point will then rise to 65°C–85°C, resulting in irreversible cell death from coagulative necrosis. Each individual ultrasound beam and energy deposition will treat a precise location. The focused waves travel through the tissue and deposit the thermal energy only at the target location. Tissue damage is similar to radiofrequency ablation in the sense that damage is both a function of the temperature the tissue is being heated to and the length of the heat exposure. The absorption coefficient of the tissue as well as the size, shape, and thermal response of the tissue play a role in determining the extent of necrosis. Focusing these acoustic waves at more than one location or by changing the focus, a therapeutic target volume can be created and ablated. Therefore, the therapeutic field is treated with multiple energy beams and is devised via a physician protocol. The typical volume of ablation after a single HIFU pulse is small and it is generally shaped like a cylinder or grain of rice, with a few millimeters in the transverse direction and about 1 cm in the height.

High acoustic intensities also create cavitation, which plays a role in the mechanical effects of HIFU. These microbubbles are created as a result of the alternating cycles of increased and reduced pressure from the propagating waves. At the time of reduced pressure, gas can be drawn out of solution and form bubbles, which then implode rapidly. This results in shock waves that can mechanically damage tissues and induce cell necrosis. The pressures achieved during the implosion of the microbubbles can be as high as 20,000–30,000 bars. In comparison, the deepest trench in the ocean has a pressure of approximately 1100 bars.

After tissue ablation and the coagulative necrosis, the cellular response at the edge of the ablation zone is the formation of granulation tissue. Histologic samples of necrotic lesions have shown that there is a sharp gradient between the tissue in the HIFU target and the surrounding area, proving that HIFU is a precise method of delivering ablative energy to the tissue. After the initial necrosis, leukocytes migrate deep into the treated tissue and the treated region is eventually replaced with proliferative repair tissue. Over time, imaging modalities have shown shrinkage of the treated areas and replacement of the tissue with fibrous scar tissue.

PRINCIPLES OF HIFU AND PROCEDURAL CONSIDERATIONS

HIFU treatment does offer some advantages over other methods of thermal ablation. It is minimally invasive and it does not rely on radiation, allowing for repetition without any long-term effects. However, as in the case of ultrasound, HIFU sound waves do not readily pass through solid structures or air. Additionally, HIFU requires the use of general anesthesia and larger glands require larger treatment times. The procedure itself involves placement of a HIFU transducer covered by a condom in the rectum. To help diminish the thermal effects on the rectum during the HIFU procedure, the rectum is generally irrigated with cold and degassed water concurrently with the real-time ultrasound. HIFU-treated lesions can become visible as hyperechoic areas in real time. Traditionally, this is a same-day procedure performed under general anesthesia that typically lasts 1–3 hours, depending on the size of the gland. Generally, the patient will have bladder drainage via a urethral catheter or suprapubic catheter for 2 weeks. If the patient has a concomitant transurethral resection of the prostate (TURP), then the urethral catheter is generally left only for a few days.

Currently, there are three systems on the market in the United States. The Sonablate® 450, which was developed by SonaCare Medical, was the first device approved in the United States. Newer models have improved upon this and added better safety features. The second main system, Ablatherm® by EDAP TMS SA has now also gained approval for ablation of prostate tissue in the United States. The Ablatherm® is the longest utilized system, with its main safety and efficacy established in Europe. Table 7.1 summarizes some of the similarities and differences between the two main systems on the market. An important difference between the two systems is the size of the ablative field, which can make one system more suited for focal, partial, or full-gland ablation. Since the ablative lesions on the Sonablate® can be stacked, the anterior-posterior limit for whole-gland ablation is <37 mm. In comparison, the anterior-posterior limit for the Ablatherm® system is fixed to <24 mm due to the way it delivers the ablative energy. Each system also includes different equipment or sensors to ensure rectal wall safety while treatment is active. The Ablatherm® allows for real-time rectal distance adjustment on each treatment slice. There are also internal controls that correct or stop treatments depending on the probe position with regard to the rectal wall. The Sonablate® system introduces the reflectivity index measurement (RIM) which analyzes real-time images of the rectal wall and digitally compares it to stored images taken prior to therapy. If the RIM score increases beyond a certain threshold, the treatment is stopped and the treating clinician is notified.

The major side effects of HIFU treatment with these two systems include urinary retention and erectile dysfunction. Regardless of the modality of energy delivery for current HIFU systems, a disadvantage is that it can be hard to target cancers in the anterior zone of the prostate or when treating

TABLE 7.1
HIFU Technology

	Ablatherm®	Sonablate®
Cost (approx.)	$750,000	$450,000
Disposables cost	$1,200	$2,400
Coupling medium	Degassed water	Proprietary gel
Type	Robotic	Manual/robotic versions available
Automated movements of probe	Transduce and probe motion	Transducer only
Type of endorectal probes	3 MHz—treatment only, 7.5 MHz	4 MHz
Real time imaging	Yes with 7.5 MHz	No
Patient positioning	Lateral	Dorsal Lithotomy
Treatment time	10 cc/hr	10 cc/hr
Fusion compatibility	None	Coming soon
Safety features	• Rectal temperature monitoring • Automatic adjustment of probe in regards to rectal wall • Automatic patient movement detection	• Rectal temperature monitoring • Rectal wall distance monitoring • Organ movement feedback
Ablation method/size		
Hemi	24 mm lesion—single row	Stackable 10 mm, 12 mm lesions
Focal	24 mm	10 mm or 12 mm
Apex sparing	4 mm safety margin required	No margin required

large glands. Also, while HIFU is a precision energy delivery system, it can be difficult to monitor the effects in real time, such as in the case of cryoablation.

INDICATIONS FOR HIFU IN PROSTATE CANCER

HIFU was initially started in a very distinct group of patients with localized prostate cancer who were not candidates for surgery.[4] But with increasing safety and efficacy data, the indications broadened to include patients who wished to undergo partial ablation for focal therapy, patients who were considered for salvage therapy in recurrent prostate cancer, as a debulking modality in patients with advanced prostate cancer, and in patients with castrate-resistant prostate cancer.[5]

As discussed previously, ablation with HIFU can be difficult in large prostates (i.e., 40 cc and above) because of the distance from the transducer to the anterior margin of the prostate. Therefore, since 2000 TURP just prior to HIFU has become routine practice for large glands. This reduces not only the size of the gland but also post-HIFU urethral sloughing/obstruction, and allows for removal of any calcifications in the transition zone that would make the HIFU treatment difficult. The increased invasiveness of a concurrent TURP is offset by the benefit of higher efficacy and reduced side effects and complications.[6,7]

Recent screening strategies have also led to earlier identification of men with small prostate tumors or with focal or unilateral disease.[8] With this shift in prostate cancer, an increased number of practitioners have started to treat focal lesions with therapies such as HIFU as a means for organ preservation.

Current contraindication for HIFU treatment includes a history of rectal fistula. Prostate size is not a contraindication as long as the volume is decreased either through the use of luteinizing hormone-releasing hormone (LHRH) agonist or concurrent or antecedent TURP with HIFU treatments. Additionally, if patients are taking anti-coagulants, then it is recommended that the medication be stopped for 10 days prior to the procedure to minimize risk of bleeding.[9]

EFFECTIVENESS/OUTCOMES OF HIFU

LOCALIZED DISEASE

To determine the effectiveness of HIFU, biochemical markers and biopsy results post-HIFU have been used as markers. However, a universal definition of biochemical failure in patients treated with HIFU remains to be created. Biochemical free survival (BFS) rates have ranged from 75% to 77%, using the Phoenix criteria (nadir PSA + 2).[10,11] Using the American Society for Radiation Oncology (ASTRO) definition, the BFS rates have ranged from 66% to 77%.[12,13] Table 7.2 also summarizes some of the current literature regarding the efficacy of HIFU. Repeat prostate biopsies were also reported in many of the studies regarding HIFU treatment, however, the timing of surveillance biopsy varied significantly. Ultimately, 8% of men had residual clinically significant disease after HIFU.[14]

Meta-analysis of previous studies has shown an increased risk of biochemical failure at 1-year follow-up in patients who underwent HIFU when compared to external beam radiotherapy (EBRT), 21% versus 1.3%.[16] However, this statistical difference was not seen at 5-year follow-up. In comparison to radical prostatectomy (RP), HIFU was noted to be at an increased risk of biochemical failure at 1 and 5 years, but again these results were not statistically significant. The predicted rates of biochemical failure in the treatment models of the meta-analysis were approximately 34% for HIFU, 13% for EBRT, and 11% for RP at 5 years.[16]

Overall survival data regarding HIFU has shown increased survival rates for HIFU when compared to EBRT at 4 years follow-up.[17,18] Estimated rates of survival were 99% for HIFU and 91% for EBRT.[16] For cancer-specific survival (CSS), a statistically significant lower rate was observed for HIFU than for EBRT at 1 year, however, there was no difference between HIFU and RP at 1 year. Predicted rates of CSS for comparison modeling at 1 year was 88% for HIFU, 95% for EBRT, and 90% for RP. One reason for this variation could be attributed to the severity of disease across the different modalities. A larger percentage of patients were Gleason 6 or less in the EBRT studies when compared to HIFU or RP. Also 50% or more patients in the HIFU and RP population represented more localized clinical stage T1 disease.[16]

HIFU AS SALVAGE THERAPY

HIFU has also been used in the past as salvage therapy in cases of advanced disease, even after modalities such as radiation, cryoablation, high-dose brachytherapy, and primary HIFU. Previous analysis has shown that in patients who experience recurrence with EBRT, the majority do not receive any local therapy. Only 3.9% of these patients undergo subsequent treatment, of which 0.9% is salvage prostatectomy and the rest cryoablation.[19] Furthermore, while salvage prostatectomy and cryoablation offer some benefits in theory, their high complexity and morbidity make it

TABLE 7.2

High-Intensity Frequency Ultrasound—Efficacy

Study	# of Patients	Mean PSA (ng/mL)	Stage	Median Follow-up (months)	Biochemical Survival	Retreatment Rate (%)
Gelet et al. (2001)[12]	102	8.38	T1-2	19	66%	78.4
Poissonnier et al. (2003)[13]	120	5.67	T1-2	27	76.9%	—
Poissonnier et al. (2007)[15]	227	7.0	T1-2	20.5	—	42.7
Blana et al. (2008)[11]	140	7.0	T1-2	76.8	77% @ 5 years	29.3
Blana et al. (2008)[10]	163	5.0—median	T1-2	57.6	75% @ 5 years	20.8

a challenging option for salvage treatment. In this scenario, salvage HIFU offers a favorable risk/benefit profile. Data regarding HIFU after radiation or surgery is sparse, but salvage HIFU after brachytherapy appears to be a viable and safe approach without a significant increase in complication when compared to primary HIFU.[4] In patients who have a recurrence post-prostatectomy, HIFU ablation of these recurrences shows negative biopsies in 77% of cases. These patients have a BFS of 91% at 5 years.[20] However, the utility of salvage HIFU in the post-prostatectomy setting relies on the ability to identify a lesion on a transrectal ultrasound and an ability to verify the lesion with a biopsy.

FOCAL THERAPY WITH HIFU

Partial gland ablation has increased in frequency as practitioners are now looking to treat localized disease while also preserving quality of life. Whole-gland HIFU has shown promising long-term function and oncologic outcomes and as imaging and ablative technologies have improved, a new shift toward partial ablation and focal therapy has been seen. Current literature includes studies that have studied short- and mid-term functional and oncologic outcomes of partial-gland HIFU in the treatment of prostate cancer. However, the current studies do not have comparison to whole-gland ablation, or with other modalities of ablation. Despite these shortcomings, a systematic review of current partial-gland ablation studies did show that CSS was 100% for the median follow-up. However, 10% of men in the primary treatment group and 37% in the salvage group had to receive additional treatment.[14] Two-year rates of biochemical recurrence ranged from 42% to 67% in the salvage therapy setting. These are comparable to biochemical failure rates following radiotherapy, which are reported as 50% at 5 years out.

Recurrences or additional treatment of patients who undergo partial-gland ablation are likely a result of missed cancers on multiparametric MRI or systematic biopsy that were not part of the initial ablative field.

ADVERSE EFFECTS

Main adverse effects of HIFU and other prostate cancer treatments include urinary incontinence, erectile dysfunction, and potential bowel issues. The risk of incontinence was largest for RP at 66%; HIFU and EBRT carried a risk of 10% and 5%, respectively.[16] Fecal incontinence was reported in a study as an adverse event for people undergoing HIFU.[21]

Erectile dysfunction (ED) in prostate cancer treatment has been heavily studied, but the outcomes assessed and measured vary widely across the studies due to differences in the definitions used and the types of data studied. Analysis of data comparing ED showed a reduced rate of ED following HIFU when compared to RP at a 1-year follow-up. However, this was not statistically significant. Predicted rates of ED with comparison models at a 1-year timeframe were 23% for HIFU and 33% for RP. The authors of this model were unable to estimate the rate of ED for people treated with EBRT.[16]

Short-term adverse events related to HIFU include dysuria, urinary retention, bladder spasms, infection, urethral stricture, bladder neck contracture, rectal bleeding, and rectal fistula. The reported rate on rectal fistulas ranged from 0%[22] to 5%.[23] Bladder neck contracture rates were also widely varied and were as high as 14%.[23,24] Urethral stricture rates were reported to be up to 16.6%.[25] Urinary infection rates ranged from 0.6% to as high as 45% of the study population.[23,26]

Two studies have reported about a variety of quality-of-life outcomes of patients undergoing HIFU. In one study, validated questionnaires such as the I-PSS, IIEF-15, and the UCLA-EPIC urinary incontinence scale were used. After HIFU therapy, 89% of studied patients achieved pad-free continence, erections sufficient for intercourse, and cancer control.[27]

FUTURE DIRECTIONS WITH HIFU

Given that HIFU is a precise method of delivering ablative energy, to increase its efficacy as a therapeutic tool for prostate cancer it will be necessary to improve imaging modalities that can help to better image and localize the tumor and concerning lesions. In addition to improvement in precision diagnostic technology, HIFU is being investigated with several advancements. This includes the use of multiparametric MRI, high-resolution ultrasound, contrast-enhanced or Doppler ultrasound, and lastly being able to fuse previous imaging with real-time HIFU.

Beyond the technological advancements, HIFU is increasingly being considered for focal therapy and in other settings. There are many ongoing trials reflecting the interest in focal therapy. One such trial is NCT02265159 that is actively recruiting participants to determine the oncologic safety of focal HIFU treatment. Additional trials are also combining imaging modalities and HIFU such as the FOcal RECurrent Assessment and Salvage Treatment (FORECAST) trial. This trial assesses accuracy of whole-body MRI as well as safety of focal salvage therapy.

HIFU may well become a form of curative therapy in localized disease or as a viable option for adjuvant therapy in advanced disease. Imaging improvements will only enhance the efficacy of HIFU and as results from ongoing clinical trials are published, it may become a more widespread treatment option for prostate cancer.

REFERENCES

1. Madersbacher S, Pedevilla M, Vingers L, Susani M, Marberger M. Effect of high-intensity focused ultrasound on human prostate cancer in vivo. *Cancer Res.* 1995;55:3346–3351.
2. Gelet A, Chapelon JY, Bouvier R et al. Treatment of prostate cancer with transrectal focused ultrasound: Early clinical experience. *Eur Urol.* 1996;29:174–183.
3. Murat FJ, Gelet A. Current status of high-intensity focused ultrasound for prostate cancer: Technology, clinical outcomes, and future. *Curr Urol Rep.* 2008;9:113–121.
4. Chaussy C, Thuroff S, Rebillard X, Gelet A. Technology insight: High-intensity focused ultrasound for urologic cancers. *Nat Clin Pract Urol.* 2005;2:191–198.
5. Gelet A, Chapelon JY, Poissonnier L et al. Local recurrence of prostate cancer after external beam radiotherapy: Early experience of salvage therapy using high-intensity focused ultrasonography. *Urology.* 2004;63:625–629.
6. Chaussy CG, Thuroff S. [Transrectal high-intensity focused ultrasound for local treatment of prostate cancer. 2009 Update]. *Urologe A.* 2009;48:710–718.
7. Vallancien G, Prapotnich D, Cathelineau X, Baumert H, Rozet F. Transrectal focused ultrasound combined with transurethral resection of the prostate for the treatment of localized prostate cancer: Feasibility study. *J Urol.* 2004;171:2265–2267.
8. Mouraviev V, Mayes JM, Polascik TJ. Pathologic basis of focal therapy for early-stage prostate cancer. *Nat Rev Urol.* 2009;6:205–215.
9. Hummel S, Paisley S, Morgan A, Currie E, Brewer N. Clinical and cost-effectiveness of new and emerging technologies for early localised prostate cancer: A systematic review. *Health Technol Assess.* 2003;7:iii, ix–x, 1–157.
10. Blana A, Murat FJ, Walter B et al. First analysis of the long-term results with transrectal HIFU in patients with localised prostate cancer. *Eur Urol.* 2008;53:1194–1201.
11. Blana A, Rogenhofer S, Ganzer R et al. Eight years' experience with high-intensity focused ultrasonography for treatment of localized prostate cancer. *Urology.* 2008;72:1329–1333; discussion 1333–1324.
12. Gelet A, Chapelon JY, Bouvier R, Rouviere O, Lyonnet D, Dubernard JM. Transrectal high intensity focused ultrasound for the treatment of localized prostate cancer: Factors influencing the outcome. *Eur Urol.* 2001;40:124–129.
13. Poissonnier L, Gelet A, Chapelon JY et al. [Results of transrectal focused ultrasound for the treatment of localized prostate cancer (120 patients with PSA < or + 10 ng/mL]. *Prog Urol.* 2003;13:60–72.
14. Golan R, Bernstein AN, McClure TD et al. Partial gland treatment of prostate cancer utilizing high-intensity focused ultrasound in the primary and salvage setting: A systematic review. *J Urol.* 2017;198:1000–1009.

15. Poissonnier L, Chapelon JY, Rouviere O et al. Control of prostate cancer by transrectal HIFU in 227 patients. *Eur Urol.* 2007;51:381–387.
16. Ramsay CR, Adewuyi TE, Gray J et al. Ablative therapy for people with localised prostate cancer: A systematic review and economic evaluation. *Health Technol Assess.* 2015;19:1–490.
17. Pinkawa M, Asadpour B, Piroth MD et al. Health-related quality of life after permanent I-125 brachytherapy and conformal external beam radiotherapy for prostate cancer—a matched-pair comparison. *Radiother Oncol.* 2009;91:225–231.
18. Misrai V, Roupret M, Chartier-Kastler E et al. Oncologic control provided by HIFU therapy as single treatment in men with clinically localized prostate cancer. *World J Urol.* 2008;26:481–485.
19. Agarwal PK, Sadetsky N, Konety BR, Resnick MI, Carroll PR. Cancer of the Prostate Strategic Urological Research E. Treatment failure after primary and salvage therapy for prostate cancer: Likelihood, patterns of care, and outcomes. *Cancer.* 2008;112:307–314.
20. Chaussy C, Thuroff S, Bergsdorf T. [Local recurrence of prostate cancer after curative therapy. HIFU (Ablatherm) as a treatment option]. *Urologe A.* 2006;45:1271–1275.
21. Uchida T, Ohkusa H, Yamashita H et al. Five years experience of transrectal high-intensity focused ultrasound using the Sonablate device in the treatment of localized prostate cancer. *Int J Urol.* 2006;13:228–233.
22. Inoue Y, Goto K, Hayashi T, Hayashi M. Transrectal high-intensity focused ultrasound for treatment of localized prostate cancer. *Int J Urol.* 2011;18:358–362.
23. Koch MO, Gardner T, Cheng L, Fedewa RJ, Seip R, Sanghvi NT. Phase I/II trial of high intensity focused ultrasound for the treatment of previously untreated localized prostate cancer. *J Urol.* 2007;178:2366–2370; discussion 2370–2361.
24. Sumitomo M, Asakuma J, Sato A, Ito K, Nagakura K, Asano T. Transurethral resection of the prostate immediately after high-intensity focused ultrasound treatment for prostate cancer. *Int J Urol.* 2010;17:924–930.
25. Uchida T, Shoji S, Nakano M et al. Transrectal high-intensity focused ultrasound for the treatment of localized prostate cancer: Eight-year experience. *Int J Urol.* 2009;16:881–886.
26. Mearini L, D'Urso L, Collura D et al. Visually directed transrectal high intensity focused ultrasound for the treatment of prostate cancer: A preliminary report on the Italian experience. *J Urol.* 2009;181:105–111; discussion 111–102.
27. Ahmed HU, Freeman A, Kirkham A et al. Focal therapy for localized prostate cancer: A phase I/II trial. *J Urol.* 2011;185:1246–1254.

8 Current Role of Cryotherapy in the Treatment of Prostate Cancer

Adnan Dervishi and Murali K. Ankem

CONTENTS

INTRODUCTION

Prostate cancer is the second most common cancer and third leading cause of death in American men. In 2017 alone, the American Cancer Society estimated about 161,360 new cases and 26,730 deaths from prostate cancer (1). Current modalities include but are not limited to radical surgery, radiotherapy, cryotherapy, high-intensity focused ultrasound (HIFU), and active surveillance.

The concept of destroying tissues by freezing was described by Arnott et al. in 1851 (2), but urologic application was initiated by Gonder and Soanes in 1966 (2). The first perineal probes were used by Magalli et al. in 1974 and are widely considered as first-generation cryosystem (2). This was abandoned due to high incidence of incontinence, impotence, urethral necrosis, and rectoure-thral fistulae. The second-generation cryosystems were popularized by Onik et al. in 1988 (2,3). Transrectal guidance for perineal placement of cryoprobes and real-time monitoring of the ice ball with concurrent use of intraurethral warming catheters reduced the complication rates. The currently available systems are third-generation cryosystems. They use the Joule-Thompson principle with argon for freezing, helium for thawing, small 17G cryo-needles, temperature sensors, and ure-thral warming catheters which have led to excellent results with low morbidity.

Traditionally cryotherapy was used in salvage setting for radiotherapy failures and in patients who are high-risk surgical candidates. Of late it is being offered as primary modality for low-risk prostate cancer in the form of focal or whole-gland ablation. Primary cryotherapy offers 5-year bio-chemical disease-free survival (bDFS) rates of 77% (2) while salvage cryotherapy achieved 58.9% with acceptable morbidity (4).

The American Urological Association recognized cryotherapy as a therapeutic option for prostate cancer in 1996. As the demand for minimally invasive effective therapies increases, with advances in imaging and ablating technology, we forecast these options will be offered more in the near future.

CRYOBIOLOGY

Cryotherapy induces cell death by vascular thrombosis and destruction of cell membrane and organelles. The intracellular formation of ice crystals causes mechanical disruption of membranes and freezing temperatures cause malfunction of proteins leading to irreversible damage. The standard double freeze and thaw process adds additional insult in the form of reperfusion injury. Chosy et al. showed that temperatures of −19.4°C are needed for complete necrosis (5). Within 24 hours coagulative necrosis ensues with infiltration of macrophages, plasma cells, and lymphocytes with eventual scar formation.

CRYOTHERAPY TECHNIQUE

We use a similar setup and technique that we use for prostate brachytherapy. This includes a standard 2D ultrasonography unit with a transrectal probe, laptop computer, perineal template, and a rotational mover device attached to the operating table. Under general or spinal anesthesia, the patient is placed in the lithotomy position. The transrectal ultrasonography probe is then inserted into the rectum until the prostate can be clearly seen in the transverse and sagittal views. A template is displayed in the transverse view and we plan the respective probe positions, leaving appropriate distances between probes, to the lateral aspect, base, and apex of the prostate, to the urethra, and to anterior rectal wall. We typically place approximately six cryo-needles, and verify their positions in the transverse and sagittal views. Three thermocouples are then inserted under guidance, at the apex, pre-rectal, and intraprostatic locations. Flexible cystoscopy is performed to verify the intraurethral/bladder placement of the cryo-needles, and once appropriate position is confirmed, a urethral warming device is then inserted. Argon gas is used as a cooling source and helium as the rewarming (thawing) source. As the freezing process commences, the progress of the ice ball formation is monitored in real time. This allows cautious monitoring of the freezing process, coverage of target area, rectal wall, and external sphincter. A standard double freeze-thaw cycle is utilized. A suprapubic catheter is then placed routinely and the patient is admitted for 23 hours observation. The suprapubic catheter is removed once the post-void residual urine is less than 150 mL.

PRIMARY WHOLE GLAND THERAPY

There are no randomized controlled studies (RCTs) comparing primary therapies for localized prostate cancer. A systematic review of literature by Wilt and associates showed a low level of evidence supporting cryotherapy as a primary modality (6). In the absence of RCTs the data is difficult to interpret because of the different study designs, criteria for failure, and use of dissimilar generations of cryosystems in various studies. Currently, post-cryotherapy failure is determined based on either American Society for Radiation Oncology (ASTRO) or Phoenix criteria. Some studies take levels equal to or above 0.5 ng/dL as evidence of recurrence. These varied definitions make it difficult to establish a successful outcome. Nevertheless, Ritch et al. observed that cryotherapy has similar short-term bDFS rates compared to other primary treatment modalities (7). Cohen et al. reported a 10-year bDFS rate of 56.01% (ASTRO) and 62.36% (Phoenix) (8). When they looked at subsets based on the risk (low, intermediate, high) the bDFS was 80.56%, 74.16%, and 45.54% respectively. The study also showed an overall survival rate of 73.81% for patients with negative biopsy status (9). To enhance understanding of the efficacy of primary cryotherapy, the Cryo Online Database (COLD) registry was initiated; it includes four academic centers and 34 community urology groups.

Five-year data from the COLD registry demonstrated bDFS rates of 77.1% (ASTRO) and 72.9% (Phoenix) for the entire group (2,4). Risk stratification and analysis showed bDFS rates of 84.7%, 73.4%, and 75.3% (ASTRO) for low-, intermediate-, and high-risk patients respectively (2,4,10). This could reflect the improvements in technology as well as the experience of the treating physicians.

One area of significant improvement is the reduction of complication rates after cryotherapy. The downtrend in complication rates has been attributed to the development of third-generation cryosystems, and has rekindled the interest in this form of therapy. In a multicenter study ($n = 106$), Han and colleagues (11) noted urethral sloughing (5%), incontinence (3%), urge incontinence (5%), urinary retention (3.3%), rectal pain (2.6%), and rectourethral fistula (0%). Hubosky et al. reported even lower rates of complications in the 2% range, and when compared to brachytherapy cohort cryotherapy patients had better urinary function (9). Although there has been an overall decrease in complications rates in whole-gland cryotherapy, the high incidence of erectile dysfunction, with only 20% of patients achieving any meaningful erections at 1 year, is discouraging (7).

SALVAGE CRYOTHERAPY

External beam radiation therapy (EBRT) is a standard primary treatment for localized prostate cancer. Even in conformal EBRT with image guidance and dose escalation technique about 20%–50% develop biochemical recurrence in 10 years (12). Post-EBRT prostate biopsy demonstrates that most failures are secondary to recurrence/residual disease. Failure to treat local recurrence might lead to debilitating urinary symptoms, possible distant spread, and poor quality of life. Despite potential benefits of salvage treatment most of the patients are usually managed by observation or androgen deprivation treatment (ADT). Post-radiation therapy failures are often treated with salvage prostatectomy (open/robotic), salvage cryotherapy, salvage HIFU, and re-radiation. Open salvage prostatectomy is technically difficult with major complication rates. Recently salvage robotic radical prostatectomy has been promising due to two-thirds of patients with bDFS rate with continence rate of 60% and potency rates of 20% in short-term (36 months) follow-up (12). Cryotherapy is a logical choice since it's inherently less invasive and has a low complication rate. Izawa et al. noted 3% incontinence and 2% fistula after salvage cryotherapy (13). Pisters and associates (4) studied COLD registry patients who underwent salvage cryotherapy ($n = 279$) and found a 5-year bDFS rate of 59% using ASTRO criteria. Izawa et al. (13) reported a post-salvage cryotherapy biopsy positive rate of less than 23%, and Chin et al. found a lower positive biopsy rate of 14.2% (14). This is not surprising because it is almost impossible to achieve a total kill of all the prostate epithelial cells. This is especially true with periurethral glands, which are protected by a urethral warming device, and lethal dose is not delivered at this site. Izawa et al. found transurethral biopsy positive rates as high as 17% (13).

An area of concern is the use of ADT along with salvage cryotherapy. This makes comparison between various studies perplexing, and the results should be accepted with caution. Most often, ADT is added to downsize the prostate to enhance the delivery of freezing temperatures to the whole gland. About 8.2% of the COLD registry patients were on ADT and some reported even higher number of patients (32%) on ADT (2,4). However, upon evaluation of outcomes of salvage cryotherapy in patients who had not received neoadjuvant hormonal ablative therapy ($n = 156$), from the COLD registry, Spiess et al. found that for 1-, 2-, and 3-year bDFS in patients with a pre-salvage PSA < 5 ng/mL were 95.3%, 86.7%, and 78.3%, respectively, versus 81.4%, 58.4%, and 52.9%, respectively, for the subgroup with a pre-salvage PSA 5 ng/mL (3). This study highlights the important prognostic role of a patient's pre-treatment PSA level and emphasizes the importance of a prompt referral once local failure is suspected (3). Salvage therapy is well tolerated, with a urinary incontinence rate of 4% and a fistula rate of 1.2% as shown in the COLD registry (4). Recent technological advances in cryosystems have led to lower urinary incontinence rates from 83% to 9% (3). The incidence of erectile dysfunction post

TABLE 8.1

Review of Outcomes from Focal Salvage Cryotherapy for Recurrent Prostate Cancer after Radiotherapy

Study (year)	Patients (n)	Pretreatment PSA (ng/mL)	Median Follow-up (Months)	bDFS Definition	bDFS (%)	Ref.
Li (2015)	91	4.8	15	Phoenix	95.1% 1 year 72.4% 3 years 46.5% 5 years	(15)
De Castro Abreu et al. (2013)	25	2.8	31	Phoenix	68%	(16)
Eisenberg et al. (2008)	19	3.3	18	ASTRO	89% 1 year 67% 2 years 50% 3 years	(17)

Abbreviations: ASTRO: American Society for Radiology and Oncology; bDFS: biochemical disease-free survival; PSA: prostate-specific antigen; Ref.: reference.

salvage therapy is very high, in the range of 90%, due to collateral damage to the neurovascular bundles. More work needs to be done in order to protect future sexual function (Table 8.1).

FOCAL CRYOTHERAPY

Focal cryotherapy is a novel approach to achieve oncologic control with preservation of quality of life. Primary treatment options for localized prostate cancer are too aggressive with significant morbidity. In select patients focal ablative techniques can be utilized to preserve potency by sparing the neurovascular bundles. Multiparametric magnetic resonance imaging (mpMRI) has enhanced the diagnosis, localization, and delivery of ablative therapy. In this area, more work is being reported in the form of MRI-guided focal cryotherapy, laser ablation, and HIFU. The limiting factor is that not all localized prostate cancers are truly localized to one small area, and the natural history of the disease is unpredictable, so this approach should be used with caution in select patient populations. Nevertheless, the quest to develop a truly minimally invasive option with minimal side effects continues and more results are being reported in the literature.

Early studies showed enough evidence to pursue this approach. Katz et al. (18) reported a bDFS rate of 84% at 3 years with preservation of potency in 68% of patients. Onik and colleagues (19) found 95% had a stable PSA at 2 years with no post-treatment positive biopsy at 1 year; 90% maintained potency as well. However, four patients underwent a whole-gland ablation as the PSA never reached nadir. This highlights one important finding that the cancer should be localized to one site or side. More information was reported by Ellis et al. (20), Bahn et al. (21), and Lambert et al. (22) with similar short-term results with preservation of potency anywhere between 70% and 88.9%. Potency was defined as erections sufficient for penetration with or without aid. None of the studies reported any significant urinary issues or bowel symptoms; however, the selection criteria varied between the studies. Lambert et al. used standard 12-core biopsies and Ellis's group recruited liberally across the board. Onik and his associates used a 3D transperineal mapping biopsy with no restrictions on the PSA or Gleason score. These results underscore the need for stricter uniform selection criteria with in-depth 3D or MRI mapping to identify occult and multifocal lesions. Eggener and colleagues (23) attempted to define the ideal selection criteria which include prostate cancers with stage T1–T2a, PSA less than 10, PSA density less than 0.15, PSA velocity less than 2 ng/dL, no Gleason 4 or 5, and no evidence of extra-prostatic extension with single lesion. Overall, focal cryotherapy lives up to the promise of satisfactory cancer control in the short term and excellent functional outcomes, however, significant challenges remain in this field of focal ablation of prostate cancer. First, some might argue these patients are ideal candidates for active surveillance in the contemporary practice. Second, there is a lack of uniform selection criteria, follow-up, and insufficient long-term data. Finally, acceptable biopsy strategy needs to be determined as well.

In summary, even though there is enough interest in this approach, its rationale is questioned in the background of active surveillance which is rapidly gaining popularity. Whether there is a super-select population at high risk for active surveillance who could be offered focal ablative option needs to be determined in the future (Tables 8.2 and 8.3).

TABLE 8.2
Outcome of Focal Cryotherapy of Localized Prostate Cancer

Study (year)	Patients (n)	Median Age	Pretreatment PSA	Median Follow-up	Definition bDFS	bDFS (%)	Ref.
Barqawi et al. (2014)	62	60.5	NA	28 months	PSA > pre-op PSA	71	(24)
Barrett et al. (2013)	50	66.5	6.1	9 months	PSA Median = 2.5 at 12 months	NA	(25)
Bahn et al. (2012)	73	64	5.9	3.7 years	NA	NA	(26)
Ward et al. (2012)	1149	67.8		21.1 months	ASTRO	75.7	(10)
Truesdale et al. (2010)	77	69.5	6.54	24 months	Phoenix	72.7	(27)
Lambert et al. (2007)	25	68	6.0	28 months	50% of pre-op PSA	84	(22)
Ellis et al. (2007)	60	69	7.2	12 months	ASTRO	80.4	(20)
Onik et al. (2007)	55	NA	8.3	3.6 years	ASTRO	93	(19)
Bahn et al. (2006)	31	63	4.95	70 months	ASTRO	92.8	(21)

Abbreviations: ASTRO: American Society for Radiology and Oncology; bDFS: biochemical disease-free survival; NA: not available; PSA: prostate-specific antigen; Ref: reference.

TABLE 8.3
Side Effects Secondary to Focal Cryotherapy

Study (year) (Ref.)	Side Effects		
	Incontinence (%)	ED (%)	Fistula (%)
Barqawi et al. (2014) (24)	0	0	0
Barrett et al. (2013) (25)	0	0	2
Bahn et al. (2012) (26)	0	26 (1 year) 14 (2.4 years)	0
Ward et al. (2012) (10)	1.6	42	0.01
Lambert et al. (2007) (22)	0	29	0
Ellis et al. (2007) (20)	3.6	29.4	0
Onik et al. (2007) (19)	1	15	0
Bahn et al. (2006) (21)	0	11.9	0

Abbreviations: ED: erectile dysfunction; Ref.: reference.

FOLLOW-UP AFTER CRYOTHERAPY

There is no standard follow-up protocol after any form of cryotherapy. Most groups have attempted to use radiation therapy follow-up protocols. Both radiation and ablative techniques aim to destroy the whole gland or part of the gland. ASTRO and Phoenix criteria are still used to report oncologic efficacy. This approach is problematic at multiple levels. First, whole-gland cryotherapy aims to destroy the prostate, however, the periurethral glands are spared due to use of a urethral warming system. These periurethral glands continue to secrete PSA, and thus some level of post-ablation PSA is expected. However, this acceptable PSA level is yet to be determined. It is even more disputable in the focal ablation as it is not clear what the acceptable PSA will be. Second, the use of post-ablation prostate biopsy and its timing and duration are not clear either. Even though it appears to be a promising follow-up strategy, it may not be desirable for the patients to have biopsies on a regular basis as biopsy is invasive and can have complications. Third, post-ablation interpretation of biopsy is complex due to ablative changes, concurrent ADT, and the fact that some patients continue to have residual cancer. No uniform opinion exists about how to deal with persistent positive biopsy with low PSA. Multicenter clinical trials and large databases like COLD will be able to provide answers in the near future.

COST ANALYSIS

Very little information is available in the literature regarding the cost comparison between cryotherapy and other modalities. Benoit et al. (38) reported overall cost reduction of 27% when compared to radical prostatectomy, and Schmidt et al. (29) found that at a cost of $13,000, cryotherapy is half the cost of radical prostatectomy. These are initial hospital costs and didn't take into consideration subsequent follow-up, interventions for complications, and recurrence of disease. It is desirable to dig deep into cost-effective analysis by head-to-head comparison of available standard treatment modalities.

FUTURE

It is indisputable that cryotherapy has evolved in the last 150 years and this is mainly due to availability of new generation cryosystems and demand for minimally invasive approaches. Availability of mpMRI in the pre-, peri-, and postoperative settings will increase the accuracy of diagnosis, treatment, and follow-up (30). New strides are being made in the field of combined modalities, that is, cryotherapy with chemo and immunotherapeutic approaches. Even though they are investigational at this time, the future holds much promise. Multicenter randomized clinical trials and analyzing COLD registry are desirable. Although it is not a standard therapy at this time, focal ablation may play an important role as a complementary therapy to active surveillance in patients with low-risk prostate cancer.

CONCLUSION

Durable PSA response with negative post-treatment biopsy rates after cryotherapy with preserved quality of life is appealing to patients and providers alike. Current data demonstrates that focal ablation bDFS are comparable to whole-gland treatment. Although erectile dysfunction remains problematic after whole-gland ablation, focal therapy has demonstrated to have a lower risk for ED. Due to its favorable outcomes and lower side effect profile, focal cryotherapy has a promising future as an alternative to whole-gland treatment for primary localized low-risk prostate cancer, as well as for recurrent cancer after radiotherapy.

In addition to establishing optimal criteria for proper patient selection, and lessening complications, further research is needed for accurate localization, delivery of ablative energy, follow-up strategies, long-term outcomes, and combined modalities such as chemo/immunotherapies.

REFERENCES

1. https://www.cancer.org/cancer/prostate-cancer/about/key-statistics.html
2. Jones JS, Rewcastle JC, Donnelly B et al. Whole gland primary prostate cryoablation: Initial results from the cryo on-line data registry. *J Urol* 2008;180:554–558.
3. Spiess PE, Levi DA, Pisters LL et al. Outcomes of salvage prostate cryotherapy stratified by pre-treatment Psa: Update from the cold registry. *World J Urol* 2013;31(6):1321–1325.
4. Pisters LL, Rewcastle JC, Donnelly B et al. Salvage prostate cryoablation: Initial results from the cryo on-line data registry. *J Urol* 2008;180:559–564.
5. Chosy SG, Nakada SY, Lee FT Jr, Warner TF. Monitoring renal cryosurgery: Predictors of tissue necrosis in swine. *J Urol* 1998;159(4):1370–1374.
6. Wilt TJ, MacDonald R, Rutks I et al. Systematic review: Comparative effectiveness and harms of treatments for clinically localized prostate cancer. *Ann Intern Med* 2008;148:435–448.
7. Ritch CR, Katz AE. Update on cryotherapy for localized prostate cancer. *Curr Urol Rep* 2009;10(3):206–211.
8. Cohen JK, Miller RJ, Ahmed S et al. Ten-year biochemical disease control for patients with prostate cancer treated with cryosurgery as primary therapy. *Urology* 2008;71:515–518.
9. Hubosky SG, Fabrizio MD, Schellhammer PF et al. Single center experience with third generation cryosurgery for management of organ-confined prostate cancer: Critical evaluation of short-term outcomes, complications and patient quality of life. *J Endourol* 2007;21:1521–1531.
10. Ward JF, Jones JS. Focal cryotherapy for localized prostate cancer: A report from the national Cryo On-Line Database (COLD) Registry. *BJU Int* 2012;109(11):1648–1654.
11. Han KR, Belldegrun AS. Third-generation cryosurgery for primary and recurrent prostate cancer. *BJU Int* 2004;93(1):14–18.
12. Zargar HH. Salvage robotic prostatectomy for radio recurrent prostate cancer: Technical challenges and outcome analysis. *Minerva Urol Nefrol* 2017;69(1):1827–1758.
13. Izawa JI, Perrotte P, Greene G et al. Local tumor control with salvage cryotherapy for locally recurrent prostate cancer after external beam radiotherapy. *J Urol* 2001;165:867–870.
14. Chin JL, Touma N, Pautler SE et al. Serial histopathology results pf salvage cryoablation for prostate cancer after radiation failure. *J Urol* 2003;170:1199–1202.
15. Li YH, Elshafei A, Agarwal G, Ruckle H, Powsang J, Jones JS. Salvage focal prostate cryoablation for locally recurrent prostate cancer after radiotherapy: Initial results from the cryo on-line data registry. *Prostate* 2015;75(1):1–7.
16. de Castro Abreu AL, Bahn D, Leslie S et al. Salvage focal and salvage total cryoablation for locally recurrent prostate cancer after primary radiation therapy. *BJU Int* 2013;112(3):298–307.
17. Eisenberg ML, Shinohara K. Partial salvage cryoablation of the prostate for recurrent prostate cancer after radiotherapy failure. *Urology* 2008;72(6):1315–1318.
18. Katz AE, Kacker R. Focal treatment for low-risk prostate cancer. *BJU Int* 2008;102:158–159.
19. Onik G, Vaughan D, Lotenfoe R et al. The "male lumpectomy": Focal therapy for prostate cancer using cryoablation results in 48 patients with at least 2 year follow up. *Urol Oncol* 2008;26:500–505.
20. Ellis DS, Manny TB Jr, Rewcastle JC. Focal cryosurgery followed by penile rehabilitation as primary treatment for localized prostate cancer: Initial results. *Urology* 2007;70:9–15.
21. Bahn DK, Silverman P, Lee F Sr et al. Focal prostate cryoablation: Initial results show cancer control and potency preservation. *J Endourol* 2006;20:688–692.
22. Lambert EH, Bolte K, Masson P et al. Focal cryosurgery: Encouraging health outcomes for unifocal prostate cancer. *Urology* 2007;69:1117–1120.
23. Eggener S, Scardino P, Carroll P et al. Focal therapy for localized prostate cancer: A critical appraisal of rationale and modalities. *J Urol* 2007;178:2260–2267.
24. Barqawi AB, Stoimenova D, Krughoff K et al. Targeted focal therapy in the management of organ confined prostate cancer. *J Urol* 2014;192(3):749–753.

25. Barret E, Ahallal Y, Sanchez-Salas R et al. Morbidity of focal therapy in the treatment of localized prostate cancer. *Eur Urol* 2013;63(4):618–622.
26. Bahn D, de Castro Abreu A, Gill I et al. Focal cryotherapy for clinically unilateral, low-intermediate risk prostate cancer in 73 men with a median follow-up of 3.7 years. *Eur Urol* 2012;62:55–63.
27. Truesdale MD, Cheetham PJ, Hruby GW et al. An evaluation of patient selection criteria on predicting progression-free survival after primary focal unilateral nerve-sparing cryoablation for prostate cancer: Recommendations for follow up. *Cancer J* 2010;16(5):544–549.
28. Benoit RM, Cohen JK, Miller RJ Jr. Comparison of the hospital costs for radical prostatectomy and cryosurgical ablation of the prostate. *Urology* 1998;52(5):820–824.
29. Schmidt JD, Doyle J, Larison S. Prostate cryoablation: Update 1998. *CA: Cancer J Clin* 1998;48(4):239–253.
30. Valerio MM, Shah TT, Shah P et al. Magnetic resonance imaging-transrectal ultrasound fusion focal cryotherapy of the prostate: A prospective development study. *Urol Oncol* 35(4):150.e1–150.e7.

9 Transperineal Mapping of the Prostate for Biopsy Strategies

Daniel Kaplon and Winston Barzell

CONTENTS

INTRODUCTION

Prostate cancer (PCa) has traditionally been regarded as a multifocal disease, yet radical prostatectomy specimens have shown that 20%–30% of men with PCa may have unilateral or unifocal cancer. The concept of an *index cancer* was recently introduced to describe the largest cancer within a prostate, almost always the highest-grade cancer present, and the one likely to penetrate the capsule. In multifocal disease, *the index cancer* is the presumed main driver of progression, outcome, and prognosis, leading to the hypothesis that small secondary cancers might be clinically irrelevant if the index lesion is treated. Ohori (1) reported that in patients with multifocal cancer, 80% of the tumor load arose from the index cancer, and that extracapsular extension, present in 28% of patients, almost always originated from the index lesion. Herein, the focus is on mapping the prostate in clinical scenarios where the prostate cancer is on surveillance protocol or on an active focal therapy treatment regimen.

Therapeutic dilemmas leading to a decision to perform transperineal biopsy of the prostate may be encountered in two patient populations: active surveillance (AS) candidates and focal therapy (FT) candidates.

ACTIVE SURVEILLANCE

Patients meeting criteria for active surveillance have minimal low-grade cancer on transrectal ultrasound (TRUS)-guided prostate biopsy. The patients meet strict criteria (less than 1 mm of Gleason score 6 or less in one biopsy core on transrectal biopsy) and have a 50% probability of having an "insignificant" cancer. Theoretically, these patients can be managed with watchful waiting as the cancer is considered to have no impact on morbidity or survival. Because up to 50% of these patients may upstage their disease, transperineal biopsy at set follow-up intervals is advised.

FOCAL THERAPY GROUP

This group is comprised of patients who appear to have limited unilateral disease as defined on initial diagnosis or with recurrence after failed primary therapy. These patients may be considered for focal therapies such as salvage "remedial" brachytherapy following prior suboptimal implant or unilateral cryotherapy as primary treatment. Other scenarios include relapse from primary external beam radiation, brachytherapy, or cryoablation. In all these cases, mapping the location and extent of the cancer is essential for rational management.

The concept of FT has been criticized on the basis that prostate cancer is frequently multifocal. Furthermore, the efficacy of FT is unproven, and validated criteria for identifying patients who can safely be managed by this modality do not exist. Consequently, it is important that the selection process for patients undergoing FT excludes patients with cancer outside the area destined to be treated while precisely locating the targeted area to be selectively ablated.

Given the limitations of our existing imaging modalities, the selection of patients for FT is currently best achieved by a comprehensive re-staging biopsy procedure.

This chapter explores the various re-staging biopsy strategies, including saturation transrectal ultrasound biopsies (TRBx), and transperineal template guided 3-dimensional pathologic mapping biopsies (3-DPM). The technique of 3-DPM is illustrated, and the advantages and disadvantages of saturation TRBx versus 3-DPM are discussed as they relate to the process of patient selection.

TRANSRECTAL BIOPSY STRATEGIES

TRANSRECTAL SYSTEMATIC BIOPSIES

Systematic sextant biopsies under transrectal ultrasound guidance (TRBx) were introduced into clinical practice in 1989 by Hodge and remained the gold standard for several years. Because of the high false negative rate of these sextant biopsies, extended biopsy protocols were introduced by many to maximize PCa detection rates. Eskew (2) described a 5-region technique incorporating lateral and midline biopsies with traditional sextant cores (total 13) which enhanced the detection rate to 40%. The improved cancer detection rates using a 12-core biopsy strategy, which includes the classic sextant distribution with another set of sextant biopsies directed more laterally, provide the basis for the current wide use of this biopsy scheme (3).

TRANSRECTAL SATURATION BIOPSIES

Several authors have proposed a technique of "saturation" biopsies to increase cancer detection and to better estimate the tumor extent and grade (4,5). When saturation TRBx is used as a repeat diagnostic procedure, the cancer detection rate is around 30%–40% (6). While saturation biopsies appear to detect more cancers than extended biopsies, the accuracy with which any TRBx scheme can determine the size, location, extent, and grade of cancer remains to be demonstrated (7). In an effort to solve the latter shortcoming a novel 3-dimensional TRUS biopsy system (The TargetScan®) has been described recently. This system uses a 3D imaging and targeting system to biopsy the prostate in a template fashion. Preliminary studies reported a 47.6% of cancer detection rate in patients with no previous biopsies; furthermore, this approach appears superior to conventional TRUS biopsy in terms of characterizing tumor size, location, and Gleason score (8).

TRANSPERINEAL BIOPSY STRATEGIES

The efficacy of FT remains unproven, and validated criteria for identifying patients who can safely be managed by this modality do not exist. It is therefore incumbent upon us to exclude patients who may unknowingly harbor more extensive significant cancer than predicted by the initial office TRBx. In our opinion, this is currently best accomplished by proceeding with a comprehensive re-staging procedure prior to selective ablation.

For many reasons, we prefer a transperineal template guided 3-DPM approach for re-staging (9,10), a perspective shared by Onik (11,12) and Crawford (13). Advantages of the transperineal approach include a ready access to the anterior apical areas of the prostate; a systematic approach to sampling that does not rely on visual 3D recall and provides a fixed reproducible set of XYZ coordinates for use in cancer mapping, treatment planning, and follow-up; and a decreased likelihood of infection and bleeding. Furthermore there are inherent difficulties in translating the findings from saturation TRBx schemes to a Cartesian coordinate transperineal grid system through which most current FT modalities are delivered. Admittedly, the disadvantages of 3-DPM are that it is tedious, requires logistical support with specimen handling and labeling, and is more costly. Additionally, it requires either a general, regional, or local anesthesia.

The 3-DPM biopsy technique has been previously described (9,10) (Figures 9.1 and 9.2). Biopsies with specific XYZ coordinates may be individually labeled and submitted, or alternatively individual biopsies may be lumped together into zones (Figure 9.3), from which a pathologic map is generated (Figure 9.4). When considering FT, and specifically hemi-gland ablation, it is important to segregate the midline biopsies (Figures 9.1 and 9.4) posterior to the urethra to prevent a "false positive" cancer reading from the side destined to be untreated. Due to the "bevel" tracking, which is a feature of most biopsy needles, a needle can inadvertently travel across the midline from a location free of cancer and sample a cancerous region on the opposite side. As this is a critical area for ablation because of its proximity to the urethra and rectal wall, separating these midline biopsies into a "neutral zone" is advisable.

Our initial practice was to leave an indwelling Foley catheter following the procedure, but in the past 100 patients a post-op catheter has not been routinely utilized. By meticulous avoidance of the

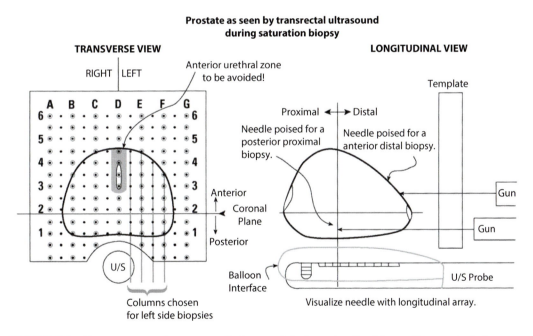

FIGURE 9.1 Prostate as seen by transrectal ultrasound during saturation biopsy. Please note that once a column is selected for biopsy, the needle should be manipulated so that its course can be visualized with the longitudinal array as illustrated. During this maneuver, it is crucial to maintain a fixed sagittal orientation of the ultrasound (US) probe. This technique prevents the needle from tracking and sampling outside the area intended for biopsy. While one is performing these biopsies, it is crucial to avoid injury to the prostatic urethra. This is accomplished by keeping a catheter in place to readily identify the urethra, and then by steering the biopsy needle away from this area. It is also important that midline biopsies are taken posterior to the urethra only because anterior midline biopsies will injure the urethra. (Reprinted from the authors Barzell, W.E., and Whitmore III, W.F., *Urol. Times*, 31, 41–42, 2003. With permission; Barzell, W.E., and Melamed, M.R., *Urology*, 70, 27–35, 2007.)

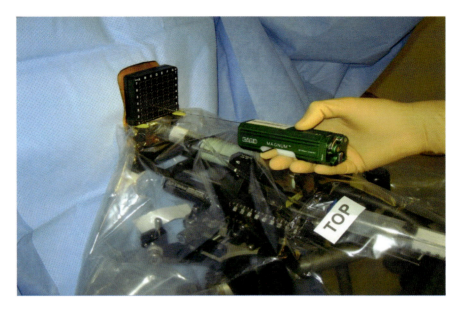

FIGURE 9.2   Operating room sterile setup.

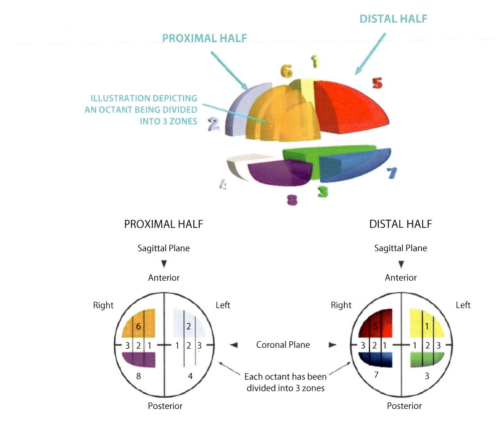

FIGURE 9.3   Specimen Organization: The prostate is divided into proximal and distal halves, and each half is divided into 4 quadrants yielding 8 octants. Each prostate octant is further divided into 3 zones, and the midline biopsies are segregated. Number of specimen jars = 24 zones + 2 midline (proximal/distal) + 2 to 8 TRUS (total = 28 to 34).

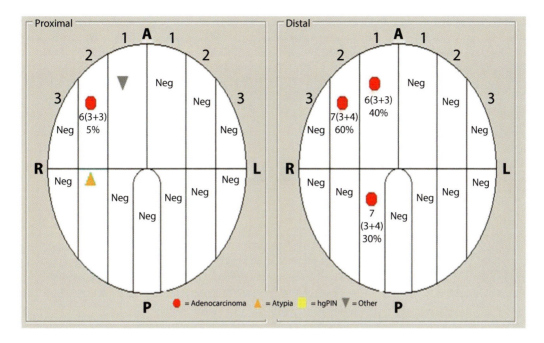

FIGURE 9.4   A sample prostate map illustrating the pathological findings after 3-DPM.

urethral and bladder mucosa in the biopsies, significant urinary bleeding should be an exceedingly rare event. Complications with 3-DPM are usually minor (9,13). In our study cited below, 12 of 140 patients (8.6%) developed minor complications (none requiring hospitalization), including urinary retention (6 of the 12), worsening lower urinary tract symptoms (LUTS) (2 of the 12), and fever, scrotal edema, significant gross hematuria, perineal ecchymosis (1 each).

In an expansion of our initial retrospective study (10), we analyzed the data on 140 patients who presented to one of the authors (WEB) between 2001 and 2009, with unilateral cancer deemed suitable for hemi-ablation based on an office TRBx. These patients underwent a re-staging procedure that included 3-DPM with a concomitant *repeat* TRBx. Patients were considered suitable for FT if there was no cancer on the side contralateral to the presenting lesion as noted on initial office TRBx. Of the 140 patients, only 67 (48%) were suitable for FT using this strict definition, a finding consistent with reports by Onik (11,12). When comparing 3-DPM to repeat TRBx in determining suitability for FT, 52% were found to be unsuitable by 3-DPM while only 6.4% were deemed unsuitable by TRBx. Additionally, repeat TRBx had a false negative rate of 52%, a sensitivity of 34%, and a negative predictive value of 28%.

Those who believe that treating the "index" cancer is sufficient, and are willing to ignore small non-index cancers, have argued that our eligibility criteria were too stringent. We have therefore considered two other definitions of suitability when the extent of cancer on the contralateral side was consistent with modified characterizations of insignificant or indolent cancer (14,15). Using these more liberal definitions of suitability, which allow potentially insignificant cancer on the side destined to be untreated, we still found that between 23% and 27% of patients presenting with unilateral small volume cancer on office TRBx were unsuitable for FT. In many patients, by relying on repeat TRBx alone, high-risk cancer on the side destined to be untreated would have been missed, and in some this "untreated" side harbored the more aggressive cancer or so-called index lesion. In the latter group, a FT treatment plan that relied solely on repeat TRBx could theoretically have targeted the "wrong" side.

While our results imply a clear superiority of 3-DPM over repeat TRBx, a word of caution is needed, as there were several biases favoring 3-DPM (10) in this study, including the limited number of repeat TRBx (average of 10/patient) in this study. Arguably, a saturation TRBx scheme would have provided a fairer comparison as discussed above (4–6), and implied by ex vivo studies (16). However, as recently demonstrated by Delongchamps (17), merely increasing the number of TRBx may not solve the inherent weakness of TRBx, indeed a 36-core biopsy scheme appeared to offer no advantage over an 18-core scheme.

Based on our own experience, validated by others (11–13), reliance on TRBx to select patients for FT may lead to an unacceptable failure rate, given the potential for significant cancer remaining undetected and thereby untreated. When significant cancer is missed by TRBx, in our experience the sites most commonly overlooked are the anterior apical regions of the prostate, a finding confirmed by Taira (18). Since the consequences of improper designation of a patient as an FT candidate may be profound, we believe that 3-DPM should be an integral component of any FT program.

CONCLUSIONS

We have chosen the transperineal approach for saturation biopsy rather than the transrectal approach as practiced by Stewart et al. (4) for both practical and theoretical reasons. First, there are physical and technical limitations of the standard transrectal approach using current equipment that limit access to the anterior and apical regions of the prostate. Second, the risk of infection and rectal bleeding is potentially higher with increasing numbers of rectal wall needle sticks. Third, inherent and inevitable inaccuracies of sampling and mapping occur when using unstabilized manual positioning of the needle guide and relying on 3D visual recall for guidance when attempting a large number of biopsies.

Conversely, the increased accuracy provided by the template-guided transperineal approach allows both a more comprehensive and systematic approach to sampling and a set of fixed reproducible coordinates to use for accurate mapping of cancer within the prostate.

The weaknesses of the transperineal route are that it requires some form of anesthesia and it is less efficient in sampling the posterior peripheral zone adjacent to the rectal wall. Although this area is perhaps the most likely to contain cancer, it is most likely also the area previously sampled by standard transrectal biopsy. For this reason, we recommend combining standard transrectal biopsy with transperineal saturation biopsy in the setting of patients who qualify under the expectant management or focal treatment indications. It is important to emphasize that, in our opinion, transperineal saturation biopsies should be done as a follow-up approach only after taking at least three negative sets of transrectal biopsies using an extended 10- to 12-biopsy regimen.

Unilateral saturation biopsies are done on the contralateral unaffected side for the focal therapy group to prove the absence of cancer on the uninvolved and what will ultimately be the untreated side. Bilateral saturation biopsies are performed in the diagnostic and expectant management groups. In the diagnostic group, they are done on those patients with a rising PSA, unacceptable and falling free PSA, or other indicators of high risk who have had at least three prior sets of negative extended ultrasound-guided systematic transrectal needle biopsies. In the expectant management group, they are performed when low Gleason score and low-volume disease are suspected and patients are being considered for a watchful waiting approach. In this latter instance, the primary purpose is to avoid the risk of undersampling leading to underdiagnosis that exists if only transrectal biopsies are done. To be conservative, we also recommend combining repeat transrectal biopsies with saturation transperineal biopsies in this setting.

Until such time that newer imaging modalities can more accurately and reliably identify small foci of PCa, 3-DPM offers an accuracy in tumor localization that is crucial not only for proper patient selection and treatment planning (9–13), but also for follow-up biopsy validation of the efficacy of FT ablation, especially when considering novel technologies.

A vital key to the success of selective FT of the prostate is proper patient selection. Currently, this is best achieved by a re-staging procedure that can exclude patients with cancer outside the area destined to be treated while precisely locating the targeted area to be selectively ablated. A re-staging procedure that uses 3-DPM fulfills these criteria and should be used in the appropriate selection of patients for FT.

REFERENCES

1. Ohori M, Eastham JA, Koh H et al. Is focal therapy reasonable in patients with early stage prostate cancer (CaP)—an analysis of radical prostatectomy (RP) specimens (abstract). *J Urol.* 2006;175:507.
2. Eskew LA, Bare RL, McCullough DL. Systematic 5 region prostate biopsy is superior to sextant method for diagnosing carcinoma of the prostate. *J Urol.* 1997;157(1):199–202; discussion 3.
3. Presti JC, Jr., Chang JJ, Bhargava V, Shinohara K. The optimal systematic prostate biopsy scheme should include 8 rather than 6 biopsies: Results of a prospective clinical trial. *J Urol.* 2000;163(1):163–166; discussion 6–7.
4. Stewart CS, Leibovich BC, Weaver AL, Lieber MM. Prostate cancer diagnosis using a saturation needle biopsy technique after previous negative sextant biopsies. *J Urol.* 2001;166(1):86–91; discussion 2.
5. Jones JS. Saturation biopsy for detecting and characterizing prostate cancer. *BJU Int.* 2007;99(6):1340–1344.
6. Jones JS, Patel A, Schoenfield L, Rabets JC, Zippe CD, Magi-Galluzzi C. Saturation technique does not improve cancer detection as an initial prostate biopsy strategy. *J Urol.* 2006;175(2):485–488.
7. Sartor AO, Hricak H, Wheeler TM et al. Evaluating localized prostate cancer and identifying candidates for focal therapy. *Urology.* 2008;72(6 Suppl):S12–S24.
8. Megwalu II, Ferguson GG, Wei JT et al. Evaluation of a novel precision template-guided biopsy system for detecting prostate cancer. *BJU Int.* 2008;102(5):546–550.
9. Barzell W, Whitmore III, WF. Transperineal template guided saturation biopsy of the prostate: Rationale, indications, and technique. *Urol Times.* 2003;31:41–42.
10. Barzell WE, Melamed MR. Appropriate patient selection in the focal treatment of prostate cancer: The role of transperineal 3-dimensional pathologic mapping of the prostate: A 4-year experience. *Urology.* 2007;70(6A):27–35.
11. Onik G, Barzell W. Transperineal 3D mapping biopsy of the prostate: An essential tool in selecting patients for focal prostate cancer therapy. *Urol Oncol-Semin Ori.* 2008;26(5):506–510.
12. Onik G, Miessau M, Bostwick DG. Three-dimensional prostate mapping biopsy has a potentially significant impact on prostate cancer management. *J Clin Oncol.* 2009;27(26):4321–4326.
13. Crawford ED, Barqawi A. Targeted focal therapy: A minimally invasive ablation technique for early prostate cancer. *Oncology (Williston Park).* 2007;21(1):27–32; discussion 3–4, 9.
14. Goto Y, Ohori M, Arakawa A, Kattan MW, Wheeler TM, Scardino PT. Distinguishing clinically important from unimportant prostate cancers before treatment: Value of systematic biopsies. *J Urol.* 1996;156(3):1059–1063.
15. Epstein JI, Walsh PC, Carmichael M, Brendler CB. Pathologic and clinical findings to predict tumor extent of nonpalpable (stage T1c) prostate cancer. *JAMA.* 1994;271(5):368–374.
16. Epstein JI, Sanderson H, Carter HB, Scharfstein DO. Utility of saturation biopsy to predict insignificant cancer at radical prostatectomy. *Urology.* 2005;66(2):356–360.
17. Delongchamps NB, de la Roza G, Jones R, Jumbelic M, Haas GP. Saturation biopsies on autopsied prostates for detecting and characterizing prostate cancer. *BJU Int.* 2009;103(1):49–54.
18. Taira AV, Merrick GS, Galbreath RW et al. Performance of transperineal template-guided mapping biopsy in detecting prostate cancer in the initial and repeat biopsy setting. *Prostate Cancer Prostatic Dis.* 2009;13(1):71–77.

10 Computer-Aided Diagnosis Systems for Prostate Cancer Detection
Challenges and Methodologies

Guillaume Lemaître, Robert Martí, and Fabrice Meriaudeau

CONTENTS

INTRODUCTION

PROSTATE ANATOMY

The prostate is an exocrine gland of the male reproductive system having an inverted pyramidal shape, which is located below the bladder and in front of the rectum. It measures approximately 3 cm in height by 2.5 cm in depth and its weight is estimated from 7 to 16 g for an adult [1]. The prostate size increases at two distinct stages during physical development: initially at puberty to reach its normal size, then again after 60 years of age leading to benign prostatic hyperplasia (BPH) [2].

A zonal classification of the prostate has been suggested by McNeal [3]. Subsequently, this categorization has been widely accepted in the literature [2,4–6] and is used during all medical examinations (e.g., biopsy, MRI screening). The classification is based on dividing the gland into three distinct regions: (i) the central zone (CZ), accounting for 20%–25% of the whole prostate gland; (ii) the transitional zone (TZ), standing for 5%; and (iii) the peripheral zone (PZ), representing the 70%. In MRI images, tissues of CZ and TZ are difficult to distinguish and are usually merged into a common region, denominated central gland (CG). As part of this classification, the prostate is divided into three longitudinal portions: base, median gland, and apex.

PROSTATE CARCINOMA

Prostate cancer (CaP) has been reported on a worldwide scale to be the second most frequently diagnosed cancer of men, accounting for 13.6% [7]. Statistically, in 2008, the number of new diagnosed cases was estimated to be 899,000, with no less than 258,100 deaths [7]. In United States, aside from skin cancer, CaP is the most commonly diagnosed cancer among men, implying that approximately 1 in 6 men will be diagnosed with CaP during their lifetime and 1 in 36 will die from this disease, causing CaP to be the second most common cause of cancer death among men [8,9].

Despite active research to determine the causes of CaP, a fuzzy list of risk factors has arisen [10]. The etiology has been linked to the following factors [10]: (i) family history [11,12], (ii) genetic factors [13–15], (iii) race/ethnicity [11,16], (iv) diet [11,17,18], and (v) obesity [11,19]. This list of risk factors alone cannot be used to diagnose CaP and, in this way, screening enables early detection and treatment.

CaP growth is characterized by two main types of evolution [20]. Slow-growing tumors, accounting for up to 85% of all CaPs [21], progress slowly and usually stay confined to the prostate gland. For such cases, treatment can be substituted with active surveillance. In contrast, the second variant of CaPs develops rapidly and metastases from prostate gland to other organs, primarily the bones [22]. Bone metastases, being an incurable disease, significantly affects the morbidity and mortality rate [23]. Hence, the results of the surveillance have to be trustworthy to distinguish aggressive from slow-growing CaP.

CaP is more likely to come into being in specific regions of the prostate. In that respect, around 70%–80% of CaPs originate in the PZ, whereas 10%–20% originate in the TZ [24–26]. Only about 5% of CaPs occur in the CZ [25,27]. However, those cancers appear to be more aggressive and more likely to invade other organs due to their locations [27].

CaP Screening and Imaging Techniques

Current CaP screening consists of three different stages. First, prostate-specific antigen (PSA) control is performed to distinguish between low- and high-risk CaP. To assert such diagnosis, samples are taken during prostate biopsy and finally analyzed to evaluate the prognosis and the stage of CaP. In this section, we present a detailed description of the current screening as well as its drawbacks.

Since its introduction in mid-1980s, PSA is widely used for CaP screening [28]. A higher-than-normal level of PSA can indicate an abnormality of the prostate either as BPH or cancer [29]. However, other factors can lead to an increased PSA level such as prostate infections, irritations, a recent ejaculation, or a recent rectal examination [2]. PSA is found in the bloodstream in two different forms: free PSA accounting for about 10% and one linked to another protein for the remaining 90%. A level of PSA higher than 10 ng mL^{-1} is considered to be at risk [2]. If the PSA level ranges from 4 to 10 ng mL^{-1}, the patient's risk is considered as suspicious [30]. In that case, the ratio of free PSA to total PSA is computed; if the ratio is higher than 15%, the case is considered as pathological [2].

A transrectal ultrasound (TRUS) biopsy is carried out for cases that are considered pathological. At least six different samples are taken randomly from the right and left parts of the three different prostate zones: apex, median, and base. These samples are further evaluated using the Gleason grading system [31]. The scoring scheme to characterize the biopsy sample is composed of five different patterns that correspond to grades ranging from 1 to 5. A higher grade is associated with a poorer prognosis [32]. Then, in the Gleason system, 2 scores are assigned corresponding to (i) the grade of the most present tumor pattern, and (ii) the grade of the second most present tumor pattern [32]. A higher Gleason score (GS) indicates a more aggressive tumor [32]. Also, it should be noted that biopsy is an invasive procedure that can result in serious infection or urine retention [33,34].

Although PSA screening has been shown to improve early detection of CaP [34], its lack of reliability motivates further investigations using MRI-based computer-aided detection and diagnosis (CAD). Two reliable studies—carried out in the United States [35] and in Europe [36,37]—have attempted to assess the impact of early detection of CaP, with diverging outcomes [34,38]. The study carried out in Europe[1] concluded that PSA screening reduces CaP-related mortality by 21%–44% [36,37], while the American[2] trial found no such effect [35]. However, both studies agree that PSA screening suffers from low specificity, with an estimated rate of 36% [39]. Both studies also agree that overtreatment is an issue: decision making regarding treatment is further complicated by difficulties in evaluating the aggressiveness and progression of CaP [40].

Hence, new screening methods should be developed with improved specificity of detection and more accurate risk assessment (i.e., aggressiveness and progression). Current research is focused on identifying new biological markers to replace PSA-based screening [41–43]. Until such research comes to fruition, these needs can be met through an active-surveillance strategy using multiparametric MRI (mpMRI) techniques [29,44]. CAD systems, which is an area of active research and forms the focus of this chapter, can be incorporated into this screening strategy to allow for more systematic and rigorous follow-up.

Another weakness of the current screening strategy is due to the untrustworthy results provided by TRUS biopsy. Due to its "blind" nature, there is a chance of missing aggressive tumors or detecting microfocal "cancers," which influences the aggressiveness-assessment procedure [45]. As a consequence, overdiagnosis is estimated at up to 30% [46], while missing clinically significant CaP is estimated at up 35% [47]. In an effort to solve both issues, alternative biopsy approaches have been explored. MRI/ultrasound (UTS)-guided biopsy has been shown to outperform standard TRUS biopsy [48]. There, mpMRI images are fused with UTS images in order to improve localization and aggressiveness assessment to carry out biopsies. Human interaction plays a major role in biopsy sampling which can lead to low repeatability; by reducing potential human errors at this stage, the CAD framework can improve repeatability of examination. CaP detection and diagnosis can benefit from the use of MRI-based CADs.

In an effort to improve the current stage of CaP diagnosis and detection, this chapter intends to review the principles of a mpMRI-CAD system starting with a description of the MRI modalities in the section titled "MRI Techniques."

CAD Systems for CaP

During the last century, physicists have focused on constantly innovating in terms of imaging techniques assisting radiologists to improve cancer detection and diagnosis. However, human diagnosis still suffers from low repeatability, synonymous with erroneous detection or interpretations of abnormalities throughout clinical decisions [49,50]. These errors are driven by two majors causes [49]: observer limitations (e.g., constrained human visual perception, fatigue, or distraction) and the complexity of the clinical cases themselves, for instance due to imbalanced data—the number of healthy cases is more abundant than malignant cases—or overlapping structures.

Computer vision has given rise to many promising solutions, but instead of focusing on fully automatic computerized systems, researchers have aimed at providing computer image analysis techniques to aid radiologists in their clinical decisions [49]. In fact, these investigations brought about both concepts of computer-aided detection (CADe) and computer-aided diagnosis (CADx) grouped under the acronym CAD. Since those first steps, evidence has shown that CAD systems enhance the diagnosis performance of radiologists. Chan et al. reported a significant 4% improvement in breast cancer detection [51], which has been confirmed in later

---

[1] The European Randomized Study of Screening for Prostate Cancer (ERSSPC) started in the 1990s in order to evaluate the effect of PSA screening on mortality rate.
[2] The Prostate, Lung, Colorectal, and Ovarian (PLCO) Cancer Screening Trial is carried out in the United States and intends to ascertain the effects of screening on mortality rate.

studies [52]. Similar conclusions have been drawn in the case of lung nodule detection [53], colon cancer [54], or CaP as well [50]. Chan et al. also hypothesized that CAD systems will be even more efficient assisting inexperienced radiologists than senior radiologists [51]. That hypothesis has been tested by Hambrock et al. and confirmed in case of CaP detection [50]. In this particular study, inexperienced radiologists obtained equivalent performance to senior radiologists, both using CAD whereas the accuracy of their diagnosis was significantly poorer without CAD's help.

In contradiction with the aforementioned statement, CAD for CaP is a young technology due to the fact that is based on a still young imaging technology: MRI [55]. Indeed, four distinct MRI modalities are employed in CaP diagnosis which have been mainly developed after the mid-1990s: (i) T2-weighted (T2-W)-MRI [56], (ii) dynamic contrast-enhanced (DCE)-MRI [57], (iii) magnetic resonance spectroscopy imaging (MRSI) [58], and (iv) diffusion weighted (DW)-MRI [59]. In addition, the increase of magnetic field strength in clinical settings, from 1.5 T to 3 T, and the development of endorectal coils, both improved image spatial resolution [60] needed to perform more accurate diagnosis. It is for this matter that the development of CAD for CaP is still lagging behind the fields stated above.

The following sections aim first to provide an overview of the current state of the art of CAD for CaP and, later, according to the drawn conclusions, to propose a CAD which takes advantages of mpMRI modalities. A review of the current proposed CAD for CaP is presented in the section titled "Review of CAD Systems for CaP."

MRI TECHNIQUES

MRI promises overcome the drawbacks of current clinical screening techniques mentioned in the introductory section. Unlike TRUS biopsy, MRI examination is a noninvasive protocol and has been shown to be the most accurate and harmless technique currently available [61]. In this section, we review different MRI imaging techniques developed for CaP detection and diagnosis. Features strengthening each modality will receive particular attention together with their drawbacks. Commonly, these features form the basis for developing analytic tools and automatic algorithms. However, we refer the reader to "CADx: Feature Detection" for more details on automatic feature detection methods since they are part and parcel of the CAD framework.

T2-W-MRI

T2-W-MRI was the first MRI modality used to perform CaP diagnosis [56]. Nowadays, radiologists make use of it for CaP detection, localization, and staging purposes. This imaging technique is well suited to render zonal anatomy of the prostate [30].

This modality relies on a sequence based on setting a long repetition time (TR), reducing the T1 effect in nuclear magnetic resonance (NMR) signal measured, and fixing the echo time (TE) to sufficiently large values in order to enhance the T2 effect of tissues. Thus, PZ and CG tissues are well perceptible in these images. The former is characterized by an intermediate/high-signal intensity (SI) while the latter is depicted by a low SI [4]. An example of a healthy prostate is shown in Figure 10.1a

In the PZ, round or ill-defined low-SI masses are synonymous with CaPs [56] as shown in Figure 10.1b. Detecting CaP in CG is more challenging. Both normal CG tissue and malignant tissue have a low SI in T2-W-MRI, reinforcing difficulties in distinguishing among them. However, CaPs in CG appear often as homogeneous mass having ill-defined edges with lenticular or "water-drop" shapes [30,62] as depicted in Figure 10.1c.

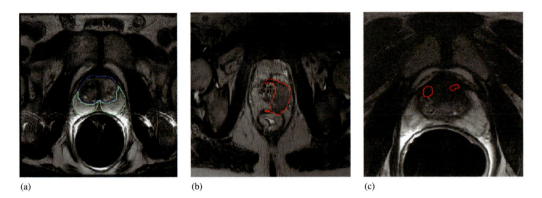

(a)   (b)   (c)

FIGURE 10.1 Rendering of T2-W-MRI prostate image with both 1.5 T and 3 T MRI scanner. (a) T2-W-MRI slice of a healthy prostate acquired with a 1.5 T MRI with an endorectal coil. The blue contour represents the CG while the PZ corresponds to the green contour. (b) T2-W-MRI slice of a prostate with a CaP highlighted in the PZ using a 3 T MRI scanner without an endorectal coil. (c) T2-W-MRI slice of a prostate with a CaP highlighted in the CG using a 1.5 T MRI scanner with an endorectal coil.

CaP aggressiveness has been shown to be inversely correlated with SI. Indeed, CaPs assessed with a GS of 4–5 implied lower SI than the one with a GS of 2–3 [63].

In spite of the availability of these useful and encouraging features, the T2-W modality lacks reliability [29,64]. Sensitivity is affected by the difficulties in detecting cancers in CG [64] while specificity rate is highly affected by outliers [30]. In fact, various conditions emulate patterns of CaP, such as BPH, post-biopsy hemorrhage, atrophy, scars, and post-treatment [4,30,59,65,66]. These issues are partly addressed using more innovative and advanced modalities.

T2 MAP

As previously mentioned, T2-W-MRI modality shows low sensitivity. Moreover, T2-W-MRI images are a composite of multiple effects [55]. However, T2 values alone have been shown to be more discriminative [67] and highly correlated with citrate concentration, a biological marker in CaP [68,69]. T2 values are computed using the characteristics of transverse relaxation which is formalized as follows in Equation 10.1:

$$M_{xy}(t) = M_{xy}(0) \exp\left(-\frac{t}{T_2}\right), \tag{10.1}$$

where $M_{xy}(0)$ is the initial value of $M_{xy}(t)$ and T2 is the relaxation time.

By rearranging Equation 10.1, the T2 map is computed by performing a linear fitting on the model presented in Equation 10.2 using several TE, $t = \{TE_1, TE_2, \ldots, TE_m\}$.

$$\ln\left[\frac{M_{xy}(t)}{M_{xy}(0)}\right] = -\frac{t}{T_2}. \tag{10.2}$$

The Fast Spin-Echo (FSE) sequence has been shown to be particularly well suited in order to build a T2 map and obtain accurate T2 values [70]. Similar to T2-W-MRI, T2 values associated with CaP are significantly lower than those of healthy tissues [68,71].

DCE-MRI

DCE-MRI is an imaging technique that exploits the vascularity characteristic of tissues. Contrast media, usually gadolinium-based, is injected intravenously into the patient. The media extravasates from vessels to extravascular-extracellular space (EES) and is released back into the vasculature before being eliminated by the kidneys [72]. Furthermore, the diffusion speed of the contrast agent may vary due to several parameters: the permeability of the micro-vessels, their surface area, and the blood flow [73].

Healthy PZ is mainly made up of glandular tissue, around 70% [74], which implies a reduced interstitial space restricting exchanges between vessels and EES [75,76]. Normal CG has a more disorganized structure, composed of mainly fibrous tissue [29,74], which facilitates the arrival of the contrast agent in EES [77]. To understand the difference between contrast media kinetic in malignant tumors and the two previous behaviors mentioned, one has to focus on the process known as angiogenesis [78]. In order to ensure growth, malignant tumors produce and release angiogenic promoter substances [78]. These molecules stimulate the creation of new vessels toward the tumor [78]. However, the new vessel networks in tumors differ from those present in healthy tissue [72]. They are more porous due to the larger number of "openings" in their capillary walls [72,74]. In contrast to healthy cases, this increased vascular permeability results in increased contrast agent exchanges between vessels and EES [79].

By making use of the previous aspects, DCE-MRI is based on an acquisition of a set of T1-W-MRI images over time. The gadolinium-based contrast agent shortens T1 relaxation time enhancing contrast in T1-W-MRI images. The aim is to post-analyze the pharmacokinetic behavior of the contrast media concentration in prostate tissues [79]. The image analysis is carried out in two dimensions: (i) in the spatial domain on a pixel-by-pixel basis and (ii) in the time domain corresponding to the consecutive images acquired with the MRI. Thus, for each spatial location, a signal linked to contrast media concentration is measured as shown in Figure 10.2b [80].

By taking the above remarks into account, CaPs is characterized by a signal having an earlier and faster enhancement and an earlier washout—that is, the rate of the contrast agent flowing out of the tissue—as shown in Figure 10.2b [79]. Three different approaches exist to analyze these signals with the aim of labeling them as corresponding to either normal or malignant tissues.

Qualitative analysis is based on a qualitative assessment of the signal shape [29]. Quantitative approaches consist of inferring pharmocokinetic parameter values [80]. Those parameters are part of mathematical-pharmacokinetic models that are directly based on physiological exchanges

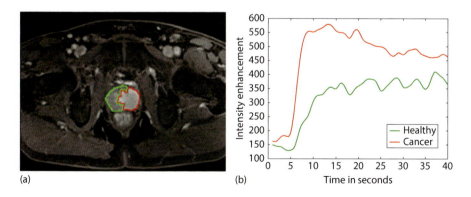

(a)   (b)

FIGURE 10.2   Illustration of typical enhancement signal observed in DCE-MRI analysis collected with a 3 T MRI scanner. (a) T1-W-MRI image where the cancer is delimited by the red contour. The green area was still not invaded by the CaP. (b) Enhancement curve computed during the DCE-MRI analysis. The red curve is typical from CaP cancer while the green curve is characteristic of healthy tissue.

between vessels and EES. Several pharmacokinetic models have been proposed such as the Kety model [81], the Tofts model [82], and mixed models [83,84]. The last family of methods mixes both approaches, grouped together under the heading of semi-quantitative methods. They rely on shape characterization using mathematical modeling to extract a set of parameters such as wash-in gradient, washout, integral under the curve, maximum signal intensity, time-to-peak enhancement, and start of enhancement [29,79]. These parameters are depicted in Figure 10.16. It has been shown that semi-quantitative and quantitative methods improve localization of CaP when compared with qualitative methods [85]. the section titled "CADx: Feature Detection" provides a full description of quantitative and semi-quantitative approaches.

DCE-MRI combined with T2-W-MRI has shown to enhance sensitivity compared to T2-W-MRI alone [86–89]. Despite this fact, DCE-MRI possesses some drawbacks. Due to its "dynamic" nature, patient motions during the image acquisition lead to spatial mis-registration of the image set [79]. Furthermore, it has been suggested that malignant tumors are difficult to distinguish from prostatitis located in PZ and BPH located in CG [29,79]. These pairs of tissues tend to have similar appearances. Later studies have shown that CaPs in CG do not always manifest in homogeneous fashion. Indeed, tumors in this zone can present both hypo-vascularization and hyper-vascularization which illustrates the challenge of CaP detection in CG [77].

DW-MRI

As previously mentioned in the introduction, DW-MRI is the most recent MRI imaging technique aiming at CaP detection and diagnosis [59]. This modality exploits the variations in the motion of water molecules in different tissues [90,91].

The distinction between healthy and CaP in DW-MRI rests on the following physiological bases. On the one hand, PZ, as previously mentioned, is mainly a glandular and tubular structure allowing water molecules to move freely [29,74]. On the other hand, CG is made up of muscular or fibrous tissue causing the motion of the water molecules to be more constrained and heterogeneous than in PZ [29]. Then, CaP growth leads to the destruction of normal glandular structure and is associated with an increase in cellular density [29,91,92]. Furthermore, these factors both have been shown to be inversely correlated with water diffusion [91,92]: higher cellular density implies a restricted water diffusion. Thus, water diffusion in CaP will be more restricted than both healthy PZ and CG [29,91].

From the NMR principle side, DW-MRI sequence produces contrasted images due to variation of water molecules' motion. The method is based on the fact that the signal in DW-MRI images is inversely correlated to the degree of random motion of water molecules [93]. In fact, gradients are used in DW-MRI modality to encode spatial location of nuclei temporarily. Simplifying the problem in only one direction, a gradient is applied in that direction, dephasing the spins of water nuclei. Hence, the spin phases vary along the gradient direction depending of the gradient intensity at those locations. Then, a second gradient is applied aiming at canceling the spin dephasing. Thus, the immobile water molecules will be subject to the same gradient intensity as the initial one, while moving water molecules will be subject to a different gradient intensity. Thus, spins of moving water molecules will stay dephased, whereas spins of immobile water molecules will come back in phase. As a consequence, a higher degree of random motion results in a more significant signal loss, whereas a lower degree of random motion is synonymous with lower signal loss [93]. Under these conditions, the MRI signal is measured as follows:

$$M_{x,y}(t, b) = M_{x,y}(0)\exp\left(-\frac{t}{T_2}\right)S_{\text{ADC}}(b),$$

(10.3)

$$S_{\text{ADC}}(b) = \exp(-b \times \text{ADC}),$$

(10.4)

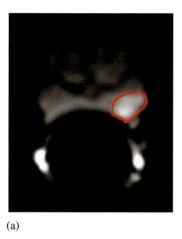

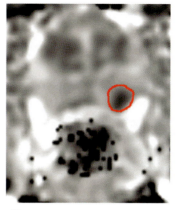

(a)   (b)

FIGURE 10.3 Illustration of DW-MRI and ADC map. The signal intensity corresponding to cancer are inversely correlated on these modalities. (a) DW-MRI image acquired with a 1.5 T MRI scanner. The cancer corresponds to the high-SI region highlighted in red. (b) ADC map computer after acquisition of DW-MRI images with 1.5 T MRI scanner. The cancer corresponds to the low-SI region highlighted in red.

where S_{ADC} refers to signal drop due to diffusion effect, ADC is the apparent diffusion coefficient, and b is the attenuation coefficient depending only on of the gradient intensity and the gradient duration [94].

By using this formulation, image acquisition with a parameter b equal to $0\,s\,mm^{-2}$ corresponds to a T2-W-MRI acquisition. Then, increasing the attenuation coefficient b—that is, increase gradient intensity and duration—enhances the contrast in DW-MRI images.

To summarize, in DW-MRI, CaPs are characterized by high SI compared to normal tissues in PZ and CG as shown in Figure 10.3a [30]. However, some tissues in CG looks similar to CaP with higher SI [30].

Diagnosis using DW-MRI combined with T2-W-MRI has shown a significant improvement compared with T2-W-MRI alone and provides highly contrasted images [74,95,96]. As drawbacks, this modality suffers from poor spatial resolution and specificity due to false positive detection [74]. With a view to eliminate these drawbacks, radiologists use quantitative maps extracted from DW-MRI, which is presented in the next section.

ADC MAP

The NMR signal measured for DW-MRI images is not only affected by diffusion as shown in Equation 10.3. However, the signal drop—Equation 10.4—is formulated such that the only variable is the acquisition parameter b [94]. The ADC is considered a "pure" diffusion coefficient and is extracted to build a quantitative map known as the ADC map. From Equation 10.3, it is clear that performing multiple acquisitions only varying b will not have any effect on the term $M_{x,y}(0)\exp(-\frac{t}{T_2})$. Thus, Equation 10.3 can be rewritten as follows:

$$S(b) = S_0 \exp(-b \times ADC). \tag{10.5}$$

To compute the ADC map, a minimum of two acquisitions are necessary: (i) for b equal to $0\,s\,mm^{-2}$, where the measured signal is equal to S_0; and (ii) b_1 greater than $0\,s\,mm^{-2}$, typically $1000\,s\,mm^{-2}$. Then, the ADC map can be computed as:

$$ADC = -\frac{\ln\left(\frac{S(b_1)}{S_0}\right)}{b_1}. \tag{10.6}$$

More accurate ADC maps are computed by acquiring a set of images with different values for the parameter b and fitting linearly a semi-logarithm function using the model presented in Equation 10.5.

Regarding the appearance of the ADC maps, it has been previously stated that by increasing the value of b, the signal of CaP tissue increases significantly. Considering Eq. (6), the tissue appearance in the ADC map is the inverse of DW-MRI images. Then, CaP tissue is associated with low SI, whereas healthy tissue appears brighter as depicted in Figure 10.3b [30].

Similar to the gain achieved by DW-MRI, diagnosis using ADC map combined with T2-W-MRI significantly outperforms T2-W-MRI alone [74,97]. Moreover, it has been shown that ADC coefficient is correlated with GS [98–100].

However, some tissues of the CG mimic CaP with low-SI [64] and image distortion can arise due to hemorrhage [74]. It has also been noted that a high variability of the ADC occurs between different patients making it difficult to define a static threshold to distinguish CaP from nonmalignant tumors [74].

Magnetic Resonance Spectroscopy Imaging (MRSI)

CaP induces metabolic changes in the prostate compared with healthy tissue. Thus, CaP detection can be carried out by tracking changes of metabolite concentration in prostate tissue. MRSI is an NMR-based technique that generates spectra of relative metabolite concentration in a region of interest (ROI).

In order to track changes of metabolite concentration, it is important to know which metabolites are associated with CaP. To address this question, clinical studies identified three biological markers: (i) citrate, (ii) choline, and (iii) polyamines composed mainly of spermine, and in less abundance of spermidine and putrescine [101–103].

Citrate is involved in the production and secretion of the prostatic fluid, and the glandular prostate cells are associated with a high production of citrate enabled by zinc accumulation by these same cells [102]. However, the metabolism allowing the accumulation of citrate requires a large amount of energy [102]. In contrast, malignant cells do not have high zinc levels leading to lower citrate levels due to citrate oxidization [102]. Furthermore, this change results in a more energy-efficient metabolism enabling malignant cells to grow and spread [102].

An increased concentration of choline is related to CaP [101]. Malignant cell development requires epigenetic mechanisms resulting in metabolic changes and relies on two mechanisms: deoxyribonucleic acid (DNA) methylation and phospholid metabolism, which both result in choline uptake, explaining its increased level in CaP tissue [101]. Spermine is also considered as a biological marker in CaP [103,104]. In CaP, reduction of the ductal volume due to shifts in polyamine homeostasis might lead to a reduced spermine concentration [104].

To determine the concentration of these biological markers, one has to focus on the MRSI modality. In theory, in presence of a homogeneous magnetic field, identical nuclei precesses at the same operating frequency known as the Lamor frequency [105]. However, MRSI is based on the fact that identical nuclei will slightly precess at different frequencies depending on the chemical environment in which they are immersed [105], a phenomenon known as the chemical shift effect (CSE) [2]. Given this property, metabolites are identified and their concentrations are determined. In this regard, the Fourier transform is used to obtain the frequency spectrum of the NMR signal [2,105]. In this spectrum, each peak is associated with a particular metabolite and the area under each peak corresponds to the relative concentration of this metabolite, as illustrated in Figure 10.4 [2].

Two different quantitative approaches are used to decide whether or not the spectra of a ROI is associated with CaP: (i) relative quantification or (ii) absolute quantification [106]. In relative quantification, the ratio of choline-polyamines-creatine to citrate is computed. The integral of the

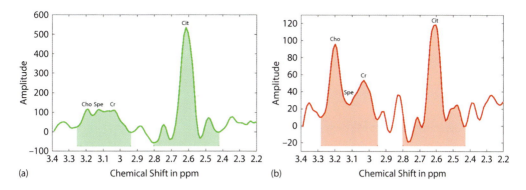

FIGURE 10.4 Illustration of an MRSI spectrum for both healthy and cancerous voxels with a 3 T MRI. The highlighted areas correspond to the related concentration of the metabolites which is computed by integrating the area under each peak. Acronyms: choline (Cho), spermine (Spe), creatine (Cr), and citrate (Cit). (a) Illustration of an MRSI spectrum of a healthy voxel acquired with a 3 T MRI. (b) Illustration of an MRSI spectrum of a cancerous voxel acquired with a 3 T MRI.

signal is computed from choline to creatine—that is, from 3.21 to 3.02 ppm—because the peaks in this region can be merged at clinical magnetic field strengths [29,104], as depicted in Figure 10.4. Considering the previous assumptions that choline concentration rises and citrate concentration decreases in the presence of CaP, the ratio computed should be higher in malignant tissue than in healthy tissue.

In contrast with relative quantification, absolute quantification measures molar concentrations by normalizing relative concentrations using water as reference [106]. In this case, "true" concentrations are directly used to differentiate malignant from healthy tissue. However, this method is not commonly used as it requires an additional step of acquiring water signals, inducing time and cost acquisition constraints.

MRSI allows examination with high specificity and sensitivity compared to other MRI modalities [74]. Furthermore, it has been shown that combining MRSI with MRI improves detection and diagnosis performance [107–109]. Citrate and spermine concentrations are inversely correlated with the GS, allowing us to distinguish low- from high-grade CaPs [103]. However, choline concentration does not provide the same properties [103].

Unfortunately, MRSI also presents several drawbacks. First, MRSI acquisition is time consuming which prevents this modality from being used in daily clinical practice [30]. In addition, MRSI suffers from low spatial resolution due to the fact that signal-to-noise (SNR) is linked to the voxel size. However, this issue is addressed by developing new scanners with higher magnetic field strengths such as 7.5 T [103]. Finally, a high variability of the relative concentrations between patients has been observed [74]. The same observation has been made depending on the zones studied (i.e., PZ, CG, base, mid-gland, apex) [106,110]. Due to this variability, it is difficult to use a fixed threshold to differentiate CaP from healthy tissue.

SUMMARY AND CONCLUSIONS

Table 10.1 provides an overview of the different modalities presented in the previous section. Indeed, each MRI modality alone provides a different discriminative level to distinguish CaP from healthy tissue. However, a recurrent theme in the literature is that the ability to combine these MRI modalities would lead to the best diagnosis performance. In this regard, we will present in the next section automatic tools which have been developed to design mpMRI CAD systems for the detection of CaP.

TABLE 10.1

Overview of the Features Associated with Each MRI Modality Used for Medical Diagnosis by Radiologists

Modality	Significant Features	CaP	Healthy Tissue	GS Correlation
T2-W-MRI	SI	Low SI in PZ [4]	Intermediate to high SI in PZ [4]	+ [63]
	Shape	Round or ill-defined mass in PZ [56]		0
	SI	Low SI in CG [30,62]	Low SI in CG [30,62]	0
	Shape	Homogeneous mass with ill-defined edges in CG [30,62]		0
T2 map	SI	Low SI [68,71]	Intermediate to high SI [68,71]	+ [67–69]
DCE MRI	Semi-quantitative features [79]:			
	• Wash-in	Faster	Slower	0
	• Washout	Faster	Slower	0
	• Integral under the curve	Higher	Lower	0
	• Maximum signal intensity	Higher	Lower	0
	• Time-to-peak enhancement	Faster	Slower	0
	Quantitative features (Tofts parameters [80]):			
	• k_{ep}	Higher	Lower	0
	• K^{trans}	Higher	lower	0
DW-MRI	SI	Higher SI [30,93]	Lower SI [30,93]	+
ADC map	SI	Low SI [30]	High SI [30]	+ [98–100]
MRSI	Metabolites:			
	• Citrate (2.64 ppm) [111]	Lower concentration [101,102,104]	Higher concentration [101,102,104]	+ [103]
	• Choline (3.21 ppm) [111]	Higher concentration [101,102,104]	Lower concentration [101,102,104]	0 [103]
	• Spermine (3.11 ppm) [111]	Lower concentration [101,102,104]	Higher concentration [101,102,104]	+ [103]

Notes: +: significantly correlated; 0: no correlation.
Abbreviations: Prostate cancer (PCa); signal intensity (SI); Gleason score (GS).

REVIEW OF CAD SYSTEMS FOR CaP

As previously mentioned, CADs are developed to advise and back up radiologists in their tasks of CaP detection and diagnosis, but not to provide fully automatic decisions [49]. CADs can be divided into two different subgroups: either as CADe, with the purpose to highlight probable lesions in MRI images, or CADx, which focuses on differentiating malignant from nonmalignant tumors [49]. Moreover, an intuitive approach, motivated by developing a framework combining detection and diagnosis, is to mix both CADe and CADx by using the output of the former as a input of the latter. Although the outcomes of these two systems should differ, the framework of both CAD systems is similar. A general CAD work-flow is presented in Figure 10.5.

MRI modalities mentioned in the section "MRI Techniques" are used as inputs of CAD for CaP. These images acquired from the different modalities show a large variability between patients: the prostate organ can be located at different positions in images—due to patient motion, variation of acquisition plan—and the SI can be corrupted with noise or artifacts during the acquisition process

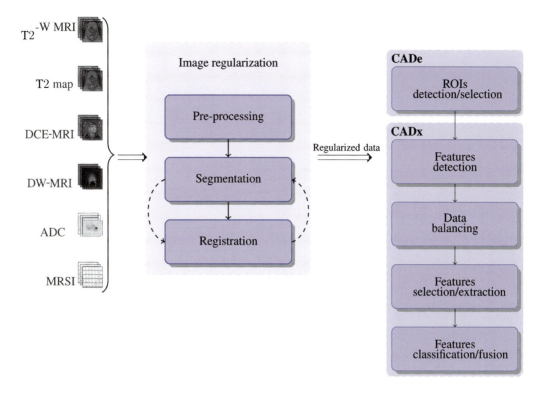

FIGURE 10.5 Common CAD framework based on MRI images used to detect CaP.

caused by the magnetic field non-homogeneity or the use of an endorectal coil. To address these issues, the first stage of CAD is to pre-process mpMRI images to reduce noise, remove artifacts, and standardize the SI. Subsequently, most of the later processes focus only on the prostate organ; therefore it is necessary to segment the prostate in each MRI modality to define it as a ROI. However, data may suffer from misalignment due to patient motions or different acquisition parameters. Therefore, a registration step is usually performed so that all the previously segmented MRI images are in the same reference frame. Registration and segmentation can be swapped depending on the strategy chosen.

Some studies do not fully apply the methodology depicted in Figure 10.5. Details about those can be found in Table 10.2. Some studies bypass the pre-processing stages to proof the robustness of their approaches to noise or other artifacts, by using directly the raw data as inputs of their CAD systems. In some cases, prostate segmentation is performed manually as well as registration. Sometimes, it is also assumed that no patient motions occur during the acquisition, removing the need of registering the mpMRI images.

Once the data are regularized, it becomes possible to extract features and classify the data to obtain the location of possible lesions (i.e., CADe) or/and the malignancy nature of these lesions (i.e., CADx).

In a CADe framework, *possible lesions are segmented automatically* and further used as input of a CADx. Nevertheless, some works also used a fusion of CADe-CADx framework in which voxel-based features are directly used, and in which the location of the malignant lesions are obtained as results. On the other hand, manual lesions segmentation is not considered to be part of CADe.

CADx is composed of the processes that allow *malignant tumors to be distinguished from nonmalignant tumors*. Here, CaP malignancy is defined using the grade of the GS determined after biopsy or prostatectomy. As presented in Figure 10.5, CADx is usually composed of the three common steps used in a classification framework: (i) features detection, (ii) feature extraction/selection, and (iii) feature classification.

TABLE 10.2

Overview of the Different Studies Reviewed with Their Main Characteristics

Index	Study	# Cases	MRI Modality				Strength of Field		Studied Zones		CAD Stages		
			T2-W	DCE	DW	MRSI	1.5 T	3 T	PZ	CG	Reg.	CADe	CADx
[112,113]	Ampeliotis et al.	25	✓	✓	✗	✗	✓	✗	✓	✗	✓	✗	✓
[114]	Antic et al.	53	✓	✗	✓	✗	✓	✗	✓	✓	✗	✗	✓
[115]	Artan et al.	10	✓	✓	✓	✗	✓	✗	✓	✗	✗	✓	✓
[116]	Artan et al.	21	✓	✓	✓	✗	✓	✗	✓	✗	✓	✓	✓
[117,118]	Cameron et al.	5/13	✓	✗	✓	✗	✗	✓	✓	✗	✗	✓	✓
[119]	Chan et al.	15	✓	✗	✓	✗	✓	✗	✓	✓	✗	✗	✓
[120]	Chung et al.	20	✓	✗	✓	✗	✗	✓	✓	✓	✗	✓	✓
[121,122]	Giannini et al.	10/56	✓	✓	✓	✓	✓	✗	✓	✗	✓	✓	✓
[123]	Kelm et al.	24	✓	✗	✓	✗	✓	✓	✓	✓	✓	✓	✓
[124]	Khalvati et al.	20	✓	✗	✓	✗	✗	✗	✓	✗	✗	✓	✓
[125]	Langer et al.	25	✓	✓	✓	✗	✓	✗	✓	✗	✓	✗	✓
[126]	Lehaire et al.	35	✓	✓	✓	✗	✓	✗	✓	✗	✓	✓	✓
[127]	Lemaitre	17	✓	✓	✓	✓	✗	✓	✓	✓	✓	✓	✓
[128]	Litjens et al.	188	✓	✓	✓	✗	✗	✓	✓	✗	✓	✓	✓
[129]	Litjens et al.	288	✓	✓	✓	✗	✓	✓	✓	✓	✓	✓	✓
[130]	Litjens et al.	347	✓	✓	✗	✗	✓	✗	✓	✓	✓	✓	✓
[131]	Liu et al.	11	✓	✓	✓	✗	✗	✓	✓	✗	✓	✗	✓
[132]	Liu et al.	54	✓	✗	✗	✗	✓	✓	✓	✓	✓	✓	✓
[133]	Lopes et al.	27	✓	✗	✗	✗	✓	✗	✓	✗	✓	✓	✓
[134]	Lv et al.	55	✓	✗	✗	✗	✓	✓	✓	✓	✓	✗	✓
[135]	Matulewicz et al.	18	✗	✗	✗	✓	✗	✗	✓	✗	✗	✓	✓
[136]	Mazzetti et al.	10	✗	✓	✓	✗	✓	✗	✓	✗	✓	✓	✓
[137,138]	Niaf et al.	23/30	✓	✓	✓	✗	✓	✗	✓	✗	✓	✗	✓
[139,140]	Ozer et al.	20	✓	✓	✓	✗	✓	✗	✓	✓	✓	✓	✓
[141]	Parfait et al.	22	✗	✗	✗	✓	✗	✓	✓	✓	✓	✓	✓
[100]	Peng et al.	48	✓	✓	✓	✗	✗	✓	✓	✓	✗	✗	✓

(Continued)

TABLE 10.2 (Continued)
Overview of the Different Studies Reviewed with Their Main Characteristics

Index	Study	# Cases	MRI Modality				Strength of Field		Studied Zones		CAD Stages		
			T2-W	DCE	DW	MRSI	1.5 T	3 T	PZ	CG	Reg.	CADe	CADx
[142]	Puech et al.	100	✗	✓	✗	✗	✓	✗	✓	✓	✗	✗	✓
[143,144]	Rampun et al.	45	✓	✗	✗	✗	✓	✗	✓	✗	✗	✗	✓
[143,145,146]	Rampun et al.	45	✓	✗	✗	✗	✓	✗	✓	✗	✓'	✓	✓
[147]	Samarasinghe et al.	40	✗	✓	✗	✗	✗	✓	✓	✗	✓'	✗	✓
[148]	Sung et al.	42	✗	✓	✗	✓	✗	✓	✓	✓	✗	✓	✓
[149]	Tiwari et al.	14	✗	✗	✗	✓	✓	❖	✗	✓	✓'	✓	✓
[150]	Tiwari et al.	18	✗	✗	✗	✓	✓	✗	✓	✓	✓'	✓	✓
[151]	Tiwari et al.	18	✗	✗	✗	✓	✓	✗	✓	✓	✓'	✓	✓
[152]	Tiwari et al.	15	✓	✗	✗	✓	✓	✗	✓	✓	✓'	✓	✓
[153]	Tiwari et al.	19	✓	✗	✗	✓	✓	✗	✓	✓	✗	✓	✓
[154]	Tiwari et al.	36	✓	✗	✗	✓	✓	✗	✓	✓	✓'	✓	✓
[155]	Tiwari et al.	29	✓	✗	✗	✓	✓	✓	✓	✓	✓'	✓	✓
[156,157]	Trigui et al.	34	✓	✓	✓	✓	✗	✓	✓	✓	✓'	✓	✓
[158]	Viswanath et al.	16	✓	✗	✗	✓	✓	✗	✓	✓	✗	✓	✓
[159]	Viswanath et al.	6	✓	✓	✗	✗	✗	✓	✓	✓	✓'	✓	✓
[160]	Viswanath et al.	6	✓	✓	✗	✗	✗	✗	✗	✗	✓'	✗	✗
[161]	Viswanath et al.	12	✓	✓	✓	✗	✗	✓	✓	✓	✓'	✓	✓
[162]	Viswanath et al.	22	✓	✗	✗	✗	✗	✓	✓	✓	✓'	✓	✓
[163]	Vos et al.	29	✓	✓	✗	✗	✓	✗	✓	✗	✓'	✗	✓
[164]	Vos et al.	29	✗	✓	✗	✗	✓	✗	✓	✗	✓'	✗	✓
[165]	Vos et al.	29	✓	✓	✗	✗	✓	✗	✓	✗	✓'	✗	✓
[166]	Vos et al.	NA	✓	✓	✓	✗	✗	✓	✓	✗	✓'	✓	✓

Notes: ✗: not used or not implemented; ✓': partially implemented; ✓: used or implemented.
Acronyms: Number (#); image regularization (Reg.).

This chapter is organized using the methodology presented in Figure 10.5. Methods embedded in the image regularization framework are presented initially to subsequently focus on the image classification framework, being divided into CADe and CADx. Finally, we present a summary of the results reported in the state-of-the-art as well as a discussion that follows. Table 10.2 summarizes the 56 different CAD studies reviewed in this section. The first set of information reported is linked to the data acquisition such as the number of patients included in the study, the modalities acquired as well as the strength of the field of the scanner used. Subsequently, information about the prostate zones considered in the CAD analysis—that is, PZ or CG—are reported since detecting CaP in the CG is a more challenging problem and has received particular attention only in the recent publications.

The papers have been selected by investigating referenced international peer-reviewed journals as well as international peer-reviewed conferences. Additionally, a breadth-search (or snowball sampling) was first used to refine missing publications. Only studies proposing CAD systems specifically for CaP have been reviewed.

PRE-PROCESSING

Three different groups of pre-processing methods are commonly applied to images as initial stage in CADs for CaP. These methods are explained for both MRI and MRSI modalities.

MRI Modalities

Noise Filtering

The NMR signal, measured and acquired in the k-space, is affected by noise. This noise obeys a complex Gaussian white noise mainly due to thermal noises in the patient [167]. Furthermore, MRI images visualized by radiologists are in fact the magnitude images resulting from the complex Fourier transform of the k-space data. The complex Fourier transform does not affect the Gaussian noise characteristics since this is a linear and orthogonal transform [167]. However, the calculation of the magnitude is a nonlinear transform—that is, the square root of the sum of squares of the real and imaginary parts—implying that the noise distribution is no longer Gaussian; it indeed follows a Rician distribution making the de-noising task more challenging. Briefly, a Rician distribution is characterized as follows: in a low-SI region (low SNR), it can be approximated with a Rayleigh distribution, while in a high-SI region (high SNR), it is similar to a Gaussian distribution [168]. Refer to Figure 10.6 to observe the difference between a Gaussian and a Rayleigh distribution. Comprehensive reviews regarding denoising methods can be found in [169,170].

Median filtering is the simplest approach used to address the de-noising issue in MRI images [139,140]. In both studies, Ozer et al. [139,140] used a square-shaped kernel of size 5×5 px.

More recently, Rampun et al. used a combination of median and anisotropic diffusion filter [143–146], proposed in [171]. In low-SNR images, the gradients generated by an edge and noise can be similar, making the de-noising by diffusion more challenging. In this condition, the threshold allowing to locally differentiate a noise gradient from an edge gradient needs to be increased, at the cost of blurring edges after filtering. Therefore, Ling and Bovik [171] proposed to apply a standard anisotropic diffusion filter with a low threshold followed by a median filtering to remove spikes.

Samarasinghe et al. filtered DCE-MRI images with a sliding 3D Gaussian filter [147]. However, from a theoretical point of view, this simple filtering method is not well formalized to address the noise distribution in MRI images. That is why more complex approaches have been proposed to overcome this problem. Another common method used to de-noise MRI images is based on wavelet decomposition and shrinkage. This filtering exploits the sparsity property of the wavelet decomposition. The projection of a noisy signal from the spatial domain to the wavelet domain implies that only few wavelet coefficients contribute to the "signal-free noise," while all wavelet coefficients contribute to the noise [172]. Therefore, insignificant wavelet coefficients are thresholded/attenuated to enforce the sparsity in the wavelet domain, which results to a de-noising process in the spatial

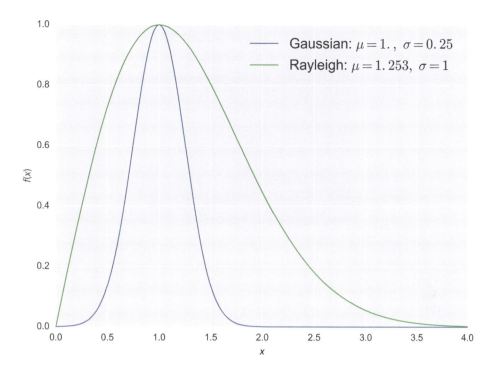

FIGURE 10.6 Illustration of a Gaussian and Rayleigh distribution. Although the mode of these distributions are identical, it can be noted that the Rayleigh distribution ($\mu = 1.253$) is suffering of a bias term when compared with the Gaussian distribution ($\mu = 1$).

domain. Investigations focus on the strategies to perform the most adequate coefficient shrinkage (e.g., thresholding, singularity property, or Bayesian framework) [173]. Ampeliotis et al. de-noised the magnitude MRI images [112,113]—that is, T2-W-MRI and DCE-MRI—by wavelet shrinkage, using thresholding techniques [174]. However, since the wavelet transform is an orthogonal transform, the Rician distribution of the noise is preserved in the wavelet domain. Hence, for low-SNR, the wavelet and scaling coefficients still suffer from a bias due to this specific noise distribution [167]. That is why, Lopes et al. filtered T2-W-MRI images [133], using the method proposed in [175] based on joint detection and estimation theory. In this approach, the wavelet coefficients "free of noise" are estimated from the noisy wavelet coefficients using a maximum a posteriori (MAP) estimate. Furthermore, the designed estimator takes spatial context into account by including both local and global information in the prior probabilities. The different probabilities needed by the MAP are empirically estimated by using mask images, representing the locations of the significant wavelet coefficients. These mask images are computed by thresholding the detail images obtained from the wavelet decomposition. To remove the bias from the wavelet and scaling coefficients, the squared magnitude MRI image is computed instead of the magnitude MRI image as proposed in [167]. This involves changing the Rician distribution to a scaled non-central Chi-squared distribution. It implies that the wavelet coefficients are also unbiased estimators and the scaling coefficients are unbiased estimators but up to a constant C as defined in Equation 10.7 which needs to be subtracted from each scaling coefficient such as:

$$C = 2^{(J+1)}\hat{\sigma}^2, \tag{10.7}$$

where J is the number of levels of the wavelet decomposition and $\hat{\sigma}$ is an estimate of the noise standard deviation.

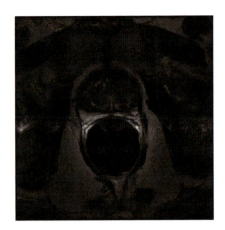

FIGURE 10.7   Example of artifacts with high SI due to perturbation from the endorectal coil which create non-homogeneity.

Bias Correction

Besides being corrupted by noise, MRI images are also affected by the inhomogeneity of the MRI field commonly referred to as bias field [176]. This bias field results in a smooth variation of the SI through the image. When an endorectal coil is used, a resulting artifact of an hyperintense signal is observed around the coil as depicted in Figure 10.7. As a consequence, the SI of identical tissues varies depending on their spatial location in the image making further processes such as segmentation, registration, or classification more challenging [177,178]. A comprehensive review of bias correction methods is proposed in Vovk et al. [178].

The model of image formation is usually formalized as follows:

$$s(\mathbf{x}) = o(\mathbf{x})b(\mathbf{x}) + \eta(\mathbf{x}), \tag{10.8}$$

where $s(\mathbf{x})$ is the corrupted SI at the pixel for the image coordinates $\mathbf{x} = \{x, y\}$, $o(\mathbf{x})$ is the "noise-free signal," $b(\mathbf{x})$ is the bias field function, and $\eta(\mathbf{x})$ is an additive white Gaussian noise. Hence, the task of bias correction involves estimating the bias function $b(\mathbf{x})$ in order to infer the "signal-free bias" $o(\mathbf{x})$.

Viswanath et al. corrected this artifact on T2-W-MRI images [160], using the model proposed in [176], in which Styner et al. model the bias field function by using a linear combination of Legendre polynomials f_i as:

$$\hat{b}(\mathbf{x}, \mathbf{p}) = \sum_{i=0}^{m-1} p_i f_i(\mathbf{x})$$

$$= \sum_{i=0}^{l}\sum_{j=0}^{l-i} p_{ij} P_i(x) P_j(y), \tag{10.9}$$

where $\hat{b}(\cdot)$ is the bias estimation with the image coordinates $\mathbf{x} = \{x, y\}$ and the m coefficients of the linear combination $\mathbf{p} = p_{11}, ..., p_{ij}$; m can be defined as $m = (l+1)((l+2)/2)$, where l is the degree of Legendre polynomials chosen; and $P_i(\cdot)$ denotes a Legendre polynomial of degree i.

This family of functions allows the bias function to be modeled as a smooth inhomogeneous function across the image. To estimate the set of parameters $\mathbf{p}$, a cost function is defined which relies on the following assumptions: (i) an image is composed of k regions with a mean μ_k and a variance

σ_k^2 for each particular class, and (ii) each noisy pixel belongs to one of the k regions with its SI value close to the class mean μ_k. Hence, the cost function is defined as follows:

$$C(\mathbf{p}) = \sum_{\mathbf{x}} \prod_{k} \rho_k (s(\mathbf{x}) - \hat{b}(\mathbf{x}, \mathbf{p}) - \mu_k), \tag{10.10}$$

$$\rho_k(x) = \frac{x^2}{x^2 + 3\sigma_k^2}, \tag{10.11}$$

where $\rho_k(\cdot)$ is a M-estimator allowing estimations to be less sensitive to outliers than the usual squared distance [179].

Finally, the parameters $\mathbf{p}$ are estimated by finding the minimum of the cost function $C(\mathbf{p})$, which was optimized using the nonlinear $(1 + 1)$ evolution strategy (ES) optimizer [180].

In a later publication, Viswanath et al. [162] as well as Giannini et al. [122] corrected T2-W-MRI using the well-known N3 algorithm [181] in which Sled et al. infer the bias function using the PDFs of the signal and bias. Taking advantage of the logarithm property, the model in Equation 10.8 becomes additive as expressed in Equation 10.12.

$$\log s(\mathbf{x}) = \log b(\mathbf{x}) + \log \left(o(\mathbf{x}) + \frac{\eta(\mathbf{x})}{b(\mathbf{x})} \right),$$
$$\approx \log b(\mathbf{x}) + \log \hat{o}(\mathbf{x}), \tag{10.12}$$

where $\hat{o}(\mathbf{x})$ is the signal only degraded by noise. Sled et al. show that Equation 10.12 is related to PDFs such that

$$S(s) = B(s) * O(s), \tag{10.13}$$

where $S(\cdot)$, $B(\cdot)$, and $O(\cdot)$ are the PDFs of $s(\cdot)$, $b(\cdot)$, and $o(\cdot)$, respectively.

The corrupted signal s is restored by finding the multiplicative field b which maximizes the frequency content of the distribution O. Sled et al. [181] argued that a brute-force search through all possible fields b and selecting the one which maximizes the high frequency content of O is possible but far too complex. By assimilating the bias field distribution to be a near Gaussian distribution as a priori, it is then possible to infer the distribution O using the Wiener deconvolution given B and S and later to estimate the corresponding smooth field b.

Lv et al. corrected the non-homogeneity in T2-W-MRI images [134] by using the method proposed by Madabhushi et al. [182] to correct the MRI images by detecting the image foreground via generalized scale (g-scale) in an iterative manner and estimating a bias field function based on a second-order polynomial model. First, the background of the MRI image is eliminated by thresholding, in which the threshold value is commonly equal to the mean SI of the considered image. Then, a seeded region growing algorithm is applied in the image foreground, considering every thresholded pixel as a potential seed. However, pixels already assigned to a region are no longer considered as potential seeds. As in seeded region growing algorithm [183], two criteria are taken into account to expand a region. First, the region grows using a connected neighborhood, initially defined by the user. Then, the homogeneity of SI is based on a fuzzy membership function taking into account the absolute difference of two pixel SI. Depending on the membership value—corresponding to a threshold which needs to be defined—the pixel considered is or is not merged to the region. Once this segmentation is performed, the largest region R is used as a mask to select pixels of the original image and the mean SI, μ_R, is computed. The background variation $b(\mathbf{x})$ is estimated as follows:

$$b(\mathbf{x}) = \frac{s(\mathbf{x})}{\mu_R}, \ \forall \mathbf{x} \in R, \tag{10.14}$$

where $s(\mathbf{x})$ is the original MRI image.

Finally, a second-order polynomial $\hat{b}_\Theta(\mathbf{x})$ is fitted in a least-squares sense as in Equation 10.15,

$$\hat{\Theta} = \arg \min_\Theta |b(\mathbf{x}) - \hat{b}_\Theta(\mathbf{x})|^2, \ \forall \mathbf{x} \in R. \tag{10.15}$$

Finally, the whole original MRI image is corrected by dividing it by the estimated bias field function $\hat{b}_\Theta(\mathbf{x})$. The convergence is reached when the number of pixels in the largest region R does not change significantly between two iterations.

SI Normalization/Standardization

As discussed in a later section, segmentation or classification tasks are usually composed of a learning stage using a set of training patients. Hence, one can emphasize the desire to perform automatic diagnosis with a high repeatability or in other words, one would be sure to obtain consistent SI of tissues across patients of the same group—that is, healthy patients versus patients with CaP—for each MRI modality. However, it is a known fact that variability between patients occurs during MRI examinations even when using the same scanner, protocol, or sequence parameters [184]. Hence, the aim of normalization or standardization of the MRI data is to remove the variability between patients and enforce the repeatability of the MRI examinations. These standardization methods are categorized either as statistical-based standardization or organ SI-based standardization.

Artan et al. [115,116], Ozer et al. [139,140], and Rampun et al. [143–146,185] standardized T2-W-MRI, DCE-MRI, and DW-MRI images by computing the *standard score* (also called *z-score*) of the pixels of the PZ as follows:

$$I_s(\mathbf{x}) = \frac{I_r(\mathbf{x}) - \mu_{pz}}{\sigma_{pz}}, \ \forall \mathbf{x} \in \text{PZ}, \tag{10.16}$$

where $I_s(\mathbf{x})$ is the standardized SI with the image coordinates $\mathbf{x} = \{x, y\}$, $I_r(\mathbf{x})$ is the raw SI, μ_{pz} is the mean SI of the PZ, and σ_{pz} is the SI standard deviation in the PZ. This transformation enforces the image PDF to have a zero mean and a unit standard deviation. In a similar way, Liu et al. normalized T2-W-MRI by making use of the median and inter-quartile range for all the pixels [132].

Lemaitre et al. proposed using the a priori that the underlying data distribution follows a Rician distribution instead of a Gaussian distribution [186]. The data are standardized by removing the mean and scaled by dividing by the standard deviation, empirically computed as follows:

$$\mu_r = \sigma \sqrt{\frac{\pi}{2}} L_{1/2}\left(-\frac{v^2}{2\sigma^2}\right), \tag{10.17}$$

$$\sigma_r = 2\sigma^2 + v^2 - \frac{\pi\sigma^2}{2} L_{1/2}^2\left(\frac{-v^2}{2\sigma^2}\right), \tag{10.18}$$

where v and σ are the distance between the reference point and the center of the bivariate distribution and the scale, respectively; and $L_{1/2}$ denotes a Laguerre polynomial.

Lv et al. scaled the SI of T2-W-MRI images using the method proposed by Nyul et al. [187], based on PDF matching [134]. This approach is based on the assumption that MRI images from the same sequence should share the same PDF appearance. Hence, one can approach this issue by transforming and matching the PDFs using some statistical landmarks such as quantiles. Using a training set, these statistical landmarks—such as minimum, 25th percentile, median, 75th percentile, and maximum—are extracted for N training images:

$$\Phi_0 = \{\phi_0^1, \phi_0^2, \cdots, \phi_0^N\},$$

$$\Phi_{25} = \{\phi_{25}^1, \phi_{25}^2, \cdots, \phi_{25}^N\},$$

$$\Phi_{50} = \{\phi_{50}^1, \phi_{50}^2, \cdots, \phi_{50}^N\}, \quad \text{(10.19)}$$

$$\Phi_{75} = \{\phi_{75}^1, \phi_{75}^2, \cdots, \phi_{75}^N\},$$

$$\Phi_{100} = \{\phi_{100}^1, \phi_{100}^2, \cdots, \phi_{100}^N\},$$

where ϕ_{nth}^{ith} is the nth percentile of the ith training image.

Lemaitre et al. extended the use of non-parametric transformation using an elastic transformation instead of a piecewise-linear transformation [186]. They proposed to use a generic method to register functional data based on the square-root slope function (SRSF) representation [188] which transforms the Fisher-Rao metric into the conventional $\mathbb{L}^2$ metric, and thus allows definition of a cost function corresponding to a Euclidean distance between two functions in this new representation.

Then, the mean of each statistical landmarks $\{\bar{\Phi}_0, \bar{\Phi}_{25}, \bar{\Phi}_{50}, \bar{\Phi}_{75}, \bar{\Phi}_{100}\}$ is also calculated. Once this training stage is performed, a piecewise linear transformation $\mathcal{T}(\cdot)$ is computed as in Equation 10.20. For each test image t, this transformation maps each statistical landmark $\varphi_{(\cdot)}{}^t$ of the image t to the pre-learned statistical landmarks $\bar{\Phi}_{(\cdot)}$. An example of such piecewise linear function is depicted in Figure 10.8.

$$\mathcal{T}(s(\mathbf{x})) = \begin{cases} \left\lceil \bar{\Phi}_0 + (s(\mathbf{x}) - \varphi_0^t)\left(\dfrac{\bar{\Phi}_{25} - \bar{\Phi}_0}{\varphi_{25}^t - \varphi_0^t}\right)\right\rceil, & \text{if } \varphi_0^t \le s(\mathbf{x}) < \varphi_{25}^t, \\[3mm] \left\lceil \bar{\Phi}_{25} + (s(\mathbf{x}) - \varphi_{25}^t)\left(\dfrac{\bar{\Phi}_{50} - \bar{\Phi}_{25}}{\varphi_{50}^t - \varphi_{25}^t}\right)\right\rceil, & \text{if } \varphi_{25}^t \le s(\mathbf{x}) < \varphi_{50}^t, \\[3mm] \left\lceil \bar{\Phi}_{50} + (s(\mathbf{x}) - \varphi_{50}^t)\left(\dfrac{\bar{\Phi}_{75} - \bar{\Phi}_{50}}{\varphi_{75}^t - \varphi_{50}^t}\right)\right\rceil, & \text{if } \varphi_{50}^t \le s(\mathbf{x}) < \varphi_{75}^t, \\[3mm] \left\lceil \bar{\Phi}_{75} + (s(\mathbf{x}) - \varphi_{75}^t)\left(\dfrac{\bar{\Phi}_{100} - \bar{\Phi}_{75}}{\varphi_{100}^t - \varphi_{75}^t}\right)\right\rceil, & \text{if } \varphi_{75}^t \le s(\mathbf{x}) \le \varphi_{100}^t, \end{cases} \quad \text{(10.20)}$$

Viswanath et al. used a variant of the piecewise linear normalization presented in Madabhushi et al. [189], to standardize T2-W-MRI images [160–162]. Instead of computing the PDF of an entire image, a pre-segmentation of the foreground is carried out via g-scale which has been discussed in the bias correction section. Once the foreground is detected, the largest region is extracted, and the regular piecewise linear normalization is applied.

The standardization problem can be tackled by normalizing the MRI images using the SI of some known organs present in these images. Niaf et al. and Lehaire et al. normalized T2-W-MRI images by dividing the original SI of the images by the mean SI of the bladder [126,137,138], which is depicted in Figure 10.9a. Giannini et al. also normalized the same modality but using the signal intensity of the obturator muscle [122]. Likewise, Niaf et al. standardized the T1-W-MRI images using the arterial input function (AIF) [137]. They computed the AIF by taking the mean of the SI in the most enhanced part of the common femoral arteries—refer to Figure 10.9b—as proposed in

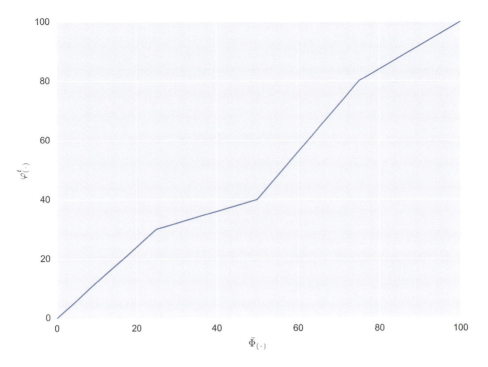

FIGURE 10.8 Example of piecewise linear normalization as proposed by Nyul et al. [187].

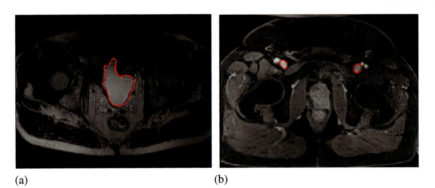

(a)   (b)

FIGURE 10.9 Illustration of the two organs used in Niaf et al. [137,138] to normalize T2-W-MRI and T1-W-MRI images. (a) Illustration and location of the bladder on a T2-W-MRI image acquired with a 3 T MRI scanner. (b) Illustration and location of the femoral arteries on a T1-W-MRI image acquired with a 3 T MRI scanner.

Wiart et al. [190]. Along the same line, Samarasinghe et al. normalized the SI of lesion regions in T1-W-MRI using the mean intensity of the prostate gland in the same modality [147].

MRSI Modality

As presented in the section titled "Clinical Aspects of TRUS Prostate Biopsy," MRSI is a modality related to a one-dimensional signal. Hence, specific pre-processing steps for this type of signal have been applied instead of standard signal processing methods.

Phase Correction

Acquired MRSI spectra suffer from zero-order and first-order phase misalignment [191,192] as depicted in Figure 10.10. Parfait et al. and Trigui et al. used a method proposed by Chen et al. where

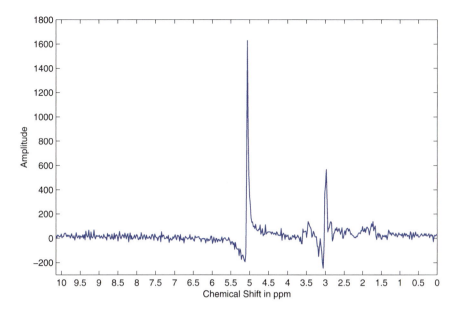

FIGURE 10.10 Illustration of phase misalignment in an MRSI spectra acquired with a 3 T MRSI scanner. Note the distortion of the signal specially visible for the water and citrate peaks visible at 5 and 3 ppm, respectively.

the phase of MRSI signal is corrected based on entropy minimization in the frequency domain [141,156,157]. The corrected MRSI signal $o(\xi)$ can be expressed as follows:

$$\Re(o(\xi)) = \Re(s(\xi))\cos(\Phi(\xi)) - \Im(\xi)\sin(\Phi(\xi)),$$

$$\Im(o(\xi)) = \Im(s(\xi))\cos(\Phi(\xi)) + \Re(\xi)\sin(\Phi(\xi)), \qquad (10.21)$$

$$\Phi(\xi) = \phi_0 + \phi_1\frac{\xi}{N},$$

where $\Re(\cdot)$ and $\Im(\cdot)$ are the real and imaginary part of the complex signal, respectively; $s(\xi)$ is the corrupted MRSI signal; ϕ_0 and ϕ_1 are the zero-order and first-order phase correction terms, respectively; and N is the total number of samples of the MRSI signal.

Chen et al. tackled this problem as an optimization in which ϕ_0 and ϕ_1 have to be inferred. Hence, the simplex Nelder-Mead optimizer [193] is used to minimize the following cost function based on the *Shannon entropy* formulation:

$$\widehat{\Phi} = \arg\min_{\Phi}\left[-\sum\Re(s'(\xi))\ln\Re(s'(\xi)) + \lambda\,\|\,\Re(s(\xi))\,\|_2\right], \qquad (10.22)$$

where $s'(\xi)$ is the first derivative of the corrupted signal $s(\xi)$ and λ is a regularization parameter. Once the best parameter Φ vector is obtained, the MRSI signal is corrected using Equation 10.21.

Water and Lipid Residuals Filtering

The water and lipid metabolites occur in much higher concentrations than the metabolites of interest, namely choline, creatine, and citrate [192,194]. Fortunately, specific MRSI sequences have been developed in order to suppress water and lipid metabolites using pre-saturation techniques [194]. However, these techniques do not perfectly remove water and lipids peaks and some residuals are still present in the MRSI spectra as illustrated in Figure 10.11. Therefore, different post-processing

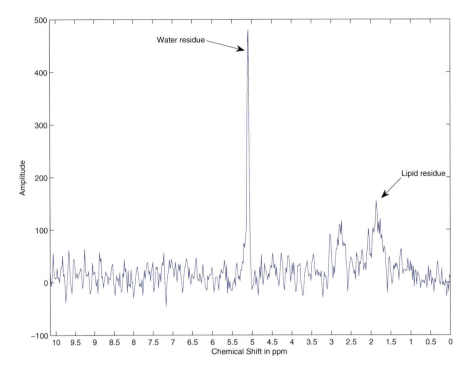

FIGURE 10.11   Illustration of the residues of water and fat even after their suppression during the acquisition protocol. The acquisition has been carried out with a 3 T MRI.

methods have been proposed to enhance the quality of the MRSI spectra by removing these residuals. For instance, Kelm et al. [123] used the HSVD algorithm proposed by Pijnappel et al. [195] which models the MRSI signal by a sum of exponentially damped sine waves in the time domain as in Equation 10.23.

$$s(t) = \sum_{k=1}^{K} a_k \exp(i\phi_k) \exp(-d_k + i2\pi f_k)\, t + \eta(t), \tag{10.23}$$

where a_k is the amplitude proportional to the metabolite concentration with a resonance frequency f_k, d_k represents the damping factor of the exponential, ϕ_k is the first-order phase, and $\eta(t)$ is a complex white noise.

The "noise-free signal" can be found using the singular value decomposition (SVD) decomposition [195]. Therefore, the noisy signal is reorganized inside a Hankel matrix H. It can be shown that the signal is considered "noise-free" if the rank of H is equal to rank K. However, due to the presence of noise, H is in fact a full rank matrix. Thus, to recover the "noise-free signal," the rank of H is truncated to K using its SVD decomposition. Hence, knowing the cut-off frequencies of water—that is, 4.65 ppm—and lipid—that is, 2.2 ppm—metabolites, their corresponding peaks are reconstructed and subtracted from the original signal [196].

Baseline Correction

Sometimes, the problem discussed in the above section regarding the lipid molecules is not addressed simultaneously with water residuals suppression. Lipids and macro-molecules are known to affect the baseline of the MRSI spectra, causing errors while quantifying metabolites, especially the citrate metabolite.

Parfait et al. compared two different methods to detect the baseline and correct the MRSI spectra [141] which are based on Lieber and Mahadevan-Jansen [197] and Devos et al. [198]. Lieber and Mahadevan-Jansen corrected the baseline in the frequency domain by fitting a low-degree polynomial $p(x)$—for example, second or third degree—to the MRSI signal $s(x)$ in a least-squares sense [197]. Then, the values of the fitted polynomial are re-assigned as:

$$p_f(x) = \begin{cases} p(x), & \text{if } p(x) \le s(x), \\ s(x), & \text{if } p(x) > s(x). \end{cases} \qquad (10.24)$$

Finally, this procedure of fitting and re-assignment is repeated on $p_f(x)$ until a stopping criterion is reached. The final polynomial function is subtracted from the original signal $s(x)$ to correct it. Parfait et al. [141] modified this algorithm by convolving a Gaussian kernel to smooth the MRSI signal instead of fitting a polynomial function, keeping the rest of the algorithm identical. Unlike Lieber and Mahadevan-Jansen [197], Devos et al. [198] corrected the baseline in the time domain by multiplying the MRSI signal by a decreasing exponential function as follows:

$$c(t) = \exp(-\beta t), \qquad (10.25)$$

with a typical β value of 0.15. However, Parfait et al. concluded that the method proposed by Lieber and Mahadevan-Jansen [197] outperformed the one by Devos et al. [198]. The later study of Trigui et al. used this conclusion and adopted the same method [156,157].

The previous baseline correction methods do not provide an optimal solution since the iterative low-pass filter enforces the smoothness of the baseline too much. Xi and Rocke proposed a baseline detection derived from a parametric smoothing model [199]. The NMR signal is formalized as a sum of a pure signal, the baseline function, and an additive Gaussian noise such as follows:

$$y_i = b_i + \mu_i e^{n_i} + \varepsilon_i, \qquad (10.26)$$

where y_i is the NMR signal, b_i is the baseline, μ_i is the true signal, and n_i and ε_i are Gaussian noises.

Xi and Rocke proposed to find the baseline function through an iterative optimization by maximizing the following cost function:

$$F(b) = \sum_{i=1}^{N} b_i - \frac{A^* N^4}{\sigma} \sum_{i=1}^{N} (b_{i+1} + b_{i-1} - 2b_i)^2 - \frac{1.25 B^*}{\sigma} \sum_{i=1}^{N} (b_i - \gamma_i)^2 g(b_i - \gamma_i), \qquad (10.27)$$

where $g(b_i - \gamma_i)$ is the Heaviside function; A^* and B^* are the terms controlling the smoothness and negative penalties, respectively; σ is an estimation of the standard deviation of the noise; and N is the total number of points in the MRSI signal.

The standard deviation of the noise σ is estimated as in Xi and Rocke [199], and the A^* and B^* are empirically set to 5×10^{-6} and 100, respectively, for all the MRSI signal. This method was used in the work of Lemaitre [127].

In the contemporary work of Tiwari et al. [154], the authors detected the baseline using a local nonlinear fitting method avoiding regions with significant peaks, which have been detected using an experimentally parametric signal-to-noise ratio set to a value larger than 5 dB.

Frequency Alignment

Due to variations of the experimental conditions, a frequency shift is commonly observed in the MRSI spectra [191,192] as depicted in Figure 10.12. Tiwari et al. [154] corrected this frequency shift by first detecting known metabolite peaks such as choline, creatine, or citrate and minimizing the frequency error between the experimental and theoretical values for each of these peaks [154].

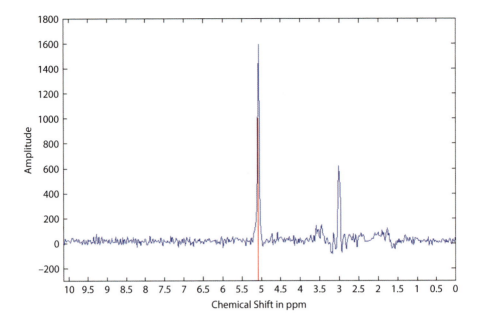

FIGURE 10.12 Illustration of frequency misalignment in a MRSI spectra acquired with a 3 T MRSI scanner. The water peak is known to be aligned at 4.65 ppm. However, it can be seen that the peak on this spectra is aligned at around 5.1 ppm.

Normalization

The NMR spectra is subject to variations due to intra-patient variations and non-homogeneity of the magnetic field. As in Devos et al. [198], Parfait et al. compared two methods to normalize MRSI signal [141]. In each method, the original MRSI spectra is divided by a normalization factor, similar to the intensity normalization described earlier. The first approach consists of estimating the water concentration from an additional MRSI sequence where the water has not been suppressed. The estimation is performed using the previously HSVD algorithm. The second approach does not require any additional acquisition and is based on the L_2 norm of the MRSI spectra $\| s(\xi) \|_2$. It should be noted that both Parfait et al. and Devos et al. concluded that the L_2 normalization is the most efficient method [141]. Lately, Trigui et al. used the L_2 normalization in their framework [156,157].

The different pre-processing methods are summarized in Table 10.3.

SEGMENTATION

The segmentation task consists of delineating the prostate boundaries in the MRI and is of particular importance for focusing the posterior processing on the organ of interest [200]. In this section, only the segmentation methods used in CAD for CaP are presented. An exhaustive review of prostate segmentation methods in MRI is available in Ghose et al. [200].

Manual Segmentation

To highlight the importance of prostate segmentation task in CAD systems, it is interesting to note the large number of studies which manually segment the prostate organs [115,116,126,135,137–140,142,156,157,163,164]. In all the cases, the boundaries of the prostate gland are manually defined in order to limit further processing only to this area. This approach ensures the right delineation of the organ, although it is subjective and prone to rater variability; nevertheless, this procedure is highly time consuming and should be performed by a radiologist.

TABLE 10.3

Overview of the Pre-Processing Methods Used in CAD Systems

Pre-Processing Operations	References
MRI Pre-Processing	
Noise Filtering	
• Anisotropic median-diffusion filtering	[143–146,185]
• Gaussian filtering	[147]
• Median filtering	[139,140]
• Wavelet-based filtering	[112,113,133]
Bias Correction	
• Parametric methods	[122,134,160]
• Nonparametric methods	[161]
Standardization	
• Statistical-based normalization	[115,116,127,134,139,140,143–146,160–162,185]
• Organ SI-based normalization	[126,137,138,147]
MRSI Pre-Processing	
Phase correction	[127,141,156,157]
Water and lipid residuals filtering	[123]
Baseline correction	[127,141,154,156,157]
Frequency alignment	[127,154,156,157]
Normalization	[127,141,156,157]

Region-Based Segmentation

Litjens et al. used a multi-atlas-based segmentation using multimodal images—that is, T2-W-MRI and ADC map—to segment the prostate with an additional pattern recognition method to differentiate CG and PZ [129], as proposed in Litjens et al. [201]. This method consists of three different steps: (i) the registration between each atlas and the multimodal images, (ii) the atlas selection, and finally (iii) the classification of the prostate voxels into either CG or PZ classes. Each atlas and the MRI images are registered through two successive registrations: a rigid registration to roughly align the atlases and the MRI images, followed by an elastic registration using a B-spline transformation. The cost function driving the registration is defined as the weighted sum of the mutual information (MI) of both T2-W-MRI and ADC map. The final atlas is selected using either a majority voting or the simultaneous truth and performance level estimation (STAPLE) approach [202]. Subsequently, each voxel within the prostate is classified either as CG or PZ using a linear discriminant analysis (LDA) classifier. Three types of features are considered to characterize the voxels: (i) anatomy, (ii) intensity, and (iii) texture. The relative position and the relative distance from the voxel to the border of the prostate encode the anatomical information. The intensity features consist of the intensity of the voxel in the ADC coefficient and the T2 map. The texture features are composed of five different features: homogeneity, correlation [203], entropy, texture strength [204], and local binary pattern (LBP) [205]. Finally, the final segmentation is obtained by removing artifacts and smoothing the contour between the zones using the thin plate spline (TPS) [206].

Litjens et al. used an almost identical algorithm in [130], initially proposed for the PROMISE12 challenge [207]. Their segmentation method is also based on multi-atlas multimodal images, but the SIMPLE method [208] is used instead, to combine labels after the registration of the different atlas to obtain the final segmentation.

Finally, Rampun et al. recurrently used a method to segment the PZ [143–146,185], which is proposed by Rampun et al. [209]. The PZ is modeled using a quadratic function driven by the center of the prostate and the left-most and the right-most coordinates of the prostate boundaries.

Model-Based Segmentation

Viswanath et al. [159,160] used the MANTRA method [210]. Multi-attribute non-initializing texture reconstruction-based active shape model (MANTRA) [210] is closely related to the active shape model (ASM) from Cootes et al. [211]. This algorithm consists of two stages: (i) a training stage where a shape and an appearance model are generated and (ii) the actual segmentation based on the learned model. For the training stage, a set of landmarks is defined and the shape model is generated as in the original ASM method [211]. Then, to model the appearance, a set of K texture images $\{I_1, I_2, \cdots, I_k\}$ based on first- and second-order statistical texture features is computed. For a given landmark l with its given neighborhood $\mathcal{N}(l)$, its feature matrix extracted is expressed as follows:

$$f_l = \{I_1(\mathcal{N}(l)), I_2(\mathcal{N}(l)), \cdots, I_k(\mathcal{N}(l))\}, \tag{10.28}$$

where $I_k(\mathcal{N}(l))$ represents a feature vector obtained by sampling the kth texture map using the neighborhood $\mathcal{N}(l)$. Therefore, multiple landmarks are generated followed by a decomposition using principal components analysis (PCA) [212] to learn the appearance variations as in ASM.

For the segmentation stage, the mean shape learned previously is initialized in the test image. The same associated texture images as in the training stage are computed. For each landmark l, a neighborhood of patches is used to sample the texture images and a reconstruction is obtained using the appearance model previously trained. The new landmark location will be defined as the position where the MI is maximal between the reconstructed and original values. This scheme is performed in a multiresolution manner as in Cootes et al. [211].

Subsequently, Viswanath et al. [162] used the weighted ensemble of regional image textures for active shape model segmentation (WERITAS) method also proposed in Toth et al. [213]. Similar to MANTRA, WERITAS is also based on the ASM formulation. It differs in the last stage of the algorithm in which the Mahalanobis distance is used, instead of the MI metric, to adapt the positions of new landmarks. In the training stage, the Mahalanobis distance is computed between landmarks and neighbor patches for each of the features. Subsequently, a new metric is proposed as a linear weighted combination of those Mahalanobis distances that maximizes the correlation with the Euclidean distance between the patches and the true landmarks. In the segmentation step, this metric is then computed between the initialized landmarks and neighboring patches in order to update landmark positions, in a similar fashion to other active contour model (ACM) models.

Litjens et al. [128] as well as Vos et al. [166] used an approach proposed by Huisman et al. [214] in which the bladder, the prostate, and the rectum are segmented. The segmentation task is performed as an optimization problem taking three parameters into account linked to organ characteristics such as: (i) the shape (i.e., an ellipse), (ii) the location, and (iii) the respective angles between them. Furthermore, Litjens et al. used only the ADC map to encode the appearance [128], whereas Vos et al. used both ADC and T2 maps [166]. The cost function, defined as the sum of the deviations, is minimized using a quasi-Newton optimizer. This rough segmentation is then used inside a Bayesian framework to refine the segmentation.

Giannini et al. segmented the prostate with a multi-Otsu thresholding [215] in ADC images [122]. Further morphological operations are applied to improve the segmentation.

Only the work of Tiwari et al. used the MRSI modality to segment the prostate organ [151]. The prostate is segmented based on an unsupervised hierarchical spectral clustering. First, each MRSI spectrum is projected into a lower-dimensional space using graph embedding [216]. To proceed, a similarity matrix W is computed using a Gaussian similarity measure from Euclidean distance [217] such that

$$W(\mathbf{x}, \mathbf{y}) = \begin{cases} \exp\left(\dfrac{\| s(\mathbf{x}) - s(\mathbf{y}) \|_2^2}{\sigma^2} \right), & \text{if } \| \mathbf{x} - \mathbf{y} \|_2 < \epsilon, \\ 0, & \text{if } \| \mathbf{x} - \mathbf{y} \|_2 > \epsilon. \end{cases} \tag{10.29}$$

where $s(\mathbf{x})$ and $s(\mathbf{y})$ are the MRSI spectra for the voxels $\mathbf{x}$ and $\mathbf{y}$, respectively; σ is the standard deviation of the Gaussian similarity measure; and ϵ is the parameter to defined an ϵ-neighborhood.

The projection can be performed as a generalized eigenvector problem such that

$$Lu = \lambda Du,$$

$$D(\mathbf{x}, \mathbf{x}) = \sum_y W(\mathbf{x}, \mathbf{y}), \qquad (10.30)$$

$$L = D - W,$$

where D is the diagonal weight matrix, L is the Laplacian matrix, λ and u represent the eigenvalues and eigenvectors. Once the MRSI spectra are projected into the lower-dimensional space, a replicate k-means clustering method is used to define 2 clusters. Subsequently, the data corresponding to the largest cluster is assumed to belong to the non-prostate voxels and thus these voxels are eliminated from the processing. The full procedure is repeated until the total number of voxels left is inferior to a given threshold experimentally set.

The segmentation algorithms used in CAD system for the detection of CaP are summarized in Table 10.4.

REGISTRATION

Image registration plays a vital role in CAD systems using mpMRI images. The features detected in each modality are grouped depending of their spatial location, requiring a perfect alignment of the mpMRI ahead of the classification.

Image registration is the procedure consisting of aligning an unregistered image—also called moving image—into a template image—also called fixed image—via a geometric transformation. This problem is usually addressed as depicted in Figure 10.13. An iterative procedure takes place to infer the geometric transformation, parametric or non-parametric, via an optimizer which maximizes the similarity between the two images. In the following, a review of the different components of a typical registration framework—transformation model, similarity metric, optimizer, and interpolation—are presented. To conclude a summary is given focusing on the registration approaches applied in CAD for CaP systems. Exhaustive reviews covering all registration methods in computer science and medical fields are available [218–220].

Geometric Transformation Models

As previously mentioned, the registration process is equivalent to finding a geometric transformation that minimizes the difference between two images. From all CAD systems reviewed, only parametric

---

TABLE 10.4

Overview of the Segmentation Methods Used in CAD Systems

Segmentation Methods	References
MRI-Based Segmentation	
Manual segmentation	[115,116,126,127,135,137–140,142,156,157,163–166]
Region-based segmentation	[129,130,143–146,185]
Model-based segmentation	[122,128,159–161,166]
MRSI-Based Segmentation	
Clustering	[151]

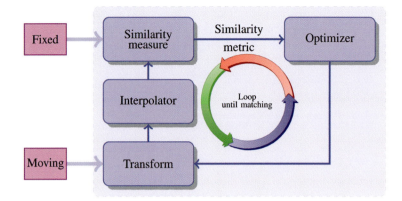

FIGURE 10.13 Typical framework involved to solve the registration problem.

methods have been implemented. Three different groups of parametric transformation models have been used—rigid, affine, and elastic—each of them characterized by a specific degree of freedom.

The simplest transformation used in terms of degrees of freedom is usually referred to as rigid transformation. This type of transformation is only composed of a rotation and a translation. Therefore, for the 2D case where $\mathbf{x} = (x, y) \in \mathbb{R}^2$, a rigid transformation $\mathcal{T}_R$ is formalized as follows:

$$
\begin{aligned}
\mathcal{T}_R(\mathbf{x}) &= \begin{bmatrix} R & \mathbf{t} \\ \mathbf{0}^{\mathrm{T}} & 1 \end{bmatrix} \mathbf{x}, \\
&= \begin{bmatrix} \cos\theta & -\sin\theta & t_x \\ \sin\theta & \cos\theta & t_y \\ 0 & 0 & 1 \end{bmatrix} \begin{bmatrix} x \\ y \\ 1 \end{bmatrix},
\end{aligned}
\tag{10.31}
$$

where θ is the rotation angle and $\{t_x, t_y\}$ represents the translation along $\{x, y\}$, respectively. In the case of 3D registration using volume, an additional component z is introduced such that $\mathbf{x} = (x, y, z)$. Thus, the rotation matrix $\mathbf{R}$ becomes of size 3×3 whereas the translation vector $\mathbf{t}$ consists of a vector of three variables. The geometric transformation $\mathcal{T}_R(\cdot)$ is embedded into a matrix of size 4×4.

The affine transformation provides additional degrees of freedom, providing rotation, translation—as with the rigid transformations—and also shearing and scaling. Hence, for a 2D space where $\mathbf{x} = (x, y) \in \mathbb{R}^2$, an affine transformation $\mathcal{T}_A$ is formalized as

$$
\begin{aligned}
\mathcal{T}_A(\mathbf{x}) &= \begin{bmatrix} A & \mathbf{t} \\ \mathbf{0}^{\mathrm{T}} & 1 \end{bmatrix} \mathbf{x}, \\
&= \begin{bmatrix} a_{11} & a_{12} & t_x \\ a_{21} & a_{22} & t_y \\ 0 & 0 & 1 \end{bmatrix} \begin{bmatrix} x \\ y \\ 1 \end{bmatrix}.
\end{aligned}
\tag{10.32}
$$

where the 4 parameters $\{a_{11}, a_{12}, a_{21}, a_{22}\}$ of the affine matrix and $\{t_x, t_y\}$ of the translation encode the deformation. As in the rigid registration case, in 3D the affine transformation $\mathcal{T}_A(\cdot)$ is of size 4×4 but now with 12 parameters involved.

Finally, the last group of transformations is known as elastic transformations and offers the advantage of handling local distortions. In the reviewed CAD systems, the radial basis functions are used to formalize the local distortions such as

$$\mathcal{T}_E(\mathbf{x}) = \frac{a_{11}x - a_{12}y + t_x + \sum_i c_i g(\|\mathbf{x} - p_i\|)}{a_{21}x + a_{22}y + t_y + \sum_i c_i g(\|\mathbf{x} - p_i\|)}, \tag{10.33}$$

where $\mathbf{x}$ are the control points in both images and $g(\cdots)$ is the actual radial basis function.

Two radial basis functions are used: (i) the TPS and (ii) the B-splines. Apart from the formalism, these two approaches have a main difference: with B-splines, the control points are usually uniformly and densely placed on a grid, whereas with TPS, the control points correspond to some detected or selected key points. By using TPS, Mitra et al. obtained more accurate and time-efficient results than with the B-splines strategy [221].

It is reasonable to point out that usually only rigid or affine registrations are used to register mpMRI from a same protocol. Elastic registration methods are more commonly used to register multi-protocol images such as histopathology with MRI images [210,213].

Similarity Measure

The most naive similarity measure used in reviewed registration framework is the mean squared error (MSE) of the SI of MRI images. For a pair of images I and J, the MSE is formalized as follows:

$$\text{MSE} = \frac{1}{N} \sum_x \sum_y [I(x, y) - J(x, y)]^2, \tag{10.34}$$

where N is the total number of pixels. This metric is not well suited when mpMRI images are involved due to the tissue appearance variations between the different modalities.

In this regard, MI was introduced as a similarity measure in registration framework in the late 1990s by Pluim et al. [222]. The MI measure finds its foundation in the assumption that a homogeneous region in the first modality image should also appear as a homogeneous region in the second modality, even if their SIs are not identical. Thus, those regions share information and the registration task is achieved by maximizing this common information. Hence, MI of two images A and B is defined as

$$MI(A; B) = S(A) + S(B) - S(A, B), \tag{10.35}$$

where $S(A)$, $S(B)$, and $S(A, B)$ are the marginal entropies of A and B and the joint entropy, respectively. Therefore, maximizing the MI is the equivalent of minimizing the joint entropy. The joint entropy measure is related to the degree of uncertainty or dispersion of the data in the joint histogram of the images A and B. As shown in Figure 10.14, the data in the joint histogram are concentrated in the case of aligned images (see Figure 10.14a), while they are more randomly distributed in the case of misaligned images (see Figure 10.14b). The entropy is computed based on an estimation of the PDF of the images and thus histogram or Parzen window methods are a common way to estimate these PDFs.

A generalized form of MI, combined mutual information (CMI), has been proposed by Chappelow et al. [223]. CMI encompasses interdependent information such as texture and gradient information into the metric. Hence, for both of images A and B, the image ensembles ϵ_n^A and ϵ_m^B are generated and composed of n and m images based on the texture and gradient. Then, the CMI is formulated such as

$$CMI(\epsilon_n^A; \epsilon_m^B) = S(\epsilon_n^A) + S(\epsilon_m^B) - S(\epsilon_n^A, \epsilon_m^B). \tag{10.36}$$

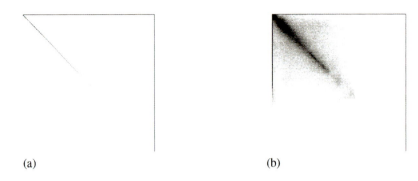

(a)   (b)

FIGURE 10.14   Difference observed in joint histogram between aligned and misaligned images. The joint measure will be more concentrated of the histogram in the case that the images are aligned and more randomly distributed in the case that both images are more misaligned. (a) Illustration of a joint histogram between two aligned images. (b) Illustration of a joint histogram between two misaligned images.

From Equation 10.36, note that CMI is estimated from high-dimensional data and as a consequence the histogram-based methods to estimate the PDFs are no longer suitable [223]. However, other alternative approaches are used, such as the one employed in Staring et al. [224] to compute the α-MI [225].

Optimization Methods

Registration is usually regarded as an optimization problem where the parameters of the geometric transformation model have to be inferred by minimizing/maximizing the similarity measure. Iterative optimization methods are commonly used, the most common methods being the L-BFGS-B quasi-Newton method [226] and the gradient descent [227]. During our review, we noticed that authors do not usually linger over optimizer choice.

Interpolation

The registration procedure involves transforming an image and pixels mapped to non-integer points must be approximated using interpolation methods. As for the optimization methods, we notice that little attention has been paid on the choice of those interpolations methods. However, commonly used methods are bi-linear, nearest-neighbor, bi-cubic, spline, and inverse-distance weighting method [228].

Registration Methods Used in CAD Systems

Table 10.5 summarizes the framework used to register mpMRI images in CAD for CaP.

Ampeliotis et al. did not use the framework as presented in Figure 10.13 to register 2D T2-W-MRI and DCE-MRI images [112,113]. By using image symmetries and the MSE metric, they found the parameters of an affine transformation but without using a common objective function. The scale factor, the rotation, and the translation are independently and sequentially estimated.

Giannini et al. used also a in-house registration method for 2D T2-W-MRI and DW-MRI images using an affine model [121,122]. The bladder is first segmented in both modalities in order to obtain its contours, which are then used as a metric function (i.e., distance between contours) for registration.

Giannini et al. and also Vos et al. used a framework based on finding an affine transformation to register the T2-W-MRI and DCE-MRI images using MI [121,165,229]. Then, an elastic registration using B-spline takes place using the affine parameters to initialize the geometric model with the same similarity measure. However, the two approaches differ regarding the choice of the optimizer since Giannini et al. used a gradient descent [121] and Vos et al. used a quasi-Newton method [165]. Moreover, Giannini et al. applied a 2D registration, whereas Vos et al. registered 3D volumes.

Viswanath et al. as well as Vos et al. registered T2-W-MRI and DCE-MRI images using an affine registration and a MI metric [159,160,163]. However, the choice of the optimizer has not been

TABLE 10.5

Classification of the Different Registration Methods Used in the CAD Systems Reviewed

Study Index	Modality Registered	Type	Geometric Model		Similarity Measure			Optimizer	
			Affine	Elastic	MSE	MI	CMI	GD	L-BFGS-B
[112,113]	T2-W - DCE	2D	✓	—	✓	—	—	—	—
[121,122]	T2-W - DW	2D	✓	✓	—	—	—	—	—
[121,122]	T2-W - DCE	2D	✓	✓	—	✓	—	✓	—
[159,160]	T2-W - DCE	2D	✓	—	—	✓	—	—	—
[161]	T2-W - DCE - DW	3D	✓	—	—	—	✓	✓	—
[163]	T2-W - DCE	3D	✓	—	—	✓	—	—	—
[165]	T2-W - DCE	3D	✓	✓	—	✓	—	—	✓
[127]	T2-W - DCE - DW	3D	✓	✓	✓	✓	—	✓	—

Notes: —: not used or not mentioned; ✓: used or implemented.

Abbreviations: Mean squared error (MSE); mutual information (MI); combined mutual information (CMI); gradient descent (GD); limited-memory Broyden-Fletcher-Goldfarb-Shannon box constraints (L-BFGS-B).

specified. Furthermore, Viswanath et al. focused on 2D registration [159,160], while Vos et al. performed 3D registration [163].

Finally, Viswanath et al. performed a 3D registration with the three modalities, T2-W-MRI, DCE-MRI, and DW-MRI, using an affine transformation model combined with the CMI similarity measure [161]. Moreover, in this latter work, the authors employed a gradient descent approach [223] to solve this problem but suggested that the Nelder-Mead simplex and the quasi-Newton methods are other possible solutions.

Lemaitre also registered T2-W-MRI, DCE-MRI, and DW-MRI images [127]. The intra-patient motions occurring during DCE-MRI is corrected by rigidly registering all series to the first series using MI and a gradient descent optimizer. Once the intra-patient motions are corrected, T2-W-MRI and the DCE-MRI are co-registered. For that matter, the prostate has been segmented in both modalities—T2-W-MRI and DCE-MRI—to create two binary masks. Therefore, these 3D binary masks are directly registered using the MSE metric and a gradient descent with an elastic registration based on B-splines. The T2-W-MRI and ADC map acquisitions are registered using the same approach as for the registration of the T2-W-MRI and the DCE-MRI modalities.

CADe: ROIs Detection/Selection

As discussed in the introduction and shown in Figure 10.5, the image classification framework is often composed of a CADe and a CADx. In this section, we focus on studies that embed a CADe in their framework. Two approaches are considered to define a CADe: (i) voxel-based delineation and (ii) lesion segmentation. These methods are summarized in Table 10.6. The first strategy is in fact linked to the nature of the classification framework and concerns the majority of the studies reviewed [115,116,121,123,124,126,127,131,133,135,136,139–141,143–146,148–162,185]. Each voxel

TABLE 10.6

Overview of the CADe Strategies Employed in CAD Systems

CADe: ROIs Selection Strategy	References
All voxels-based approach	[115,116,121,123,124,126,127,131,133,135,136,139–141,143–146,148–162,185]
Lesions candidate detection	[117,118,128–130,166]

is a possible candidate and will be classified as cancerous or healthy. The second group of methods is composed of method implementing a lesion segmentation algorithm to delineate potential candidates to further obtain a diagnosis through the CADx. This approach is borrowed from other application areas such as breast cancer. These methods are in fact very similar to the classification framework used in CADx later.

Regarding lesion candidate detection, Vos et al. highlighted lesion candidates by detecting blobs in the ADC map [166]. These candidates are filtered using some a priori criteria such as SI or diameter. As mentioned in the section "Clinical Aspects of TRUS Prostate Biopsy" and Table 10.1, low SI in ADC map can be linked to potential CaP. Hence, blob detectors are suitable to highlight these regions. Blobs are detected in a multiresolution scheme, by computing the three main eigenvalues $\{\lambda_{\sigma,1}, \lambda_{\sigma,2}, \lambda_{\sigma,3}\}$ of the Hessian matrix, for each voxel location of the ADC map at a specific scale σ [230]. The probability p of a voxel $\mathbf{x}$ being a part of a blob at the scale σ is given by

$$P(\mathbf{x}, \sigma) = \begin{cases} \dfrac{\|\lambda_{\sigma,3}(\mathbf{x})\|^2}{\|\lambda_{\sigma,1}(\mathbf{x})\|}, & \text{if } \lambda_{\sigma,k}(\mathbf{x}) > 0 \text{ with } k = \{1, 2, 3\}, \\ 0, & \text{otherwise.} \end{cases} \quad (10.37)$$

The fusion of the different scales is computed as

$$L(\mathbf{x}) = \max P(\mathbf{x}, \sigma), \forall \sigma. \quad (10.38)$$

The candidate blobs detected are then filtered depending on their appearances—that is, maximum of the likelihood of the region, diameter of the lesion—and their SI in ADC and T2-W-MRI images. The detected regions are then used as inputs for the CADx. Cameron et al. used a similar approach by automatically selecting low-SI connected regions in the ADC map with a size larger than 1 mm^2 [117,118].

Litjens et al. used a pattern recognition approach to delineate the ROIs [128]. A blobness map is computed in the same manner as in Vos et al. [165] using the multiresolution Hessian blob detector on the ADC map, T2-W, and pharmacokinetic parameters maps (see Section 3.5.2 for details about those parameters). Additionally, the position of the voxel $\mathbf{x} = \{x, y, z\}$ is used as a feature as well as the Euclidean distance of the voxel to the prostate center. Hence, each feature vector is composed of eight features and a support vector machine (SVM) classifier is trained using a radial basis function (RBF) kernel (see Section 3.8 for more details).

Subsequently, Litjens et al. modified this approach by including only features related to the blob detection on the different maps as well as the original SIs of the parametric images [129]. Two new maps are introduced based on texture and a k-nearest neighbor (k-NN) classifier is used instead of a SVM classifier. The candidate regions are then extracted by performing a local maxima detection followed by post-processing region growing and morphological operations.

CADx: Feature Detection

Discriminative features that help to recognize CaP from healthy tissue first need to be detected. This processing is known in computer vision as feature extraction. However, feature extraction also refers to the name given in pattern recognition to some types of dimension reduction methods which are presented later. In order to avoid confusion between these two aspects, in this survey, the procedure "detecting" or "extracting" features from images and signals is defined as feature detection. This section summarizes the different features used in CAD for CaP.

Image-Based Features

This section focuses on image-based features which can be categorized into two categories: (i) voxelwise detection and (ii) region-wise detection.

Voxelwise Detection in MRI

This strategy refers to the fact that a feature is extracted at each voxel location. As discussed in the section "MRI Techniques," CaP has an influence on the SI in mpMRI images. Therefore, intensity-based feature is the most commonly used feature [112,113,115–122,124–131,137–140,143,144,156,157,163]. This feature consists of the extraction of the intensity of the MRI modality of interest.

Edge-based features have also been used to detect SI changes but bring additional information regarding the SI transition. Each feature is computed by convolving the original image with an edge operator. Three operators are commonly used: (i) Prewitt operator [231], (ii) Sobel operator [232], and (iii) Kirsch operator [233]. These operators differ due to the kernel used which attenuates more or less the noise. Multiple studies have used the resulting magnitude and orientation of the edges computed in their classification frameworks [120,124,126,127,137,138,145,146,152,153,155,158,161,185].

Gabor filters [234,235] offer an alternative to the usual edge detector, with the possibility to tune the direction and the frequency of the filter to encode a specific pattern. A Gabor filter is defined by the modulation of a Gaussian function with a sine wave which can be further rotated and is formalized as in Equation 10.39:

$$g(x, y; \theta, \psi, \sigma, \gamma) = \exp\left(-\frac{x'^2 + \gamma^2 y'^2}{2\sigma^2}\right) \cos\left(2\pi \frac{x'}{\lambda} + \psi\right), \quad (10.39)$$

with

$$x' = s\left(x\cos\theta + y\sin\theta\right),$$

$$y' = s\left(-x\sin\theta + y\cos\theta\right),$$

where λ is the wavelength of the sinusoidal factor, θ represents the orientation of the Gabor filter, ψ is the phase offset, σ is the standard deviation of the Gaussian envelope, γ is the spatial aspect ratio, and s is the scale factor. In an effort to characterize pattern and texture, a bank of Gabor filters is usually created with different angles, scale, and frequency—refer to Figure 10.15—and then convolved with the image. Viswanath et al. [162], Tiwari et al. [154], and more recently Khalvati et al. [124] and Chung et al. [120] have designed a bank of Gabor filters to characterize texture and edge information in T2-W-MRI and DW-MRI modalities.

Lemaitre [127] used a 3D Gabor filters bank. 3D Gabor filters [236] are not commonly used and we recall their formulation in Equation 10.40:

$$g(\mathbf{x}; \sigma, f, \theta, \phi) = \hat{g}(\mathbf{x}; \sigma)\exp\left(j2\pi f\left(x\sin\theta\cos\phi + y\sin\theta\sin\phi + z\cos\theta\right)\right), \quad (10.40)$$

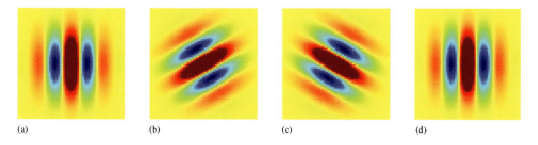

(a) (b) (c) (d)

FIGURE 10.15 Illustration of four different Gabor filters varying their orientations θ. (a) $\theta = 0°$, (b) $\theta = 60°$, (c) $\theta = 120°$, (d) $\theta = 180°$.

where,

$$\hat{g}(\mathbf{x}; \sigma) = \frac{1}{(2\pi)^{\frac{3}{2}}} \exp\left(-\frac{1}{2}\left(\frac{x^2}{\sigma_x^2} + \frac{y^2}{\sigma_y^2} + \frac{z^2}{\sigma_z^2}\right)\right), \tag{10.41}$$

where $\mathbf{x}$ is the position vector $\{x, y, z\}$, σ is the standard deviation vector $\{\sigma_x, \sigma_y, \sigma_z\}$ of the 3D Gaussian envelope, f is the radial center frequency of the sine wave, θ is the elevation angle, and ϕ is the azimuth angle.

Additionally, Lemaitre [127] features based on phase congruency as proposed by Kovesi are computed [237]. Therefore, from a log-Gabor filter bank, the orientation image, the local weighted mean phase angle, and the phase angle are estimated at each voxel.

Texture-based features provide other characteristics discerning CaP from healthy tissue. The most common texture analysis for image classification is based on the gray-level co-occurrence matrix (GLCM) with their related statistics which have been proposed by Haralick et al. [238]. In a neighborhood around a central voxel, a GLCM is built considering each voxel pair defined by a specific distance and angle. Then, using the GLCM, a set of statistical features is computed as defined in Table 10.7 and assigned to the location of the central voxel. Therefore, N—up to 14—statistical maps are derived from the GLCM analysis, one per statistics presented in Table 10.7. GLCM is commonly used in CAD systems, on the different MRI modalities, namely T2-W-MRI, DCE-MRI, or DW-MRI [114,117,118,120,124,126,127,137,138,145,146,152,153,155,156,158,160–162,185]. However, the statistics extracted from the GLCM vary across studies. Along the same line, Rampun et al. extracted from T2-W-MRI [145,185] Tamura features [239] composed of three features to characterize texture: (i) coarseness, (ii) contrast, and (iii) directionality.

Lopes et al. used fractal analysis, and more precisely a local estimation of the fractal dimension [240], to describe the texture roughness at a specific location. The fractal dimension is estimated through a wavelet-based method in multiresolution analysis. They showed that cancerous tissues have a higher fractal dimension than healthy tissue.

Chan et al. described texture using the frequency signature via the discrete cosine transform (DCT) [241], defining a neighborhood of 7×7 px for modalities used, namely T2-W-MRI and DW-MRI. The DCT allows to decompose a portion of an image into a coefficient space, where few of these coefficients encode the significant information. The DCT coefficients are computed such as

$$C_{k_1, k_2} = \sum_{m=0}^{M-1} \sum_{n=0}^{N-1} p_{m,n} \cos\left[\frac{\pi}{M}\left(m + \frac{1}{2}\right)k_1\right] \cos\left[\frac{\pi}{N}\left(n + \frac{1}{2}\right)k_2\right], \tag{10.42}$$

where C_{k_1, k_2} is the DCT coefficient at the position k_1, k_2, M and N are the dimension of the neighborhood and $p_{m,n}$ is the pixel SI at the position $\{m, n\}$.

Lemaitre [127] incorporated those features in a CAD system.

Regarding other features, Viswanath et al. projected T2-W-MRI images into the wavelet space, using the Haar wavelet, and used the resulting coefficients as features [162]. Litjens et al. computed the texture map based on T2-W-MRI images using a Gaussian filter bank [128]. Likewise, Rampun et al. employed a rotation invariant filter bank proposed in Leung and Malik [242]. The bank is composed of 48 filters including Gaussian filters, first and second derivatives of Gaussian filters, as well as Laplacian of Gaussian.

Region-Wise Detection in MRI

Unlike the previous section, another strategy is to study a region instead of each pixel independently. Usually, the feature maps are computed using the method presented in voxel-based approach followed by a step in which features are computed in some specific delineated regions to characterize them.

TABLE 10.7

The 14 Statistical Features for Texture Analysis Commonly Computed From the GLCM p as Presented by Haralick et al. [238]

Statistical Features	Formula
Angular second moment	$\sum_i \sum_j p(i,j)^2$
Contrast	$\sum_{n=0}^{N_g-1} n^2 \left[\sum_{i=1}^{N_g-1} \sum_{j=1}^{N_g-1} p(i,j) \right], \lvert i-j \rvert = n$
Correlation	$\dfrac{\sum_i \sum_j (ij) p(i,j) - \mu_x \mu_y}{\sigma_x \sigma_y}$
Variance	$\sum_i \sum_j (i-\mu)^2 p(i,j)$
Inverse difference moment	$\sum_i \sum_j \dfrac{1}{1+(i-\mu)^2} p(i,j)$
Sum average	$\sum_{i=2}^{2N_g} i p_{x+y}(i)$
Sum variance	$\sum_{i=2}^{2N_g} (i-f_s)^2 p_{x+y}(i)$
Sum entropy	$-\sum_{i=2}^{2N_g} p_{x+y}(i) \log p_{x+y}(i)$
Entropy	$-\sum_i \sum_j p(i,j) \log p(i,j)$
Difference variance	$\sum_{i=0}^{N_g-1} i^2 p_{x-y}(i)$
Difference entropy	$-\sum_{i=0}^{N_g-1} p_{x-y}(i) \log p_{x-y}(i)$
Info. measure of corr. 1	$\dfrac{S(X;Y) - S_1(X;Y)}{\max(S(X),S(Y))}$
Info. measure of corr. 2	$\sqrt{\left(1 - \exp\left[-2(H_2(X;Y) - H(X;Y))\right]\right)}$
Max. corr. coeff.	$\sqrt{\lambda_2}$, of $Q(i,j) = \sum_k \dfrac{p(i,k) p(j,k)}{p_x(i) p_y(k)}$

The most common feature type is based on statistics and more specifically the statistic-moments such as mean, standard deviation, kurtosis, and skewness [100,112–114,117,118,120,124,126,128–130,137,138,145,146,152,153,155,158,160–162,185]. Additionally, some studies extract additional statistical landmarks based on percentiles [100,114,126,128–130,137,138,164–166]. The percentiles to use are manually determined by observing the PDF of the features and checking which values allow the best to differentiate malignant from healthy tissue.

Further statistics are computed through the use of histogram-based features. Liu et al. introduced four different types of histogram-based features to characterize hand-delineated lesions [132]. The first type corresponds to the histogram of the SI of the image. The second type is the histogram of oriented gradient (HOG) [243] which encodes the local shape of the object of interest by using the distribution of the gradient directions. This descriptor is extracted mainly in three steps. First, the gradient image and its corresponding magnitude and direction are computed. Then, the ROI is divided into cells and an oriented-based histogram is generated for each cell. At each pixel location, the orientation of the gradient votes for a bin of the histogram and this vote is weighted by the magnitude of the same gradient. Finally, the cells are grouped into blocks and each block is normalized. The third histogram-based type used by Liu et al. [132] is the shape context introduced by Belongie et al. [244]. The shape context is also a way to describe the shape of an object of interest. First, a set of points defining edges have to be detected and for each point of each edge, a log-polar-based histogram is computed using the relative points distribution. The last set of histogram-based feature extracted is based on the framework described in Zhao et al. [245] that uses the Fourier transform of the histogram created via local binary pattern (LBP) [205]. LBP is generated by comparing the value of the central pixel with its neighbors, defined through a radius and the number of connected neighbors. Then, in the ROI, the histogram of the LBP distribution is computed. The discrete Fourier transform (DFT) of the LBP histogram is used to make the feature invariant to rotation.

Another subset of features are anatomical-based features, which have been used in various studies [117,118,129,130,135]. Litjens et al. computed the volume, compactness, and sphericity related to the given region [129,130]. Additionally, Litjens et al. introduced a feature based on symmetry in which they computed the mean of a candidate lesion as well as its mirrored counterpart and computed the quotient as feature [130]. Lemaitre [127] incorporated those features in their CAD system. Matulewicz et al. introduced four features corresponding to the percentage of tissue belonging to the PZ, CG, periurethral region, or outside the prostate region for the considered ROI [135]. Finally, Cameron et al. defined four features based on morphology and asymmetry: (i) the difference of morphological closing and opening of the ROI, (ii) the difference of the initial perimeter and the one after removing the high-frequency components, (iii) the difference between the initial ROI and the one after removing the high-frequency components, and (iv) the asymmetry by computing the difference of the two areas splitting the ROI by its major axes [117,118].

The last group of region-based features is based on fractal analysis. This group of features is based on estimating the fractal dimension, which is a statistical index representing the complexity of the analyzed texture. Lv et al. proposed two features based on fractal dimension: (i) texture fractal dimension and (ii) histogram fractal dimension [134]. The first feature is based on estimating the fractal dimension on the SI of each image and thus this feature is a statistical characteristic of the image roughness. The second fractal dimension is estimated using the PDF of each image and characterizes the complexity of the PDF. Lopes et al. proposed a 3D version to estimate the fractal dimension of a volume using a wavelet decomposition [133].

DCE-Based Features

DCE-MRI is more commonly based on a SI analysis over time as presented in the section "Prostate Anatomy and Histological Architecture." In this section, the specific features extracted for DCE-MRI analysis are presented.

Whole-Spectra Approach

Some studies use the whole DCE time series as a feature vector [112,113,127,154,158,159]. In some cases, the high-dimensional feature space is reduced using dimension reduction methods.

Semi-Quantitative Approach

Semi-quantitative approaches are based on mathematically modeling the DCE time series. The parameters modeling the signal are commonly used, mainly due to the simplicity of their computation [122,126,127,136–138,142,147,148,156,157]. Parameters included in semi-quantitative analysis are summarized in Table 10.8 and are also graphically depicted in Figure 10.16. A set of time features corresponding to specific amplitude level (start, maximum, and end) are extracted. Then, derivative and integral features are also considered as discriminative and are commonly computed.

TABLE 10.8

Parameters Used as Features for a DCE Semi-Quantitative Analysis in CAD Systems

Semi-Quantitative Features	Explanations
Amplitude Features	
S_0	Amplitude at the onset of the enhancement
S_{max}	Amplitude corresponding to 95% of the maximum amplitude
S_p	Amplitude corresponding to the maximum amplitude
S_f	Amplitude at the final time point
Time Features	
t_0	Time at the onset of the enhancement
t_{max}	Time corresponding to 95% of the maximum amplitude
t_p	Time corresponding to the maximum amplitude
t_f	Final time
t_{tp}	Time to peak which is the time from t_0 to t_p
Derivatives and Integral Features	
WI	Wash-in rate corresponding to the signal slope from t_0 to t_m or t_p
WO	Washout rate corresponding to the signal slope from t_m or t_p to t_p
IAUC	Initial area under the curve which is the area between t_0 to t_f

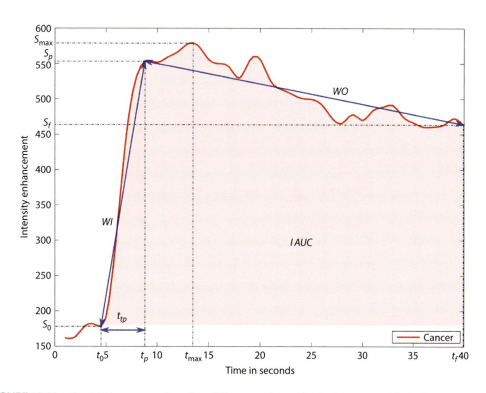

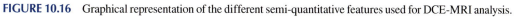

FIGURE 10.16   Graphical representation of the different semi-quantitative features used for DCE-MRI analysis.

Quantitative Approach

As presented in the section "MRI Techniques," quantitative approaches correspond to mathematical-pharmacokinetic models based on physiological exchanges. Four different models have been used in CAD for CaP systems. The most common model reviewed is the *Brix model* [115,116,127,131,139,140,148]. This model is formalized as follows:

$$\frac{S(t)}{S(0)} = 1 + Ak_{ep}\left(\frac{\exp(-k_{ep}t) - \exp(-k_{el}t)}{k_{el} - k_{ep}}\right), \tag{10.43}$$

where $S(\cdot)$ is the DCE signal, A is the parameter simulating the tissue properties, k_{el} is the parameter related to the first-order elimination from the plasma compartment, and k_{ep} is the parameter of the transvascular permeability. The parameters k_{ep}, k_{el}, and A are computed from the MRI data and used as features.

Another model is Tofts model [82] which has been used in a number of studies [121,122,125–127,136–138]. In this model, the DCE signal relative to the concentration is presented as

$$C_t(t) = v_p C_p(t) + K_{trans}\int_0^t C_p(\tau)\exp(-k_{ep}(t-\tau))\,d\tau, \tag{10.44}$$

where $C_t(\cdot)$ is the concentration of the medium, $C_p(\cdot)$ is the AIF which has to be estimated independently, K_{trans} is the parameter related to the diffuse transport of media across the capillary endothelium, k_{ep} is the parameter related to the exchanges back into the vascular space, and v_e is the extravascular-extracellular space fraction defined such that $v_e = 1 - v_p$. In this model, parameters K_{trans}, k_{ep}, and v_e are computed and used as features.

Mazzetti et al., Giannini et al., and Lemaitre used the Weibull function [121,122,127,136] which is formalized as

$$S(t) = At\exp(-t^B), \tag{10.45}$$

where A and B are the two parameters which have to be inferred.

They also used another empirical model which is based on the West-like function and named the phenomenological universalities (PUN) [246], formalized as

$$S(t) = \exp\left[rt + \frac{1}{\beta}a_0 - r\left(\exp(\beta t) - 1\right)\right], \tag{10.46}$$

where the parameters β, a_0, and r are inferred. For all these models, the parameters are inferred using an optimization curve fitting approach.

MRSI-Based Features

Whole Spectra Approach in MRSI

As in the case of DCE analysis, one common approach is to incorporate the whole MRSI spectra in the feature vector for classification [123,127,135,141,149,151–153,155–157,159]. Sometimes postprocessing involving dimension reduction methods is performed to reduce the complexity during the classification as it will be presented in Section 3.7.2.

Quantification Approach in MRSI

We can reiterate that in MRSI only few biological markers—that is, choline, creatine, and citrate metabolites—are known to be useful to discriminate CaP and healthy tissue. Therefore, only the concentrations of these metabolites are considered as a feature prior to classification. In order to perform this quantification, four different approaches have been used. Kelm et al. [123] used the following models: QUEST [247], AMARES [248], and VARPRO [249]. They are all time-domain quantification methods varying by the type of pre-knowledge embedded and the optimization approaches used to solve the quantification problem. Unlike the time-domain quantification approaches, Parfait et al. used the LcModel approach proposed in Provencher [250], which solves the optimization problem in the frequency domain. Although Parfait et al. and Lemaitre used each metabolite relative concentration individually [127,141], other authors such as Kelm et al. proposed to compute relative concentrations as the ratios of metabolites as shown in Equations 10.47 and 10.48.

$$R_1 = \frac{[\text{Cho}] + [\text{Cr}]}{[\text{Cit}]} \tag{10.47}$$

$$R_2 = \frac{[\text{Cit}]}{[\text{Cho}] + [\text{Cr}] + [\text{Cit}]}, \tag{10.48}$$

where Cit, Cho, and Cr are the relative concentrations of citrate, choline, and creatine, respectively.

Recently, Trigui et al. used an absolute quantification approach from which water sequences are acquired to compute the absolute concentration of the metabolites [156,157]. Absolute quantification using water as reference is based on the fact that the fully relaxed signal from water or metabolites is proportional to the number of moles of the molecules in the voxel [251].

Wavelet Decomposition Approach in MRSI

Tiwari et al. performed a wavelet packet decomposition [252] of the spectra using the Haar wavelet basis function and its coefficients as features.

The feature detection methods used in CAD are summarized in Table 10.9.

FEATURE BALANCING

Data imbalance is a recurrent issue in classification, notably in medical data. The problem of imbalanced datasets lies in the fact that one of the class has a smallest number of data—that is, in medical data, the class corresponding to patients with a disease—compared with the other classes. Therefore, solving the problem of imbalance is equivalent to under- or over-sampling part of the dataset to obtain an equal number of samples in the different classes. Recently, Lemaitre used balancing methods during the learning stage to tackle this issue [253].

Undersampling

Techniques that reduce the number of samples of the majority class to be equal to the number of samples of minority class are referred to as undersampling (US) techniques.

Nearmiss (NM) offers three different methods to undersample the majority class [254]. In nearmiss-1 (NM-1), samples from the majority class are selected such that for each sample, the average distance to the k nearest neighbor (NN) samples from the minority class is minimum. Nearmiss-2 (NM-2) diverges from NM-1 by considering the k farthest neighbors samples from the minority class. In nearmiss-3 (NM-3), a subset M containing samples from the majority class is generated by finding the m NN from each sample of the minority class. Then, samples from the subset M are selected such that for each sample, the average distance to the k NN samples from the minority class is maximum.

Instance-hardness-threshold (IHT) select samples with a high hardness threshold [255]. Hardness indicates the likelihood of misclassification rate for each sample. The notation

TABLE 10.9

Overview of the Feature Detection Methods Used in CAD Systems

Feature Detection Methods	Indexes
MRI Image	
Voxelwise Detection	
Intensity-based	✓−−[112,113,143,144,163] −−✓[121] ✓−✓[115–120,122,124,125, 128–131,139,140,156,157] ✓✓✓[126,127,137,138]
Edge-based	
• Prewitt operator	✓−−[152,153,155,158] ✓−✓[127]
• Sobel operator	✓−−[145,146,152,153,155,158,160–162,185] ✓−✓[127] ✓✓✓[126,137,138]
• Kirsch operator	✓−−[152,153,155,158,160–162] ✓−✓[120,124,127] [126,137,138]
• Gabor filtering	✓−−[154,158,162] ✓−✓[120,124,127]
• Phase congruency	✓−✓[127]
Texture-based	
• Haralick features	✓−−[114,145,146,152,153,155,156,158,160,162,185] ✓✓−[161] ✓−✓[117,118,120,124] ✓✓✓[126,129,137,138]
• Tamura features	✓−−[145,146,185]
• Fractal analysis	✓−−[133,134]
• DCT	✓✓✓[119]
• Wavelet-based features	✓−−[162]
• Gaussian filter bank	✓−−[130,145,146,185]
• Laplacian of Gaussian filter bank	✓−−[145,146,185]
Position-based	[119,128–130]
Region-Wise Detection	
Statistical-based	
• Percentiles	−✓✓[164] −−✓[100,114] ✓✓−[165] ✓✓✓[126,128–130,137,138,166]
• Statistical-moments	✓−−[112,113,145,146,152,153,155,158,160,162,185] −−✓[114] −✓✓[161] ✓−✓[100,117,118,120,124] ✓✓✓[126,128–130,137,138]
Histogram-based	
• PDF	[132]
• HOG	✓✓✓[132]
• Shape context	✓✓✓[132]
• LBP	✓✓✓[132,127]
Anatomical-based	[117,118,129,130,135]
Fractal-based	[133,134]
DCE Signal	
Whole spectra approach	[112,113,127]
Semi-quantitative approach	✓ᵗ[142] [122,126,127,136–138,147,148,156,157]
Quantitative approach	
• Toft model	✓ᵗ[100,132] [121,122,125–130,136–138]
• Brix model	✓ᵗ[115,116,139,140] [127,131,148]
• Weibull function	[121,122,127,136]
• PUN	[121,122,127,136]
MRSI Signal	
Whole spectra approach	[123,127,135,141,149–153,155,158]
Quantification approach	[123,127,141,156,157]
Wavelet-based approach	[154]

Notes: (✓-✓-✓-): triplet stating the implementation or not of the feature for respectively T2-W-MRI images, DCE-MRI images, DCE-MRI images; ✓: used or implemented; ✓ᵗ: partially implemented.

of instance hardness is drawn through the decomposition of $p(h|t)$ using Bayes' theorem, where h represent the mapping function used to map input features to their corresponding labels and t represents the training set.

$$IH_h(\langle x_i, y_i \rangle) = 1 - p(y_i | x_i, h). \tag{10.49}$$

Therefore, undersampling is performed by keeping the most probable samples—that is, filtering the samples with high hardness value—through k-fold cross-validation (k-CV) training sets while considering specific threshold for filtering.

Oversampling

In contrast to US techniques, data can be balanced by oversampling (OS) in which the new samples belonging to the minority class are generated, aiming at equalizing the number of samples in both classes.

Synthetic minority oversampling technique (SMOTE) is a method to generate new synthetic samples [256]. Define x_i as a sample belonging to the minority class, and define x_{nn} as a randomly selected sample from the k-NN of x_i, with k set to 3. A new sample x_j is generated such that $x_j = x_i + \sigma(x_{nn} - x_i)$, where σ is a random number in the interval $[0,1]$.

SMOTE-borderline1 (SMOTE-b1) oversamples the minority class samples similarly to SMOTE [257]. However, instead of using all the minority samples, it focuses on the borderline samples of the minority class. Borderline samples simply indicate the samples that are closer to the other class. First, the borderline samples of the minority class are detected. A sample x_i belongs to borderline samples if more than half of its k-NN samples belong to the majority class. Synthetic data is then created based on the SMOTE method for borderline samples by selecting them. Then, s-NN of the minority class are selected to generate synthetic sample similarly to SMOTE.

SMOTE-borderline2 (SMOTE-b2) performs similarly to SMOTE-b1 [257]. However, the s-NN are not computed by considering only the minority class but by considering both classes. The same generation rules as SMOTE are used.

The data balancing used in CAD systems are summarized in Table 10.10.

CADx: FEATURE SELECTION AND FEATURE EXTRACTION

As presented in the previous section, it is a common practice to extract a wide variety of features. While dealing with mpMRI, the feature space created is a high-dimensional space which might mislead or corrupt the classifier during the training phase. Therefore, it is of interest to reduce the number of dimensions before proceeding to the classification task. The strategies used can be

TABLE 10.10

Overview of the Data Balancing Methods Used in CAD Systems

Balancing Methods	References
Under-Sampling	
Nearmiss-1 and nearmiss-2 and nearmiss-3	[127]
Instance-hardness-threshold	[127]
Over-Sampling	
SMOTE and SMOTE-b1 and SMOTE-b2	[127]

grouped as: (i) feature selection and (ii) feature extraction. In this section only the methods used in CAD for CaP systems are presented.

Feature Selection

The feature selection strategy is based on selecting the most discriminative feature dimensions of the high-dimensional space. Thus, the low-dimensional space is then composed of a subset of the original features detected. In this section, methods employed in CAD for CaP detection are presented; a more extensive review specific to feature selection is available in Saeys et al. [258].

Niaf et al. make use of the p-value by using the independent two-sample t-test with equal mean for each feature dimension [137,138]. In this statistical test, there are two classes: CaP and healthy tissue. Hence, for each particular feature, the distribution of each class is characterized by their means $\bar{X}_1$ and $\bar{X}_2$ and standard deviation s_{X_1} and s_{X_2}. Therefore, the null hypothesis test is based on the fact that both distribution means are equal. The t-statistic used to verify the null hypothesis is formalized such that

$$t = \frac{\bar{X}_1 - \bar{X}_2}{s_{X_1 X_2} \cdot \sqrt{\dfrac{1}{n_1} + \dfrac{1}{n_2}}}, \tag{10.50}$$

$$s_{X_1 X_2} = \sqrt{\frac{(n_1 - 1)s_{X_1}^2 + (n_2 - 1)s_{X_2}^2}{n_1 + n_2 - 2}},$$

where n_1 and n_2 are the number of samples in each class. From Equation 10.50, the more the means of the class distribution diverge, the larger the t-statistic will be, implying that this particular feature is more relevant and able to make the distinction between the two classes.

The p-value statistic is deduced from the t-test and corresponds to the probability of obtaining such an extreme test assuming that the null hypothesis is true [259]. Hence, the smaller the p-value, the more likely the null hypothesis is to be rejected and the more relevant the feature is likely to be. Finally, the features are ranked and the most significant features are selected. However, this technique suffers from a main drawback in that it assumes each feature is independent, which is unlikely to happen, and introduces a high degree of redundancy in the features selected.

Vos et al. [166] employed a similar feature ranking approach but make use of the Fisher discriminant ratio to compute the relevance of each feature dimension. Taking the aforementioned formulation, the Fisher discriminant ratio is formalized as the ratio of the interclass variance to the intraclass variance as follows:

$$F_r = \frac{(\bar{X}_1 - \bar{X}_2)^2}{s_{X_1}^2 + s_{X_2}^2} \tag{10.51}$$

Therefore, a relevant feature dimension is selected when the interclass variance is maximum and the intraclass variance in minimum. Once the features are ordered, the authors select the feature dimensions with the largest Fisher discriminant ratio.

Lemaitre used the one-way analysis of variance (ANOVA) test [127]. This test is based on computing the F-test which is the ratio of the between-group variability over the within group variability. The F-value is computed for each pair of features and the K feature dimensions corresponding to the largest F-values are kept.

MI is a possible metric to use for selecting a subset of feature dimensions. This method has previously been presented in Section 3.3 and expressed in Equation 10.35. Peng et al. [260] introduced two main criteria to select the feature dimensions based on MI: (i) maximal relevance and (ii) minimum redundancy. The maximal relevance criterion is based on the paradigm that the classes and the feature dimension which has to be selected have to share a maximal MI; it is formalized as follows:

$$\operatorname{argmax} Rel(\mathbf{x}, c) = \frac{1}{|\mathbf{x}|} \sum_{x_i \in \mathbf{x}} MI(x_i, c), \qquad (10.52)$$

where $\mathbf{x} = \{x_i; i = 1, \cdots, d\}$ is a feature vector of d dimensions and c is the class considered. As in the previous method, using maximal relevance criterion alone implies an independence between each feature dimension. The minimal redundancy criterion enforces the selection of a new feature dimension which shares as little as possible MI with the previously selected feature dimensions such that

$$\operatorname{argmin} Red(\mathbf{x}) = \frac{1}{|\mathbf{x}|^2} \sum_{x_i, x_j \in \mathbf{x}} MI(x_i, x_j). \qquad (10.53)$$

Combining these two criteria is known as the minimum redundancy maximum relevance (mRMR) algorithm [260]. Two combinations are usually used: (i) the difference or (ii) the quotient. This method has been used on several occasions for selecting a subset of features prior to classification [120,124,126,137,138,162].

Random forest (RF) provides information regarding the importance of each feature using the metric based on the Gini index. The feature importance in RF is linked with the Gini importance. In a tree classifier, the Gini impurity criterion of the child nodes is inferior to the parent node. For each individual feature, adding the decrease of the Gini impurity along the tree gives information about the feature importance: the higher, the better. Therefore, one can add the decrease of the Gini impurity across all the trees of a forest to obtain the importance of a specific feature for this forest. Subsequently, the K most important features are selected to perform the feature selection. Lemaitre used this approach to make a feature selection when training their RF [127].

Feature Extraction

The feature extraction strategy is related to dimension reduction methods but not selecting discriminative features. Instead, these methods aim at mapping the data from the high-dimensional space into a low-dimensional space to maximize the separability between the classes. As in the previous sections, only methods employed in CAD systems are reviewed in this section. We refer the reader to Fodor [261] for a full review of feature extraction techniques.

PCA is the most commonly used linear mapping method in CAD systems. PCA is based on finding the orthogonal linear transform mapping the original data into a low-dimensional space. The space is defined such that the linear combinations of the original data with the kth greatest variances lie on the kth principal components [262]. The principal components are computed by using the eigenvectors-eigenvalues decomposition of the covariance matrix. Let $\mathbf{x}$ denote the data matrix. Then, the covariance matrix and eigenvectors-eigenvalues decomposition are defined as in Equation 10.54 and Equation 10.55, respectively. The eigenvectors-eigenvalues decomposition can be formalized as

$$\Sigma = \mathbf{x}^T \mathbf{x} \qquad (10.54)$$

$$\mathbf{v}^{-1} \Sigma \mathbf{v} = \Lambda, \qquad (10.55)$$

where $\mathbf{v}$ are the eigenvectors matrix and Λ is a diagonal matrix containing the eigenvalues.

It is then possible to find the new low-dimensional space by sorting the eigenvectors using the eigenvalues and finally to select the eigenvectors corresponding to the largest eigenvalues. The total variation that is the sum of the principal eigenvalues of the covariance matrix [261], usually corresponds to the 95%–98% of the cumulative sum of the eigenvalues. Tiwari et al. used PCA in order to reduce the complexity of feature space [127,150,151,154].

Sparse-PCA is another approach for feature extraction and dimension reduction [263]. Similarly to PCA, this approach projects the data as a linear combination of input data. However, instead of using original data, it uses a sparse representation of the data, and therefore projects them as a linear combination of a few input components rather than all of them. Referring to Equation 10.55, the cost function of sparse-PCA is formulated to maximize the variance while maintaining the sparsity constraint:

$$\arg\max \quad \mathbf{v}^{-1}\Sigma\mathbf{v},$$
$$\text{subject to } \|\mathbf{v}\|_2 = 1, \tag{10.56}$$
$$\|\mathbf{v}\|_0 \leq k,$$

where k indicates that number of non-zero elements in $\mathbf{v}$.

Lemaitre used this approach to decompose the signal obtained from the DCE-MRI and MRSI acquisitions.

Similar to PCA decomposition, independent components analysis (ICA) projects data on independent components [264]. However, it does not require orthogonality of the space and does not assume Gaussian distribution for each independent source. Therefore, in contrast to PCA, it can recover uniquely the signals themselves rather than linear subspace in which the signals lie [265]. This method has been used by Lemaitre [127].

Nonlinear mapping has been also used for dimension reduction and is mainly based on Laplacian eigenmaps and locally linear embedding (LLE) methods. Laplacian eigenmaps, also referred to as spectral clustering in computer vision, aim to find a low-dimensional space in which the proximity of the data should be preserved from the high-dimensional space [216,217]. Therefore, two adjacent data points in the high-dimensional space should also be close in the low-dimensional space. Similarly, two distant data points in the high-dimensional space should also be distant in the low-dimensional space. To compute this projection, an adjacency matrix is defined as follows:

$$W(i, j) = \exp\|\mathbf{x}_i - \mathbf{x}_j\|_2, \tag{10.57}$$

where $\mathbf{x}_i$ and $\mathbf{x}_j$ are the two samples considered. Then, the low-dimensional space is found by solving the generalized eigenvectors-eigenvalues problem:

$$(D - W)\mathbf{y} = \lambda D\mathbf{y}, \tag{10.58}$$

where D is a diagonal matrix such that $D(i, i) = \sum_j W(j, i)$. Finally the low-dimensional space is defined by the k eigenvectors of the k smallest eigenvalues [217]. Tiwari et al. [149,151,152] and Viswanath et al. [158] used this spectral clustering to project their feature vector into a low-dimensional space. The feature space in these studies is usually composed of features extracted from a single or multiple modalities and then concatenated before applying the Laplacian eigenmaps dimension reduction technique.

Tiwari et al. used a slightly different approach by combining the Laplacian eigenmaps techniques with a prior multi-kernel learning strategy [151,155]. First, multiple features are extracted from multiple modalities. The features of a single modality are then mapped to a higher-dimensional space via the Kernel trick [266], namely a Gaussian kernel. Then, each kernel is linearly combined to obtain a combined kernel K and the adjacency matrix W is computed. Finally, the same scheme as in the Laplacian eigenmaps is applied. However, in order to use the combined kernel, Equation 10.58 is rewritten as

$$K(D-W)K^{T}\mathbf{y} = \lambda KDK^{T}\mathbf{y}, \tag{10.59}$$

which is solved as a generalized eigenvectors-eigenvalues problem as previously. Viswanath et al. used Laplacian eigenmaps inside a bagging framework in which multiple embeddings are generated by successively selecting feature dimensions [161].

LLE is another widely used nonlinear dimension reduction technique, first proposed in Roweis and Saul [267]. LLE is based on the fact that a data point in the feature space is characterized by its neighborhood. Thus, each data point in the high-dimensional space is transformed to represent a linear combination of its k-nearest neighbors. This can be expressed as

$$\hat{\mathbf{x}}_i = \sum_j W(i, j)\mathbf{x}_j, \tag{10.60}$$

where $\hat{\mathbf{x}}_i$ are the data points estimated using its neighboring data points $\mathbf{x}_j$, and W is the weight matrix. The weight matrix W is estimated using a least square optimization as in Equation 10.61:

$$\widehat{W} = \arg\min_{W} \sum_i |\mathbf{x}_i - \sum_j W(i, j)\mathbf{x}_j|^2,$$
$$\text{subject to } \sum_j W(i, j) = 1. \tag{10.61}$$

Then, the essence of LLE is to project the data into a low-dimensional space, while retaining the data spatial organization. Therefore, the projection into the low-dimensional space is tackled as an optimization problem:

$$\hat{\mathbf{y}} = \arg\min_{\mathbf{y}} \sum_i |\mathbf{y}_i - \sum_j W(i, j)\mathbf{y}_j|^2. \tag{10.62}$$

This optimization is solved as an eigenvectors-eigenvalues problem by finding the kth eigenvectors corresponding to the kth smallest eigenvalues of the sparse matrix $(I-W)^{T}(I-W)$.

Tiwari et al. used a modified version of the LLE algorithm in which they applied LLE in a bagging approach with multiple neighborhood sizes [150]. The different embeddings obtained were then fused using the maximum likelihood (ML) estimation.

Another way of reducing the complexity of high-dimensional feature space is to use the family of so-called dictionary-based methods. Sparse coded features (SCF) representation has become very popular in other computer vision application and has been used by Lehaire et al. [126]. The main goal of sparse modeling is to efficiently represent the images as a linear combination of a few typical patterns, called atoms, selected from a dictionary. Sparse coding consists of three main steps: sparse approximation, dictionary learning, and low-level features projection [268].

Sparse approximation: Given a dictionary $\mathbf{D} \in \mathbb{R}^{n \times K}$ composed of K atoms and an original signal $\mathbf{y} \in \mathbb{R}^n$—that is, one feature vector—the sparse approximation corresponds to find the sparest vector $\mathbf{x} \in \mathbb{R}^K$ such that

$$\arg\min_{\mathbf{x}} \|\mathbf{y} - \mathbf{D}\mathbf{x}\|_2 \quad \text{s.t.} \|\mathbf{x}\|_0 \leq \lambda, \tag{10.63}$$

where λ is a specified sparsity level.

Solving the above optimization problem is an NP-hard problem [269]. However, approximate solutions are obtained using greedy algorithms such as matching pursuit (MP) [270] or orthogonal matching pursuit (OMP) [271,272].

Dictionary learning: As stated previously, the sparse approximation is computed given a specific dictionary **D**, which involves a learning stage from a set of training data. This dictionary is learned using K-SVD which is a generalized version of K-means clustering and uses the SVD. The dictionary is built in an iterative manner by solving the optimization problem of Equation 10.64, alternatively computing the sparse approximation of **X** and the dictionary **D**:

$$\arg\min_{\mathbf{D},\,\mathbf{X}} \| \mathbf{Y} - \mathbf{DX} \|_2 \qquad \text{s.t.} \| \mathbf{x}_i \|_1 \leq \lambda, \tag{10.64}$$

where **Y** is a training set of low-level descriptors, **X** is the associated sparse coded matrix—that is, a set of high-level descriptors—with a sparsity level λ, and **D** is the dictionary with K atoms. Given **D**, **X** is computed using the batch-OMP algorithm, while given **X**, **D** is sequentially updated, one atom at a time using SVD.

Low-level features projection: Once the dictionary is learned, each set of low-level features $\mathbf{F}_l$ previously extracted is encoded using the dictionary **D**, solving the optimization problem presented in Equation 10.63 such that $\mathbf{F}_l \simeq \mathbf{DX}_l$.

The bag of words (BoW) approach offers an alternative method [273] for feature extraction. BoW was used by Rampun et al. [143,144]. This model represents the features by creating a codebook or visual dictionary from the set of low-level features. The set of low-level features are clustered using k-means to create the dictionary with k clusters known as visual words. Once the codebook is created from the training set, the low-level descriptors are replaced by their closest word within the codebook. The final descriptor is a histogram of size k which represents the codebook occurrences for a given mapping.

The feature selection and extraction used in CAD systems are summarized in Table 10.11.

TABLE 10.11

Overview of the Feature Selection and Extraction Methods Used in CAD Systems

Dimension Reduction Methods	References
Feature Selection	
Statistical test	[127,137,138,166]
MI-based methods	[120,124,126,127,137,138,163]
Correlation-based methods	[145,185]
Feature Extraction	
Linear mapping	
PCA	[150,151]
Sparse-PCA	[127]
ICA	[127]
Non-linear mapping	
Laplacian eigenmaps	[149,151–153,158,161]
LLE and LLE-based	[150,151,158,159]
Dictionary-based learning	
Sparse coding	[126]
BoW	[143,144]

CADx: Classification

Once the feature vector has been extracted and eventually the complexity reduced, it is possible to make a decision and classify this feature vector to belong to CaP or healthy tissue. A full review of classification methods used in pattern recognition is available in Bishop [274].

Rule-Based Method

Lv et al. make use of a decision stump classifier to distinguish CaP and healthy classes [134]. Puech et al. detect CaP by implementing a given set of rules and scores based on a medical support approach [142]. During the testing, the feature vector goes through these different rules, and a final score is computed resulting in a final decision.

Clustering Methods

One of the simplest supervised machine learning classification methods is k-nearest neighbor (k-NN). In this method, a new unlabeled vector is assigned to the most represented class from its k nearest neighbors in the feature space. The parameter k is usually an odd number in order to avoid any tie case. This method is used in a number of studies [137,138,144], mainly to make a comparison with different machine learning techniques. Litjens et al. used k-NN to roughly detect potential CaP voxels before performing a region-based classification [129].

The k-means algorithm is an unsupervised clustering method in which the data is partitioned into k clusters in an iterative manner. First, k random centroids are defined in the feature space and each data point is assigned to the nearest centroid. Then, the centroid position for each cluster is updated by computing the mean of all the samples belonging to this particular cluster. Both assignment and updating are repeated until the centroids are stable. The number of clusters k is usually defined as the number of classes. This algorithm can also be used for "online" learning. In case that new data has to be incorporated, the initial centroid positions correspond to the results of a previous k-means training and is followed by the assignment-updating stage previously explained. Tiwari et al. used k-means in an iterative procedure [149,151]. Three clusters were defined corresponding to CaP, healthy, and non-prostate. Tiwari et al. repeatedly applied k-means, and at each iteration, the voxels corresponding to the largest cluster were excluded under the assumption that it was assigned to "non-prostate" cluster. The algorithm stopped when the number of voxels in all remaining clusters were smaller than a given threshold. Tiwari et al. and Viswanath et al. used k-means in a repetitive manner in order to be less sensitive to the centroids initialization [150,158,159]. Thus, k clusters are generated T times and the final assignment is performed by majority voting using a co-association matrix as proposed in Fred and Jain [275].

Linear Model Classifiers

Linear discriminant analysis (LDA) is used as a classification method in which the optimal linear separation between two classes is found by maximizing the interclass variance and minimizing the intraclass variance [276]. The linear discriminant function is defined as follows:

$$\delta_k(\mathbf{x}_i) = \mathbf{x}_i^\mathsf{T} \Sigma^{-1} \mu_k - \frac{1}{2} \mu_k^\mathsf{T} \Sigma^{-1} \mu_k + \log(\pi_k), \tag{10.65}$$

where $\mathbf{x}_i = \{x_1, x_2, \ldots, x_n\}$ is an unlabeled feature vector of n features, Σ is the covariance matrix of the training data, μ_k is the mean vector of the class k, and π_k is the prior probability of class k. To perform the classification, a sample $\mathbf{x}_i$ is assigned to the class that maximizes the discriminant function as in Equation 10.66:

$$C(\mathbf{x}_i) = \arg \max_k \delta_k(\mathbf{x}_i), \tag{10.66}$$

LDA has been used in numerous studies [114,119,137,138,166].

Logistic regression is also used to perform binary classification and provides the probability of an observation to belong to a class. The posterior probability of one of the classes, c_1 is written as

$$p(c_1 \mid \mathbf{x}_i) = \frac{1}{1 + \exp(-\mathbf{w}^T \mathbf{x}_i)}, \tag{10.67}$$

with $p(c_2 \mid \mathbf{x}_i) = 1 - p(c_1 \mid \mathbf{x}_i)$ and where $\mathbf{w}$ is the vector of the regression parameters allowing to obtain a linear combination of the input feature vector $\mathbf{x}_i$. Thus, an unlabeled observation $\mathbf{x}_i$ is assigned to the class that maximizes the posterior probability as shown in Equation 10.68:

$$C(\mathbf{x}_i) = \arg \max_k p(C = k \mid \mathbf{x}_i). \tag{10.68}$$

From Equation 10.67, one can see that the key to classification using a logistic regression model is to infer the set of parameters $\mathbf{w}$ through a learning stage using a training set. This vector of parameters $\mathbf{w}$ is inferred by estimating the maximum likelihood. This step is performed through an optimization scheme, using a quasi-Newton method [226], which seeks in an iterative manner for the local minimum in the derivative of Equation 10.67. This method has been used to create a linear probabilistic model in several studies [123,126,142,185].

Nonlinear Model Classifier

Viswanath et al. used quadratic discriminant analysis (QDA) instead of LDA [162]. Unlike LDA in which one assumes that the class covariance matrix Σ is identical for all classes, a covariance matrix Σ_k specific to each class is computed. Thus, Equation 10.65 becomes

$$\delta_k(\mathbf{x}_i) = \mathbf{x}_i^T \Sigma_k^{-1} \mu_k - \frac{1}{2} \mu_k^T \Sigma_k^{-1} \mu_k + \log(\pi_k), \tag{10.69}$$

where $\mathbf{x}_i$ has additional terms corresponding to the pairwise products of individual features such as $\{x_1, x_2, \ldots, x_n, x_1^2, x_1 x_2, \ldots x_n^2\}$. The classification scheme in the case of the QDA is identical to Equation 10.66.

Probabilistic Classifiers

The most commonly used classifier is the naive Bayes classifier which is a probabilistic classifier assuming independence between each feature dimension [277]. This classifier is based on Bayes' theorem:

$$p(C = k \mid \mathbf{x}) = \frac{p(C) p(\mathbf{x} \mid C)}{p(\mathbf{x})}, \tag{10.70}$$

where $p(C = k \mid \mathbf{x})$ is the posterior probability, $p(C)$ is the prior probability, $p(\mathbf{x} \mid C)$ is the likelihood, and $p(\mathbf{x})$ is the evidence. However, the evidence term is usually discarded since it is not class dependent and plays the role of a normalization term. Hence, in a classification scheme, an unlabeled observation is classified to the class which maximizes the posterior probability as

$$C(\mathbf{x}_i) = \arg \max_k p(C = k \mid \mathbf{x}_i), \tag{10.71}$$

$$p(C = k \mid \mathbf{x}_i) = p(C = k) \prod_{j=1}^{n} p(x_{ij}, \mid C = k), \tag{10.72}$$

where d is the number of dimensions of the feature vector $\mathbf{x}_i = \{x_{i1}, \cdots, x_{id}\}$. Usually, a model includes both the prior and likelihood probabilities, and it is common to use an equal prior probability for each class or eventually a value based on the relative frequency derived from the training set. Regarding the likelihood probability, it is common to choose a Gaussian distribution to characterize each class. Thus, each class is characterized by two parameters: (i) the mean and (ii) the standard deviation. These parameters are inferred from the training set by using the maximum likelihood estimation (MLE) approach. The naive Bayes classifier has been used in numerous studies [117,118,121,136–138,143–145,185].

Ensemble Learning Classifiers

AdaBoost (AdB) is an adaptive method based on an ensemble learning method, initially proposed by Freund and Schapire [278]. AdB linearly combines several weak learners resulting in a final strong classifier. A weak learner is defined as a classification method performing slightly better than a random classifier. Popular choices regarding the weak learner classifiers are decision stump or decision tree learners such as iterative dichotomiser 3 (ID3) [279], C4.5 [280], and classification and regression tree (CART) [281].

AdB is considered an adaptive method in the way that the weak learners are selected. The selection is performed in an iterative manner. At each iteration t, the weak learner selected h_t corresponds to the one minimizing the classification error on a distribution of weights D_t, which is associated with the training samples. Each weak learner is assigned a weight α_t as follows:

$$\alpha_t = \frac{1}{2} \ln \frac{1 - \epsilon_t}{\epsilon_t}, \tag{10.73}$$

where ϵ_t corresponds to the classification error rate of the weak learner on the distribution of weight D_t.

Before performing a new iteration, the distribution of weight D_t is updated such that the weights associated with the misclassified samples by h_t increase and the weights of well-classified samples decrease as shown in Equation 10.74:

$$D_{t+1}(i) = \frac{D_t(i) \exp(-\alpha_t \, y_i \, h_t(\mathbf{x}_i))}{Z_t}, \tag{10.71}$$

where $\mathbf{x}_i$ is the ith sample corresponding to class y_i and Z_t is a normalization factor forcing D_{t+1} to be a probability distribution. This procedure allows to select a weak learner at the next iteration $t+1$ which will classify in priority the previous misclassified samples. Thus, after T iterations, the final strong classifier corresponds to the linear combination of the weak learners selected and the classification is performed such that

$$C(\mathbf{x}_i) = \text{sign}\left(\sum_{t=1}^{T} \alpha_t h_t(\mathbf{x}_i)\right). \tag{10.75}$$

Lopes et al. made use of the AdB classifier to perform their classification [133], while Litjens et al. used the GentleBoost variant [282] which provides a modification of the function affecting the weight at each weak classifier [130].

Gradient boosting (GB) is an ensemble classifier [283] which similarly formulated to AdB as in Equation 10.76:

$$F(x) = \sum_{m=1}^{M} \gamma_m \, h_m(x), \tag{10.76}$$

where $h_m(x)$ is a weak learner with its associated weight γ_m. As with AdB, $h_m(x)$ is chosen to minimize a loss function using the additive model F_{m-1}. The difference between AdB and GB lies in the fact that this minimization is tackled as a numerical optimization problem using the steepest descent. Lemaitre used the GB as a meta-classifier to fuse several RF classifiers [127].

RF is a classification method which is based on creating an ensemble of decision trees and was introduced by Breiman [284]. In the learning stage, multiple decision tree learners [281] are trained. However, each decision tree is trained using a different dataset. Each of these datasets corresponds to a bootstrap sample generated by randomly choosing n samples with replacement from the initial N samples available [285]. Then, randomization is also part of the decision tree growth. At each node of the decision tree, from the bootstrap sample of D dimensions, a number of $d \ll D$ dimensions are randomly selected. Finally, the dth dimension in which the classification error is minimum is used. This best "split" classifier is often evaluated using MI or the Gini index. Finally, each tree is grown as much as possible without using any pruning procedure. In the prediction stage, the unlabeled sample is introduced in each tree and each of them is assigned a class. Finally, it is common to use a majority voting approach to choose the final class label. The RF classifier has been used in a number of studies [123,127,130,143–145,147,154–157,160,185].

Probabilistic boosting-tree is another ensemble learning classifier which shares principles with AdB but uses them inside a decision tree [286]. In the training stage, the probabilistic boosting-tree method grows a decision tree and at each node, a strong classifier is learned in an almost comparable scheme to AdB. Once the strong learner is trained, the training set is split into two subsets which are used to train the next strong classifiers in the next descending nodes. Thus, three cases are conceivable to decide in which branch to propagate each sample training $\mathbf{x}_i$:

- If $q(+1, \mathbf{x}_i) - 1/2 > \epsilon$ then $\mathbf{x}_i$ is propagated to the right branch set and a weight $w_i = 1$ is assigned.
- If $q(-1, \mathbf{x}_i) - 1/2 > \epsilon$ then $\mathbf{x}_i$ is propagated to the left branch set and a weight $w_i = 1$ is assigned.
- Else $\mathbf{x}_i$ will be propagated in both branches with $w_i = q(+1, \mathbf{x}_i)$ in the right branch and $w_i = q(-1, \mathbf{x}_i)$ in the left branch.

With $\mathbf{w} = w_i, i = \{1, \cdots, N\}$ corresponding to distribution of weights, N the number of samples as in AdB and $q(\cdot)$ is defined as

$$q(+1, \mathbf{x}_i) = \frac{\exp(2H(\mathbf{x}_i))}{1 + \exp(2H(\mathbf{x}_i))}, \tag{10.77}$$

$$q(-1, \mathbf{x}_i) = \frac{\exp(-2H(\mathbf{x}_i))}{1 + \exp(-2H(\mathbf{x}_i))}. \tag{10.78}$$

Employing such a scheme tends to divide the data in such a way that positive and negative samples are naturally split as shown in Figure 10.17. In the classification stage, the unlabeled sample $\mathbf{x}$ is propagated through the tree, where at each node, it is classified by each strong classifier previously learned and where an estimation of the posterior distribution is computed. The posterior distribution corresponds to the sum of the posterior distribution at each node of the decision tree. The probabilistic boosting-tree classifier has been used in several studies [152–154,161].

Kernel Method

A Gaussian process for classification is a kernel method in which it is assumed that the data can be represented by a single sample from a multivariate Gaussian distribution [287]. In the case of linear logistic regression for classification, the posterior probability is expressed as

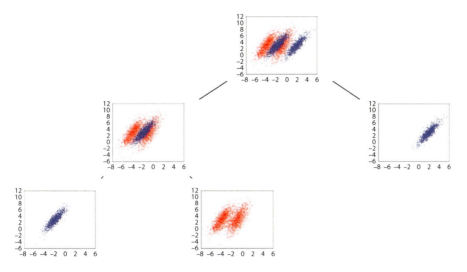

FIGURE 10.17 Representation of the capabilities of the probabilistic boosting-tree algorithm to split the positive and negative samples at each node of the tree.

$$p(y_i | \mathbf{x}_i, \mathbf{w}) = \sigma(y_i \, f(\mathbf{x}_i)), \tag{10.79}$$

$$f(\mathbf{x}_i) = \mathbf{x}_i^\mathsf{T} \mathbf{w},$$

where $\sigma(\cdot)$ is the logistic function and $\mathbf{w}$ are the parameters vector of the model. Thus, the classification using Gaussian processes is based on assigning a Gaussian process prior over the function $f(\mathbf{x})$ which is characterized by a mean function $\bar{f}$ and covariance function K. Therefore, in the training stage, the best mean and covariance functions have to be inferred in regard to our training data using a Newton optimization and a Laplacian approximation. The prediction stage is performed in two stages. First, for a new observation $\mathbf{x}_*$, the corresponding probability $p(f(\mathbf{x}_*) | f(\mathbf{x}))$ is computed such that

$$p(f(x_*) | f(x)) = \mathcal{N}(K_* K^{-1} \bar{f}, K_{**} - K_* (K')^{-1} K_*^T),$$

$$K' = K + W^{-1}, \tag{10.80}$$

$$W = \nabla\nabla \log p(y | f(x)),$$

where K_{**} is the covariance function $k(\mathbf{x}_*, \mathbf{x}_*)$ the testing sample $\mathbf{x}_*$, and K_* is the covariance function $k(\mathbf{x}, \mathbf{x}_*)$ of training-testing samples $\mathbf{x}$ and $\mathbf{x}_*$. Then, the function $f(\mathbf{x}_*)$ is squashed using the sigmoid function and the probability of the class membership is defined such that

$$C(x_*) = \sigma\left(\frac{\bar{f}(x_*)}{\sqrt{1 + \mathrm{var}(f(x_*))}} \right). \tag{10.81}$$

Only Kelm et al. used Gaussian process for classification of MRSI data [123].

Sparse Kernel Methods

In a classification scheme using Gaussian processes, when a prediction is performed, the whole training data are used to assign a label to the new observations. That is why this method is also called a kernel method. The sparse kernel category is composed of methods that rely on only a few labeled observations of the training set to assign the label of new observations [274].

SVM is a sparse kernel method aimed at finding the best linear hyper-plane—nonlinear separation is discussed further—which separates two classes such that the margin between the two classes is maximized [288]. The margin is in fact the region defined by two hyper-planes splitting the two classes, such that there are no points lying in between. The distance between these two hyper-planes is equal to $\frac{2}{\|\mathbf{w}\|}$ where $\mathbf{w}$ is the normal vector of the hyper-plane splitting the classes. Thus, maximizing the margin is equivalent to minimizing the norm $\|\mathbf{w}\|$. Hence, this problem is solved by an optimization approach and formalized as

$$\underset{\mathbf{w}}{\arg\min} \quad \frac{1}{2}\|\mathbf{w}^2\|, \tag{10.82}$$
$$\text{subject to} \quad y_i(\mathbf{w}.\mathbf{x}_i - b) \geq 1, i = \{1, \dots, N\},$$

where $\mathbf{x}_i$ is a training sample with is corresponding class label y_i. From Equation 10.82, it is important to notice that only few points from the set of N points are selected which later define the hyper-plane. This constraint is imposed in the optimization problem using Lagrange multipliers α. All points that are not lying on the margin are assigned a corresponding $\alpha_i = 0$, which is formalized as Equation 10.83:

$$\underset{\mathbf{w},b}{\arg\min}\underset{\alpha\geq0}{\max}\left\{\frac{1}{2}\|\mathbf{w}\|^2 - \sum_{i=1}^{n}\alpha_i[y_i(\mathbf{w}\cdot\mathbf{x}_i - b) - 1]\right\}. \tag{10.83}$$

The different parameters are inferred using quadratic programming. This version of SVM is known as hard-margin since no points can lie in the margin area. However, it is highly probable not to find any hyper-plane splitting the classes such as specified previously. Thus, a soft-margin optimization approach has been proposed [289], where points have the possibility to lie on the margin but at the cost of a penalty ξ_i which is minimized in the optimization process such that

$$\underset{w,\xi,b}{\arg\min}\underset{\alpha,\beta}{\max}\left\{\frac{1}{2}\|\mathbf{w}\|^2 + C\sum_{i=1}^{n}\xi_i - \sum_{i=1}^{n}\alpha_i[y_i(\mathbf{w}\cdot\mathbf{x}_i - b) - 1 + \xi_i] - \sum_{i=1}^{n}\beta_i\xi_i\right\}. \tag{10.84}$$

The decision to assign the label to a new observation $\mathbf{x}_i$ is taken such that

$$C(\mathbf{x}_i) = \text{sign}\left(\sum_{n=1}^{N}\alpha_n(\mathbf{x}_n.\mathbf{x}_i) + b_0\right), \tag{10.85}$$

where $\mathbf{x}_n | n = \{1, \cdots, S\}$, S being the support vectors.

SVM can also be used as a nonlinear classifier by performing a Kernel trick [290]. The original data $\mathbf{x}$ is projected to a high-dimensional space in which it is assumed that a linear hyper-plane splits the two classes. Different kernels are popular such as the RBF kernel, polynomial kernels, or sigmoid kernels. In CAD for CaP systems, SVM is the most popular classification method and has been used in a multitude of research works [100,115,116,119,120,122,124,126,128,129,132,133,137–141,148,154,157,163–166].

Relevant vector machine (RVM) is a sparse version of Gaussian process previously presented, proposed by Tipping [291]. RVM is identical to a Gaussian process with the following covariance function [292]:

$$K_{\text{RVM}}(\mathbf{x}_p, \mathbf{x}_q) = \sum_{j=1}^{M}\frac{1}{\alpha_j}\Phi_j(\mathbf{x}_p)\Phi_j(\mathbf{x}_q), \tag{10.86}$$

where $\phi(\cdot)$ is a Gaussian basis function, $\mathbf{x}_i | i = \{1, \cdots, N\}$ are the N training points, and a are the weights vector. As mentioned in Quinonero-Candela [292], the sparsity regarding the relevance vector arises for some j, the weight $\alpha_j^{-1} = 0$. The set of weights a is inferred using the expectation maximization algorithm. Ozer et al. used RVM to make a comparison with SVM for the task of CaP detection [139,140].

Neural Network

Multilayer perceptron is a feed-forward neural network considered as the most successful model of this kind in pattern recognition [274]. The most well-known model used is based on two layers where a prediction of an observation is computed as

$$C(\mathbf{x}_n, w_{ij}^{(1)}, w_{kj}^{(2)}) = \sigma \left[\sum_{j=0}^{M} w_{kj}^{(2)} h \left(\sum_{i=0}^{D} w_{ij}^{(1)} x_{in} \right) \right], \tag{10.87}$$

where $h(\cdot)$ and $\sigma(\cdot)$ are two activation functions, usually nonlinear, and $w_{ij}^{(1)}$ and $w_{kj}^{(2)}$ are the weights associated with the linear combination with the input feature $\mathbf{x}_n$ and the hidden unit.

A graphical representation of this network is presented in Figure 10.18. Relating Figure 10.18 with Equation 10.87, it can be noted that this network is composed of some successive nonlinear mapping of the input data. First, a linear combination of the input vector $\mathbf{x}_n$ is mapped into some hidden units through a set of weights $w_{ij}^{(1)}$. This combination becomes nonlinear by the use of the activation function $h(\cdot)$, which is usually chosen to be a sigmoid function. Then, the output of the networks consists of a linear combination of the hidden units and the set of weights $w_{kj}^{(2)}$. This combination is also mapped nonlinearly using an activation function $\sigma(\cdot)$, which is usually a logistic function. Thus, the training of such a network resides in finding the best weights $w_{ij}^{(1)}$ and $w_{kj}^{(2)}$, which model the best the training data. The error of this model is computed as

$$E(w_{ij}^{(1)}, w_{kj}^{(2)}) = \frac{1}{2} \sum_{n=1}^{N} \left(C(\mathbf{x}_n, w_{ij}^{(1)}, w_{kj}^{(2)}) - y(\mathbf{x}_n) \right)^2, \tag{10.88}$$

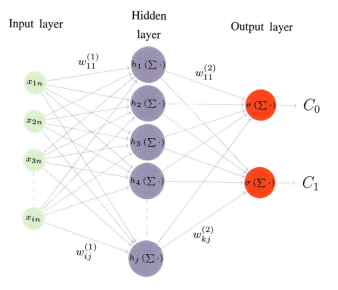

FIGURE 10.18 Representation of a neural network of the multilayer perceptron family.

where $\mathbf{x}_n | n = \{1, \cdots, N\}$ are the N training vectors with their corresponding class label $y(\mathbf{x}_n)$.

Therefore, the best set of weights is inferred in an optimization framework where the error $E(\cdot)$ needs to be minimized. This optimization is performed using a gradient descent method where the derivative of Equation 10.88 is computed using the backpropagation algorithm proposed by [293]. This type of network has been used multiple times [135,141,145,156,157].

Probabilistic neural networks are another type of feed-forward network that is derived from the multilayer perceptron case and has been proposed by Specht [294]. This classifier is modeled by changing the activation function $h(\cdot)$ in Equation 10.87 to an exponential function such that

$$h(\mathbf{x}_n) = \exp\left(-\frac{(\mathbf{w}_j - \mathbf{x})^{\mathrm{T}}(\mathbf{w}_j - \mathbf{x})}{2\sigma^2}\right), \tag{10.89}$$

where σ is a free parameter set by the user.

The other difference of the probabilistic neural networks compared with the multilayer perceptron networks resides in the architecture as shown in Figure 10.19. This network is formed by two hidden layers. The first hidden layer consists of the pattern layer, in which the mapping is done using Equation 10.89. This pattern layer is subdivided into a number of groups corresponding to the number of classes. The second hidden layer corresponds to the summation layer which simply sums the output of each subgroup of the pattern layer. This method is used in several studies [112,113,161].

Graphical Model Classifiers

Markov random field (MRF) is used as a lesion segmentation method to detect CaP. First, let define s as a pixel that belongs to a certain class denoted by ω_s. The labeling process is defined as $\omega = \{\omega_s, s \in I\}$, where I is the set of all the pixels inside the image. The observations corresponding to SI in the image are noted $\mathcal{F} = \{f_s | s \in I\}$. Thus, the image process $\mathcal{F}$ represents the deviation

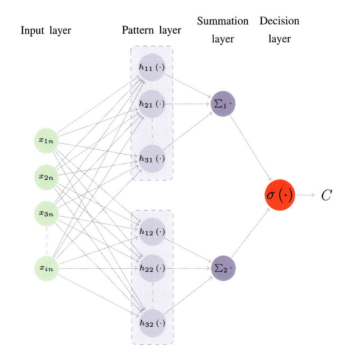

FIGURE 10.19 Representation of a neural network of the probabilistic neural network family.

from the labeling process ω [295]. Hence, lesion segmentation is equivalent to estimating the best $\hat{\omega}$ which maximizes the posterior probability $p(\omega|\mathcal{F})$. Thus, using a Bayesian approach, this problem is formulated such that

$$p(\omega|\mathcal{F}) = \arg\max_{\omega} \prod_{s\in I} p(f_s|\omega_s)\, p(\omega). \tag{10.90}$$

It is generally assumed that $p(f_s|\omega_s)$ follows a Gaussian distribution and that the pixels classes $\lambda = \{1, 2\}$ for a binary classification are characterized by their respective mean μ_λ and standard deviation σ_λ. Then, ω is a Markov random field, thus

$$p(\omega) = \frac{1}{Z}\exp\left(-U(\omega)\right), \tag{10.91}$$

where Z is a normalization factor to obtain a probability value, and $U(\cdot)$ is the energy function.

Thus, the segmentation problem is solved as an optimization problem where the energy function $U(\cdot)$ has to be minimized. There are different possibilities to define the energy function $U(\cdot)$. However, it is common to define the energy function such that it combines two types of potential function: (i) a local term relative to the pixel itself and (ii) a smoothing prior that embeds neighborhood information which penalizes the energy function affecting the region homogeneity. This optimization of such a function can be performed using an algorithm such as iterated conditional modes [295]. Liu et al. and Ozer et al. used MRF as an unsupervised method to segment lesions in mpMRI images [131,140]. Artan et al. and Chung et al. used conditional random fields instead of MRF for MRI segmentation [115,116,120]. The difference between these two methods resides in the fact that conditional probabilities are defined as

$$p(\omega|\mathcal{F}) = \frac{1}{Z}\exp\left[-\sum_{s\in I}V_{C1}(\omega_s\,|\,\mathcal{F}) - \sum_{\{s,\,r\}\in C}V_{C2}(\omega_s,\omega_r|\mathcal{F})\right]. \tag{10.92}$$

$V_{C1}(\cdot)$ is the state (or partition) feature function and $V_{C2}(\cdot)$ is the transition (or edge) feature function [296].

Classification methods used to distinguish CaP from healthy tissue in CAD systems are summarized in Table 10.12.

MODEL VALIDATION

In pattern recognition, the use of model validation techniques to assess the performance of a classifier plays an important role in reporting results. Two techniques are broadly used in the development of CAD systems and are summarized in Table 10.13. The most popular technique used in CAD systems is the leave-one-out cross-validation (LOOCV) technique. From the whole data, one patient is kept for validation and the other cases are used for training. This manipulation is repeated until each patient has been used for validation. This technique is popular when working with a limited number of patients, allowing for training on a representative number of cases even with a small dataset. However, LOOCV suffers from a large variance and is considered as an unreliable estimate [297].

The other technique is the k-CV technique which is based on splitting the dataset into k subsets where the samples are randomly selected. Then, one fold is kept for testing and the remaining

TABLE 10.12

Overview of the Classifiers Used in CAD Systems

Classifier	References
Rule-Based Method	[134,142]
Clustering Methods	
k-means clustering	[149–151]
k-NN	[129,137,138,144]
Linear Model Classifiers	
LDA	[114,119,130,137,138,166]
Logistic regression	[123,125,126,185]
Nonlinear Classifier	
QDA	[162]
Probabilistic Classifier	
Naive Bayes	[117,118,121,136–138,143–145,185]
Ensemble Learning Classifiers	
AdB	[130,133]
GB	[127]
RF	[123,127,130,143–145,147,154–157,160,185]
Probabilistic boosting tree	[151,153,154]
Kernel Method	
Gaussian processes	[123]
Sparse Kernel Methods	
SVM	[100,115,116,119,120,122,124,126,128,129,132,133,137–141,148,154,157,163–166]
RVM	[139,140]
Neural Network	
Multiple layer perceptron	[135,141,145,156,157]
Probabilistic neural network	[112,113,161]
Graphical Model Classifiers	
Markov random field	[131,140]
Conditional random field	[115,116,120]

TABLE 10.13

Overview of the Model Validation Techniques Used in CAD Systems

Model Validation Techniques	References
LOOCV	[100,112–121,123,124,126,129,130,136–140,142,155,161,163,165]
k-CV	[128,141,143–146,151–154,156,157,160,162,166,185]

subsets are used for training. The classification is then repeated as in the LOOCV technique. In fact LOOCV is a particular case of k-CV when k equals the number of patients. In the reviewed papers, the typical values used for k have been set to 3 and 5. k-CV is regarded as more appropriate than LOOCV, but the number of patients in the dataset needs to be large enough for the results to be meaningful.

TABLE 10.14

Overview of the Evaluation Metrics Used in CAD Systems

Evaluation Metrics	References
Accuracy	[115,116,131,148,154]
Sensitivity—specificity	[100,115–118,121,124,131,133,136,139,140,141,147,150,151,156–159]
ROC—AUC	[100,113,114,119,121–123,125,126,132–138,143–146,152–155,160–165,185]
FROC	[128,129,166]
Dice's coefficient	[115,116,131,139]

EVALUATION MEASURES

Several metrics are used in order to assess the performance of a classifier and are summarized in Table 10.14. Voxels in the MRI image are classified into healthy or malign tissue and compared with a ground-truth. This allows to compute a confusion matrix by counting true positive (TP), true negative (TN), false positive (FP), and false negative (FN) samples. From this analysis, different statistics are extracted.

The first statistic used is the accuracy which is computed as the ratio of true detection to the number of samples. However, depending on the strategy employed in the CAD work-flow, this statistic is highly biased by a high number of true negative samples which boost the accuracy score, overestimating the actual performance of the classifier. That is why, the most common statistics computed are sensitivity and specificity defined in Equations 10.93 and 10.94, respectively. The metrics give a full overview of the performance of the classifier.

$$SE = \frac{TP}{TP + FN},$$ (10.93)

$$SP = \frac{TN}{TN + FP}.$$ (10.94)

These statistics are also used to compute the receiver operating characteristic (ROC) curves [298], which give information about voxelwise classification. This analysis represents graphically the sensitivity as a function of $(1 - \text{specificity})$, which is in fact the false positive rate, by varying the discriminative threshold of the classifier. By varying this threshold, more true negative samples are found but often at the cost of detecting more false negatives. However, this fact is interesting in CAD since it is possible to obtain a high sensitivity and to ensure that no cancers are missed even if more false alarms have to be investigated or the opposite. A statistic derived from ROC analysis is the area under the curve (AUC) which corresponds to the area under the ROC and is a measure used to make comparisons between models.

The free-response receiver operating characteristic (FROC) extends the ROC analysis but to a lesion-based level. The same confusion matrix is computed where the sample is not pixels but lesions. However, it is important to define what is a true positive sample in that case. Usually, a lesion is considered as a true positive sample if the region detected by the classifier overlaps "sufficiently" the one delineated in the ground-truth. However, "sufficiently" is a subjective measure defined by each researcher and can correspond only to one pixel. However, an overlap of 30%–50% is usually adopted. Finally, in addition to the overlap measure, Dice's coefficient is often computed to evaluate the accuracy of the lesion localization. This coefficient consists of the ratio between twice the number of pixels in common and the sum of the pixels of the lesions in the ground-truth GT and the output of the classifier S, defined as shown in Equation 10.95:

$$Q_D = \frac{2|GT \cap S|}{|GT| + |S|}.$$ (10.95)

DISCUSSION

RESULTS REPORTED

As discussed previously in section "Evaluation Measures," different metrics have been used to report results. A comparison of the different methods reviewed is given depending on the metric used in field of research as well as the type of MRI scanner used, that is, 1.5 T or 3 T. For each field, the *best classification performance* obtained in each study have been reported in these figures. The results in terms of AUC-ROC are depicted in Figure 10.20. The results vary from 71% to 97% for some experiments with a 1.5 T MRI scanner and from 77% to 95% with a 3 T MRI scanner.

The results with regard to sensitivity and specificity are reported in Figure 10.21. In the case of data collected with a 1.5 T MRI scanner, the sensitivity ranges from 74% to 100% and the specificity from 43% to 93%. For experiments carried out with a 3 T MRI scanner, the sensitivity varies from 60% to 99% and the specificity from 66% to 100%. Four studies also use FROC analysis to report their results and are reported in Figure 10.22.

COMPARISON

We would like to stress the following findings drawn during the review of the different studies:

1. Quantitatively, it is difficult to make a fair comparison between the different studies reviewed. Different factors come into play to elucidate this fact. Mainly a lack of standardization has to be pointed out in regard to experimental evaluation: (i) different datasets are used during the evaluation of the frameworks developed, hindering an inter-study comparison (the same conclusion has been recently drawn by Litjens et al. [130] supporting this

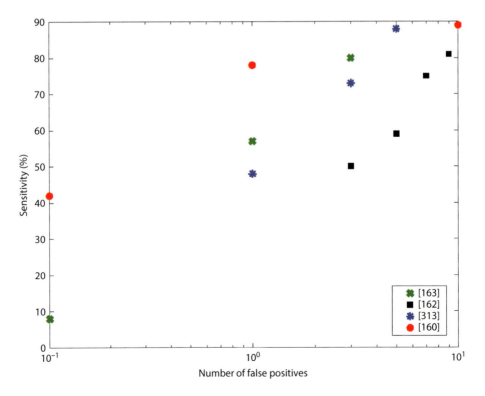

FIGURE 10.20 Comparison in terms of FROC of the methods using data from 3 T MRI scanner.

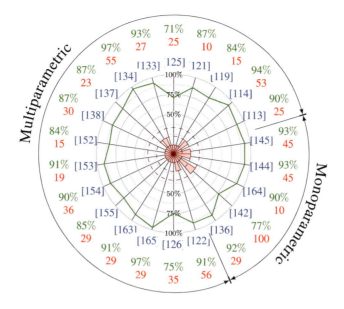

(a)

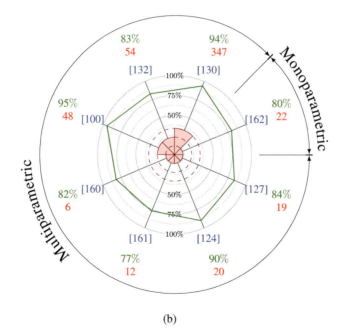

(b)

FIGURE 10.21 Numerical and graphical comparison of the results in terms of AUC for 1.5 T (a) and 3 T (b) MRI scanners. The green values represent the metric and are graphically reported in the green curve in the center of the figure. The red values and areas correspond to the number of patients in the dataset. The numbers between brackets in blue correspond to the reference as reported in Table 10.2.

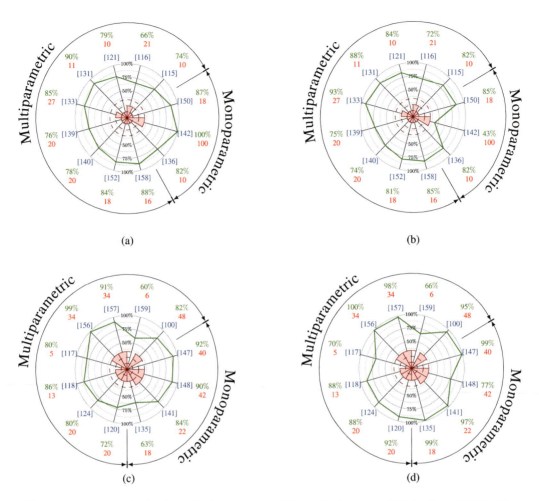

FIGURE 10.22 Numerical and graphical comparison of the results in terms of SE (a), (c) and SP (b), (d) for 1.5 T and 3 T MRI scanners. The values in green represent the metric and are graphically reported in the green curve in the center of the figure. The red values and areas correspond to the number of patients in the dataset. The numbers between brackets in blue correspond to the reference as reported in Table 10.2.

argument); and (ii) the experimental results are not reported with a common metric which leads to the inability to compare the different studies.

2. However, multiple studies reported some performance improvements using mpMRI techniques instead of monoparametric imaging techniques. Considering only the most recent studies proposing CADe-CADx frameworks, the following results can be highlighted. Viswanath et al. obtained an AUC of 77% using an ensemble learning approach combining the features from the three MRI modalities, that is, T2-W-MRI, DCE–MRI, and DW-MRI, while the results obtained as stand-alone modalities range from 62% to 65% [161]. Tiwari et al. draw similar conclusions by using T2-W-MRI and MRSI modalities as in both stand-alone and multiparametric frameworks with an improved AUC ranging from 57%–76% to 85% [155]. The most recent work of Litjens et al. obtained an improved AUC metric from 71% to 76% considering each modality separately, that is, T2-W-MRI, DCE-MRI, and DW-MRI—to 89% in their mpMRI framework.

3. The studies comparing particular combinations of more than a single modality give rise to the same fact [128,130,132,140]: using three modalities led to better performances than using any combination of two modalities.

4. Unlike remark 2, no straightforward conclusions can be given regarding the classification performance using each modality in a stand-alone framework. With the modalities being processed by different methods, it does not allow us to conclude if a particular modality by itself is more suitable than another. However, we are able to distinguish some interesting trends which deserve the attention of the community. Tiwari et al. observed that MRSI is a more suitable modality than T2-W to highlight CaP [152,154,155]. Moreover, ADC maps have demonstrated a better discriminative power than T2-W as well [100,125,161]. Lately, Litjens et al. observed that the DW-MRI modality is more suitable than both DCE-MRI and T2-W-MRI to distinguish CaP in their CADx system [130]. Recently, Rampun et al. showed, however, some promising results using T2-W-MRI only in conjunction with textons and BoW; this study should be transposed to other MRI modalities [144].

5. Furthermore, mpMRI has attracted the attention of both radiologists and computer vision researchers. Indeed, pioneer research groups included new modalities over years when at the same time, new research groups directly introduced mpMRI CAD systems. These facts lead us to think that CaP researches will benefit from mpMRI techniques.

6. When focusing on the different modalities used, it can be pointed out that only Trigui et al. reported the use of all modalities in a single framework by incorporating the MRSI modality [156,157]. Although the results reported are promising, the detection has been performed at MRSI scale. Lemaitre performed a similar study but at a finer resolution (i.e., T2-W-MRI) [127]. They concluded that MRSI was significantly improving the classification performance for CaP detection.

7. Lately, three studies focused on developing a region-based classification in which the PZ will be analyzed separately [129,130,162]. The promising results obtained indicate that this strategy should be further investigated.

8. Recent studies are using quantitative features in addition to SI. It seems that these quantitative features provide uncorrelated information with respect to SI features and should lead to better classification performance when combined all together.

9. Regarding the methods used in the "image regularization"—that is, pre-processing, segmentation, and registration—it is particularly difficult to distinguish the benefit of one method over another since none of the studies focus on comparing these processing stages. The focus is usually entirely based on the "image classification" framework where different methods are directly compared. Note that the performance of a classifier is highly linked with the features vector extracted from particular data. Hence, one cannot conclude that one machine learning method is more appropriate than another, but we can identify a trend in which SVM as well as ensemble learning classifiers—that is, AdaBoost, GentleBoost, and RF—seem to perform better than neural network, LDA, or naive Bayes.

10. We would like to draw the attention of the reader to the feature extraction/selection stage. This processing could reduce the complexity and support finding a better feature space for classification. However, few studies are performing such approaches. Niaf et al., Khalvati et al., Chung et al., Rampun et al., and Lemaitre are successfully applying a scheme to reduce the number of dimensions by selecting the most discriminative features [120,124,127,137,138,145,185]. It allows them to obtain improved performances compared with a classification performed with their initial feature vector. Another group of studies also applied different feature extraction methods [126,127,143,144,149–151,153–155,158,159,162]. In these specific cases, no comparison is performed against the original data.

11. Currently, only the work of Lemaitre has tackled the problem of balancing in datasets. They found that balancing can have a positive effect on the classification performance. In our humble opinion, classification performance would benefit from further investigation in this area.

CONCLUSION

This chapter leads to some general discussions which could direct to future avenues for research. As previously mentioned, no open mpMRI is currently available. This fact leads to an impossibility to fairly compare the different algorithms designed over years. Also, the availability of a full mpMRI dataset, could lead to the development of algorithms that use all the different modalities currently available. Recalling Table 10.2, it can be noted that a single research work provides a solution using the four different modalities at the same time. Also, all the algorithms are focused only on one type of scanner, either 1.5 T and 3 T. A dataset including both these types of imaging could allow development of more generic algorithms.

Analyzing the different stages of the CAD work-flow, it is seen that the current CAD systems do not include all the pre-processing steps. It could be interesting to evaluate the improvement using these pre-processing steps on the final results. Regarding segmentation and registration of the prostate, CAD systems could greatly benefit from specific research in these areas which could lead to a better automation of those systems.

Additionally, few research works focus on the problem of imbalanced datasets. While classifying at the voxel level, the medical datasets are highly imbalanced regarding the frequencies of CaP against healthy samples. Imbalanced data substantially compromises the learning process since most of the standard machine learning algorithms expect balanced class distribution or an equal misclassification cost [299]. Therefore, it seems important to investigate this field of pattern recognition to improve the classification performance while developing CAD systems.

REFERENCES

1. K. H. Leissner and L. E. Tisell, "The weight of the human prostate," *Scand. J. Urol. Nephrol.*, vol. 13, no. 2, pp. 137–142, 1979.
2. S. Parfait, "Classification de spectres et recherche de biomarqueurs en spectroscopie par résonqnce magnétique nucléaire du proton dans les tumeurs prostatiques," PhD dissertation, Université de Bourgogne, 2010.
3. J. E. McNeal, "The zonal anatomy of the prostate," *Prostate*, vol. 2, pp. 35–49, 1981.
4. H. Hricak, G. C. Dooms, J. E. McNeal, A. S. Mark, M. Marotti, A. Avallone, M. Pelzer, E. C. Proctor, and E. A. Tanagho, "MR imaging of the prostate gland: Normal anatomy," *Am. J. Roentgenol.*, vol. 148, pp. 51–58, 1987.
5. A. Villers, A. Steg, and L. Boccon-Gibod, "Anatomy of the prostate: Review of the different models," *Eur. Urol.*, vol. 20, pp. 261–268, 1991.
6. F. V. Coakley and H. Hricak, "Radiologic anatomy of the prostate gland: A clinical approach," *Radiol. Clin. North Am.*, vol. 38, pp. 15–30, 2000.
7. J. Ferlay, H. R. Shin, F. Bray, D. Forman, C. Mathers, and D. M. Parkin, "Estimates of worldwide burden of cancer in 2008: GLOBOCAN 2008,"*Int. J. Cancer*, vol. 127, no. 12, pp. 2893–2917, 2010.
8. R. Siegel, D. Naishadham, and A. Jemal, "Cancer statistics, 2013," *CA Cancer J. Clin.*, vol. 63, no. 1, pp. 11–30, 2013.
9. American Cancer Society, "Cancer facts and figures 2013," https://www.cancer.org/research/cancer-facts-statistics/all-cancer-facts-figures/cancer-facts-figures-2013.html, 2013, accessed August 1, 2013.
10. American Cancer Society, "Cancer facts and figures 2010," https://www.cancer.org/research/cancer-facts-statistics/all-cancer-facts-figures/cancer-facts-figures-2010.html, 2010, accessed August 1, 2013.
11. E. Giovannucci, Y. Liu, E. A. Platz, M. J. Stampfer, and W. C. Willett, "Risk factors for prostate cancer incidence and progression in the health professionals follow-up study,"*Int. J. Cancer*, vol. 121, no. 7, pp. 1571–1578, 2007.
12. G. D. Steinberg, B. S. Carter, T. H. Beaty, B. Childs, and P. C. Walsh, "Family history and the risk of prostate cancer," *Prostate*, vol. 17, no. 4, pp. 337–347, 1990.
13. M. L. Freedman, C. A. Haiman, N. Patterson, G. J. McDonald, A. Tandon, A. Waliszewska, K. Penney et al., "Admixture mapping identifies 8q24 as a prostate cancer risk locus in African-American men," *Proc. Natl. Acad. Sci. U.S.A.*, vol. 103, no. 38, pp. 14068–14073, 2006.

14. L. T. Amundadottir, P. Sulem, J. Gudmundsson, A. Helgason, A. Baker, B. A. Agnarsson, A. Sigurdsson et al., "A common variant associated with prostate cancer in European and African populations," *Nat. Genet.*, vol. 38, no. 6, pp. 652–658, 2006.

15. I. Agalliu, R. Gern, S. Leanza, and R. D. Burk, "Associations of high-grade prostate cancer with BRCA1 and BRCA2 founder mutations," *Clin. Cancer Res.*, vol. 15, no. 3, pp. 1112–1120, 2009.

16. R. M. Hoffman, F. D. Gilliland, J. W. Eley, L. C. Harlan, R. A. Stephenson, J. L. Stanford, P. C. Albertson, A. S. Hamilton, W. C. Hunt, and A. L. Potosky, "Racial and ethnic differences in advanced-stage prostate cancer: The Prostate Cancer Outcomes Study," *J. Natl. Cancer Inst.*, vol. 93, no. 5, pp. 388–395, 2001.

17. R. W. Ma and K. Chapman, "A systematic review of the effect of diet in prostate cancer prevention and treatment," *J. Hum. Nutr. Diet*, vol. 22, no. 3, pp. 187–199, 2009.

18. D. D. Alexander, P. J. Mink, C. A. Cushing, and B. Sceurman, "A review and meta-analysis of prospective studies of red and processed meat intake and prostate cancer," *Nutr. J.*, vol. 9, p. 50, 2010.

19. C. Rodriguez, S. J. Freedland, A. Deka, E. J. Jacobs, M. L. McCullough, A. V. Patel, M. J. Thun, and E. E. Calle, "Body mass index, weight change, and risk of prostate cancer in the Cancer Prevention Study II Nutrition Cohort," *Cancer Epidemiol. Biomarkers Prev.*, vol. 16, no. 1, pp. 63–69, 2007.

20. S. Strum and D. Pogliano, "What every doctor who treats male patients should know," *PCRI Insights*, vol. 8, no. 2, pp. 4–5, 2005.

21. G. L. Lu-Yao, P. C. Albertsen, D. F. Moore, W. Shih, Y. Lin, R. S. DiPaola, M. J. Barry, A. Zietman, M. O'Leary, E. Walker-Corkery, and S. L. Yao, "Outcomes of localized prostate cancer following conservative management," *JAMA*, vol. 302, no. 11, pp. 1202–1209, 2009.

22. G. Oster, L. Lamerato, A. G. Glass, K. E. Richert-Boe, A. Lopez, K. Chung, A. Richhariya, T. Dodge, G. G. Wolff, A. Balakumaran, and J. Edelsberg, "Natural history of skeletal-related events in patients with breast, lung, or prostate cancer and metastases to bone: A 15-year study in two large US health systems," *Support Care Cancer*, vol. 21, no. 12, pp. 3279–3286, 2013.

23. L. Ye, H. G. Kynaston, and W. G. Jiang, "Bone metastasis in prostate cancer: Molecular and cellular mechanisms (Review)," *Int. J. Mol. Med.*, vol. 20, no. 1, pp. 103–111, 2007.

24. C. L. Carrol, F. G. Sommer, J. E. McNeal, and T. A. Stamey, "The abnormal prostate: MR imaging at 1.5 T with histopathologic correlation," *Radiology*, vol. 163, no. 2, pp. 521–525, 1987.

25. J. E. McNeal, E. A. Redwine, F. S. Freiha, and T. A. Stamey, "Zonal distribution of prostatic adenocarcinoma. Correlation with histologic pattern and direction of spread," *Am. J. Surg. Pathol.*, vol. 12, no. 12, pp. 897–906, 1988.

26. T. A. Stamey, A. N. Donaldson, C. E. Yemoto, J. E. McNeal, S. Sozen, and H. Gill, "Histological and clinical findings in 896 consecutive prostates treated only with radical retropubic prostatectomy: Epidemiologic significance of annual changes," *J. Urol.*, vol. 160, no. 6 Pt 2, pp. 2412–2417, 1998.

27. R. J. Cohen, B. A. Shannon, M. Phillips, R. E. Moorin, T. M. Wheeler, and K. L. Garrett, "Central zone carcinoma of the prostate gland: A distinct tumor type with poor prognostic features," *J. Urol.*, vol. 179, no. 5, pp. 1762–1767, 2008.

28. R. Etzioni, D. F. Penson, J. M. Legler, D. di Tommaso, R. Boer, P. H. Gann, and E. J. Feuer, "Overdiagnosis due to prostate-specific antigen screening: Lessons from U.S. prostate cancer incidence trends," *J. Natl. Cancer Inst.*, vol. 94, no. 13, pp. 981–990, 2002.

29. C. M. Hoeks, J. O. Barentsz, T. Hambrock, D. Yakar, D. M. Somford, S. W. Heijmink, T. W. Scheenen et al., "Prostate cancer: Multiparametric MR imaging for detection, localization, and staging," *Radiology*, vol. 261, no. 1, pp. 46–66, 2011.

30. J. O. Barentsz, J. Richenberg, R. Clements, P. Choyke, S. Verma, G. Villeirs, O. Rouviere, V. Logager, and J. J. Futterer, "ESUR prostate MR guidelines 2012," *Eur. Radiol.*, vol. 22, no. 4, pp. 746–757, 2012.

31. D. F. Gleason, "The Veteran's Administration Cooperative Urologic Research Group: Histologic grading and clinical staging of prostatic carcinoma," in *Urologic Pathology: The Prostate*, M. Tannenbaum (Ed.), Philadelphia, PA: Lea & Febiger, pp. 171–198, 1977.

32. J. I. Epstein, W. C. Allsbrook, M. B. Amin, and L. L. Egevad, "The 2005 International Society of Urological Pathology (ISUP) consensus conference on Gleason grading of prostatic carcinoma," *Am. J. Surg. Pathol.*, vol. 29, no. 9, pp. 1228–1242, 2005.

33. N. Hara, M. Okuizumi, H. Koike, M. Kawaguchi, and V. Bilim, "Dynamic contrast-enhanced magnetic resonance imaging (DCE-MRI) is a useful modality for the precise detection and staging of early prostate cancer," *Prostate*, vol. 62, no. 2, pp. 140–147, 2005.

34. R. Chou, J. M. Croswell, T. Dana, C. Bougatsos, I. Blazina, R. Fu, K. Gleitsmann et al., "Screening for prostate cancer: A review of the evidence for the U.S. Preventive Services Task Force," *Ann. Intern. Med.*, vol. 155, no. 11, pp. 762–771, 2011.

35. G. L. Andriole, E. D. Crawford, R. L. Grubb, S. S. Buys, D. Chia, T. R. Church, M. N. Fouad et al., "Mortality results from a randomized Prostate-cancer screening trial," *N. Engl. J. Med.*, vol. 360, no. 13, pp. 1310–1319, 2009.

36. F. H. Schröder, J. Hugosson, M. J. Roobol, T. L. Tammela, S. Ciatto, V. Nelen, M. Kwiatkowski et al., "Prostate-cancer mortality at 11 years of follow-up," *N. Engl. J. Med.*, vol. 366, no. 11, pp. 981–990, 2012.

37. J. Hugosson, S. Carlsson, G. Aus, S. Bergdahl, A. Khatami, P. Lodding, C. G. Pihl, J. Stranne, E. Holmberg, and H. Lilja, "Mortality results from the Göteborg randomised population-based prostate-cancer screening trial," *Lancet Oncol.*, vol. 11, no. 8, pp. 725–732, 2010.

38. A. Heidenreich, P. A. Abrahamsson, W. Artibani, J. Catto, F. Montorsi, H. Van Poppel, M. Wirth, and N. Mottet, "Early detection of prostate cancer: European Association of Urology recommendation," *Eur. Urol.*, vol. 64, no. 3, pp. 347–354, 2013.

39. F. H. Schroder, H. B. Carter, T. Wolters, R. C. van den Bergh, C. Gosselaar, C. H. Bangma, and M. J. Roobol, "Early detection of prostate cancer in 2007. Part 1: PSA and PSA kinetics," *Eur. Urol.*, vol. 53, no. 3, pp. 468–477, 2008.

40. C. Delpierre, S. Lamy, M. Kelly-Irving, F. Molinie, M. Velten, B. Tretarre, A. S. Woronoff et al., "Life expectancy estimates as a key factor in over-treatment: The case of prostate cancer," *Cancer Epidemiol.*, vol. 37, no. 4, pp. 462–468, 2013.

41. A. Bourdoumis, A. G. Papatsoris, M. Chrisofos, E. Efstathiou, A. Skolarikos, and C. Deliveliotis, "The novel prostate cancer antigen 3 (PCA3) biomarker," *Int. Braz. J. Urol.*, vol. 36, no. 6, pp. 665–668, 2010.

42. R. Morgan, A. Boxall, A. Bhatt, M. Bailey, R. Hindley, S. Langley, H. C. Whitaker et al., "Engrailed-2 (EN2): A tumor specific urinary biomarker for the early diagnosis of prostate cancer,"*Clin. Cancer Res.*, vol. 17, no. 5, pp. 1090–1098, 2011.

43. J. Brenner, A. Chinnaiyan, and S. Tomlins, "ETS fusion genes in prostate cancer," in *Prostate Cancer*, ser. Protein Reviews, Vol. 16, D. J. Tindall (Ed.), New York: Springer, pp. 139–183, 2013.

44. C. M. Moore, A. Ridout, and M. Emberton, "The role of MRI in active surveillance of prostate cancer," *Curr. Opin. Urol.*, vol. 23, no. 3, pp. 261–267, 2013.

45. M. Noguchi, T. A. Stamey, J. E. McNeal, and C. M. Yemoto, "Relationship between systematic biopsies and histological features of 222 radical prostatectomy specimens: Lack of prediction of tumor significance for men with nonpalpable prostate cancer," *J. Urol.*, vol. 166, no. 1, pp. 104–109, 2001.

46. G. P. Haas, N. B. Delongchamps, R. F. Jones, V. Chandan, A. M. Serio, A. J. Vickers, M. Jumbelic, G. Threatte, R. Korets, H. Lilja, and G. de la Roza, "Needle biopsies on autopsy prostates: Sensitivity of cancer detection based on true prevalence," *J. Natl. Cancer Inst.*, vol. 99, no. 19, pp. 1484–1489, 2007.

47. A. V. Taira, G. S. Merrick, R. W. Galbreath, H. Andreini, W. Taubenslag, R. Curtis, W. M. Butler, E. Adamovich, and K. E. Wallner, "Performance of transperineal template-guided mapping biopsy in detecting prostate cancer in the initial and repeat biopsy setting," *Prostate Cancer Prostatic Dis.*, vol. 13, no. 1, pp. 71–77, 2010.

48. N. B. Delongchamps, M. Peyromaure, A. Schull, F. Beuvon, N. Bouazza, T. Flam, M. Zerbib, N. Muradyan, P. Legman, and F. Cornud, "Prebiopsy magnetic resonance imaging and prostate cancer detection: Comparison of random and targeted biopsies," *J. Urol.*, vol. 189, no. 2, pp. 493–499, 2013.

49. M. L. Giger, H. P. Chan, and J. Boone, "Anniversary paper: History and status of CAD and quantitative image analysis: The role of Medical Physics and AAPM," *Med. Phys.*, vol. 35, no. 12, pp. 5799–5820, 2008.

50. T. Hambrock, P. C. Vos, C. A. Hulsbergen-van de Kaa, J. O. Barentsz, and H. J. Huisman, "Prostate cancer: Computer-aided diagnosis with multiparametric 3-T MR imaging–effect on observer performance," *Radiology*, vol. 266, no. 2, pp. 521–530, 2013.

51. H. P. Chan, B. Sahiner, M. A. Helvie, N. Petrick, M. A. Roubidoux, T. E. Wilson, D. D. Adler, C. Paramagul, J. S. Newman, and S. Sanjay-Gopal, "Improvement of radiologists' characterization of mammographic masses by using computer-aided diagnosis: An ROC study," *Radiology*, vol. 212, no. 3, pp. 817–827, 1999.

52. J. C. Dean and C. C. Ilvento, "Improved cancer detection using computer-aided detection with diagnostic and screening mammography: Prospective study of 104 cancers," *Am. J. Roentgenol.*, vol. 187, no. 1, pp. 20–28, 2006.

53. F. Li, M. Aoyama, J. Shiraishi, H. Abe, Q. Li, K. Suzuki, R. Engelmann, S. Sone, H. Macmahon, and K. Doi, "Radiologists' performance for differentiating benign from malignant lung nodules on high-resolution CT using computer-estimated likelihood of malignancy," *Am. J. Roentgenol.*, vol. 183, no. 5, pp. 1209–1215, 2004.

54. N. Petrick, M. Haider, R. M. Summers, S. C. Yeshwant, L. Brown, E. M. Iuliano, A. Louie, J. R. Choi, and P. J. Pickhardt, "CT colonography with computer-aided detection as a second reader: Observer performance study," *Radiology*, vol. 246, no. 1, pp. 148–156, 2008.

55. J. V. Hegde, R. V. Mulkern, L. P. Panych, F. M. Fennessy, A. Fedorov, S. E. Maier, and C. M. Tempany, "Multiparametric MRI of prostate cancer: An update on state-of-the-art techniques and their performance in detecting and localizing prostate cancer," *J. Magn. Reson. Imaging*, vol. 37, no. 5, pp. 1035–1054, 2013.

56. H. Hricak, R. D. Williams, D. B. Spring, K. L. Moon, M. W. Hedgcock, R. A. Watson, and L. E. Crooks, "Anatomy and pathology of the male pelvis by magnetic resonance imaging," *Am. J. Roentgenol.*, vol. 141, no. 6, pp. 1101–1110, 1983.

57. R. A. Huch Boni, J. A. Boner, U. M. Lutolf, F. Trinkler, D. M. Pestalozzi, and G. P. Krestin, "Contrast-enhanced endorectal coil MRI in local staging of prostate carcinoma," *J. Comput. Assist. Tomogr.*, vol. 19, no. 2, pp. 232–237, 1995.

58. J. Kurhanewicz, D. B. Vigneron, H. Hricak, P. Narayan, P. Carroll, and S. J. Nelson, "Three-dimensional H-1 MR spectroscopic imaging of the in situ human prostate with high (0.24-0.7-cm^3) spatial resolution," *Radiology*, vol. 198, no. 3, pp. 795–805, 1996.

59. J. Scheidler, R. Petsch, U. Muller-Lisse, A. Heuck, and M. Reiser, "Echo-planar diffusion-weighted MR imaging of the prostate," in *Proceedings of the 7th Annual Meeting of ISMRM Philadelphia*, p. 1103, 1999.

60. M. G. Swanson, D. B. Vigneron, T. K. Tran, N. Sailasuta, R. E. Hurd, and J. Kurhanewicz, "Single-voxel oversampled J-resolved spectroscopy of in vivo human prostate tissue," *Magn. Reson. Med.*, vol. 45, no. 6, pp. 973–980, 2001.

61. B. Turkbey and P. L. Choyke, "Multiparametric MRI and prostate cancer diagnosis and risk stratification," *Curr. Opin. Urol.*, vol. 22, no. 4, pp. 310–315, 2012.

62. O. Akin, E. Sala, C. S. Moskowitz, K. Kuroiwa, N. M. Ishill, D. Pucar, P. T. Scardino, and H. Hricak, "Transition zone prostate cancers: Features, detection, localization, and staging at endorectal MR imaging," *Radiology*, vol. 239, no. 3, pp. 784–792, 2006.

63. L. Wang, Y. Mazaheri, J. Zhang, N. M. Ishill, K. Kuroiwa, and H. Hricak, "Assessment of biologic aggressiveness of prostate cancer: Correlation of MR signal intensity with Gleason grade after radical prostatectomy," *Radiology*, vol. 246, no. 1, pp. 168–176, 2008.

64. A. P. Kirkham, M. Emberton, and C. Allen, "How good is MRI at detecting and characterising cancer within the prostate?" *Eur. Urol.*, vol. 50, no. 6, pp. 1163–1174, 2006.

65. L. E. Quint, J. S. Van Erp, P. H. Bland, S. H. Mandell, E. A. Del Buono, H. B. Grossman, G. M. Glazer, and P. W. Gikas, "Carcinoma of the prostate: MR images obtained with body coils do not accurately reflect tumor volume," *Am. J. Roentgenol.*, vol. 156, no. 3, pp. 511–516, 1991.

66. M. Cruz, K. Tsuda, Y. Narumi, Y. Kuroiwa, T. Nose, Y. Kojima, A. Okuyama, S. Takahashi, K. Aozasa, J. O. Barentsz, and H. Nakamura, "Characterization of low-intensity lesions in the peripheral zone of prostate on pre-biopsy endorectal coil MR imaging," *Eur. Radiol.*, vol. 12, no. 2, pp. 357–365, 2002.

67. W. Liu, B. Turkbey, J. Senegas, S. Remmele, S. Xu, J. Kruecker, M. Bernardo, B. J. Wood, P. A. Pinto, and P. L. Choyke, "Accelerated T2 mapping for characterization of prostate cancer," *Magn. Reson. Med.*, vol. 65, no. 5, pp. 1400–1406, 2011.

68. G. P. Liney, M. Lowry, L. W. Turnbull, D. J. Manton, A. J. Knowles, S. J. Blackband, and A. Horsman, "Proton MR T2 maps correlate with the citrate concentration in the prostate," *NMR Biomed.*, vol. 9, no. 2, pp. 59–64, 1996.

69. G. P. Liney, L. W. Turnbull, M. Lowry, L. S. Turnbull, A. J. Knowles, and A. Horsman, "In vivo quantification of citrate concentration and water T2 relaxation time of the pathologic prostate gland using 1H MRS and MRI," *Magn. Reson. Imaging*, vol. 15, no. 10, pp. 1177–1186, 1997.

70. G. P. Liney, A. J. Knowles, D. J. Manton, L. W. Turnbull, S. J. Blackband, and A. Horsman, "Comparison of conventional single echo and multi-echo sequences with a fast spin-echo sequence for quantitative T2 mapping: Application to the prostate," *J. Magn. Reson. Imaging*, vol. 6, no. 4, pp. 603–607, 1996.

71. P. Gibbs, D. J. Tozer, G. P. Liney, and L. W. Turnbull, "Comparison of quantitative T2 mapping and diffusion-weighted imaging in the normal and pathologic prostate," *Magn. Reson. Med.*, vol. 46, no. 6, pp. 1054–1058, 2001.

72. I. Gribbestad, K. Gjesdal, G. Nilsen, S. Lundgren, M. Hjelstuen, and A. Jackson, "An introduction to dynamic contrast-enhanced MRI in oncology," in *Dynamic Contrast-Enhanced Magnetic Resonance Imaging in Oncology*, ser. Medical Radiology, A. Jackson, D. Buckley, and G. Parker (Eds.), Berlin, Germany: Springer, pp. 1–22, 2005.

73. A. R. Padhani, "Dynamic contrast-enhanced MRI in clinical oncology: Current status and future directions," *J. Magn. Reson. Imaging*, vol. 16, no. 4, pp. 407–422, 2002.

74. Y. J. Choi, J. K. Kim, N. Kim, K. W. Kim, E. K. Choi, and K. S. Cho, "Functional MR imaging of prostate cancer," *Radiographics*, vol. 27, pp. 63–75, 2007.

75. D. L. Buckley, C. Roberts, G. J. Parker, J. P. Logue, and C. E. Hutchinson, "Prostate cancer: Evaluation of vascular characteristics with dynamic contrast-enhanced T1-weighted MR imaging–initial experience," *Radiology*, vol. 233, no. 3, pp. 709–715, 2004.

76. C. G. van Niekerk, J. A. van der Laak, M. E. Borger, H. J. Huisman, J. A. Witjes, J. O. Barentsz, and C. A. Hulsbergen-van de Kaa, "Computerized whole slide quantification shows increased microvascular density in pT2 prostate cancer as compared to normal prostate tissue," *Prostate*, vol. 69, no. 1, pp. 62–69, 2009.

77. C. G. van Niekerk, J. A. Witjes, J. O. Barentsz, J. A. van der Laak, and C. A. Hulsbergen-van de Kaa, "Microvascularity in transition zone prostate tumors resembles normal prostatic tissue," *Prostate*, vol. 73, no. 5, pp. 467–475, 2013.

78. P. Carmeliet and R. K. Jain, "Angiogenesis in cancer and other diseases," *Nature*, vol. 407, no. 6801, pp. 249–257, 2000.

79. S. Verma, B. Turkbey, N. Muradyan, A. Rajesh, F. Cornud, M. A. Haider, P. L. Choyke, and M. Harisinghani, "Overview of dynamic contrast-enhanced MRI in prostate cancer diagnosis and management," *Am. J. Roentgenol.*, vol. 198, no. 6, pp. 1277–1288, 2012.

80. P. Tofts, "T1-weighted DCE imaging concepts: Modelling, acquisition and analysis," in *Magneton Flash*, Germany: Siemens, 2010.

81. S. Kety, "The theory and applications of the exchange of inert gas at the lungs and tissues," *Pharmacol. Rev.*, vol. 3, no. 1, pp. 1–41, 1951.

82. P. S. Tofts, "Modeling tracer kinetics in dynamic Gd-DTPA MR imaging," *J. Magn. Reson. Imaging*, vol. 7, no. 1, pp. 91–101, 1997.

83. H. B. Larsson, T. Fritz-Hansen, E. Rostrup, L. Sondergaard, P. Ring, and O. Henriksen, "Myocardial perfusion modeling using MRI," *Magn. Reson. Med.*, vol. 35, no. 5, pp. 716–726, 1996.

84. K. S. St Lawrence and T. Y. Lee, "An adiabatic approximation to the tissue homogeneity model for water exchange in the brain: I. Theoretical derivation," *J. Cereb. Blood Flow Metab.*, vol. 18, no. 12, pp. 1365–1377, 1998.

85. A. B. Rosenkrantz, A. Sabach, J. S. Babb, B. W. Matza, S. S. Taneja, and F. M. Deng, "Prostate cancer: Comparison of dynamic contrast-enhanced MRI techniques for localization of peripheral zone tumor," *Am. J. Roentgenol.*, vol. 201, no. 3, pp. W471–W478, 2013.

86. G. J. Jager, E. T. Ruijter, C. A. van de Kaa, J. J. de la Rosette, G. O. Oosterhof, J. R. Thornbury, S. H. Ruijs, and J. O. Barentsz, "Dynamic TurboFLASH subtraction technique for contrast-enhanced MR imaging of the prostate: Correlation with histopathologic results," *Radiology*, vol. 203, no. 3, pp. 645–652, 1997.

87. J. K. Kim, S. S. Hong, Y. J. Choi, S. H. Park, H. Ahn, C. S. Kim, and K. S. Cho, "Wash-in rate on the basis of dynamic contrast-enhanced MRI: Usefulness for prostate cancer detection and localization," *J. Magn. Reson. Imaging*, vol. 22, no. 5, pp. 639–646, 2005.

88. H. P. Schlemmer, J. Merkle, R. Grobholz, T. Jaeger, M. S. Michel, A. Werner, J. Rabe, and G. van Kaick, "Can pre-operative contrast-enhanced dynamic MR imaging for prostate cancer predict microvessel density in prostatectomy specimens?" *Eur. Radiol.*, vol. 14, no. 2, pp. 309–317, 2004.

89. B. Zelhof, M. Lowry, G. Rodrigues, S. Kraus, and L. Turnbull, "Description of magnetic resonance imaging-derived enhancement variables in pathologically confirmed prostate cancer and normal peripheral zone regions," *BJU Int.*, vol. 104, no. 5, pp. 621–627, 2009.

90. D. Le Bihan, E. Breton, D. Lallemand, M. L. Aubin, J. Vignaud, and M. Laval-Jeantet, "Separation of diffusion and perfusion in intravoxel incoherent motion MR imaging," *Radiology*, vol. 168, no. 2, pp. 497–505, 1988.

91. D. M. Koh and D. J. Collins, "Diffusion-weighted MRI in the body: Applications and challenges in oncology," *Am. J. Roentgenol.*, vol. 188, no. 6, pp. 1622–1635, 2007.

92. D. M. Somford, J. J. Futterer, T. Hambrock, and J. O. Barentsz, "Diffusion and perfusion MR imaging of the prostate," *Magn. Reson. Imaging Clin. N. Am.*, vol. 16, no. 4, pp. 685–695, 2008.

93. T. A. Huisman, "Diffusion-weighted imaging: Basic concepts and application in cerebral stroke and head trauma,"*Eur. Radiol.*, vol. 13, no. 10, pp. 2283–2297, 2003.

94. D. Le Bihan, E. Breton, D. Lallemand, P. Grenier, E. Cabanis, and M. Laval-Jeantet, "MR imaging of intravoxel incoherent motions: Application to diffusion and perfusion in neurologic disorders," *Radiology*, vol. 161, no. 2, pp. 401–407, 1986.

95. R. Shimofusa, H. Fujimoto, H. Akamata, K. Motoori, S. Yamamoto, T. Ueda, and H. Ito, "Diffusion-weighted imaging of prostate cancer," *J. Comput. Assist. Tomogr.*, vol. 29, no. 2, pp. 149–153, 2005.

96. A. R. Padhani, "Integrating multiparametric prostate MRI into clinical practice," *Cancer Imaging*, vol. 11, Spec No A, pp. 27–37, 2011.

97. K. W. Doo, D. J. Sung, B. J. Park, M. J. Kim, S. B. Cho, Y. W. Oh, Y. H. Ko, and K. S. Yang, "Detectability of low and intermediate or high risk prostate cancer with combined T2-weighted and diffusion-weighted MRI," *Eur. Radiol.*, vol. 22, no. 8, pp. 1812–1819, 2012.

98. T. Hambrock, D. M. Somford, H. J. Huisman, I. M. van Oort, J. A. Witjes, C. A. Hulsbergen-van de Kaa, T. Scheenen, and J. O. Barentsz, "Relationship between apparent diffusion coefficients at 3.0-T MR imaging and Gleason grade in peripheral zone prostate cancer," *Radiology*, vol. 259, no. 2, pp. 453–461, 2011.

99. Y. Itou, K. Nakanishi, Y. Narumi, Y. Nishizawa, and H. Tsukuma, "Clinical utility of apparent diffusion coefficient (ADC) values in patients with prostate cancer: Can ADC values contribute to assess the aggressiveness of prostate cancer?" *J. Magn. Reson. Imaging*, vol. 33, no. 1, pp. 167–172, 2011.

100. Y. Peng, Y. Jiang, C. Yang, J. Brown, T. Antic, I. Sethi, C. Schmid-Tannwald, M. Giger, S. Eggener, and A. Oto, "Quantitative analysis of multiparametric prostate MR images: Differentiation between prostate cancer and normal tissue and correlation with Gleason score–a computer-aided diagnosis development study," *Radiology*, vol. 267, no. 1, pp. 787–796, 2013.

101. H. M. Awwad, J. Geisel, and R. Obeid, "The role of choline in prostate cancer," *Clin. Biochem.*, vol. 45, no. 18, pp. 1548–1553, 2012.

102. L. C. Costello and R. B. Franklin, "The clinical relevance of the metabolism of prostate cancer; zinc and tumor suppression: Connecting the dots," *Mol. Cancer*, vol. 5, p. 17, 2006.

103. G. F. Giskeodegard, H. Bertilsson, K. M. Selnaes, A. J. Wright, T. F. Bathen, T. Viset, J. Halgunset, A. Angelsen, I. S. Gribbestad, and M. B. Tessem, "Spermine and citrate as metabolic biomarkers for assessing prostate cancer aggressiveness," *PLoS ONE*, vol. 8, no. 4, p. e62375, 2013.

104. M. van der Graaf, R. G. Schipper, G. O. Oosterhof, J. A. Schalken, A. A. Verhofstad, and A. Heerschap, "Proton MR spectroscopy of prostatic tissue focused on the detection of spermine, a possible biomarker of malignant behavior in prostate cancer," *MAGMA*, vol. 10, no. 3, pp. 153–159, 2000.

105. E. Haacke, R. Brown, M. Thompson, and R. Venkatesan, *Magnetic Resonance Imaging: Physical Principles and Sequence Design*. Hoboken, NJ: Wiley, 1999.

106. G. Lemaître, "Absolute quantification at 3 T," Master's thesis, Université de Bourgogne, Heriot-Watt University, Universitat de Girona, 2011.

107. J. Scheidler, H. Hricak, D. B. Vigneron, K. K. Yu, D. L. Sokolov, L. R. Huang, C. J. Zaloudek, S. J. Nelson, P. R. Carroll, and J. Kurhanewicz, "Prostate cancer: Localization with three-dimensional proton MR spectroscopic imaging–clinicopathologic study," *Radiology*, vol. 213, no. 2, pp. 473–480, 1999.

108. Y. Kaji, J. Kurhanewicz, H. Hricak, D. L. Sokolov, L. R. Huang, S. J. Nelson, and D. B. Vigneron, "Localizing prostate cancer in the presence of postbiopsy changes on MR images: Role of proton MR spectroscopic imaging," *Radiology*, vol. 206, no. 3, pp. 785–790, 1998.

109. J. C. Vilanova, J. Comet, C. Barceló-Vidal, J. Barceló, E. López-Bonet, A. Maroto, M. Arzoz, À. Moreno, and J. Areal, "Peripheral zone prostate cancer in patients with elevated PSA levels and low free-to-total PSA ratio: Detection with MR imaging and MR spectroscopy," *Radiology*, vol. 253, no. 1, pp. 135–143, 2009.

110. P. Walker, G. Crehange, S. Parfait, A. Cochet, P. Maignon, L. Cormier, and F. Brunotte, "Absolute quantification in 1H MRSI of the prostate at 3T," in *ISMRM Annual Meeting 2010*, 2010.

111. S. Verma, A. Rajesh, J. J. Futterer, B. Turkbey, T. W. Scheenen, Y. Pang, P. L. Choyke, and J. Kurhanewicz, "Prostate MRI and 3D MR spectroscopy: How we do it," *Am. J. Roentgenol.*, vol. 194, no. 6, pp. 1414–1426, 2010.

112. D. Ampeliotis, A. Anonakoudi, K. Berberidis, and E. Z. Psarakis, "Computer aided detection of prostate cancer using fused information from dynamic contrast enhanced and morphological magnetic resonance images," in *IEEE International Conference on Signal Processing and Communications*, pp. 888–891, 2007.

113. D. Ampeliotis, A. Anonakoudi, K. Berberidis, E. Z. Psarakis, and A. Kounoudes, "A computer-aided system for the detection of prostate cancer based on magnetic resonance image analysis," in *International Symposium on Communications, Control and Signal Processing*, 2008.

114. T. Antic, Y. Peng, Y. Jiang, M. L. Giger, S. Eggener, and A. Oto, "A study of T2-weighted MR image texture features and diffusion-weighted MR image features for computer-aided diagnosis of prostate cancer," in *Proceedings of SPIE 8670, Medical Imaging 2013: Computer-Aided Diagnosis*, pp. 86701H–86701H–6, 2013.

115. Y. Artan, D. Langer, M. Haider, T. H. Van der Kwast, A. Evans, M. Wernick, and I. Yetik, "Prostate cancer segmentation with multispectral MRI using cost-sensitive Conditional Random Fields," in *Biomedical Imaging: From Nano to Macro, 2009. ISBI'09. IEEE International Symposium on*, pp. 278–281, 2009.

116. Y. Artan, M. A. Haider, D. L. Langer, T. H. van der Kwast, A. J. Evans, Y. Yang, M. N. Wernick, J. Trachtenberg, and I. S. Yetik, "Prostate cancer localization with multispectral MRI using cost-sensitive support vector machines and conditional random fields," *IEEE Trans. Image Process.*, vol. 19, no. 9, pp. 2444–2455, 2010.

117. A. Cameron, A. Modhafar, F. Khalvati, D. Lui, M. J. Shafiee, A. Wong, and M. Haider, "Multiparametric MRI prostate cancer analysis via a hybrid morphological-textural model," in *2014 36th Annual International Conference of the IEEE Engineering in Medicine and Biology Society*. IEEE, pp. 3357–3360, 2014.

118. A. Cameron, F. Khalvati, M. A. Haider, and A. Wong, "Maps: A quantitative radiomics approach for prostate cancer detection," *IEEE Trans. Biomed. Eng.*, vol. 63, no. 6, pp. 1145–1156, 2016.

119. I. Chan, W. Wells, R. V. Mulkern, S. Haker, J. Zhang, K. H. Zou, S. E. Maier, and C. M. Tempany, "Detection of prostate cancer by integration of line-scan diffusion, T2-mapping and T2-weighted magnetic resonance imaging; a multichannel statistical classifier," *Med. Phys.*, vol. 30, no. 9, pp. 2390–2398, 2003.

120. A. Chung, F. Khalvati, M. Shafiee, M. Haider, and A. Wong, "Prostate cancer detection via a quantitative radiomics-driven conditional random field framework," *IEEE Access*, vol. 3, pp. 2531–2541, 2015.

121. V. Giannini, A. Vignati, S. Mazzetti, M. De Luca, C. Bracco, M. Stasi, F. Russo, E. Armando, and D. Regge, "A prostate CAD system based on multiparametric analysis of DCE T1-w, and DW automatically registered images," in *Proceedings of SPIE 8670, Medical Imaging 2013: Computer-Aided Diagnosis*, pp. 86703E–86703E–6, 2013.

122. V. Giannini, S. Mazzetti, A. Vignati, F. Russo, E. Bollito, F. Porpiglia, M. Stasi, and D. Regge, "A fully automatic computer aided diagnosis system for peripheral zone prostate cancer detection using multi-parametric magnetic resonance imaging," *Comput. Med. Imaging Graph.*, vol. 46, pp. 219–226, 2015.

123. B. M. Kelm, B. H. Menze, C. M. Zechmann, K. T. Baudendistel, and F. A. Hamprecht, "Automated estimation of tumor probability in prostate magnetic resonance spectroscopic imaging: Pattern recognition vs quantification," *Magn. Reson. Med.*, vol. 57, no. 1, pp. 150–159, 2007.

124. F. Khalvati, A. Wong, and M. A. Haider, "Automated prostate cancer detection via comprehensive multi-parametric magnetic resonance imaging texture feature models," *BMC Med. Imaging*, vol. 15, no. 1, p. 27, 2015.

125. D. L. Langer, T. H. van der Kwast, A. J. Evans, J. Trachtenberg, B. C. Wilson, and M. A. Haider, "Prostate cancer detection with multi-parametric MRI: Logistic regression analysis of quantitative T2, diffusion-weighted imaging, and dynamic contrast-enhanced MRI," *J. Magn. Reson. Imaging*, vol. 30, no. 2, pp. 327–334, 2009.

126. J. Lehaire, R. Flamary, O. Rouvière, and C. Lartizien, "Computer-aided diagnostic system for prostate cancer detection and characterization combining learned dictionaries and supervised classification," in *2014 IEEE International Conference on Image Processing (ICIP)*. IEEE, pp. 2251–2255, 2014.

127. G. Lemaitre, "Computer-aided diagnosis for prostate cancer using multi-parametric magnetic resonance imaging," PhD dissertation, Universitat de Girona and Université de Bourgogne, 2016.

128. G. J. S. Litjens, P. C. Vos, J. O. Barentsz, N. Karssemeijer, and H. J. Huisman, "Automatic computer aided detection of abnormalities in multi-parametric prostate MRI," in *Proceedings of SPIE 7963, Medical Imaging 2011: Computer-Aided Diagnosis*, pp. 79630T–79630T–7, 2011.

129. G. J. S. Litjens, J. O. Barentsz, N. Karssemeijer, and H. J. Huisman, "Automated computer-aided detection of prostate cancer in MR images: From a whole-organ to a zone-based approach," in *Proceedings of SPIE 8315, Medical Imaging 2012: Computer-Aided Diagnosis*, pp. 83150G–83150G–6, 2012.

130. G. Litjens, O. Debats, J. Barentsz, N. Karssemeijer, and H. Huisman, "Computer-aided detection of prostate cancer in MRI," *IEEE Trans. Med. Imaging*, vol. 33, no. 5, pp. 1083–1092, 2014.

131. X. Liu, D. L. Langer, M. A. Haider, Y. Yang, M. N. Wernick, and I. S. Yetik, "Prostate cancer segmentation with simultaneous estimation of Markov random field parameters and class," *IEEE Trans. Med. Imaging*, vol. 28, no. 6, pp. 906–915, 2009.

132. P. Liu, S. Wang, B. Turkbey, K. Grant, P. Pinto, P. Choyke, B. J. Wood, and R. M. Summers, "A prostate cancer computer-aided diagnosis system using multimodal magnetic resonance imaging and targeted biopsy labels," in *Proceedings of SPIE 8670, Medical Imaging 2013: Computer-Aided Diagnosis*, pp. 86701G–86701G–6, 2013.

133. R. Lopes, A. Ayache, N. Makni, P. Puech, A. Villers, S. Mordon, and N. Betrouni, "Prostate cancer characterization on MR images using fractal features," *Med. Phys.*, vol. 38, no. 1, pp. 83–95, 2011.

134. D. Lv, X. Guo, X. Wang, J. Zhang, and J. Fang, "Computerized characterization of prostate cancer by fractal analysis in MR images," *J. Magn. Reson. Imaging*, vol. 30, no. 1, pp. 161–168, 2009.

135. L. Matulewicz, J. F. Jansen, L. Bokacheva, H. A. Vargas, O. Akin, S. W. Fine, A. Shukla-Dave, J. A. Eastham, H. Hricak, J. A. Koutcher, and K. L. Zakian, "Anatomic segmentation improves prostate cancer detection with artificial neural networks analysis of 1H magnetic resonance spectroscopic imaging," *J. Magn. Reson. Imaging*, 2013.

136. S. Mazzetti, M. De Luca, C. Bracco, A. Vignati, V. Giannini, M. Stasi, F. Russo, E. Armando, S. Agliozzo, and D. Regge, "A CAD system based on multi-parametric analysis for cancer prostate detection on DCE-MRI," in *Proceedings of SPIE 7963, Medical Imaging 2011: Computer-Aided Diagnosis*, pp. 79633Q–79633Q–7, 2011.

137. E. Niaf, O. Rouvire, and C. Lartizien, "Computer-aided diagnosis for prostate cancer detection in the peripheral zone via multisequence MRI," in *Proceedings of SPIE 7963, Medical Imaging 2011: Computer-Aided Diagnosis*, 2011.

138. E. Niaf, O. Rouviere, F. Mege-Lechevallier, F. Bratan, and C. Lartizien, "Computer-aided diagnosis of prostate cancer in the peripheral zone using multiparametric MRI," *Phys. Med. Biol.*, vol. 57, no. 12, pp. 3833–3851, 2012.

139. S. Ozer, M. Haider, D. L. Langer, T. H. Van der Kwast, A. Evans, M. Wernick, J. Trachtenberg, and I. Yetik, "Prostate cancer localization with multispectral MRI based on Relevance Vector Machines," in *Biomedical Imaging: From Nano to Macro, 2009. ISBI'09. IEEE International Symposium on*, pp. 73–76, 2009.

140. S. Ozer, D. L. Langer, X. Liu, M. A. Haider, T. H. van der Kwast, A. J. Evans, Y. Yang, M. N. Wernick, and I. S. Yetik, "Supervised and unsupervised methods for prostate cancer segmentation with multispectral MRI," *Med. Phys.*, vol. 37, no. 4, pp. 1873–1883, 2010.

141. S. Parfait, P. Walker, G. Crhange, X. Tizon, and J. Mitran, "Classification of prostate magnetic resonance spectra using Support Vector Machine," *Biomed. Signal Process. Control*, vol. 7, no. 5, pp. 499–508, 2012.

142. P. Puech, N. Betrouni, N. Makni, A. S. Dewalle, A. Villers, and L. Lemaitre, "Computer-assisted diagnosis of prostate cancer using DCE-MRI data: Design, implementation and preliminary results," *Int. J. Comput. Assist. Radiol. Surg.*, vol. 4, no. 1, pp. 1–10, 2009.

143. A. Rampun, L. Zheng, P. Malcolm, and R. Zwiggelaar, "Classifying benign and malignant tissues within the prostate peripheral zone using textons," in *Medical Image Understanding and Analysis (MIUA 2015)*, 2015.

144. A. Rampun, B. Tiddeman, R. Zwiggelaar, and P. Malcolm, "Computer aided diagnosis of prostate cancer: A texton based approach," *Med. Phys.*, vol. 43, no. 10, pp. 5412–5425, 2016.

145. A. Rampun, L. Zheng, P. Malcolm, B. Tiddeman, and R. Zwiggelaar, "Computer-aided detection of prostate cancer in t2-weighted MRI within the peripheral zone," *Phys. Med. Biol.*, vol. 61, no. 13, pp. 4796–4825, 2016.

146. A. Rampun, L. Wang, P. Malcolm, and R. Zwiggelaar, "A quantitative study of texture features across different window sizes in prostate t2-weighted MRI," *Procedia Comput. Sci.*, vol. 90, pp. 74–79, 2016.

147. G. Samarasinghe, A. Sowmya, and D. A. Moses, "Semi-quantitative analysis of prostate perfusion MRI by clustering of pre and post contrast enhancement phases," in *Biomedical Imaging (ISBI), 2016 IEEE 13th International Symposium on*. IEEE, 2016, pp. 943–947.

148. Y. S. Sung, H. J. Kwon, B. W. Park, G. Cho, C. K. Lee, K. S. Cho, and J. K. Kim, "Prostate cancer detection on dynamic contrast-enhanced MRI: Computer-aided diagnosis versus single perfusion parameter maps," *Am. J. Roentgenol.*, vol. 197, no. 5, pp. 1122–1129, 2011.

149. P. Tiwari, A. Madabhushi, and M. Rosen, "A hierarchical unsupervised spectral clustering scheme for detection of prostate cancer from magnetic resonance spectroscopy (MRS)," *Med. Image Comput. Comput. Assist. Interv.*, vol. 10, no. Pt 2, pp. 278–286, 2007.

150. P. Tiwari, M. Rosen, and A. Madabhushi, "Consensus-locally linear embedding (C-LLE): Application to prostate cancer detection on magnetic resonance spectroscopy," *Med. Image Comput. Comput. Assist. Interv.*, vol. 11, no. Pt 2, pp. 330–338, 2008.

151. P. Tiwari, M. Rosen, and A. Madabhushi, "A hierarchical spectral clustering and nonlinear dimensionality reduction scheme for detection of prostate cancer from magnetic resonance spectroscopy (MRS)," *Med. Phys.*, vol. 36, no. 9, pp. 3927–3939, 2009.

152. P. Tiwari, M. Rosen, G. Reed, J. Kurhanewicz, and A. Madabhushi, "Spectral embedding based probabilistic boosting tree (ScEPTre): Classifying high dimensional heterogeneous biomedical data," *Med. Image Comput. Comput. Assist. Interv.*, vol. 12, no. Pt 2, pp. 844–851, 2009.

153. P. Tiwari, J. Kurhanewicz, M. Rosen, and A. Madabhushi, "Semi supervised multi kernel (SeSMiK) graph embedding: Identifying aggressive prostate cancer via magnetic resonance imaging and spectroscopy," *Med. Image Comput. Comput. Assist. Interv.*, vol. 13, no. Pt 3, pp. 666–673, 2010.

154. P. Tiwari, S. Viswanath, J. Kurhanewicz, A. Sridhar, and A. Madabhushi, "Multimodal wavelet embedding representation for data combination (MaWERiC): Integrating magnetic resonance imaging and spectroscopy for prostate cancer detection," *NMR Biomed.*, vol. 25, no. 4, pp. 607–619, 2012.

155. P. Tiwari, J. Kurhanewicz, and A. Madabhushi, "Multi-kernel graph embedding for detection, Gleason grading of prostate cancer via MRI/MRS," *Med. Image Anal.*, vol. 17, no. 2, pp. 219–235, 2013.

156. R. Trigui, J. Miteran, L. Sellami, P. Walker, and A. B. Hamida, "A classification approach to prostate cancer localization in 3T multi-parametric MRI," in *Advanced Technologies for Signal and Image Processing (ATSIP), 2016 2nd International Conference on*. IEEE, pp. 113–118, 2016.

157. R. Trigui, J. Mitéran, P. Walker, L. Sellami, and A. B. Hamida, "Automatic classification and localization of prostate cancer using multi-parametric MRI/MRS," *Biomed. Signal Process. Control*, vol. 31, pp. 189–198, 2017.

158. S. Viswanath, P. Tiwari, M. Rosen, and A. Madabhushi, "A meta-classifier for detecting prostate cancer by quantitative integration of *In Vivo* magnetic resonance spectroscopy and magnetic resonance imaging," in *Medical Imaging 2008: Computer-Aided Diagnosis*, vol. 6915. SPIE, 2008.

159. S. Viswanath, B. N. Bloch, E. Genega, N. Rofsky, R. Lenkinski, J. Chappelow, R. Toth, and A. Madabhushi, "A comprehensive segmentation, registration, and cancer detection scheme on 3 Tesla in vivo prostate DCE-MRI," *Med. Image Comput. Comput. Assist. Interv.*, vol. 11, no. Pt 1, pp. 662–669, 2008.

160. S. Viswanath, B. N. Bloch, M. Rosen, J. Chappelow, R. Toth, N. Rofsky, R. Lenkinski, E. Genega, A. Kalyanpur, and A. Madabhushi, "Integrating structural and functional imaging for computer assisted detection of prostate cancer on multi-protocol in vivo 3 Tesla MRI," in *Society of Photo-Optical Instrumentation Engineers (SPIE) Conference Series*, ser. Society of Photo-Optical Instrumentation Engineers (SPIE) Conference Series, Vol. 7260, 2009.

161. S. Viswanath, B. N. Bloch, J. Chappelow, P. Patel, N. Rofsky, R. Lenkinski, E. Genega, and A. Madabhushi, "Enhanced multi-protocol analysis via intelligent supervised embedding (EMPrAvISE): Detecting prostate cancer on multi-parametric MRI," in *Proceedings of SPIE 7963, Medical Imaging 2011: Computer-Aided Diagnosis*, 2011.

162. S. E. Viswanath, N. B. Bloch, J. C. Chappelow, R. Toth, N. M. Rofsky, E. M. Genega, R. E. Lenkinski, and A. Madabhushi, "Central gland and peripheral zone prostate tumors have significantly different quantitative imaging signatures on 3 Tesla endorectal, in vivo T2-weighted MR imagery," *J. Magn. Reson. Imaging*, vol. 36, no. 1, pp. 213–224, 2012.

163. P. C. Vos, T. Hambrock, J. O. Barentsz, and H. J. Huisman, "Combining T2-weighted with dynamic MR images for computerized classification of prostate lesions," in *Medical Imaging 2008: Computer-Aided Diagnosis*, Vol. 6915. SPIE, 2008.

164. P. C. Vos, T. Hambrock, C. A. Hulsbergen-van de Kaa, J. J. Futterer, J. O. Barentsz, and H. J. Huisman, "Computerized analysis of prostate lesions in the peripheral zone using dynamic contrast enhanced MRI," *Med. Phys.*, vol. 35, no. 3, pp. 888–899, 2008.

165. P. C. Vos, T. Hambrock, J. O. Barentsz, and H. J. Huisman, "Computer-assisted analysis of peripheral zone prostate lesions using T2-weighted and dynamic contrast enhanced T1-weighted MRI," *Phys. Med. Biol.*, vol. 55, no. 6, pp. 1719–1734, 2010.

166. P. C. Vos, J. O. Barentsz, N. Karssemeijer, and H. J. Huisman, "Automatic computer-aided detection of prostate cancer based on multiparametric magnetic resonance image analysis," *Phys. Med. Biol.*, vol. 57, no. 6, pp. 1527–1542, 2012.

167. R. Nowak, "Wavelet-based Rician noise removal for magnetic resonance imaging," *IEEE Trans. Image Process.*, vol. 8, no. 10, pp. 1408–1419, 1999.

168. J. V. Manjon, J. Carbonell-Caballero, J. J. Lull, G. Garcia-Marti, L. Marti-Bonmati, and M. Robles, "MRI denoising using non-local means,"*Med. Image Anal.*, vol. 12, no. 4, pp. 514–523, 2008.

169. A. Buades, B. Coll, and J. Morel, "A review of image denoising algorithms, with a new one," *Multiscale Model. Simul.*, vol. 4, pp. 490–530, 2005.

170. J. Mohan, V. Krishnaveni, and Y. Guo, "A survey on the magnetic resonance image denoising methods," *Biomed. Signal Process. Control*, vol. 9, pp. 56–69, 2014.

171. H. Ling and A. C. Bovik, "Smoothing low-SNR molecular images via anisotropic median-diffusion," *IEEE Trans. Med. Imaging*, vol. 21, no. 4, pp. 377–384, 2002.

172. D. L. Donoho and J. M. Johnstone, "Ideal spatial adaptation by wavelet shrinkage," *Biometrika*, vol. 81, no. 3, pp. 425–455, 1994.

173. A. Pizurica, "Image denoising using wavelets and spatial context modeling," PhD dissertation, Universiteit Gent, 2002.

174. S. Mallat, *A Wavelet Tour of Signal Processing: The Sparse Way*, 3rd ed. Orlando, FL: Academic Press, 2008.

175. A. Pizurica, W. Philips, I. Lemahieu, and M. Acheroy, "A versatile wavelet domain noise filtration technique for medical imaging," *IEEE Trans. Med. Imaging*, vol. 22, no. 3, pp. 323–331, 2003.

176. M. Styner, C. Brechbuhler, G. Szckely, and G. Gerig, "Parametric estimate of intensity inhomogeneities applied to MRI," *IEEE Trans. Med. Imaging*, vol. 19, no. 3, pp. 153–165, 2000.

177. M. Jungke, W. Von Seelen, G. Bielke, S. Meindl, M. Grigat, and P. Pfannenstiel, "A system for the diagnostic use of tissue characterizing parameters in NMR-tomography," in *Proceedings of Information Processing in Medical Imaging*, Vol. 87, pp. 471–481, 1987.

178. U. Vovk, F. Pernus, and B. Likar, "A review of methods for correction of intensity inhomogeneity in MRI," *IEEE Trans. Med. Imaging*, vol. 26, no. 3, pp. 405–421, 2007.

179. S. Z. Li, "Robustizing robust M-estimation using deterministic annealing," *Pattern Recognit.*, vol. 29, pp. 159–166, 1996.

180. M. Styner and G. Gerig, "Evaluation of 2D/3D bias correction with 1 + 1ES-optimization," ETH Zürich, Technical Report, 1997.

181. J. G. Sled, A. P. Zijdenbos, and A. C. Evans, "A nonparametric method for automatic correction of intensity nonuniformity in MRI data," *IEEE Trans. Med. Imaging*, vol. 17, no. 1, pp. 87–97, 1998.

182. A. Madabhushi, J. Udupa, and A. Souza, "Generalized scale: Theory, algorithms, and application to image inhomogeneity correction," *Comput. Vis. Image Underst.*, vol. 101, no. 2, pp. 100–121, 2006.

183. L. G. Shapiro and G. C. Stockman, *Computer Vision*. Upper Saddle River, NJ: Prentice Hall, 2001.

184. L. G. Nyul and J. K. Udupa, "On standardizing the MR image intensity scale," *Magn. Reson. Med.*, vol. 42, no. 6, pp. 1072–1081, 1999.

185. A. Rampun, L. Zheng, P. Malcolm, and R. Zwiggelaar, "Computer aided diagnosis of prostate cancer within the peripheral zone in T2-weighted MRI," in *Medical Image Understanding and Analysis (MIUA 2015)*, 2015.

186. G. Lemaitre, M. R. Dastjerdi, J. Massich, J. C. Vilanova, P. M. Walker, J. Freixenet, A. Meyer-Baese, F. Mériaudeau, and R. Marti, "Normalization of T2W-MRI prostate images using Rician a priori," in *SPIE Medical Imaging*. International Society for Optics and Photonics, pp. 529–978, 2016.

187. L. G. Nyul, J. K. Udupa, and X. Zhang, "New variants of a method of MRI scale standardization," *IEEE Trans. Med. Imaging*, vol. 19, no. 2, pp. 143–150, 2000.

188. A. Srivastava, E. Klassen, S. Joshi, and I. Jermyn, "Shape analysis of elastic curves in Euclidean spaces," *IEEE Trans. Pattern Anal. Mach. Intell.*, vol. 33, no. 7, pp. 1415–1428, 2011.

189. A. Madabhushi and J. K. Udupa, "New methods of MR image intensity standardization via generalized scale," *Med. Phys.*, vol. 33, no. 9, pp. 3426–3434, 2006.

190. M. Wiart, L. Curiel, A. Gelet, D. Lyonnet, J. Y. Chapelon, and O. Rouviere, "Influence of perfusion on high-intensity focused ultrasound prostate ablation: A first-pass MRI study," *Magn. Reson. Med.*, vol. 58, no. 1, pp. 119–127, 2007.

191. L. Chen, Z. Weng, L. Goh, and M. Garland, "An efficient algorithm for automatic phase correction of {NMR} spectra based on entropy minimization," *J. Magn. Reson.*, vol. 158, no. 12, pp. 164–168, 2002.

192. M. Osorio-Garcia, A. Croitor Sava, D. M. Sima, F. Nielsen, U. Himmelreich, and S. Van Huffel, Quantification improvements of 1H MRS Signals, in *Magnetic Resonance Spectroscopy*, InTech, pp. 1–27, 2012.

193. J. A. Nelder and R. Mead, "A simplex method for function minimization," *Comput. J.*, vol. 7, no. 4, pp. 308–313, 1965.

194. H. Zhu, R. Ouwerkerk, and P. B. Barker, "Dual-band water and lipid suppression for MR spectroscopic imaging at 3 Tesla," *Magn. Reson. Med.*, vol. 63, no. 6, pp. 1486–1492, 2010.

195. W. Pijnappel, A. van den Boogaart, R. de Beer, and D. van Ormondt, "SVD-based quantification of magnetic resonance signals," *J. Magn. Reson. (1969)*, vol. 97, no. 1, pp. 122–134, 1992.

196. T. Laudadio, N. Mastronardi, L. Vanhamme, P. V. Hecke, and S. V. Huffel, "Improved Lanczos algorithms for blackbox {MRS} data quantitation," *J. Magn. Reson.*, vol. 157, no. 2, pp. 292–297, 2002.

197. C. A. Lieber and A. Mahadevan-Jansen, "Automated method for subtraction of fluorescence from biological Raman spectra," *Appl. Spectrosc.*, vol. 57, no. 11, pp. 1363–1367, 2003.

198. A. Devos, L. Lukas, J. A. Suykens, L. Vanhamme, A. R. Tate, F. A. Howe, C. Majos, A. Moreno-Torres, M. van der Graaf, C. Arus, and S. Van Huffel, "Classification of brain tumours using short echo time 1H MR spectra," *J. Magn. Reson.*, vol. 170, no. 1, pp. 164–175, 2004.

199. Y. Xi and D. M. Rocke, "Baseline correction for NMR spectroscopic metabolomics data analysis," *BMC Bioinformatics*, vol. 9, no. 1, p. 1, 2008.

200. S. Ghose, A. Oliver, R. Marti, X. Llado, J. C. Vilanova, J. Freixenet, J. Mitra, D. Sidibe, and F. Meriaudeau, "A survey of prostate segmentation methodologies in ultrasound, magnetic resonance and computed tomography images," *Comput. Methods Programs Biomed.*, vol. 108, no. 1, pp. 262–287, 2012.

201. G. Litjens, O. Debats, W. van de Ven, N. Karssemeijer, and H. Huisman, "A pattern recognition approach to zonal segmentation of the prostate on MRI," *Med. Image Comput. Comput. Assist. Interv.*, vol. 15, no. Pt 2, pp. 413–420, 2012.

202. S. K. Warfield, K. H. Zou, and W. M. Wells, "Simultaneous truth and performance level estimation (STAPLE): An algorithm for the validation of image segmentation," *IEEE Trans. Med. Imaging*, vol. 23, no. 7, pp. 903–921, 2004.

203. M. Amadasun and R. King, "Textural features corresponding to textural properties," *IEEE Trans. Syst. Man Cybern.*, vol. 19, no. 5, pp. 1264–1274, 1989.

204. H. Li, M. L. Giger, O. I. Olopade, A. Margolis, L. Lan, and M. R. Chinander, "Computerized texture analysis of mammographic parenchymal patterns of digitized mammograms," *Acad. Radiol.*, vol. 12, no. 7, pp. 863–873, 2005.

205. T. Ojala, M. Pietikäinen, and D. Harwood, "A comparative study of texture measures with classification based on featured distributions," *Pattern Recognit.*, vol. 29, no. 1, pp. 51–59, 1996.

206. F. L. Bookstein, "Principal warps: Thin-plate splines and the decomposition of deformations," *IEEE Trans. Pattern Anal. Mach. Intell.*, vol. 11, no. 6, pp. 567–585, 1989.

207. G. Litjens, R. Toth, W. van de Ven, C. Hoeks, S. Kerkstra, B. van Ginneken, G. Vincent et al., "Evaluation of prostate segmentation algorithms for MRI: The PROMISE12 challenge," *Med. Image Anal.*, vol. 18, no. 2, pp. 359–373, 2014.

208. T. R. Langerak, U. A. van der Heide, A. N. Kotte, M. A. Viergever, M. van Vulpen, and J. P. Pluim, "Label fusion in atlas-based segmentation using a selective and iterative method for performance level estimation (simple)," *IEEE Trans. Med. Imaging*, vol. 29, no. 12, pp. 2000–2008, 2010.

209. A. Rampun, P. Malcolm, and R. Zwiggelaar, "Detection and localisation of prostate cancer within the peripheral zone using scoring algorithm," in *Irish Machine Vision and Image Processing*, 2014.

210. R. Toth, J. Chappelow, M. Rosen, S. Pungavkar, A. Kalyanpur, and A. Madabhushi, "Multi-attribute non-initializing texture reconstruction based active shape model (MANTRA)," *Med. Image Comput. Comput. Assist. Interv.*, vol. 11, no. Pt 1, pp. 653–661, 2008.

211. T. F. Cootes, C. J. Taylor, D. H. Cooper, and J. Graham, "Active shape models—Their training and application," *Comput. Vis. Image Underst.*, vol. 61, no. 1, pp. 38–59, 1995.

212. K. Pearson, "On lines and planes of closest fit to systems of points in space," *Philos. Mag.*, vol. 2, no. 6, pp. 559–572, 1901.

213. R. Toth, S. Doyle, S. Pungavkar, A. Kalyanpur, and A. Madabhushi, "A boosted ensemble scheme for accurate landmark detection for active shape models," in *SPIE Medical Imaging*, Vol. 7260, Orlando, FL, 2009.

214. H. Huisman, P. Vos, G. Litjens, T. Hambrock, and J. Barentsz, "Computer aided detection of prostate cancer using T2, DWI and DCE MRI: Methods and clinical applications," in *Proceedings of the 2010 International Conference on Prostate Cancer Imaging: Computer-Aided Diagnosis, Prognosis, and Intervention*, ser. MICCAI'10. Berlin, Germany: Springer-Verlag, pp. 4–14, 2010.

215. N. Otsu, "A threshold selection method from gray-level histograms," *Automatica*, vol. 11, no. 285–296, pp. 23–27, 1975.

216. J. Shi and J. Malik, "Normalized cuts and image segmentation," *IEEE Trans. Pattern Anal. Mach. Intell.*, vol. 22, no. 8, pp. 888–905, 2000.

217. M. Belkin and P. Niyogi, "Laplacian eigenmaps and spectral techniques for embedding and clustering," in *Advances in Neural Information Processing Systems 14*. MIT Press, pp. 585–591, 2001.

218. J. B. Maintz and M. A. Viergever, "A survey of medical image registration," *Med. Image Anal.*, vol. 2, no. 1, pp. 1–36, 1998.

219. B. Zitová and J. Flusser, "Image registration methods: A survey," *Image Vis. Comput.*, vol. 21, no. 11, pp. 977–1000, 2003.

220. J. Mitra, R. Marti, A. Oliver, X. Llado, J. C. Vilanova, and F. Meriaudeau, "A comparison of thin-plate splines with automatic correspondences and B-splines with uniform grids for multimodal prostate registration," in *Society of Photo-Optical Instrumentation Engineers (SPIE) Conference Series*, ser. Society of Photo-Optical Instrumentation Engineers (SPIE) Conference Series, Vol. 7964, 2011.

221. J. Mitra, Z. Kato, R. Marti, A. Oliver, X. Llado, D. Sidibe, S. Ghose, J. C. Vilanova, J. Comet, and F. Meriaudeau, "A spline-based non-linear diffeomorphism for multimodal prostate registration," *Med. Image Anal.*, vol. 16, no. 6, pp. 1259–1279, 2012.

222. J. Pluim, J. Maintz, and M. Viergever, "Mutual-information-based registration of medical images: A survey," *IEEE Trans. Med. Imaging*, vol. 22, no. 8, pp. 986–1004, 2003.

223. J. Chappelow, B. N. Bloch, N. Rofsky, E. Genega, R. Lenkinski, W. DeWolf, and A. Madabhushi, "Elastic registration of multimodal prostate MRI and histology via multiattribute combined mutual information," *Med. Phys.*, vol. 38, no. 4, pp. 2005–2018, 2011.

224. M. Staring, U. A. van der Heide, S. Klein, M. A. Viergever, and J. P. Pluim, "Registration of cervical MRI using multifeature mutual information," *IEEE Trans. Med. Imaging*, vol. 28, no. 9, pp. 1412–1421, 2009.

225. A. Hero, B. Ma, O. Michel, and J. Gorman, "Applications of entropic spanning graphs," *IEEE Signal Process. Mag.*, vol. 19, no. 5, pp. 85–95, 2002.

226. R. H. Byrd, P. Lu, J. Nocedal, and C. Zhu, "A limited memory algorithm for bound constrained optimization," *SIAM J. Sci. Comput.*, vol. 16, no. 5, pp. 1190–1208, 1995.

227. P. Viola and W. M. Wells, III, "Alignment by maximization of mutual information," *Int. J. Comput. Vision*, vol. 24, no. 2, pp. 137–154, 1997.

228. J. Mitra, "Multimodal image registration applied to magnetic resonance and ultrasound prostatic images," PhD dissertation, Universitat de Girona and Université de Bourgogne, 2012.

229. D. Rueckert, L. I. Sonoda, C. Hayes, D. L. Hill, M. O. Leach, and D. J. Hawkes, "Nonrigid registration using free-form deformations: Application to breast MR images," *IEEE Trans. Med. Imaging*, vol. 18, no. 8, pp. 712–721, 1999.

230. Q. Li, S. Sone, and K. Doi, "Selective enhancement filters for nodules, vessels, and airway walls in two- and three-dimensional CT scans," *Med. Phys.*, vol. 30, no. 8, pp. 2040–2051, 2003.

231. J. Prewitt, Object enhancement and extraction, in *Picture Processing and Psychohistories*, B. Lipkin and A. Rosenfeld (Eds.), New York: Academic Press, pp. 75–149, 1970.

232. I. Sobel, "Camera models and machine perception," DTIC Document, Technical Report, 1970.

233. R. Kirsch, "Computer determination of the constituent structure of biological images," *Comput. Biomed. Res.*, vol. 4, no. 3, pp. 315–328, 1971.

234. D. Gabor, "Theory of communication. Part 1: The analysis of information," *J. Inst. Electr. Eng.*, vol. 93, no. 26, pp. 429–441, 1946.

235. J. G. Daugman, "Uncertainty relation for resolution in space, spatial frequency, and orientation optimized by two-dimensional visual cortical filters," *J. Opt. Soc. Am. A*, vol. 2, no. 7, pp. 1160–1169, 1985.

236. Y. Wang and C.-S. Chua, "Face recognition from 2D and 3D images using 3D Gabor filters,"*Image Vis. Comput.*, vol. 23, no. 11, pp. 1018–1028, 2005.

237. P. Kovesi, "Image features from phase congruency," *Videre: J. Comput. Vis. Res.*, vol. 1, no. 3, pp. 1–26, 1999.

238. R. Haralick, K. Shanmugam, and I. Dinstein, "Textural features for image classification," *IEEE Trans. Syst. Man Cybern.*, vol. SMC-3, no. 6, pp. 610–621, 1973.

239. H. Tamura, S. Mori, and T. Yamawaki, "Textural features corresponding to visual perception," *IEEE Trans. Syst. Man Cybern.*, vol. 8, no. 6, pp. 460–473, 1978.

240. A. Benassi, S. Cohen, and J. Istas, "Identifying the multifractional function of a Gaussian process," *Stat. Probabil. Lett.*, vol. 39, no. 4, pp. 337–345, 1998.

241. N. Ahmed, T. Natarajan, and K. Rao, "Discrete cosine transform," *IEEE Trans. Comput.*, vol. C-23, no. 1, pp. 90–93, 1974.

242. T. Leung and J. Malik, "Representing and recognizing the visual appearance of materials using three-dimensional textons," *Int. J. Comput. Vis.*, vol. 43, no. 1, pp. 29–44, 2001.

243. N. Dalal and B. Triggs, "Histograms of oriented gradients for human detection," in *Computer Vision and Pattern Recognition, 2005. CVPR 2005. IEEE Computer Society Conference on*, vol. 1, pp. 886–893, 2005.

244. S. Belongie, J. Malik, and J. Puzicha, "Shape matching and object recognition using shape contexts," *IEEE Trans. Pattern Anal. Mach. Intell.*, vol. 24, no. 4, pp. 509–522, 2002.

245. G. Zhao, T. Ahonen, J. Matas, and M. Pietikainen, "Rotation-invariant image and video description with local binary pattern features," *IEEE Trans. Image Process.*, vol. 21, no. 4, pp. 1465–1477, 2012.

246. P. Castorina, P. P. Delsanto, and C. Guiot, "Classification scheme for phenomenological universalities in growth problems in physics and other sciences," *Phys. Rev. Lett.*, vol. 96, p. 188701, 2006.

247. H. Ratiney, M. Sdika, Y. Coenradie, S. Cavassila, D. van Ormondt, and D. Graveron-Demilly, "Time-domain semi-parametric estimation based on a metabolite basis set," *NMR Biomed.*, vol. 18, no. 1, pp. 1–13, 2005.

248. L. Vanhamme, A. van den Boogaart, and S. Van Huffel, "Improved method for accurate and efficient quantification of MRS data with use of prior knowledge," *J. Magn. Reson.*, vol. 129, pp. 35–45, 1997.

249. T. Coleman and Y. Li, "An interior trust region approach for nonlinear minimization subject to bounds," Cornell University, Technical Report, 1993.

250. S. W. Provencher, "Estimation of metabolite concentrations from localized in vivo proton NMR spectra," *Magn. Reson. Med.*, vol. 30, no. 6, pp. 672–679, 1993.

251. C. Gasparovic, T. Song, D. Devier, H. J. Bockholt, A. Caprihan, P. G. Mullins, S. Posse, R. E. Jung, and L. A. Morrison, "Use of tissue water as a concentration reference for proton spectroscopic imaging," *Magn. Reson. Med.*, vol. 55, no. 6, pp. 1219–1226, 2006.

252. R. Coifman and M. Wickerhauser, "Entropy-based algorithms for best basis selection," *IEEE Trans. Inf. Theory*, vol. 38, no. 2, pp. 713–718, 1992.

253. G. Lemaître, F. Nogueira, and C. K. Aridas, "Imbalanced-learn: A python toolbox to tackle the curse of imbalanced datasets in machine learning," *J. Mach. Learn. Res.*, vol. 18, no. 17, pp. 1–5, 2017. Available: http://jmlr.org/papers/v18/16-365.html

254. I. Mani and I. Zhang, "KNN approach to unbalanced data distributions: A case study involving information extraction," in *Proceedings of Workshop on Learning from Imbalanced Datasets*, 2003.

255. M. R. Smith, T. Martinez, and C. Giraud-Carrier, "An instance level analysis of data complexity," *Mach. Learn.*, vol. 95, no. 2, pp. 225–256, 2014.

256. N. V. Chawla, K. W. Bowyer, L. O. Hall, and W. P. Kegelmeyer, "Smote: Synthetic minority over-sampling technique," *J. Artif. Intell. Res.*, pp. 321–357, 2002.

257. H. Han, W. Y. Wang, and B. H. Mao, "Borderline-smote: A new over-sampling method in imbalanced data sets learning," in *International Conference on Intelligent Computing*, Springer, pp. 878–887, 2005.

258. Y. Saeys, I. Inza, and P. Larranaga, "A review of feature selection techniques in bioinformatics," *Bioinformatics*, vol. 23, no. 19, pp. 2507–2517, 2007.

259. S. N. Goodman, "Toward evidence-based medical statistics. 1: The P value fallacy,"*Ann. Intern. Med.*, vol. 130, no. 12, pp. 995–1004, 1999.

260. H. Peng, F. Long, and C. Ding, "Feature selection based on mutual information criteria of max-dependency, max-relevance, and min-redundancy," *IEEE Trans. Pattern Anal. Mach. Intell.*, vol. 27, no. 8, pp. 1226–1238, 2005.

261. I. Fodor, "A survey of dimension reduction techniques," Technical Report, Lawrence Livermore National Laboratory, Livermore, CA, 2002.

262. I. T. Jolliffe, *Principal Component Analysis*, 2nd ed. New York: Springer, 2002.

263. H. Zou, T. Hastie, and R. Tibshirani, "Sparse principal component analysis," *J. Comput. Graph. Stat.*, vol. 15, no. 2, pp. 265–286, 2006.

264. P. Comon, "Independent component analysis, a new concept?" *Signal Process.*, vol. 36, no. 3, pp. 287–314, 1994.

265. K. P. Murphy, *Machine Learning: A Probabilistic Perspective*. Cambridge, MA: MIT Press, 2012.

266. M. A. Aizerman, E. A. Braverman, and L. Rozonoer, "Theoretical foundations of the potential function method in pattern recognition learning," in *Automation and Remote Control*, no. 25, pp. 821–837, 1964.

267. S. T. Roweis and L. K. Saul, "Nonlinear dimensionality reduction by locally linear embedding," *Science*, vol. 290, no. 5500, pp. 2323–2326, 2000.

268. R. Rubinstein, M. Zibulevsky, and M. Elad, "Efficient implementation of the K-SVD algorithm using batch orthogonal matching pursuit," *CS Technion.*, vol. 40, no. 8, pp. 1–15, 2008.

269. M. Elad, *Sparse and Redundant Representations: From Theory to Applications in Signal and Image Processing*, 1st ed. New York: Springer, 2010.

270. S. G. Mallat and Z. Zhang, "Matching pursuits with time-frequency dictionaries," *IEEE Tran. Signal Process.*, vol. 41, no. 12, pp. 3397–3415, 1993.

271. Y. C. Pati, R. Rezaiifar, and P. Krishnaprasad, "Orthogonal matching pursuit: Recursive function approximation with applications to wavelet decomposition," in *Signals, Systems and Computers, 1993. 1993 Conference Record of the Twenty-Seventh Asilomar Conference on*. IEEE, pp. 40–44, 1993.

272. G. Davis, S. Mallat, and M. Avellaneda, "Adaptive greedy approximations," *Constr. Approx.*, vol. 13, no. 1, pp. 57–98, 1997.

273. J. Sivic and A. Zisserman, "Video google: A text retrieval approach to object matching in videos," in *IEEE ICCV*, pp. 1470–1477, 2003.

274. C. M. Bishop, *Pattern Recognition and Machine Learning*. Secaucus, NJ: Springer-Verlag, 2006.

275. A. Fred and A. Jain, "Combining multiple clusterings using evidence accumulation," *IEEE Trans. Pattern Anal. Mach. Intell.*, vol. 27, no. 6, pp. 835–850, 2005.

276. J. Friedman, "Regularized discriminant analysis," *J. Am. Stat. Assoc.*, vol. 84, no. 405, pp. 165–175, 1989.

277. I. Rish, "An empirical study of the naive Bayes classifier," in *Proceedings of IJCAI 2001 Workshop on Empirical Methods in Artificial Intelligence*, Vol. 3, New York, pp. 41–46, 2001.

278. Y. Freund and R. Schapire, "A decision-theoretic generalization of on-line learning and an application to boosting," *J. Comput. Syst. Sci.*, vol. 55, no. 1, pp. 119–139, 1997.

279. J. Quinlan, "Induction of decision trees," *Mach. Learn.*, vol. 1, no. 1, pp. 81–106, 1986.

280. J. Quinlan, *C4.5: Programs for Machine Learning.* San Francisco, CA: Morgan Kaufmann Publishers, 1993.

281. L. Breiman, J. Friedman, R. Olshen, and C. Stone, *Classification and Regression Trees.* Monterey, CA: Wadsworth & Brooks, 1984.

282. J. Friedman, T. Hastie, and R. Tibshirani, "Additive logistic regression: A statistical view of boosting," *Ann. Stat.*, vol. 28, p. 2000, 1998.

283. J. H. Friedman, "Greedy function approximation: A gradient boosting machine," *Ann. Stat.*, pp. 1189–1232, 2001.

284. L. Breiman, "Random forests," *Mach. Learn.*, vol. 45, no. 1, pp. 5–32, 2001.

285. B. Efron, "Bootstrap methods: Another look at the jackknife," *Ann. Stat.*, vol. 7, no. 1, pp. 1–26, 1979.

286. Z. Tu, "Probabilistic boosting-tree: Learning discriminative models for classification, recognition, and clustering," in *Computer Vision, 2005. ICCV 2005. Tenth IEEE International Conference on*, Vol. 2, pp. 1589–1596, 2005.

287. C. Rasmussen and C. Williams, *Gaussian Processes for Machine Learning.* Cambridge, MA: MIT Press, 2005.

288. V. Vapnik and A. Lerner, "Pattern recognition using generalized portrait method," *Automat. Rem. Contr.*, vol. 24, 1963.

289. C. Cortes and V. Vapnik, "Support-vector networks," *Mach. Learn.*, vol. 20, no. 3, pp. 273–297, 1995.

290. B. E. Boser, I. M. Guyon, and V. N. Vapnik, "A training algorithm for optimal margin classifiers," in *Proceedings of the Fifth Annual Workshop on Computational Learning Theory*, ser. COLT'92. New York: ACM, pp. 144–152, 1992.

291. M. Tipping, "Sparse Bayesian learning and the relevance vector machine," *J. Mach. Learn. Res.*, vol. 1, pp. 211–244, 2001.

292. J. Quinonero-Candela, A. Girard, and C. Rasmussen, "Prediction at an Uncertain Input for Gaussian processes and relevance vector machines application to multiple-step ahead time-series forecasting," DTU Informatics, Technical Report, 2002.

293. D. E. Rumelhart, G. E. Hinton, and R. J. Williams, "Learning internal representations by error propagation," in *Neurocomputing: Foundations of Research*, J. A. Anderson and E. Rosenfeld (Eds.), Cambridge, MA: MIT Press, pp. 673–695, 1988.

294. D. F. Specht, "Probabilistic neural networks for classification, mapping, or associative memory," in *Neural Networks, 1988, IEEE International Conference on*, Vol. 1, pp. 525–532, 1988.

295. Z. Kato and T. Pong, "A Markov random field image segmentation model using combined color and texture features," in *Computer Analysis of Images and Patterns*, ser. Lecture Notes in Computer Science, Vol. 2124, W. Skarbek (Ed.), Berlin, Germany: Springer, pp. 547–554, 2001.

296. Z. Kato and J. Zerubia, *Markov Random Fields in Image Segmentation. Collection Foundation and Trends in Signal Processing.* Now Editor, World Scientific, 2012.

297. B. Efron, "Estimating the error rate of a prediction rule: Improvement on cross-validation," *J. Am. Stat. Assoc.*, vol. 78, no. 382, pp. 316–331, 1983.

298. C. E. Metz, "Receiver operating characteristic analysis: A tool for the quantitative evaluation of observer performance and imaging systems," *J. Am. Coll. Radiol.*, vol. 3, no. 6, pp. 413–422, 2006.

299. H. He and E. Garcia, "Learning from imbalanced data," *IEEE Trans. Knowl. Data Eng.*, vol. 21, no. 9, pp. 1263–1284, 2009.

11 Early Diagnosis and Staging of Prostate Cancer Using Magnetic Resonance Imaging
State of the Art and Perspectives

Ruba Alkadi, Fatma Taher, Ayman El-Baz, and Naoufel Werghi

CONTENTS

INTRODUCTION

Prostate cancer is the second most common cancer among men in the United States after skin cancer [1]. It is estimated that 1 in every 7 men will be suspected with prostate cancer in his lifetime. According to the American Cancer Society, prostate cancer caused 26,730 deaths in the United States in 2017 [1]. Although it can be a serious disease, early diagnosis of prostate cancer can significantly prevent the growth of cancerous cells.

In fact, there are several types of tumors that may occur in the prostatic gland. These tumors can be benign or malignant. Some malignant tumors grow fast, but most of them grow slowly and are localized in the prostate gland [2]. Approximately 85% of diagnosed prostate cancers (CaP) are confined in the prostate gland [3]. According to McNeal et al. [4], 68% of diagnosed CaP is present in the peripheral zone (PZ) and those are considered less aggressive, while 32% is present in the central gland (CG) which are considered more aggressive.

In general, CaP can be treated by surgery, therapy, or most commonly active surveillance [2]. In active surveillance, the treatment option is deferred until some symptoms start to occur or until the cancer cells develop in an irregular manner that necessitates medical intervention [3]. This option is usually favored for two reasons: (a) it avoids the side effects of other treatment options such as therapy and surgical intervention, and (b) most of the localized CaPs do not effect patients during their lifetime because they either do not progress or they progress slowly [5]. Thus only aggressive and fast-growing cancers are candidates for medical intervention. In fact, studies show that many older men who died because of other causes also had CaP that did not affect them during their lifetime [2].

Several tests are considered in the daily clinical routine to diagnose a patient with prostate cancer. Usually, a blood test is conducted to check the prostate-specific antigen (PSA) level. An increased PSA level may be symptomatic for prostate cancer. However, this increase is also related to other common health issues such as benign prostatic hyperplasia (BPH) and prostatitis. Recently, the United State Preventive Services Task Force (USPSTF) recommended against PSA-based CaP screening in an attempt to reduce the overdiagnosis and overtreatment associated with this screening tool [5]. The USPSTF highlights the fact that PSA screening is unable to accurately select patients who may benefit from treatment and others who would benefit more from active surveillance.

After a positive PSA blood test, a transrectal ultrasound (TRUS) guided biopsy (GB) is carried out to further confirm the presence of prostate cancer. TRUS is an imaging technique that depends on measuring the echoes of initially sent ultrasound waves. It is used to guide a needle to take small samples of the prostatic tissue [1]. The samples are then analyzed and given a score called the Gleason score (GS). Due to its "blind" nature, TRUS-GB often leads to overdiagnosis and hence overtreatment [6,7]. Also, significant tumors in the prostate may be missed by the biopsy for the same reason. Surprisingly, prostate cancer is still the only solid organ cancer that is diagnosed by randomized sampling biopsies [6].

In the past few years, the use of magnetic resonance imaging (MRI) was proposed by the CaP research community as the most accurate noninvasive screening tool for prostate cancer diagnosis and staging [8]. Especially in the case of active surveillance, MRI can greatly assist doctors in disease monitoring and treatment management [9]. MRI is an imaging technique that uses the fundamentals of nuclear magnetic resonance (NMR) phenomenon to produce images that describe internal physical and chemical characteristics of an object [10]. By nature, some atoms such as hydrogen (H) possess a random nuclear spin (Figure 11.1a). However, when exposed to an external magnetic field (B0), these spins are aligned to produce a net magnetic moment (Figure 11.1b). The MRI technique depends on measuring the time needed by these spins to return to their original orientations after turning off the aligning magnetic field B0 as in Figure 11.1c.

The most common measurable quantities are the longitudinal relaxation time T1 and the transverse relaxation time T2 [11]. These quantities differ between human tissues making it meaningful to be used as a medical imaging tool. Table 11.1 shows how the T2 values differ between different

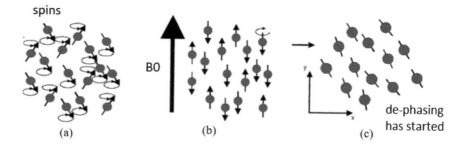

spins

BO

(a)   (b)   (c)

de-phasing has started

FIGURE 11.1 (a) Natural random nuclear spin, (b) spins align due to the magnetic field B0, (c) spins de-phasing after removing the effect of B0. (From Toennies, K., *Guide to Medical Image Analysis: Methods and Algorithms*, Springer, London, UK, 2012.)

TABLE 11.1

T2 Values of Some Tissues

Tissue	T2 (msec)
Muscle	47
Fat	85
Kidney	58
Liver	43

tissue types [11]. These values are used on a grayscale intensity values to create the T1-weighted (T1W) MRI and the T2-weighted (T2W) MRI, respectively.

T2W-MRI is the standard MRI modality that shows the anatomy of the scanned organ. In contrary, T1W-MRI produces a greyscale image that complements the T2W-MRI. In other words, the black matters in the former appear in white in the latter, and vice versa. Usually T1W images are acquired in a time series one after another to show the functionality of an organ. Because of their dynamic appearance, these images are called the dynamic contrast-enhanced (DCE) MRI. The image quality is enhanced by the injection of a contrast agent in the body of the patient at the time of acquisition. Diffusion-weighted (DW) MRI is a third modality that uses the T2 values to show the water molecules diffusion in the screened tissue. Mathematically, DW images are T2W images multiplied by an exponential factor that depends on the apparent diffusion coefficient (ADC) of the water molecules and the attenuation coefficient of the applied gradient pulse b as shown in the following equation [12]:

$$S(b) = S_0 e^{-b \times \text{ADC}}$$

(11.1)

where $S(b)$ is the DW signal and S_0 is the T2W signal. Note that when the attenuation coefficient b is 0 sec/mm^2, the DW image is the same as the T2W image [12].

Finally, a non-imaging modality that uses the same NMR principle is magnetic resonance spectroscopy (MRS). This technique records a 2D signal for each spatial location in the scanned object which, clinically, carries information about the presence of certain metabolites in that location. More details about each modality will be provided in the following sections.

As can be noticed, the MR imaging technique does not include any ionizing radiation and thus is not harmful to the human body [10]. This is by far the main reason for the MRI becoming a daily clinical practice in many medical fields.

Although MRI has shown competitive diagnosis performance compared to PSA and TRUS-GB, it has not yet been considered as a first-line diagnosis tool. The main reason is related to the

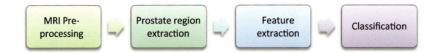

FIGURE 11.2   MRI-based CAD for CaP pipeline.

difficulties and challenges encountered by radiologists when reading and analyzing MRIs. More precisely, the 3D nature of MRI makes it difficult to analyze the full prostate volume by visual inspection, and hence it is very dependent on the radiologist's experience. Moreover, the analysis outcome is also affected by the large amount of data that needs to be analyzed simultaneously.

To resolve this issue, a multimodality MRI-based computer-aided diagnosis (CAD) system was first proposed by Chan et al. [13] in 2003. Since then, several CAD systems have been proposed by the research community targeting the issue of the deployment of a fully automated MRI-based CAD system for CaP diagnosis to overcome the limitations of reliability caused by potential human errors.

GENERAL PROCESS PIPELINE

Similar to other medical imaging CAD systems, the computer-aided diagnosis of prostate cancer using MRI framework encompasses four stages, namely: pre-processing, prostate region extraction, features extraction, and classification (see Figure 11.2). The pre-processing is a set of procedures applied on the MRI images in order to improve quality by reducing undesirable effects inferred by the images acquisition. The prostate region extraction applies segmentation techniques that aim at the correct delineation of the prostate region. The feature extraction is the process of defining and deriving from the prostate region computational entities that form a sort of prostate cancer signature. While it performs dimensionality reduction by encoding the prostate region into a compact format, the feature extraction is also meant to be discriminative, as much as possible separating the malignant and benign cases. The extracted features are then fed into the last stage, the classification, whereby they are treated and mapped into one of the aforementioned categories. Depending on the type and the discriminative power of the features, the classification method can range from basic technique, such as minimum distance classifier, to the heavy machine learning system, such as deep learning networks.

In this chapter, state-of-the-art full MRI-based CAD for CaP systems presented in the literature are reviewed. We categorize the reviewed systems based on the MRI modality used as an input for the CAD system. In the first four sections we review T2-weighted, DCE, MRS, and DW MRI-based CAD systems that are presented in a monomodality framework, respectively. In Section 11.5, we review the different fusion methods used in the multimodality MRI framework.

T2-WEIGHTED MRI

T2W is an MR imaging protocol that uses the transverse relaxation time (T2) to construct a grayscale image of the scanned object. Figure 11.3 shows a slice of a T2W-MRI obtained using a 1.5 Tesla scanner with an endorectal coil placed while acquisition to improve the image resolution [12].

Due to its increasing popularity and availability by many health providers, T2W-MR images have been an effective tool for noninvasive CaP diagnosis [14]. The reason is that normal prostatic tissues appear visually different from cancerous tissues in terms of intensity and homogeneity [7,15,16]. More precisely, malignant tissues are characterized by lower signal intensity in the PZ of the prostate and a more homogeneous appearance in both the CG and the PZ compared to the surrounding healthy tissues [12,16]. The other main advantage of this modality is that it provides the zonal anatomy of the prostate gland. That is, the CG is well distinguished from the PZ of the prostate and the surrounding non-prostatic tissues [15].

On the other hand, studies have reported the lack of reliability of T2W-MRI reflected by the low sensitivity and specificity [17]. This mainly results from the difficulty of CaP detection in the CG

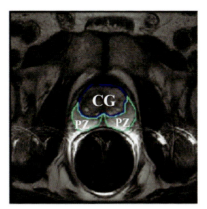

FIGURE 11.3   T2W-MRI using a 1.5 Tesla MRI scanner and an endorectal coil. The CG is delineated with blue while the green contour represents the PZ. (From Lemaitre, G., Computer-aided diagnosis for prostate cancer using multi-parametric magnetic resonance imaging, Doctoral Program in Technology, France, 2016.)

as well as the existence of some other nonmalignant diseases such as BPH that have similar visual appearance as malignant tissues in T2W-MRIs [16]. Finally, unlike DCE-MRI, T2W-MRI does not provide information about the functionality of the organ under study [18].

In fact, these limitations of T2W-MRI have been addressed by incorporating data from other MRI modalities (to be discussed later in this chapter). It is also worth noting that very few studies have used this modality as the only input for their CAD systems. Instead, many studies have suggested fusing T2-weighted imaging (T2WI) with other modalities to boost the performance of their CAD systems in general [14].

Pre-processing

T2W-MRIs suffer from artifacts and noise due to factors related to MRI acquisition, such as magnetic field inhomogeneity [19] and thermal noise [14]. The most popular artifacts that were addressed in the literature are (a) intensity scale nonlinearity [15], and (b) bias field effect which is introduced by the use of endorectal coil at the time of MRI examination [12]. In Viswanath et al. [16], the former is adjusted by the generalized scale algorithm, which aims at aligning the intensity histogram to ensure a normalized intensity scale. While the latter is corrected by the nonparametric nonuniform intensity normalization (N3) algorithm described in Sled et al. [20].

On the other hand, Rampun et al. [14] corrected the above artifacts by first applying a median filter, then normalizing the image intensity to zero mean and a unit variance and finally removing remaining noise by an anisotropic diffusion filter. They reported that this three-step process has the advantage of (i) removing noise, (ii) preserving edges, and (iii) standardizing image intensities between different patients.

To normalize the intensity values and avoid interpatient variability, Niaf et al. [21] used the mean SI of the bladder as a normalization factor to normalize the T2WI.

Lopes et al. [19] investigated the use of wavelet-based filters in the preprocessing stage; however, it was then excluded as it did not have an effect on the overall system.

Prostate Region Extraction

Identifying the region of interest (ROI) in the MR images is essential to reduce the complexity of the next stages and enhance the performance of the overall CAD system. This step could be performed either (i) manually by the radiologist or (ii) automatically by the CAD system.

Manual selection of a 12×12 pixels ROI was performed in Lv et al. [15] and manual delineation by an experienced radiologist was reported in Rampun et al. [14].

Instead, automated prostate capsule segmentation presented in Bulman et al. [22] was performed in Viswanath et al. [16] where Active Shape Model (ASM) was initialized by automatically identifying prostatic voxels inside a box that contains all the prostate volume.

FEATURE EXTRACTION AND SELECTION

As mentioned earlier, the main descriptive feature of CaP in T2W-MRI is its low signal intensity and its homogenous appearance. Most of the studies have focused on capturing these measures as the main features in their CAD systems. Lopes et al. [19] proposed the use of fractal and multifractal features to detect the unique texture of cancerous tissues. An experiment comparing *classical texture features*, including co-occurrence matrices, Gabor filters, and wavelet frame decomposition, and *fractal geometry-based features* shows the superiority of the latter in identifying prostate cancer [19].

Lv et al. [15] employed the same concept of fractal geometry with some variations in the algorithms. Texture fractal dimension was used to quantify the roughness of the texture. The intensity, along with the 2D spatial distribution, formed a 3D surface as shown in Figure 11.4b and e, at which the 3D box-counting algorithm is applied. In addition, the 2D version of the same box-counting technique is used on the intensity histogram (Figure 11.4c and f) to assess the irregularity and complexity of the intensity distribution. Note the clear difference between healthy and non-healthy tissues in terms of the intensity inhomogeneity explained above.

Furthermore, distinct textural signatures in the CG and PZ could be uniquely identified according to Viswanath et al. [16]. A total of 110 features extracted from Gabor wavelet transform, Haar wavelet transform, Haralick texture feature, and Grey-level statistical features were employed. Then, feature selection by minimum Redundancy Maximum Relevance (mRMR) is performed in order to identify the unique signatures of cancer in both the CG and PZ. Results show that CaP could be distinctively identified in the CG by Gabor filters, while it could be better distinguished by Haralick texture features in the PZ. Moreover, the optimum 15 features in the CG and 25 features in the PZ for identifying tumor were identified in Viswanath et al. [16].

Rampun et al. [14] identified a larger set of 215 features and grouped them in six classes in an attempt to investigate the performance of a CAD system that only uses the T2W-MRI. The

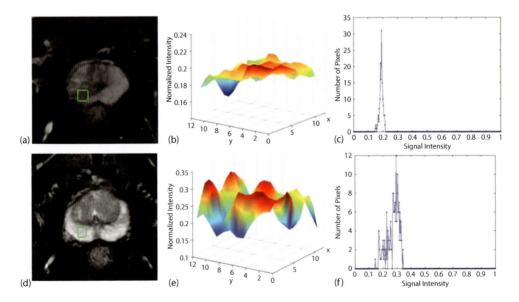

FIGURE 11.4 PZ with CaP (a) and without CaP (d) enclosed with a green box on a T2W-MRI slice; (b), (e) intensity values (z-axis) represented on their spatial locations (x, y), and (c), (f) 2D intensity histograms. (From Lv, D. et al., *J. Magn. Reson. Imaging*, 30, 161–168, 2009.)

CsfSubsetEval method was used to reduce the feature space dimensionality. It is reported that Gaussian filters, Laplacian of Gaussian filters, image magnitude of the Sobel operator, and Tamura's contrast were among the most selected features when the window size is optimum (9 × 9 voxels). Results comparable to other multimodality systems were obtained using T2W-MRI only.

CLASSIFICATION

To simply assess the distinguishing capacity of fractal features, Lv et al. [15] used a simple thresh-olding technique along with the statistical t-test. The *t* test yielded an impressive group difference ($P < 0.001$) at 95% confidence level for the histogram fractal dimension (HFD) explained above. The potential robustness of the fractal indices is also evaluated by varying the critical value of these indices. The area under curve (AUC) of the receiver operating characteristic (ROC) curve is then determined. HFD yielded an AUC of 0.966.

Lopes et al. [19] made use of the same fractal and multifractal dimensions, estimated by the Variance method and the multifractional Brownian motion (mBm), respectively. Nonetheless, the authors proposed a classification framework instead of the simple thresholding used by Lv et al. [15]. Support vector machine (SVM) and Adaptive Boosting (AdaBoost) classifiers were both tested on a voxel-based scheme. The SVM yielded a sensitivity of 0.83 and a specificity of 0.91, while a slightly better performance was noted for the AdaBoost where a sensitivity and specificity of 0.85 and 0.93, respectively, were achieved.

Quadratic discriminant analysis (QDA) was performed by Viswanath et al. [16] on the 110 features described above to highlight the effectiveness of uniquely identifying region-based features in the prostate gland. The AUC was obtained by varying the threshold of the QDA function and eventually yielded a value of 0.86.

Rampun et al. [14] reported the performance of 9 popular classifiers and two meta-voting classifiers, where the decisions of the two and three best-performing classifiers were combined, respectively. Keeping all parameters in the default setting, the meta-vote (best 2) classifier outperformed all the other 10 classifiers with an AUC of 92.7% ± 7.4%, an accuracy of 85.5% ± 7.2%, and a sensitivity of 93.3% ± 9.1%. This classifier combined the results of the Bayesian networks (BNets) and the alternating decision tree (ADTree) using the average probability combination rule. It is important to note that some classifiers are very sensitive to parameter settings and thus, their performances could be greatly improved by tuning these parameters instead of keeping them on the default setting.

SUMMARY

A summary of Section 11.2 findings is provided in Table 11.2.

TABLE 11.2
Highlights of Section 11.2

	Highlights
Pre-processing	• Three-step pre-processing by [14]. Generalized scale algorithm and N3 algorithm [16].
	• Segmentation by ASM [16].
	• Manual segmentation [14,15].
Feature selection and extraction	• Fractal features achieve better distinguishing capacity than classical features [15,19].
	• Tumors are characterized by unique structural and textural characteristics in the CG and PZ [16].
Classification	• AUC = 0.966 using thresholding [15].
	• AUC = 0.93 using SVM and AdaBoost [19].
	• AUC = 0.86 using QDA [16].
	• AUC = 0.93 using meta-vote (BNets, and ADTree) [14].

DYNAMIC CONTRAST-ENHANCED MRI

DCE-MRI is an imaging technique that produces a sequence of T1W-MRI images that demonstrates the behavior of a pre-injected contrast agent (usually gadolinium-based) in the targeted tissue. This introduces "time" as a fourth dimension to the 3D MRI, which in turns allows for a noninvasive access to tissue vascular characteristics [23]. The main advantage of this modality is that it realizes the microvasculature difference between healthy and cancerous tissues [17]. Basically, this difference results from the nature of malignant tumors which are well fed with blood via vessel networks that are of high capillary permeability. As a result, the rate at which the contrast media is exchanged between vessels and extravascular-extracellular space (EES) in malignant tissues is higher than the corresponding rate in healthy tissues [12,24]. Figure 11.6a and b shows an example of two slices of T1W-MRI from a DCE sequence before and after contrast agent injection.

In this context, the main aim is to plot the intensity enhancement versus time curves for each voxel or region in the prostate and eventually extract the so-called pharmacokinetic parameters from these curves [12]. Figure 11.5 shows the common parameters that are usually extracted from the signal enhancement curves. Figure 11.6c and d show the intensity enhancement curve of the two delineated foci in Figure 11.6b. The intensity enhancement curve of the tissue circled in green is shown in Figure 11.6c while the intensity enhancement curve in Figure 11.6d corresponds to the cancerous tissue in the red circle.

In the literature, more than 15 perfusion parameters have been introduced, with forward volume transfer constant (k^{trans}) and reverse reflux rate constant (k_{ep}) being the most useful clinically according to [17,25,26]. The former represents the flow rate of the contrast agent from the blood into the prostate tissue (wash-in rate), while the later represents the flow rate of the contrast agent leaving the tissue to the blood vessels (washout rate) [26].

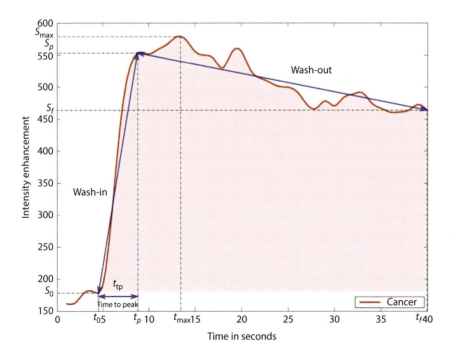

FIGURE 11.5 Typical intensity enhancement curve of a cancerous tissue. Note the wash-in rate, washout rate, time to peak (t_{tp}), contrast agent arrival time (t_0), first peak time (t_p), maximum peak time (t_{max}), and the corresponding intensities (S_0, S_p, S_{max}), respectively. (From Lemaitre, G. et al., *Comput. Biol. Med.*, 60, 8–31, 2015.)

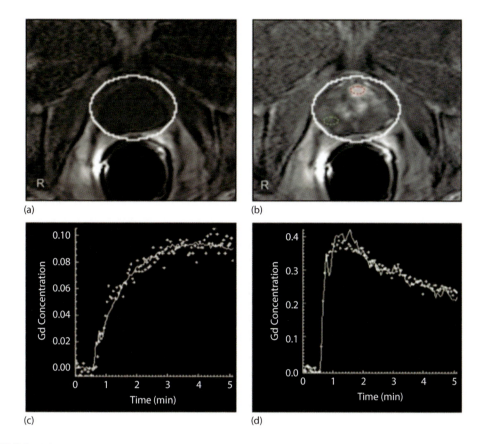

FIGURE 11.6 T1W images (a) before and (b) after the injection of a contrast agent, and the corresponding intensity enhancement curves for (c) the healthy tissue circled in green and (d) the tumor foci circled in red in the corresponding (b). Note the early wash-in and washout rates in the case of tumor in (d) compared to normal tissue in (c). (From Ocak, I. et al., *Am. J. Roentgenol.*, 189, 192–201, 2007.)

Studies have shown superiority, in terms of sensitivity and specificity, of DCE- over T2W-MRI in differentiating between healthy and cancerous tissues [17,27]. Hara et al. [28] recommended the use of DCE-MRI alone instead of biopsy for CaP diagnosis in older patients.

Although some perfusion parameters could act as relatively good discriminative features, a considerable overlap of these parameters between malignant and benign tissues is present [17]. Especially in the CG, it is still challenging to distinguish between healthy and cancerous tissues due to the fact that they could exhibit the same pharmacokinetic behavior in both cases [12,29]. Finally, due to its temporal nature, the DCE-MRI modality is affected by patient breathing and motion [30]. It is also worth noting that contrast media injection is not always suitable for patients with kidney problems [18].

PRE-PROCESSING

In the CAD system proposed by Vos et al. [24], manual lesion localization using a 3D drawing tool was used to localize the suspected lesion by a sphere on the 3D MRI. Similarly, manual delineation of the ROI was adopted in Sung et al. [17].

In Viswanath et al. [31], a multi-attribute, non-initializing, texture reconstruction based active shape model (MANTRA) segmentation algorithm which only requires a rough manual initialization is used to automatically segment the prostate gland [32]. This method depends on finding a statistical shape model of the prostate borders and statistical texture model of the area surrounding the prostate border. These two models were then used in an ASM framework.

Another novel segmentation framework is proposed by Firjani et al. [30] at which a maximum a posteriori (MAP) of a log-likelihood function is estimated. The function accounts for the shape *priori*, the spatial interaction and the specific visual appearance of the prostate in each subject. In addition, a non-rigid registration scheme is developed to account for deformation due to patient's motion during acquisition. A segmentation sensitivity of 84.6% was obtained on a dataset of 30 patients.

FEATURE EXTRACTION AND SELECTION

Sung et al. [17] extracted 13 perfusion parameters out of each signal enhancement-time curve, namely: baseline and peak signal intensities, initial slope, maximum slope during the initial 50 seconds after the contrast agent injection, time to peak, wash-in rate, washout rate, percentage of relative enhancement, percentage enhancement ratio, time of arrival, efflux rate constant indicating the trans-vascular permeability (k_{ep}), first-order rate constant for eliminating the contrast agent from the blood plasma (k_{el}), and a constant representing the size of the extravascular extracellular space (A^H).

Vos et al. [24] identified only three pharmacokinetic features which were selected based on the clinical experience. These include (i) 50% percentile T1 static value which is useful in identifying post-biopsy hemorrhage, (ii) 75% percentile k_{ep} and K^{trans} which indicate the permeability of the blood vessels that increase in inflamed and tumor tissues, (iii) 25% percentile late wash which is defined by the slope of the curve after the first wash-in and which highly correlates to malignant tumors according to Vos et al. [24]. On the other hand, the *peak perfusion* value and the *wash-in slope* were the only two parameters utilized by Firjani et al. [30] to characterize each voxel in the segmented prostate.

In contrast, the dimensionality of the intensity feature space is reduced in [31] by the nonlinear dimension reduction: locally linear embedding (LLE) algorithm. This idea of reducing the feature vector of each voxel is borrowed from Varini et al. [33] where LLE was applied on breast DCE-MRI to detect malignant lesions. Basically, this algorithm attempts to represent each data point by a linear combination of its k-nearest neighbors [12].

CLASSIFICATION

Puech et al. [29,34] used thresholding based on maximum and median wash-in and washout slopes in both the PZ and CG in order to give a suspicion score of the selected lesion. A sensitivity of 100% was obtained in both PZ and CG with a corresponding 45% and 40% specificity in the PZ and CG, respectively.

A k-NN classifier was used by Firjani et al. [30] to distinguish between malignant and benign tumors. The boundaries of the tumor were then delineated using a level-set deformable model. A classification accuracy of 100% was obtained on a 21-patients dataset.

Similarly, Viswanath et al. [31] applied consensus k-means clustering repeatedly to the reduced manifold using different values of k. A co-association matrix which represents the association between any two data points based on the number of times they appear in the same cluster throughout the iterations is then constructed. Multidimensional scaling (MDS) is then performed on the co-association matrix, followed by a k-means clustering which yielded the final stable clusters.

Another classification method is adapted as well [31], and compared to the first method. This is the 3 time point (3TP) method, where inflection points are determined in the intensity-time curves at each pixel. Mainly, these values are used to estimate the contrast agent wash-in and washout rates. An improvement in the sensitivity from 38.2% to 60.7% and the specificity from 69.1% to 83.2% when using consensus k-means clustering is reported. It is important to note that these results were obtained relative to a rigorous ground truth and that this study considered both PZ and CG.

In contrast, Vos et al. [24] fused their three features mentioned above in a SVM to classify malignant and benign lesions in the PZ. The obtained sensitivity was 83% with a corresponding specificity of 58%. These results were obtained with reference to an approximated ground truth that resulted from a roughly registered histology.

Likewise, SVM was mainly used by Sung et al. [17] to fuse all 13 previously extracted perfusion parameters. Besides, thresholding using the cut-off (optimum) point on the ROC curve was also applied to each individual perfusion parameter map besides T2WI. The individual perfusion parameter maps and T2WI were then compared using sensitivity and specificity measures. Expectedly, the SVM-based CAD system showed superior performance in the PZ with an accuracy, sensitivity, and specificity of 89%, 89%, and 89%, respectively. Nevertheless, the accuracy, sensitivity, and specificity were 77%, 91%, and 64%, respectively, in the CG. It is suggested that this difference in the performance is related to the low specificity of the perfusion parameters in the CG.

SUMMARY

A summary of Section 11.3 findings is provided in Table 11.3.

TABLE 11.3
Highlights of Section 11.3

	Highlights
Pre-processing	• Three-step pre-processing by [14]. Generalized scale algorithm and N3 algorithm [16]. • Segmentation by ASM [16]. • Manual segmentation [14,15].
Feature selection and extraction	• Thirteen parameters are extracted in [17]. • Three parameters are extracted in [24]. • Peak perfusion and wash-in slope is used in [30]. • In [31], the curve vector is reduced using LLE to obtain a feature vector.
Classification	• Sen = spec = 77% for SVM [17]. • Sen = 83%; spec = 58% for SVM [24]. • Accuracy = 100% for k-NN [30]. • Sen = 60%; spec = 83% for k-means clustering [31].

MR SPECTROSCOPY (MRS)

Complementing structural MRI, magnetic resonance spectroscopy imaging (MRSI) is a modality that provides 3D spectral information describing the metabolic concentrations in a spatial grid [12,35]. Usually, the spectral grid is superposed on a 2D slice T2W-MRI which forms the 3D modality [36,37]. An example for a 3×6 spectroscopic grid projected of the T2W-MRI is shown in Figure 11.7.

Note the low resolution of the MRS grid as each voxel in this grid can cover a $k \times k$ voxels on the T2WI. Moreover, each voxel is characterized by a complex spectrum signal at which information about several metabolites can be extracted. Hence, each spectrum at each location is analyzed individually to determine the type of the corresponding tissue which is shown in the T2W-MRI. More precisely, the area under each peak of the spectrum maps to the relative concentration of a certain metabolite [12,37,38]. Figure 11.8 shows MR spectra for a healthy and a malignant tissue in the prostate. Note the difference in the relative concentration, interpreted by the height of citrate and choline peaks, between healthy and cancerous tissues [36].

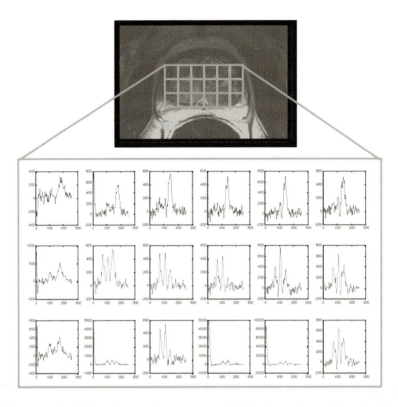

FIGURE 11.7 A sample MRS grid superimposed on a T2WI. (From Tiwari, P. et al., *Med. Phys.*, 36, 3927–3939, 2009.)

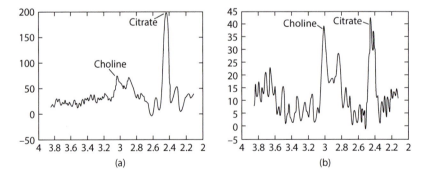

FIGURE 11.8 (a) Healthy and (b) malignant spectrum. Note that each peak corresponds to a certain metabolite. (From Trigui, R. et al., *Biomed. Signal Process. Control*, 31, 189–198, 2017.)

Clinical studies suggest that the presence of malignant cells is associated with a lower concentration of citrate and a higher concentration of choline [39]. In addition, the ratio (choline + creatine/citrate) has also been correlated to the presence of CaP [37].

Compared to other modalities, MRSI shows higher potential to differentiate between healthy and CaP tissues [39]. A study conducted by Zi-jun et al. [40] shows a significant positive correlation between the diagnostic accuracy of MRSI and the GS of CaP, which suggests the effectiveness of this modality in the evaluation of the aggressiveness of CaP [12].

On the other hand, MRSI lacks (i) spatial resolution, (ii) consistent interpatient metabolite concentrations [12], and (iii) consistent metabolite concentrations in different zones of the prostate [38]. Also, one of the drawbacks that prevents this modality from being part of the clinical routine is its long acquisition time. However, high magnetic field strength is suggested to resolve this problem [12].

PRE-PROCESSING

Parfait et al. [39] proposed a full MRSI pre-processing framework that addresses the removal of unwanted artifacts present in phase, baseline, and intensity standardization.

Phase correction is first applied using the Automated phase Correction based on Minimization of Entropy (ACME) algorithm proposed in [41]. This algorithm iterates to find two coefficients: (i) a zero-order phase coefficient and (ii) a first-order phase coefficient, by minimizing an objective function.

In addition, baseline correction is also applied in Parfait et al. [39] to remove the artifact caused by the presence of macromolecules and lipids within the tissue of interest, which causes additive wide peaks to the spectra. A Gaussian low-pass filter (LPF) was applied iteratively to the spectra to remove the assumed additive noise. Figure 11.9 shows the signal before and after baseline correction. Finally, normalization using the T2-normalization technique is considered before classification. To correct the baseline artifact, Kelm et al. [42] used time-domain selective Hankel singular values of dynamic system (HSVD) filtering which aims at removing signal components outside the frequency range of interest [43]. These two methods are essentially similar in the sense that they both filter out unwanted frequency components to correct the baseline signal.

To determine the "informative" MRS blocks that are relevant to the prostate, Tiwari et al. [37] used graph embedding, a nonlinear dimensionality reduction scheme, to reduce the space dimensionality of the whole spectra, followed by a replicated k-means clustering. This clustering algorithm yielded two stable clusters: one corresponds to prostatic voxels and the other corresponds to non-prostatic voxels. The larger cluster is then eliminated as it is assumed to correspond to non-prostatic voxels. The average sensitivity and specificity of this selection process were 97.66% and 98.87%, respectively.

Instead, Parfait et al. [39] and Matulewicz et al. [38] used manual selection of MRS blocks that lie inside the prostate.

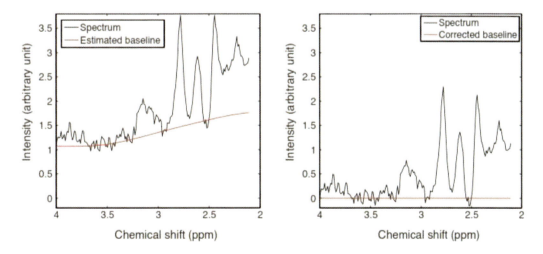

FIGURE 11.9 MRS signal before (left) and after (right) baseline correction using iterative low-pass filtering. (From Parfait, S. et al., *Biomed. Signal Process. Control*, 7, 499–508, 2012.)

FEATURE EXTRACTION AND SELECTION

Feature extraction of MRSI spectrum could be classified into two main categories [35,37]: (i) quantification-based analysis and (ii) pattern recognition-based analysis. In the first category, studies have focused on peak detection and relative concentration calculation for the purpose of detecting irregular concentrations of metabolites which are biomarkers for CaP. However, recent studies [12,42] show that the pattern recognition approach is more efficient and less sensitive to noise and artifacts. This approach relies on analyzing the whole spectra instead of performing traditional peak detection algorithms.

Kelm et al. [42] present a comparison between three quantification methods, and four pattern recognition approaches including: (i) principle component analysis (PCA), (ii) independent component analysis (ICA), (iii) nonnegative matrix factorization (NMF), and (iv) partial least squares (PLS). The authors claim no significant difference in the AUC of these four methods. However, they report a comparable performance of the studied pattern recognition approaches to that of quantitation based on the semi-parametric quantum estimation (QUEST) approach proposed in [44].

Similarly, Parfait et al. [39] have shown that the final CAD performance is significantly improved when using the whole real spectra as an input for the classifier compared to the quantification-based techniques.

CLASSIFICATION

Matulewicz et al. [38] trained an artificial neural networks (ANN), a nonlinear classifier, with one hidden layer that has the smallest possible number of neurons to avoid overtraining and poor generalization. Two models were tested, one that has the MRSI spectra as the input and another one that has the MRSI spectra plus the rough location of the voxel specified as one of four labels each corresponds to a pre-identified region in the prostate. Their results show that the second model provides an improvement in the sensitivity, specificity and AUC over the first model. Nevertheless, the maximum sensitivity achieved in this work is 62.5%, which is considered unsatisfactory compare to other MRSI-based CAD systems. However, the main contribution of their study is that it shows an improvement in the sensitivity (from 50% to 62.5%) when considering zonal anatomy of each voxel as an extra input to the ANN classifier.

While in Kelm et al. [42], the classification methods were subdivided into linear and nonlinear methods. Linear classification methods are (i) logistic regression, (ii) generalized PLS, and (iii) P-spline signal regression (PSR), while nonlinear methods considered in this study are (i) RF, (ii) SVM, and (iii) Gaussian processes (GP).

They conclude that nonlinear classification methods outperform all other combinations of linear classification methods. Also, nonlinear classifiers easily outperform quantification-based approaches. All conclusions were drawn based on the AUC measure, which yields the robustness of the particular approach. The final output of their CAD system is a tumor probability map shown in Figure 11.10.

On the other hand, Parfait et al. [39] have compared three classification methods: (i) SVM, (ii) multilayer perceptron (MLP), a family of ANN, and (iii) Bayes classification rule, which is based on thresholding the relative concentration of choline/citrate. The best performance (error rate 4.51%, sensitivity 83.57%, and specificity 98.11%) was achieved using SVM with the input spectra being pre-processed for phase, baseline, and intensity scale correction.

Besides, for the purpose of identifying cancerous spectra, Tiwari et al. [37] used four different feature extraction methods: (i) graph embedding, (ii) LLE, (iii) PCA, and (iv) z-score. They used replicated clustering (similar to the one described in Section 11.4.1) to classify the MRS signals into three classes: (i) normal, (i) suspicious, and (iii) indeterminate. A sensitivity of 81.36% with a corresponding specificity of 64.71% was obtained using LLE followed by replicated clustering.

It can be concluded that nonlinear methods are more suitable for spectral classification as the output of classification is linearly non-separable.

SUMMARY

A summary of Section 11.4 findings is provided in Table 11.4.

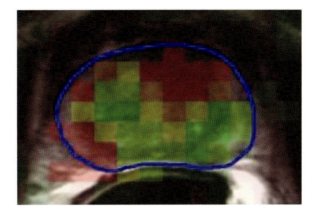

FIGURE 11.10 Tumor probability color map obtained by the CAD system presented in Kelm et al. [42]. Red, yellow and green correspond to tumor, undecided, and healthy tissues, respectively.

TABLE 11.4
Highlights of Section 11.4

	Highlights
Pre-processing	• Phase correction by ACME, baseline correction by LPF, normalization by T2- normalization [39].
	• HSVD filtering is applied in [42].
	• Graph embedding with k-means Clustering to select informative spectra [37].
Feature selection and extraction	• Pattern recognition approach is more reliable than traditional quantification-based approach [39,42].
Classification	• The inclusion of zonal anatomy with the MRS improves performance; sen = 62.5% [38].
	• Nonlinear classifiers outperform linear classifiers [42].
	• SVM outperformed MLP and Bayes classification in [39].
	• LLE followed by replicated clustering outperformed, graph embedding, PCA, and z-score classification in [37].

DIFFUSION-WEIGHTED MRI

Simply, DW-MRI is an MR imaging modality at which the motion of water molecules is reflected in each voxel intensity value. In a certain location in the image, higher intensity values imply less water diffusion, while low intensity values indicate higher diffusion of water molecules. In fact, this property allows for a better distinction between healthy and CaP tissues.

Table 11.5 summarizes the differences between these three tissues in the DW-MRI context [12,34]. DWI can be acquired at different attenuation coefficients known as the b value. This value can be changed by changing the gradient pulse intensity and duration. Figure 11.11 shows a sample DW-MRIs for the same patient but at different b values.

Although DW-MRI provides better distinction between soft tissues, CG tissues can sometimes be confused with CaP tissues as they both restrict the diffusion of water. Also, this modality lacks spatial resolution according to Lemaitre [12].

On the other hand, ADC is a parameter that can be calculated using DW-MRI acquired at two b values: (i) $b_0 = 0$ sec/mm^2 which is essentially the T2W-MRI and (ii) $b_1 > b_0$, as follows:

$$\text{ADC} = \frac{\ln\left(S(b_1)/S_0\right)}{b_1} \tag{11.2}$$

TABLE 11.5

Prostate Zonal Anatomy in the DW-MRI Modality. Note That the CG is Not Well Distinguished from Other Tissues, Which is the Main Drawback of DW-MRI.

Tissue	Physiological Property	Water Molecules Diffusion	Visual Appearance in DW-MRI	Visual Appearance in ADC Maps
PZ	Soft glandular and tubular tissue	High	Low SI	High SI
CG	Muscular and fibrous structure	Constrained and heterogeneous		—
CaP	High cellular density due to the uncontrolled growth of cells	Very restricted	High SI	Low SI

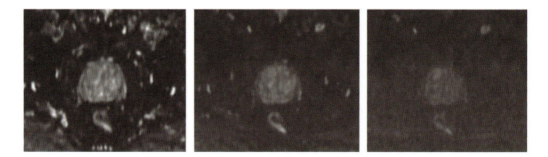

FIGURE 11.11 Example of DW-MRI obtained at different b values.

where $S(b_1)$ and S_0 are the measured signals at b_1 and b_0, respectively [12]. Note that this equation is obtained by rearranging Equation 11.1.

ADC maps could be generated at different b values using the above equation. High discriminatory performance between high, intermediate, and low GS using ADC maps was reported in the PZ [45].

An experiment conducted by Litjens et al. [46] shows that a CAD system that uses features from DWI alone performs as good as another one which uses features from the combination of T2W-, DCE- and DW-MRI.

In Reda et al. [18,47], the authors proposed a fully automated CAD system that segments the prostate using an NMF-based level set segmentation method which uses intensity, shape, and spatial features to accurately segment the prostate from the surrounding tissues. This segmentation method yielded a dice similarity coefficient (DSC) of 86.9%.

The cumulative distribution functions (CDFs) of the normalized ADC maps of the segmented prostate were then calculated and considered as the global features for differentiating between benign and malignant tissues. The CDFs for 53 patients were obtained for $b = [100\ 200\ 300\ 400\ 500\ 600\ 700]$, and were all fed to a stacked nonnegativity constraint auto-encoder (SNCAE). Results show that the ADC-CDF at $b = 700$ s/mm^2 outperforms all other alternatives including the ADC-CDFs at all b values together. Impressively, 100% accuracy, sensitivity, and specificity were obtained on a leave-one-out cross-validation of 53 patients.

A similar framework is presented by Reda et al. [48], but instead of using the ADC-CDFs at $b = 700$ s/mm^2 as the only input for the SNCAE, the authors used all the seven b values in a majority voting framework. The overall accuracy obtained is 97.6% on a dataset of 42 patients.

In the same context, Firjani et al. [49] used an intensity, shape, and spatial interaction model to segment the prostate. Nevertheless, boundaries of the suspected tumors were first delineated using a level-set-based deformable model. Later, a k-nearest neighbor classifier was used to determine the malignancy of the tumor. The mean intensity values of the DW-MRI at $b = 0$ sec/mm^2, $b = 800$ sec/mm^2 and the ADC mean intensity value were found to be the most discriminant features.

TABLE 11.6
Highlights of Section 11.5

	Highlights
Pre-processing	• Segmentation using spatial, shape, and intensity interaction models was performed in [49], [47], and [18].
Feature selection and extraction	• CDF of the ADC maps at $b = 700$ s/mm² used in [47] and [18]. • CDF of the ADC maps at $b = [100\ 200\ 300\ 400\ 500\ 600\ 700]$ s/mm² are used in [48]. • The mean intensity values of the DW-MRI at $b = 0$ sec/mm², $b = 800$ sec/mm², and the ADC mean intensity value were found to be the most discriminant features [49].
Classification	• SNCAE [18,47]. • SNCAE and majority voting [48]. • k-nearest neighbor classifier [49].

SUMMARY

A summary of Section 11.5 findings is provided in Table 11.6.

MULTIMODALITY-BASED CAD SYSTEMS

The introduction of new types of MRI modalities, obtained using different acquisition methods, and containing different information encouraged a new trend of integrating these modalities together and benefiting from their potential complementarity for the purpose of enhancing the overall interpretation and decision [50].

Indeed, several works have demonstrated the validity of the multimodality integration schemes in the context of prostate cancer diagnosis.

It has been shown that combining multiparametric MRI yields better performance in terms of the AUC. Artan et al. [51] have tested several combinations of MRI modalities using the same CAD system, the ROC curve for each combination is then plotted as shown in Figure 11.12. It is clear from

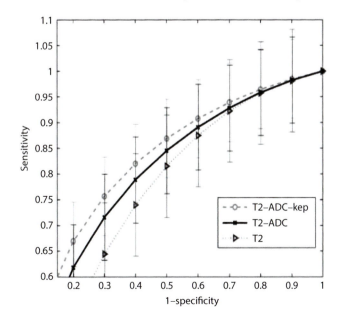

FIGURE 11.12 Average ROC curves using the same CAD system for (1) T2 maps, (2) T maps + ADC, (3) T2 maps + ADC + K_{ep} (obtained from DCE-MRI). (From Artan, Y. et al., *IEEE Trans. Image Process*, 19, 2444–2455, 2010.)

the graph that the multimodality MRI-based CAD systems achieve higher AUC compared to mono- or bi-modality systems. Other studies [52–55] have also examined and compared the performance of CAD for CaP systems that use mono- and multiparametric MRI. They reported better performance of the later in terms of several evaluation measures.

Similar to monomodality CAD systems, the pipeline of the multimodal CAD systems starts with an optional pre-processing and segmentation step, followed by extracting features from the resultant MRI and reducing the feature space if necessary. These steps are usually performed on a per-modality basis, regardless of the number of MRI modalities that are considered in the CAD system as a whole.

Within the multimodality framework, the integration of data obtained from the multiple channels can be performed at different levels, namely, *data level*, *feature level*, and *classifier level*.

Data-level fusion is a machine learning approach at which the input is simply the raw data. In the case of multimodality MRI systems, raw data may include intensity values, signal enhancement curves, and MR spectra. So far, no work has been reported in the MRI-based CAD for CaP systems regarding the data-level integration. In fact, all the multimodal approaches adopted either feature fusion or classifier fusion. However, recently a new paradigm of data fusion of MRI modalities has been proposed within a deep learning approach presented in Liu et al. [56]. In this work, four different types of MRI inputs were generated, using different combinations of DWI, ADC maps, k^{trans}, and transverse T2WI as the red, green, blue (RGB) channels to form a color image in the RGB format. This type of image is then fed into a deep learning architecture trained on input images of the same type. Impressively, the proposed system outperformed other 69 systems in the PROSTATEx challenge with an AUC, sensitivity, and specificity of 0.95, 0.89, and 0.89, respectively.

FEATURE-LEVEL FUSION

In this fusion scheme, feature vectors are extracted from each modality and then simply aggregated by concatenation to form a unique feature matrix. However, in this scenario, feature selection could be performed either before or after aggregation.

Feature-level fusion seems to be the most popular in the area of CAD for CaP systems. Full CAD systems presented in several studies [21,36,57–60] have reported the use of engineered features obtained from multimodal MRI to detect prostate cancer. That is, features are extracted from each modality and concatenated in a unique feature vector, before being fused into a certain classifier.

An example of the CAD systems that performed feature selection on per-modality basis is Tiwari et al. [57]. They presented a novel scheme for data integration from MR imaging and non-imaging (spectroscopy) channels. Initially, feature extraction took place on a per-modality basis. Then, the feature space dimension was reduced to a pre-defined number of features by PCA. This step was also essential for unifying the feature vector length for all channels. Finally, the feature vectors of both modalities were concatenated and random forest (RF) is used to classify the data and obtain the final decision. A maximum accuracy of 0.83 and an AUC of 0.89 is obtained.

On the other hand, Lemaitre et al. [12] showed that performing feature selection *after* feature aggregation yields better AUC compared to feature selection performed on per-modality basis *prior* to feature aggregation. In other words, feature selection performed on the final feature vector obtained from the multiparametric MRI outperforms selecting features from the individual modalities.

CLASSIFIER-LEVEL FUSION

Here a stand-alone classifier is trained by features obtained from each modality, and hence the final decision is made by combining the individual decisions of each classifier. In our context, ensemble learning is the most commonly used classifier fusion method to combine the interpretation of the individual per-modality learners. Lemaitre [12] refers to classifier fusion scheme as stacking. He defines stacking as a learning method that comprises three stages: (i) training the per-modality classifier, (ii) validating the overall system by another set of data, and (iii) testing the overall system. Figure 11.13 shows a schematic that explains the stacking principle [12].

Two classifier fusion methods are commonly used in the design of CAD for CaP systems. These are (i) score combination by logistic regression, and (ii) stacking by AdaBoost or Gradient Boosting (GB) as a meta-classifier.

In [46], Litjens et al. extracted voxel features from DWI, DCE, and T2WI and fused them all together in an RF classifier to give a suspicion score between 0 and 1 for each voxel. Then lesion segmentation was performed based on these scores. Again, RF was used to determine whether the obtained lesions are benign or cancerous.

The work of Litjens et al. [61] builds upon the CAD system developed earlier by Litjens et al. [46]. They used the combination by score scheme to combine the radiologist scores and the scores obtained from the CAD system presented by logistic regression [46]. They have shown the potential improvement in the performance of the combined system over the scores obtained from the radiologists and their CAD system individually.

Other studies [36,42,57] used the AdaBoost ensemble learning method. This method tries to find the best linear modal that combines multiple weak learners in order to obtain a final strong classifier [12].

In this context, it is worth noting that Lemaitre [12] has investigated three different data combination schemes to determine the most feasible one. These include (i) concatenating 331 features extracted from all the four modalities including anatomical features in a single classifier (which corresponds to feature-level fusion discussed above), (ii) stacking using AdaBoost as a meta-classifier, and (iii) stacking using GB as a meta-classifier. Results show the superiority of the feature-level aggregation scheme over the other two classifier fusion alternatives. Figure 11.14 shows the ROC analysis of three different approaches presented in [12]. The maximum obtained AUC is 0.836 which corresponds to the feature-level fusion.

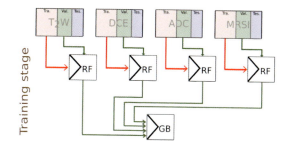

FIGURE 11.13 Stacking as a classifier fusion scheme. In the training stage, a RF classifier is trained individually for each modality (red line). Then, a validation set of MR images is provided at the input of each RF at which the probabilistic output is used to train a Meta classifier, either Gradient Boosting or AdaBoost (blue line). (From Lemaitre, G., Computer-aided diagnosis for prostate cancer using multi-parametric magnetic resonance imaging, Doctoral Program in Technology, France, 2016.)

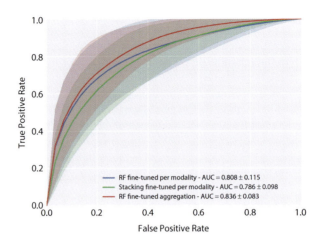

FIGURE 11.14 ROC analysis of three CAD systems: (a) RF-based CAD where selected features from each modality are combined on a unique feature matrix (blue), (b) stacking-based CAD where selected features from each modality are fed using the principle of stacking (green), and (c) RF-based CAD where all features from mp-MRI are combined and then feature selection is performed on the resulted feature matrix (red). (From Lemaitre, G., Computer-aided diagnosis for prostate cancer using multi-parametric magnetic resonance imaging, Doctoral Program in Technology, France, 2016.)

SUMMARY

A summary of the discussed fusion methods is shown in Figure 11.15.

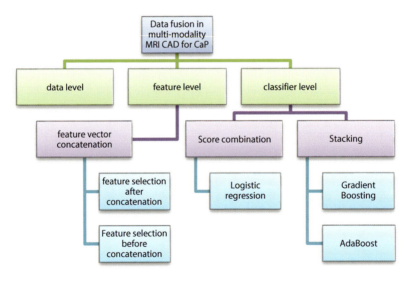

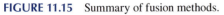
FIGURE 11.15 Summary of fusion methods.

PERSPECTIVES AND AVENUES FOR FUTURE RESEARCH

Early detection of prostate cancer is the key for an accurate diagnosis and treatment of the disease. Common screening strategies such as PSA and TRUS-GB have shown limitations in different aspects including accuracy and invasiveness. Typically, these limitations result in late or inappropriate diagnosis and treatment. Lately, several MR imaging techniques have been introduced in the area of prostate cancer detection holding the potential promise of an accurate noninvasive detection and diagnosis.

However, several problems and challenges are still present in the scene before the MRI screening becomes part of the daily clinical routine in the case of prostate cancer. One of these problems is the complexity of the MR images, especially in the case of 3D images, which makes the task of the radiologist difficult, time consuming, and prone to human errors. Also, the interpretation of MRI is highly dependent on the radiologist's experience, which results in inter-reader variability. These challenges and problems have created the need for an automated alternative that can guide and assist radiologists in their tasks and reduce the number of false positives caused by human errors. Consequently, image processing-based CAD systems are being developed to tackle these issues.

Different MRI modalities are investigated and processed through the designed systems. To date, there seems to be no consensus on the imaging modality that is best for prostate cancer detection. However, there is nearly a consensus on the fact that processing a combination of multimodality MRI gives better results compared to processing a single modality. This might be obvious as additional modalities provide additional complementary information of the subject of study. Particularly, T2WI provides the most accurate anatomical information, DCE provides the functional information, MRSI provides metabolites concentration, and DWI provides the best soft tissue contrast by measuring the water molecules diffusion. Nevertheless, concerns about time and cost are still present for the case of multimodality MRI- based CAD systems.

To the best of the authors' knowledge, only the work of Trigui et al. [36] and Lemaitre [12] have combined all the four MRI modalities in a single framework. Other studies, however, have used different combinations of two or three modalities.

Although the area of CAD for CaP has experienced an extensive research, it is difficult to aggregate these studies and draw significant conclusions regarding the best approach or the best performance. The absence of standardization in many aspects such as:

1. MRI acquisition protocol: different datasets are acquired at different setting and by different MR scanners.
2. Ground truth: some studies consider a rough ground truth that is dependent on the radiologist delineation of the prostate cancer, while others evaluate their results based on a more rigid ground truth that is obtained after a full prostatectomy (surgical removal of the prostate gland).
3. Registration (which refers to the alignment of the images): Different alignment methodologies were followed by the reviewed studies.
4. Manual verses automated segmentation: the classification stage is highly dependent on the segmentation accuracy. Usually, automatic segmentation dos not yield a perfect delineation of the ROI compared to manual segmentation. Errors in the segmentation stage may significantly affect the overall performance and robustness of the system.
5. Consideration of the CG: most of the reviewed CAD systems have focused on detecting cancer in the PZ only. Other studies however, considered the whole prostate gland.

   It is worth mentioning that, MRI lacks contrast of prostatic cancer in the CG which reduces the sensitivity in this part of the image. This in terms is suggested to reduce the overall measured accuracy of CAD systems that considered CG in their studies.
6. Inconsistency in the classes considered in the CAD systems, that is, some studies takes into account the presence of two classes (healthy/cancer) while others assume a third class which is the (abnormal/undecided) class. This class is claimed to represent other benign tumors or diseases.
7. Different measures are used in evaluating each CAD system, including AUC of the ROC curve, sensitivity, specificity, and accuracy.
8. The results of individual studies are incomparable specially that the dataset sizes vary significantly.

To tackle the problems associated with the absence of a universal validation dataset, Lemaitre et al. [7] provided the research community with an open access dataset that includes images of the four modalities for each patient with the ground truth. We refer the reader to that review for more details about this dataset.

In the case of multimodality approach, several issues are to be further investigated by the research community. Those include data-level fusion and classifier-level fusion. Based on the brief investigations provided by Lemaitre [12] and Liu et al. [56], the former provides promising results that may outperform feature-level-based CAD systems. Hopefully, deep learning networks will provide a better alternative for the engineered features to be used in a CAD framework.

REFERENCES

1. American Cancer Society, *Key Statistics for Prostate Cancer*, American Cancer Society, Atlanta, GA, 2017.
2. American Cancer Society, *Prostate Cancer*, American Cancer Society, Atlanta, GA, 2017.
3. G. Lu-Yao, P. Albertsen, D. Moore, W. Shih, Y. Lin, R. DiPaola, M. Barry et al., Outcomes of localized prostate cancer following conservative management, *JAMA*, 302(11), 1202–1209, 2009.
4. J. McNeal, E. Redwine, F. Freiha and T. Stamey, Zonal distribution of prostatic adenocarcinoma: Correlation with histologic pattern and direction of spread, *American Journal of Surgical Pathology*, 12(12), 897–906, 1988.
5. U.S. Preventive Services Task Force, Screening for prostate cancer: U.S. Preventive Services Task Force recommendation statement, *Annals of Internal Medicine*, 157(2), 120–134, 2012.
6. A. Rastinehad, B. Turkbey, S. Salami, O. Yaskiv, A. George, M. Fakhoury, K. Beecher et al., Improving detection of clinically significant prostate cancer: Magnetic resonance imaging/transrectal ultrasound fusion guided prostate biopsy, *The Journal of Urology*, 191, 1749–1754, 2014.
7. G. Lemaitre, R. Marti, J. Freixenet, J. Vilanova, P. Walker and F. Meriaudeau, Computer-aided detection and diagnosis for prostate cancer based on mono and multi-parametric MRI: A review, *Computers in Biology and Medicine*, 60, 8–31, 2015.
8. B. Turkbey and P. Choyke, Multiparametric MRI and prostate cancer diagnosis and risk stratification, *Current Opinion in Urology*, 22(4), 310–315, 2012.
9. D. Margolis, *Everything You Need to Know about Prostate MRI*, Prostate Cancer Research Institute, Los Angeles, CA, 2015.
10. H. Zhu, *Medical Image Processing Overview*, University of Calgary, Toronto, Canada, 2003.
11. K. Toennies, *Guide to Medical Image Analysis: Methods and Algorithms*, Springer, London, UK, 2012.
12. G. Lemaitre, Computer-aided diagnosis for prostate cancer using multi-parametric magnetic resonance imaging, Doctoral Program in Technology, France, 2016.
13. I. Chan, W. Wells, R. Mulern, S. Haker, J. Zheng, K. Zou, S. Maier and M. Tempany, Detection of prostate cancer by integration of line-scan diffusion, T2-mapping and T2-weighted magnetic resonance imaging; a multichannel statistical classifier, *Medical Physics*, 30(9), 2390–2398, 2003.
14. A. Rampun, L. Zheng, P. Malcolm, B. Tiddeman and R. Zwiggelaar, Computer-aided detection of prostate cancer in T2- weighted MRI within the peripheral zone, *Physics in Medicine & Biology*, 61, 4796–4825, 2016.
15. D. Lv, X. Guo, X. Wang, J. Zhang and J. Fang, Computerized characterization of prostate cancer by fractal analysis in MR images, *Journal of Magnetic Resonance Imaging*, 30, 161–168, 2009.
16. S. Viswanath, N. Bloch, J. Chappelow, R. Toth, N. Rofsky, E. Genega, R. Linkinski and A. Madabhushi, Central gland and peripheral zone prostate tumors have significantly different quantitative imaging signatures on 3 Tesla endorectal, in vivo T2-weighted magnetic resonance imagery, *Journal of Magnetic Resonance Imaging*, 36(1), 213–224, 2012.
17. Y. Sung, H.-J. Kwon, B.-W. Park, G. Cho, C. Lee, K.-S. Cho and J. Kim, Prostate cancer detection on dynamic contrast- enhanced MRI: Computer-aided diagnosis versus single perfusion parameter maps, *AJR Genitourinary Imaging*, 197, 1122–1129, 2011.
18. I. Reda, A. Shalaby, M. Elmogy, A. Abou Elfotouh, F. Khalifa, M. Abou El-Ghar, E. Hosseini-Asl, G. Gimelfarb, N. Wergi and A. El-Baz, A comprehensive non-invasive framework for diagnosing prostate cancer, *Computers in Biology and Medicine*, 81, 148–158, 2017.
19. R. Lopes, A. Ayache, N. Makni, P. Puech, A. Villers, S. Mordon and N. Betrouni, Prostate cancer characterization on MR images using fractal features, *Medical Physics*, 38(1), 83–95, 2011.
20. J. Sled, A. Zijdenbos and A. Evans, A non-parametric method for automatic correction of intensity non-uniformity in MRI data, *IEEE Transactions on Medical Imaging*, 17(1), 87–97, 1998.

21. E. Niaf, O. Rouviere, F. Mege-Lechevallier, F. Bratan and C. Lartizien, Computer-aided diagnosis of prostate cancer in the peripheral zone using multiparametric MRI, *Physics in Medicine and Biology*, 57, 3833–3851, 2012.
22. J. Bulman, R. Toth, A. Patel, N. Bloch, C. McMahon, L. Ngo, A. Madabhushi and N. Rofsky, Automated computer-derived prostate volumes from MR imaging data: Comparison with radiologist-derived MR imaging and pathologic specimen volumes, *Radiology*, 262(1), 144–151, 2012.
23. A. Padhani, Dynamic contrast-enhanced MRI in clinical oncology: Current status and future directions, *Journal of Magnetic Resonance Imaging*, 16(4), 407–422, 2002.
24. P. Vos, T. Hambrock, C. Hulsbergen, J. Futterer, J. Barentsz and H. Huisman, Computerized analysis of prostate lesions in the peripheral zone using dynamic contrast enhanced MRI, *Medical Physics*, 35(3), 888–899, 2008.
25. I. Ocak, M. Bernardo, G. Metzger, T. Barrett, P. Pinto, P. Albert and P. Choyke, Dynamic contrast-enhanced MRI of prostate cancer at 3T: A study of pharmacokinetic parameters, *American Journal of Roentgenology*, 189, 192–201, 2007.
26. P. Gao, C. Shi, L. Zhao, Q. Zhou and L. Luo, Differential diagnosis of prostate cancer and noncancerous tissue in the peripheral zone and central gland using the quantitative parameters of DCE-MRI, *Medicine*, 95(52), 1–11, 2016.
27. A. S. N. Jackson, S. A. Reinsberg, S. A. Sohaib, E. Charls-Edwards, S. Jhavar, T. J. Christmas, A. C. Thompson et al., Dynamic contrast-enhanced MRI for prostate cancer localization, *The British Journal of Radiology*, 82, 148–156, 2009.
28. N. Hara, M. Okuizumi, H. Koike, M. Kawaguchi and V. Bilim, Dynamic contrast-enhanced magnetic resonance imaging (DCE-MRI) is a useful modality for the precise detection and staging of early prostate cancer, *The Prostate*, 62, 140–147, 2004.
29. P. Puech, N. Betrouni, R. Viard, A. Villers, X. Leroy and L. Lemaitre, Prostate cancer computer-assisted diagnosis software using dynamic contrast-enhanced MRI, in *29th Annual International Conference of the IEEE EMBS*, Lyon, France, 2007.
30. A. Firjani, F. Khalifa, A. Elnakib, G. Gimelfarb, M. Abou El-Ghar, A. Elmaghraby and A. El-Baz, A novel image-based approach for early detection of prostate cancer using DCE-MRI, in *Computational Intelligence in Biomedical Imaging*, K. Suzuki (Ed.), Springer, New York, 2014, pp. 55–82.
31. S. Viswanath, N. Bloch, N. Rofsky, R. Linkinski, E. Genega, J. Chappelow, R. Toth and A. Madabhushi, A comprehensive segmentation, registration, and cancer detection scheme on 3 Tesla in vivo DCE MRI, *Med Image Comput Comput Assist Interv*, 11, 662–669, 2008.
32. R. Toth, P. Tiwari, M. Rosen, A. Kalyanpur, S. Pungavkar and A. Madabhushi, A multi-modal prostate segmentation scheme by combining spectral, in *Proceedings of SPIE Medical Imaging*, 2008.
33. C. Varini, A. Degenhard and T. Nattkemper, Visual exploratory analysis of DCE-MRI data in breast cancer by dimensional data reduction: A comparative study, *Biomedical Signal Processing and Control*, 1(1), 56–63, 2006.
34. P. Puech, N. Batrouni, N. Makni, A.-S. Dewalle, A. Villers and L. Lemaitre, Computer-assisted diagnosis of prostate cancer using DCE-MRI data: design, implementation and preliminary results, *International Journal of Computer Assisted Radiology and Surgery*, 4, 1–10, 2009.
35. P. Tiwari, A hierarchical spectral clustering and non-linear dimensionality reduction scheme for detection of prostate cancer from magnatic resonance spectroscopy, *Medical Physics*, 36, 3927–3939, 2009.
36. R. Trigui, J. Miteran, P. Walker, L. Sellami and B. Hamida, Automatic classification and localization of prostate cancer using multi-parametric MRI/MRS, *Biomedical Signal Processing and Control*, 31, 189–198, 2017.
37. P. Tiwari, M. Rosen and A. Madabhushi, A hierarchical spectral clustering and non-linear dimensionality reduction scheme for detection of prostate cancer from magnetic resonance spectroscopy, *Medical Physics*, 36(9), 3927–3939, 2009.
38. L. Matulewicz, J. Jansen, L. Bokacheva, H. Vargas, O. Akin, S. Fine, A. Shukla-Dave et al., Anatomic segmentation improves prostate cancer detection with artificial neural networks analysis of 1H MRSI, *Journal of Magnetic Resonance Imaging*, 40(6), 1414–1421, 2014.
39. S. Parfait, P. Walker, G. Crehange, X. Tizon and J. Miteran, Classification of prostate magnetic resonance spectra using Support Vector Machine, *Biomedical Signal Processing and Control*, 7, 499–508, 2012.
40. C. Zi-jun, Z. Yang, B. Mei, H. Yue and L. Xin-zi, A correlation study of Gleason score and the diagnostic accuracy of MRS in prostate cancer based on pathological section, *Journal of China Clinic Medical Imaging*, no. 12, 2012, 009.
41. L. Chen, Z. Weng, I. Goh and M. Garlan, An efficient algorithm for automatic phase correction of NMR spectra based on entropy minimization, *Journal of Magnetic Resonance*, 158(1–2), 164–168, 2002.

42. M. Kelm, B. Menze, C. Zechmann, K. Baudendistel and F. Hamprecht, *Automated Estimation of Tumor Probability in Prostate MRSI: Pattern Recognition vs. Quantification*, Interdisciplinary Center for Scientific Computing, Heidelberg, Germany, 2006.

43. W. Pijnappel, A. van den Boogaart, R. de Beer and D. van Ormondt, SVD-based quantification of magnetic resonance signals, *Journal of Magnetic Resonance Imaging*, 97(1), 122–134, 1992.

44. H. Ratiney, M. Sdika, Y. Coenradie, S. Cavassila, D. van Ormondt and D. Graveron-Demilly, Time-domain semi- parametric estimation based on a metabolite basis set, *NMR Biomed*, 18, 1–13, 2005.

45. T. Hambrock, D. Somford, H. Huisman, I. Oort, J. Witjes, C. de Kaa, T. Scheenen and J. Barentsz, Relationship between apparent diffusion coefficients at 3.0-T MR imaging and Gleason graded in peripheral zone prostate cancer, *Radiology*, 259, 453–461, 2011.

46. G. Litjens, O. Debats, J. Barentsz, N. Karssemeijer and H. Huisman, Computer-aided detection of prostate cancer in MRI, *IEEE Transactions on Medical Imaging*, 33(5), 1083–1092, 2014.

47. I. Reda, A. Shalaby, M. Abou El-Ghar, F. Khalifa, M. Elmogy, A. Aboulfotouh, E. Hosseini-Asl, N. Werghi and A. El-Baz, Computer-aided diagnostic tool for early detection of prostate cancer, in *IEEE International Conference on Image Processing*, 2016.

48. I. Reda, A. Shalaby, M. Abou El-Ghar, F. Khalifa, M. Elmogy, A. Aboulfotouh, E. Hosseini Asl, A. El-Baz and R. Keynton, A new NMF-autoencoder based CAD system for early diagnosis of prostate cancer, in *IEEE 13th International Symposium on Biomedical Imaging*, 2016.

49. A. Firjani, A. Elnakib, F. Khalifa, G. Gimelfarb, M. Abou El- Ghar, A. Elmaghraby and A. El-Baz, A diffusion-weighted imaging based diagnostic system for early detection of prostate cancer, *Journal of Biomedical Science and Engineering*, 6, 346–356, 2013.

50. D. Lahat, T. Adali and C. Jutten, Multimodal data fusion: An overview of methods, challenges and prospects, in *IEEE Multimodal Data Fusion*, 103, 1449–1477, 2015.

51. Y. Artan, M. Haider, D. Langer, T. Kwast, A. Evans, Y. Yang, M. Wernick, J. Trachtenberg and I. Yetik, Prostate cancer localization with multispectral MRI using cost-sensitive support vector machines and conditional random fields, *IEEE Transactions on Image Processing*, 19(9), 2444–2455, 2010.

52. Y. Artan and I. Yetik, Prostate cancer localization using multiparametric MRI based on semisupervised techniques with automated seed initialization, *IEEE Transactions on Information Technology in Biomedicine*, 16(6), 1313–1323, 2012.

53. I. Ocak, M. Bernardo, G. Metzger, T. Barrett, P. Pinto, P. Albert and P. Choyke, Dynamic contrast-enhanced MRI of prostate cancer at 3T: A study of pharmokinetic parameters, *American Journal of Roentgenology*, 189(4), 192–200, 2009.

54. P. Vos, T. Hambrock, J. Barentsz and H. Huisman, Computer- assisted analysis of peripheral zone prostate lesions using T2- weighted and dynamic contrast enhanced T1-weighted MRI, *Physics in Medicine and Biology*, 55, 1719–1734, 2010.

55. M. Haidar, T. van der Kwast, J. Tanguay, A. Evans, A. Hashmi, G. Lockwood and J. Trachtenberg, Combined T2-weighted and diffusion weighted MRI for localization of prostate cancer, *American Journal of Roentgenology*, 189(2), 323–328, 2009.

56. S. Liu, H. Zheng, Y. Feng and W. Li, Prostate cancer diagnosis using deep learning with 3D multiparametric MRI, in *Proceedings of SPIE*, Orlando, FL, 2017.

57. P. Tiwari, J. Kurhanewicz, S. Viswanath, A. Sridhar and A. Madabhushi, Multimodal wavelet embedding representation for data combination (MaWERiC): Integrating magnetic resonance imaging and spectroscopy for prostate cancer detection, *NMR Biomed*, 25(4), 607–619, 2012.

58. V. Pieter, T. Hambrock, J. Barentsz and H. Huisman, Computer-assisted analysis of peripheral zone prostate lesions using T2-weighted and dynamic contrast enhanced T1-weighted MRI, *Physics in Medicine and Biology*, 55, 1719–1734, 2010.

59. P. Vos, J. Barentsz, N. Karssemeijer and H. Huisman, Automatic computer-aided detection of prostate cancer based on multiparametric magnetic resonance image analysis, *Physics in Medicine and Biology*, 57, 1527–1542, 2012.

60. V. Giannini, S. Mazzetti, A. Vignati, F. Russo, E. Bollito, F. Porpiglia, M. Stasi and D. Regge, A fully automatic computer aided diagnosis system for peripheral zone prostate cancer detection using multi-parametric magnetic resonance imaging, *Computerized Medical Imaging and Graphics*, 46, 219–226, 2015.

61. G. Litjens, J. Barentsz, N. Karssemeijer and H. Huisman, Clinical evaluation of a computer-aided diagnosis system for determining cancer aggressiveness in prostate MRI, *European Radiology*, 25, 3187–3199, 2015.

62. P. Tiwari, M. Rosen and A. Madabhushi, Consensus-locally linear embedding (C-LLE): Application to prostate cancer, in *Med Image Comput Comput Assist Interv*, 11, 330–338, 2008.

12 A DCE-MRI-Based Noninvasive CAD System for Prostate Cancer Diagnosis

F. Khalifa, A. Shalaby, Mohamed Abou El-Ghar, Jasjit S. Suri, and A. El-Baz

CONTENTS

PROSTATE: ANATOMY, FUNCTION, AND DISEASES

The prostate is the largest accessory gland in the male urinary and reproductive system. It is a cone-shaped organ about the size of a walnut that weighs approximately 15–20 g and measures approximately $4 \times 2 \times 3$ centimeters in a mature male [1]. In this section, brief descriptions of the prostate anatomy and function, as well as the diseases that affect the prostate, are provided.

The prostate is located deep in the pelvis just below the urinary bladder and in front of the rectum, see Figure 12.1. It surrounds the urethra as it exits the bottom of the bladder. The prostate has two main functions. First, it stores, secretes, and controls the flow of the milky fluid, which constitutes 30% of the volume of the semen and is injected into the urethra along with sperm when a male is sexually aroused. Second, it controls the diameter of the urethra, thereby controlling the flow of urine [3]. To accomplish these functions, the prostate contains three main cell types: (i) gland cells that excrete seminal fluid, (ii) muscles cells that control the diameter of the urethra for urine flow and ejaculation, and (iii) fibrous cells that make up the supportive structure of the prostate [3].

In pathology, the prostate region is divided into different segments or zones. Each of these zones consists of different cell types and is susceptible to different types of diseases. Figure 12.2 illustrates the main glandular zones of the prostate: the peripheral zone (PZ), the central zone (CZ), and the transition zone (TZ). The PZ is the subcapsular portion of the prostate gland that surrounds the distal urethra and constitutes up to 70% of a normal prostate gland. The CZ is the second largest region of the prostate that surrounds the ejaculatory ducts and constitutes about 25% of a normal

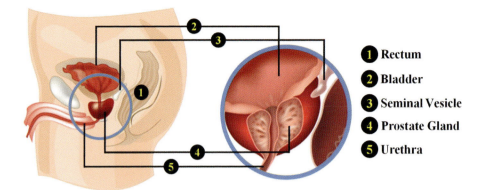

FIGURE 12.1 Schematic illustration of an anatomical view of the lower abdomen area that contains the prostate. (From HealthNews Texas, *PSA Test Reduces Prostate Cancer Deaths* [Online], http://healthnewstexas.com/5262/psa-test-reduces-prostate-cancer-deaths/.)

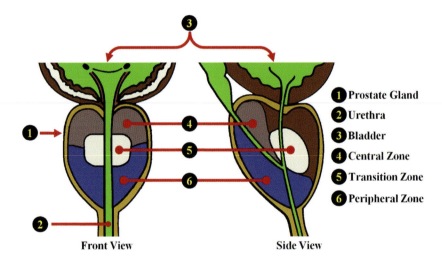

FIGURE 12.2 Schematic illustration of the front and side cross-sectional views of the prostate showing different prostate zones. (SIU School of Medicine, *Enlarged Prostate* [Online], http://www.siumed.edu/surgery/urology/bph.html.)

prostate gland. The third zone is the TZ that surrounds the urethra and is the region of the prostate that grows throughout life. The TZ comprises about 5% of a normal prostate gland [4].

The function of the prostate can be affected by various types of medical complications. The three most common prostate problems are the prostatitis, benign prostatic hyperplasia (prostate enlargement), and prostate cancer. Prostatitis is microscopic inflammation (swelling) of the tissue of the prostate gland, which affects mostly young and middle-aged men [6]. This inflammatory disease is usually caused by bacteria and is categorized into four groups based on the chronicity of symptoms [7]: Type I—acute bacterial prostatitis, Type II—chronic bacterial prostatitis, Type III—chronic abacterial prostatitis (chronic pelvic pain syndrome), and Type IV—asymptomatic inflammatory prostatitis. Type I is less likely to occur; however, it is potentially life-threatening. Type II is also relatively uncommon and occurs when bacteria find a spot on the prostate where they can survive. On the other hand, Type III is the most common and can be found in men of any age; nevertheless, it is the least understood form of prostatitis [8]. The incidence of Type IV is unknown; diagnosis is made after a biopsy and is usually correlated with the higher PSA values [9]. Benign prostatic hyperplasia, the second medical complication that affects the prostate, is caused by noncancerous enlargement of the prostate gland and is associated with aging. This condition can cause men to have some troubles, such as a frequent need to urinate and difficulty to start urination or to fully empty the bladder [10].

The last type of prostate disease is prostate cancer, which is one of the most common cancers among males. In most cases, prostate cancer has no symptoms and is only found with screening. When symptoms are present, they include pain, difficulty in urinating, and problems during sexual intercourse. Prostate cancer is a slow-growing cancer that may invade other organs if untreated. In addition, it has different occurrence rates at different zones of the prostate, due to the difference in cell types that compromise each zone. The vast majority (70%) of prostate cancer originates in the PZ, while only 25% occurs in the TZ and 5% in the CZ, which tends to be the more aggressive type [11]. In order to determine how far the cancer has spread (within the prostate or to other body parts), a staging test is performed. Staging of prostate cancer plays an important role in the choice and the success of treatment. Prostate cancer has four stages (Stages I through IV). Stage I is the earliest cancer stage in which the cancer cells are confined to a microscopic area and are too small to be either felt by a physician or seen in imaging tests. Stage II is more advanced than stage I and the cancer can be felt by a physician. Like stage I, however, the cancer is still confined only to the prostate gland. In stage III, the cancer spreads outside the prostate to nearby tissues, for example, the seminal vesicles. The final stage of prostate cancer is stage IV in which the cancer cells have spread beyond the outer layer of the prostate to the nearby organs, such as the lymph nodes, bones, rectum, or bladder.

Prostate cancer is the sixth leading cause of cancer-related death in men worldwide and is the second in the United States [12]. Therefore, it is crucial to detect/diagnose prostate cancer in its earliest stage to improve the effectiveness of treatment and increase the patient's chance of survival. In recent years, both the diagnosis and the treatment of prostate cancer continue to evolve using different techniques and methods. The next section overviews different techniques that are used for early diagnosis of prostate cancer as well as the related work on prostate cancer detection and diagnosis in the context of the proposed framework.

CURRENT DIAGNOSTIC METHODS OF PROSTATE CANCER

Prostate cancer is the most frequently diagnosed male malignancy and the second leading cause (after lung cancer) of cancer-related death in the United States, with more than 238,000 new cases and a mortality rate of about 30,000 in 2013 [13]. Early diagnosis improves the effectiveness of treatment and increases the patient's chances of survival. Compared to other types of cancers such as lung cancer, prostate cancer, when treated by removing the prostate gland, has a zero chance of recurrence. There are many techniques that are used for the diagnosis of prostate cancer. The main diagnostic tools for prostate cancer are digital rectal exam (DRE), serum concentration using prostate-specific antigen (PSA) blood test, and needle biopsy. The DRE test is carried out by a skilled physician who manually feels for any abnormalities in the prostate gland through the rectum. The DRE is inexpensive and easy to perform. However, the accuracy of a DRE examination is not high enough and depends on physician experience. Also, it can only detect tumors with sufficient volumes. Another screening test for the diagnosis of prostate cancer is performed using PSA—an enzyme that is secreted by the prostatic cells. The higher the values of PSA, the more likely the prostate gland is to have cancer. However, PSA is associated with a high risk of overdiagnosis of prostate cancer as higher PSA levels may reflect other conditions, such as an enlarged or inflamed prostate [14]. In addition, PSA screening lacks the ability to provide accurate information about the location and the extent of the cancer. If either the DRE or PSA tests raises any concern, a needle biopsy is performed to collect tissue samples from the prostate, which are analyzed in a lab to determine whether or not cancer cells are present. Biopsy remains the gold standard for diagnosis of prostate cancer, but it is the last resort because of its invasive nature, high costs, and potential morbidity rates. Additionally, the relatively small needle biopsy samples have a higher possibility of producing false positive diagnosis.

To overcome these limitations, noninvasive evaluation of prostate cancer has been clinically explored with several medical imaging tools, such as ultrasound, computed tomography (CT), and magnetic resonance imaging (MRI). These imaging methods are favorable due to their ability to provide reliable information about the size and shape of the prostate gland and can localize the cancer foci, which would improve the accuracy of diagnosis and enable more efficient treatment. Transrectal ultrasound (TRUS) is the most commonly used technique for prostate imaging. TRUS is used in estimating the volume of the prostate gland in PSA screening, and is often used in planning and guiding needle biopsies [15]. TRUS is often chosen due its inexpensive cost, ease of use, portability, and real-time nature. However, it does have several disadvantages, including low contrast and a low signal-to-noise ratio (SNR) [16]. As a result, it can be difficult to accurately detect and locate cancerous cells using TRUS images. Traditional CT imaging modality is widely used for post-therapy evaluation by physicians to assess the effectiveness of treatment [15]. However, it uses radiation and has poor soft-tissue contrast resolution, which does not allow precise distinction of the internal or external anatomy of the prostate. As an alternative for ultrasound and CT, MRI techniques are becoming increasingly attractive as new diagnostic tools for prostate cancer. Over the past years, these MRI-based techniques have shown varying degrees of success for improved visualization and localization of prostate cancer [17–30]. The key advantage of MRI is that it provides higher contrast of soft tissues, which allows for better detection of cancerous tissues. In addition to anatomical information, MRI can provide valuable functional information about the tissue by using functional acquisition techniques, such as MR spectroscopy (MRS), dynamic contrast-enhanced (DCE)-MRI, and diffusion-weighted imaging (DWI) [27].

In this chapter, the focus is on using DCE-MRI to develop a computer-aided diagnostic (CAD) system for early detection of prostate cancer. The lack of ionizing radiation, increased spatial resolution, and the ability to provide both anatomical and functional information are the key motivations for using DCE-MRI. In general, early diagnosis of prostate cancer using DCE-MRI requires intermediate image-processing steps, such as prostate registration, segmentation, and classification. The next sections introduce the related work on prostate segmentation and registration, as well as the state-of-the-art CAD systems for early detection of prostate cancer.

RELATED WORK IN PROSTATE SEGMENTATION AND REGISTRATION

Prostate segmentation, that is, the delineation of prostate borders from the surrounding tissues, is a basic step in any noninvasive CAD system for early detection of prostate cancer. However, accurate delineation of prostate borders in MR images is a challenge due to large variations of prostate shapes within a specific time series as well as across subjects; the lack of strong edges and diffused prostate boundaries; and the similar intensity profile of the prostate and surrounding tissues. Although manual outlining of the prostate border enables the prostate volume to be determined, it is time consuming and observer dependent. Moreover, traditional edge detection methods [31] are unable to extract the correct boundaries of the prostate since the gray-level distributions of the prostate and the surrounding organs are hardly distinguishable. To overcome this limitation, most successful known approaches have addressed the segmentation challenges by incorporating the prostate appearances and shapes into their segmentation techniques.

In particular, an automated framework by Allen et al. [32] was proposed for 3D prostate segmentation that consists of two steps. First, voxel classification is performed based on Gaussian probabilities of gray level. Then, a statistical shape model is used to segment the prostate region. A hybrid 2D/3D active shape model (ASM)-based methodology for global optimal segmentation of the 3D MRI prostate data was proposed by Zhu et al. [33]. Iterative segmentation was performed by a 2D ASM search on each slice, then the final surface is reconstructed from the 2D search results and updated by re-estimating the parameters of the 3D probabilistic shape model. Klein et al. [34,35] presented an atlas-based segmentation approach that utilized a localized version of mutual information (MI) to extract the prostate from MR images. The segmentation of the prostate is obtained as the average of the best-matched registered atlas set to the test image (image to be segmented). Flores-Tapia et al. [36] proposed a semi-automated edge detection technique for MRI prostate segmentation. In their framework, the prostate borders were detected by tracing four manually selected reference points on the edge of the prostate using a static wavelet transform [37] to locate the prostate edges. Toth et al. [38] presented an algorithm for the automatic segmentation of the prostate in multimodal MRI. Their algorithm starts by isolating the region of interest (ROI) from MRS data. Then, an ASM within the ROI is used to obtain the final segmentation. A semi-automated approach by Vikal et al. [39] used a priori knowledge of prostate shape to detect the contour in each slice and then refined them to form a 3D prostate surface. An unsupervised segmentation method was proposed by Liu et al. [40] for the segmentation of MR prostate images. A level set deformable model was employed and was guided by an elliptical prostate shape prior and intensity gradient was employed to refine the initial results obtained by Otsu thresholding [41]. A maximum a posteriori (MAP)-based framework was proposed by Makni et al. [42] to perform automated 3D MRI prostate segmentation. Their framework combined gray level, contextual information regarding voxels' neighborhoods using Markov random field (MRF), and statistical shape information to find optimum segmentation based on Bayesian a posteriori classification, estimated with the iterative conditional mode (ICM) algorithm. Liu et al. [43] proposed an automated approach that utilized fuzzy MRF modeling for prostate segmentation from multiparametric MRI. Their framework exploited T2-weighted image intensities, pharmacokinetic (PK) parameter k_{ep}, and apparent diffusion coefficient (ADC) values in a Bayesian approach to label prostate pixels as cancerous or noncancerous. The labeled pixels are then clustered using the k-means algorithm. The system had a specificity of 89.58%, sensitivity of 87.50%, accuracy of 89.38%, and a Dice similarity coefficient (DSC) of 62.2%. A similar approach was developed by Artan et al. [44] and located cancerous regions using cost-sensitive support vector machine (SVM). Prostate segmentation was performed using a conditional random field and the same three features in Liu et al. [43] were utilized for classification. The DSC for prostate localization and segmentation was 0.46 ± 0.26, and the area under the receiver operator characteristic (ROC) curves (A_z) of the classification was 0.79 ± 0.12. Ozer et al. [45] also developed a technique that directly segmented prostate cancers using the same three features in Liu et al. and Artan et al. [43,44]. Both the SVM and relevance vector machine (RVM) [46] classifiers were used and the system showed a specificity of 0.78 and a sensitivity of 0.74 for RVM and 0.74 and 0.79 for SVM. Gao et al. [47] proposed a shape-based technique that utilized point cloud registration of the MR images before segmenting the prostate. The final prostate border is obtained by minimizing a cost functional that incorporated both the local image statistics as well as the learned shape prior. Martin et al. [48] developed an atlas-based approach for segmenting the prostate from 3D MR images by mapping a probabilistic anatomical atlas to the test image. The resulting map is used to constrain a deformable model-based segmentation framework. Firjani et al. [49] proposed a MAP-based framework that combines a graph-cut approach and three image features (gray-level intensities, spatial interactions between the prostate pixels, and a prior shape model) for 2D DCE-MRI prostate segmentation. Their method was later extended in Firjani et al. [50] to allow for 3D segmentation from DCE-MRI volumes. It utilized both a 3D MRF to model the spatial interaction between the prostate voxels and a 3D shape prior. Recently, Dowling et al. [51] proposed an automated framework that combined dynamic multi-atlas label fusion methods. They employed the diffeomorphic demons method for the nonrigid registration using the selective and iterative method for performance level estimation (SIMPLE) technique [52]. In their framework, a pre-processing step for bias field correction, histogram equalization, and anisotropic diffusion smoothing was employed. Ghose et al. [53] proposed a probabilistic graph-cut-based framework for prostate segmentation based on the fusion of the posterior probabilities determined with a probabilistic atlas and a supervised random forest learning framework. An automated technique that first applied global registration to the prostate MRI data followed by an active appearance model (AAM)-based segmentation of the prostate tissue was proposed by Ghose et al. [54].

In summary, a tremendous number of studies have been developed for the segmentation and registration of prostate MRI data. However, in most of these approaches the segmentation and registration reliability is not very high due to the following reasons: (i) parametric shape models fail in the presence of large gray-level variability across subjects and time; (ii) edge detection methods are not suitable for discontinued objects; (iii) deformable models tend to fail in the case of excessive noise, poor image resolution, diffused boundaries, or occluded objects if they do not incorporate a priori models (e.g., shape and appearance). In addition, most of the motion correction models account only for the global motion and do not take into account the local motion of the prostate due to transmitted respiratory and peristaltic effects. Furthermore, the existing local motion correction methods are intensity-based techniques, which are prone to nonlinear intensity variations over the time series and perform poorly in pre-contrast images. Also, local motion correction methods register the original gray-level data without any prior segmentation; therefore, they do not guarantee voxel-on-voxel matches of the registered perfusion data.

RELATED WORK ON CAD SYSTEMS FOR PROSTATE CANCER

The development of CAD systems for detecting prostate cancer using MR image modalities is an ongoing area of research. Current medical studies suggest that T2-weighted MRI and DCE-MRI hold promise for improving prostate cancer detection, thereby reducing the need for prostate biopsy [18,26,55–67]. In this section, the state-of-the-art CAD systems developed for prostate cancer detection will be discussed.

To the best of our knowledge, the first semi-automated computerized MRI-based CAD system for prostate cancer diagnosis was developed by Chan et al. [55]. In their study, multimodal MRI (T2-weighted, T2-mapping, and line scan diffusion imaging) were used to estimate malignancy likelihood in the PZ of the prostate. Both statistical maps and textural features were obtained and a SVM and linear discriminant analysis (LDA) classifiers were employed for the classification. Their systems resulted in an A_z of 0.761 ± 0.043 and 0.839 ± 0.064, for SVM and LDA, respectively. Madabhushi et al. [56] proposed an automated CAD system for detecting prostatic adenocarcinoma from MR prostate images. In their method, multiple image features, including gray-level statistics (intensity values, mean, and standard deviation), intensity gradient, and Gabor filter features, were used for classifying groups of pixels as tumors. A k_n-nearest neighbor classifier and Bayesian conditional densities were used for classification, and the system achieved an A_z of 0.957. A study by Engelbrecht et al. [57] evaluated which MRI parameters would result in optimal discrimination of prostatic carcinoma from normal PZ and CZ of the prostate. Using the ROC curves, their study concluded that the relative peak enhancement was the most accurate perfusion parameter for cancer detection in the PZ and CZ of the gland. A semi-automated CAD system by Kim et al. [58] demonstrated that parametric imaging of the wash-in rate was more accurate for the detection of prostate cancer in the PZ than was T2-weighted imaging alone. However, they also observed significant overlap between the wash-in rate for cancer and normal tissue in the TZ. Fütterer et al. [26] developed a CAD system to compare the accuracies of T2-weighted MRI, DCE-MRI, and MRS imaging for prostate cancer localization. The results showed higher accuracy in DCE-MRI than were achieved with T2-weighted MRI in prostate cancer localization. A similar study was conducted by Rouvière et al. [59] for the detection of postradiotherapy recurrence of prostate cancer. Their study also concluded that DCE-MRI possesses the ability to depict the intra-prostatic distribution of recurrent cancer after therapy more accurately and with less inter-observer variability than T2-weighted MRI. Puech et al. [18,60] developed a semi-automated dynamic MRI-based CAD system for the detection of prostate cancer. Candidate lesion ROIs were selected either manually or by using a region growing technique initiated by a user-selected seed point. Lesions are classified as benign, malignant, or indeterminate based on the analysis of the median wash-in and washout values. Their CAD system demonstrated a sensitivity and specificity of 100% and 45% for the PZ, and sensitivity and specificity of 100% and 40% for the TZ. Ocak et al. [61]

developed a CAD system using PK analysis for prostate cancer diagnostics in patients with biopsy-proven lesions. In their framework, four PK parameters (K^{trans}, k_{ep}, v_e, and the area under the gadolinium concentration curve) were determined and compared for cancer, inflammation, and healthy peripheral. Their results showed improvement in prostate cancer specificity using the K^{trans} and k_{ep} parameters over that obtained using conventional T2-weighted MRI. An automated DCE-MRI CAD system for prostate cancer detection was proposed by Viswanath et al. [62]. Prostate borders were segmented using an ASM, and a nonrigid registration scheme (affine and thin plate spline) was employed to map the whole mount histological sections onto corresponding 2D DCE-MRI. In order to classify prostate tissue, a local linear embedding approach [68] was used to create a feature vector using local neighborhood intensities. Then, a k-means clustering approach was used for the classification and the system achieved an accuracy of about 77%. Their framework was later extended in Viswanath et al. [63] by combining T2-weighted features and DCE-MRI functional features. The system validation showed that the integration of both modalities (A_z of 0.815) has a better performance of either individual modalities (0.704 for T2-weighted MRI and 0.682 for DCE-MRI). A semi-automated framework by Vos et al. [64] classified prostate lesions using quantitative PK maps and T1 estimates. PK features were extracted from a user-defined ROI around the prostate and a SVM was used to estimate the likelihood of malignancy. Based on the ROC analysis, the reported results showed that the system had an accuracy of 83% in the classification of the ROIs with abnormal enhancement patterns in the PZ. Ampeliotis et al. [65] proposed a semi-automated multiparametric CAD system that used T2-weighted and DCE-MRI. The T2-weighted pixel intensities and the four low-frequency coefficients of the discrete cosine transform were used as features and probabilistic neural networks were employed as the classifier. Based on the ROC analysis (A_z of 0.898), their study concluded that the fused T2-weighted and dynamic MRI features outperform that of either modality's features alone. A similar CAD system was proposed by Litjens et al. [66] that employed an ASM to segment the prostate. In order to classify the segmented prostate voxels, the ADC, K^{trans}, and k_{ep} parameters were estimated and a SVM classifier with a radial basis function kernel was used. The validation results showed a sensitivity of 74.7% and 83.4% with seven and nine false positives (FPs) per patient, respectively. Vos et al. [67] utilized an automated CAD system for the detection of prostate cancer. Just as in Litjens et al. [66], the prostate was segmented using an ASM-based technique. Then, multiple ROIs were located within the segmented prostate using peak and mean neighborhood intensity and ADC values. These values and the differences between the peak and the mean were again used as features for ROI classification. In addition, the 25 percentile T2, 25 percentile ADC, 25 percentile washout, 50 percentile T1, 75 percentile K^{trans}, and 75 percentile v_e were used as features. The resulting feature vector was classified using an LDA classifier. This system had an A_z of 0.83 ± 0.20. A maximum A_z of 0.88 was reported for high-grade tumors, but the system had difficulty classifying lower-grade tumors, achieving a maximum A_z of 0.74. Another semi-automated multiparametric system by Peng et al. [69] utilized T2-weighted, DCE-MRI, and DWI. Candidate features, including the T2-weighted intensity skew, the K^{trans}, and the average and 10th percentile ADC, were calculated from a manually selected ROI. Then, an LDA classifier was used to differentiate prostate cancer from normal tissue in those ROIs. Their CAD system concluded that the best diagnostic performance (A_z of 0.95 ± 0.02, sensitivity [SEN] of 0.82, and specificity [SPE] of 0.953) is obtained by combining the 10th percentile ADC, average ADC, and T2-weighted intensity skewness features.

In summary, developing noninvasive CAD systems for the detection and diagnosis of prostate cancer is an area of research interest. Current CAD systems focus mainly on the initial voxel classification stage by obtaining likelihood maps that combine information from MR images using mathematical descriptors. State-of-the art studies showed that voxel basis discrimination between benign and malignant tissue is feasible with good performances. However, the majority of these studies were performed by radiologists who selected an ROI (small window) around the prostate and followed signal changes within these ROIs. In addition, the final diagnosis and patient management is left to the radiologist. Unfortunately, such approaches not only require manual interaction of the operators, but also ROI selection biases the final decision and brings up the same issue of over- or underestimating the problem in the entire gland, just as with biopsy. Moreover, manual ROI selection and function curve generation from these ROIs assume that the prostates (prostate contours) remain exactly the same from scan to scan. Nonetheless, prostate contours may not always exactly match due to patient movement or breathing effects; therefore, motion correction techniques should be applied first before ROI selection. Also, to automate the algorithm and to cancel ROI dependency, segmentation approaches that can separate the prostate from the surrounding structures are needed.

To overcome the limitations of the existing work on prostate cancer diagnosis using MR images, a novel noninvasive DCE-MRI-based framework (Figure 12.3) for early diagnosis of prostate cancer is proposed. The proposed framework performs sequentially the following processing steps. First, the prostate is segmented from the surrounding anatomical tissues based on a MAP estimate of a new likelihood function. To handle the object inhomogeneities and variability and overcome image noise, the proposed likelihood function accounts for the visual appearances of the prostate and background, 3D spatial interaction between the prostate voxels, and a learned 3D shape model. Second, in order to account for any local prostate deformations that could occur during the scanning process, a nonrigid registration algorithm is employed, which is based on deforming a target prostate object over evolving iso-contours to match a reference object. The correspondences between the target and reference objects are found by the solution of the Laplace equation. In the third step, agent kinetic curves that show the contrast agent (CA) propagation into the tissue are obtained, and then used to collect two features to distinguish between malignant and benign detected tumors using a k_n-nearest neighbor classifier. Finally, parametric map displays that illustrate the propagation of the CA into the prostate tissue are constructed for visual assessment and characterization of the physiological data. Details of the proposed framework are described in the following sections.

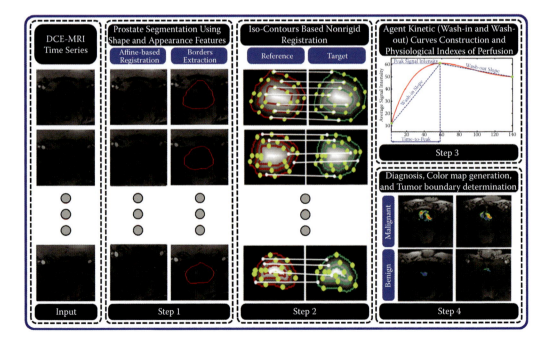

FIGURE 12.3 The proposed CAD system for early detection of prostate cancer.

PROSTATE SEGMENTATION

The segmentation of the prostate from DCE-MRI is a challenge due to the anatomical complexity of the prostate and the undistinguishable gray-level distribution of the prostate and surrounding organs. To account for these challenges, a MAP-based approach based on a learned shape model and an identifiable joint Markov-Gibbs random field (MGRF) model (Figure 12.4) is proposed. The proposed MGRF image model relates the joint probability of an image and its object- background region segmentation map, to geometric structure and to the energy of repeated patterns within the image [70]. The basic theory behind such models is that they assume that the signals associated with each voxel depend on the signals of the neighboring voxel, and thus explicitly take into account their spatial interaction and other features such as shape.

The input 3D DCE-MRI data $\mathbf{g}$ and its region map $\mathbf{m}$ are described by the joint MGRF model in Equation 12.1. The Bayesian MAP estimate of the map, given $\mathbf{g}$, $\mathbf{m}^* = \arg\max_{\mathbf{m}} L(\mathbf{g},\mathbf{m})$ maximize the log-likelihood function:

$$L(\mathbf{g},\mathbf{m}) = \log(P(\mathbf{g}\,|\,\mathbf{m})) + \log(P(\mathbf{m})) \tag{12.1}$$

where $P(\mathbf{g}\,|\,\mathbf{m})$ is a conditional distribution of the images given the map $\mathbf{m}$ and $P(\mathbf{m}) = P_{sp}(\mathbf{m})P_V(\mathbf{m})$ is an unconditional probability distribution of maps. Here, $P_{sp}(\mathbf{m})$ denotes the prostate shape prior, and $P_V(\mathbf{m})$ is a Gibbs probability distribution with potentials $\mathbf{V}$, which specifies a MGRF model of spatially homogeneous maps $\mathbf{m}$.

The specific visual appearance of the prostate in each dataset to be segmented is taken into account by modeling the marginal gray-level distribution with the LCDG model [71]. To overcome noise effect and to ensure the homogeneity of the segmentation, the spatial voxel interactions between the region labels of a given map $\mathbf{m}$ are also taken into account using the pairwise MGRF spatial model as described in this section and the nearest voxel 26-neighbors shown in Figure 12.5. In addition to voxelwise image intensities and their pairwise spatial interaction, additional constraints based on the expected shape of the prostate are introduced by co-aligning each given DCE-MRI data to a training database and using probabilistic 3D prostate shape model $P_{sp}(\mathbf{m})$, see Figure 12.6.

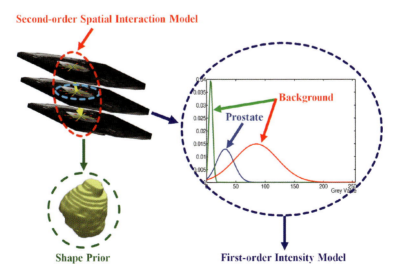

FIGURE 12.4   Illustration of the joint Markov-Gibbs random field (MGRF) image model of the prostate DCE-MRI.

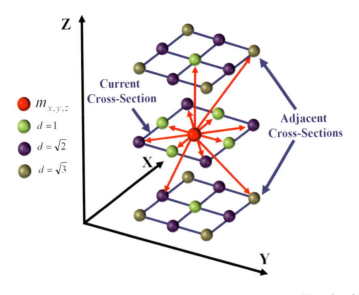

FIGURE 12.5 Three-dimensional second-order MGRF neighborhood system. Note that the reference voxel is shown in red and d represents the absolute distance between two voxels in the same and adjacent MRI slices, or cross-sections.

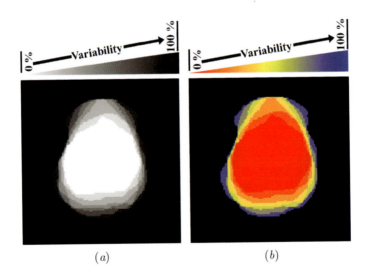

FIGURE 12.6 Gray-coded (a) and color-coded (b) axial view of the prostate shape prior.

To perform initial prostate segmentation, a given 3D DCE-MRI is aligned to one of the training data. The shape model provides the voxelwise object and background probabilities being used, together with the conditional image intensity model $P(\mathbf{g}\,|\,\mathbf{m})$, to build an initial region map. The final Bayesian segmentation is performed using the identified joint MGRF model of the DCE-MRI data and its region maps. In total, the proposed prostate segmentation approach involves the steps summarized in Algorithm 12.1.

Algorithm 12.1   Prostate Segmentation Approach

Input: 3D MRI prostate data **g** to be segmented.
Output: segmented prostate border (the final estimate **m**).

Training Phase:

1. Co-alignment of the 3D DCE-MRI training sets using a 3D affine registration in a way that maximizes their MI [72].
2. Manual delineation of the prostate borders from the co-aligned data.
3. Estimation of the voxelwise probabilities by counting how many times each voxel (x, y, z) was segmented as the prostate.

Testing Phase:

1. Perform a 3D affine alignment of a given MRI to an arbitrary prototype prostate from the training set using MI [72] as a matching metric.
2. Estimate the conditional intensity model $P(\mathbf{g} \mid \mathbf{m})$ by identifying the bimodal LCDG.
3. Use the intensity model found in Step 2 and the learned probabilistic shape model to perform an initial segmentation (region map **m**) of the prostate.
4. Use **m** to estimate the potential for the Potts MGRF model and to identify the MGRF model $P(\mathbf{m})$ of region maps.
5. Improve **m** using voxelwise stochastic relaxation (ICM [73]) through successive iterations to maximize Equation 12.1 until the log-likelihood remains almost the same for two successive iterations.
6. **Update the Shape Prior** by adding the current segmented 3D prostate data to the prior calculated shape model.

NONRIGID REGISTRATION

Due to patient breathing and local movement, accurate registration is a main issue in DCE-MRI time series. After affine registration and prostate segmentation, the Laplace-based nonrigid registration is used for local motion correction of the prostate over the time frame of image acquisition. For completeness, the main steps of the Laplace-based nonrigid registration is summarized in Figure 12.7 as follows:

1. Generation of the distance maps inside the prostate regions (Figure 12.7 a,b).
2. Generation of the iso-contours using distance maps in Step 1 (Figure 12.7 c,d).
3. Solution of the Laplace equation between respective reference and target iso-contours to co-allocate the corresponding points.

PERFUSION CHARACTERIZATION AND TUMOR BOUNDARY DETERMINATION

After the nonrigid alignment, the time-intensity or agent kinetic curves are constructed by calculating the average intensities of prostate regions for each time sequence. These curves show the response of the prostate tissue to the transient of the CA perfusing into each image section (see Figure 12.8). To characterize the physiological data, parametric map displays are constructed to illustrate the propagation of the CA into the prostate tissue. To construct the initial color maps, the changes in image signals $\Delta_{x,y,z}$ due to the CA transient are estimated (see Figure 12.8) from the constructed kinetic curves as the difference between the signals of image sequences at

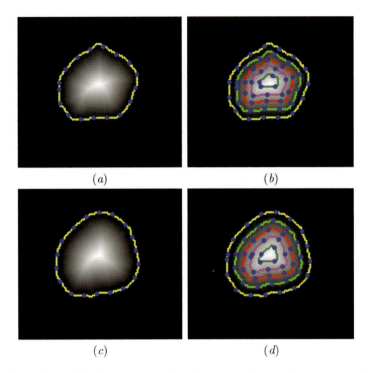

FIGURE 12.7   Generation of the iso-contours: the reference and target distance maps (a, b), and their iso-contours (c, d).

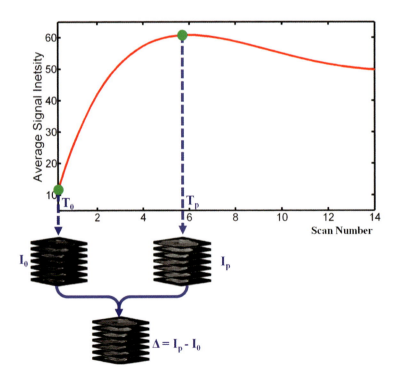

FIGURE 12.8   Estimating the changes in image signals Δ from the kinetic curve as the difference between the peak (I_p) and initial (I_0) signals of the image sequences.

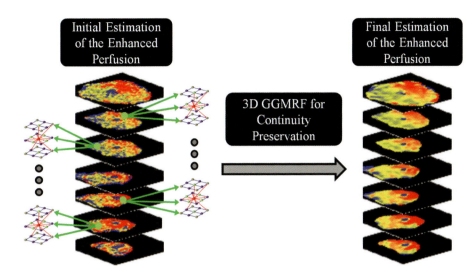

FIGURE 12.9   Enhanced perfusion estimation and continuity analysis using the 3D GGMRF image model.

peak time (T_p) and initial time (T_0). To preserve continuity (remove inconsistencies), the initial estimated $\Delta_{x,y,z}$ values are considered as samples from a generalized Gauss-Markov random field (GGMRF) image model [74] of measurements with the 26-voxel neighborhood shown in Figure 12.5. Continuity of the constructed 3D volume (see Figure 12.9) is amplified by using their MAP estimates [74]:

$$\hat{\Delta}_{\mathbf{P}} = \arg\min_{\Delta_{\mathbf{P}}}\{|\,\Delta_{\mathbf{P}} - \tilde{\Delta}_{\mathbf{P}}\,|^a + \alpha^a \chi^b \sum_{\mathbf{P}' \in \nu_{\mathbf{P}}} \Gamma_{\mathbf{P},\mathbf{P}'}\,|\,\tilde{\Delta}_{\mathbf{P}} - \Delta_{\mathbf{P}'}\,|^b\} \tag{12.2}$$

where $\Delta_{x,y,z}$ and $\tilde{\Delta}_{x,y,z}$ denote the original values and their expected estimates at the observed 3D location, $\mathbf{P} = (x,y,z)$, $\nu_{\mathbf{P}}$ is the neighborhood system (Figure 12.5), $\Gamma_{\mathbf{P},\mathbf{P}'}$ is the GGMRF potential, and α and χ are scaling factors. The parameter $b \in [1.01, 2.0]$ controls the smoothing level (e.g., smooth, $b = 2$, vs. relatively abrupt edges, $b = 1.01$). The parameter $a \in \{1,2\}$ determines the Gaussian, $a = 2$, or Laplace, $a = 1$, prior distribution of the estimator. Then, the color maps are generated based on the final estimated $\hat{\Delta}$ (see Figure 12.13).

The final step after the 3D GGMRF smoothing is the delineation of the detected tumor boundary, which is important to determine the cancer stage in case of malignancy. To achieve this, the level set deformable model [75] is applied again. The evolution of the level set is controlled by a stochastic speed function that accounts for the perfusion information and spatial interactions between the prostate voxels.

EXPERIMENTAL RESULTS

PATIENTS AND DATA ACQUISITION

The performance of the proposed framework has been evaluated by applying it on DCE-MRI prostate data that has been collected from 30 patients. These patients had biopsy-proven prostate cancer. DCE-MRI was obtained at 1.5 T using a gradient-echo T2 imaging (SIGNA Horizon, General Electric Medical Systems, Milwaukee, WI) using an additional pelvic coil. Images were taken at a 7 mm thickness with an interslice gap of 0.5 mm; T_R was 50 msec; T_E was minimum; flip angle at 60°; band width was 31.25 kilohertz (kHz); field-of-view (FOV) was 28 cm; and the number of slices was 7. The DCE-MRI process started with a series of MRI scans that were used to establish a baseline in image intensity. These scans were performed without the administration of the CA so that the tissue's non-enhanced image intensity could be established. In the next stage, 10 cubic centimeter (cc) of gadoteric acid (Dotarem 0.5 millimole/milliliter [mmol/mL]; Guerbet, France) was administered intravenously at a rate of 3 mL/sec. At this point, a series of MRI scans was performed every 10 sec for approximately 3 min, and every series contained 7 slices. Note that all the subjects were diagnosed using a biopsy (ground truth).

SEGMENTATION RESULTS

The proposed segmentation approach has been tested on DCE-MRI sequences for 30 independent subjects. Figure 12.10 shows some segmentation results of the prostate region at selected image sections for different subjects and their associated FP and false negative (FN) segmentation errors, with respect to the ground truth segmentation. The ground truths were obtained by manual delineation of the prostate borders by an MR imaging expert. The positive predictive value (PPV), SEN, and DSC statistics for the proposed approach are summarized in Table 12.1.

To highlight the advantage of the proposed segmentation approach, all time series images have been segmented using the shape-based (SB) approach proposed by Tsai et al. [76]. The comparative results for a few of them are shown in Figure 12.11 and Table 12.2 summarizes the segmentation

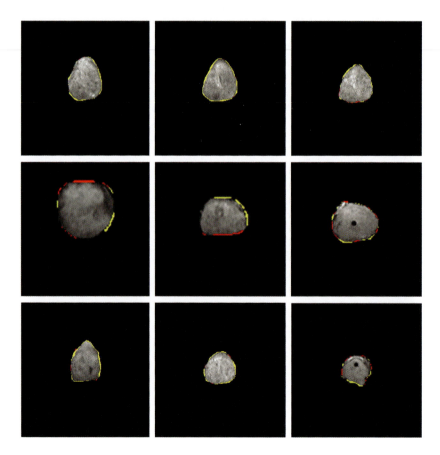

FIGURE 12.10 Sample segmentation results of the proposed segmentation approach for different subjects at different cross-sections. The false negative (FN) and false positive (FP) error referenced to the ground truth **G** are shown in yellow and red, respectively.

TABLE 12.1

Error Statistics of the Proposed Segmentation Approach

	Performance Metric		
	PPV	SEN	DSC
Mean ± SD	0.982 ± 0.004	0.846 ± 0.004	0.923 ± 0.004

Abbreviation: SD: standard deviation.

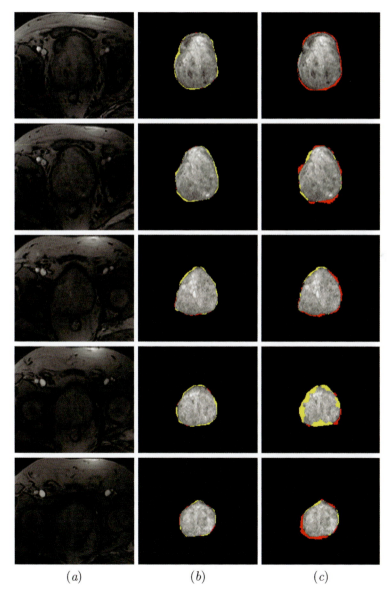

(a) (b) (c)

FIGURE 12.11 Comparative segmentation results: (a) DCE-MRI of the prostate, (b) proposed segmentation, and (c) segmentation with [76]. The false negative (FN) and false positive (FP) errors referenced to the ground truth **G** are shown in yellow and red, respectively.

TABLE 12.2

Comparative Segmentation Accuracies of the Proposed Prostate Segmentation Against the Shape-Based (SB) Approach [76] in Comparison to the Expert's Ground Truth

	Segmentation Technique	
	Proposed Approach	**SB Approach [76]**
Mean ± SD (%)	0.53 ± 0.33	5.91 ± 4.44
Two-tailed P-value	0.0001	

Abbreviation: SD: standard deviation.

error statistics of the proposed approach and the SB approach with respect to ground truth. The differences between the mean errors of the proposed approach and the SB approach are shown to be statistically significant by the unpaired t-test (the two-tailed value P is less than 0.0001).

DIAGNOSTIC RESULTS

The ultimate goal of the proposed framework is to successfully distinguish between malignant and benign detected tumors by constructing the time-intensity curves from the DCE-MRI sequences. The curves show the response of the prostate tissues as the CA perfuses. The malignant subjects show an abrupt increase of the signal intensity and the benign subjects show a delay in reaching their peak (see Figure 12.12). From these curves, it is conclude that the peak signal value and the wash-in slope are the two major features that can be extracted for the classification of prostate cancer. To distinguish between benign and malignant cases, a k_n-nearest neighbor classifier is used to learn the statistical characteristics of both benign and malignant cases from the time-intensity curves of the training sets. Nine datasets were used for the training and the other 21 datasets were used for testing. The diagnostic accuracy of the k_n classifier was 100% for all training and testing datasets.

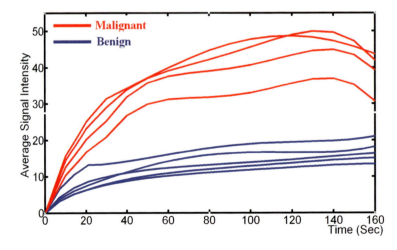

FIGURE 12.12 Normalized signal intensity, averaged over the entire prostate, with respect to the timing of contrast agent delivery for selected malignant (red) and benign (blue) subject.

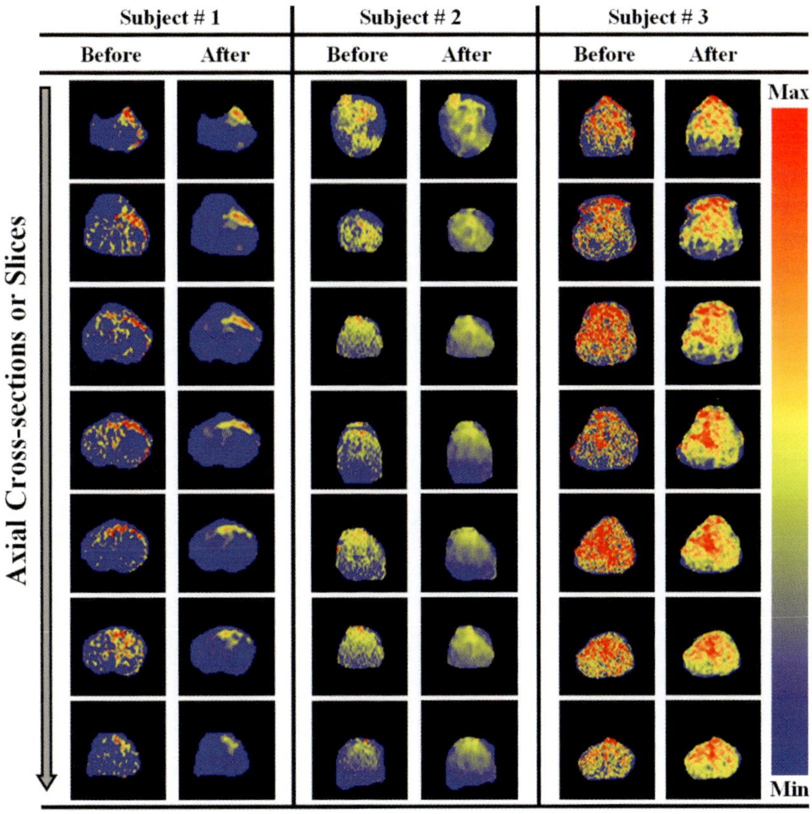

FIGURE 12.13 Color-coded maps for three subjects before and after the 3D GGMRF smoothing using $\alpha = 1$, $\chi = 5$, $b = 1.01$, $a = 2$, and $\Gamma_{P,P'} = \sqrt{2}$. The red and blue ends of the color scale relate to the maximum and minimum changes, respectively.

Following the classification, a visual assessment is performed using color-coded maps. Figure 12.13 presents the color-coded maps over all image sections before and after applying the 3D GGMRF smoothing for three independent subjects. Figure 12.14 show two examples of the tumor contours determination for one benign and one malignant subject.

CONCLUSIONS

In this chapter, a noninvasive framework for detecting prostate cancer using DCE-MRI is proposed. The framework includes delineation of the prostate region, local motion correction, and k_n-classification. The proposed framework has the documented ability to reliably distinguish benign from malignant prostate cancer, in a biopsy proven preliminary cohort of 30 patients. To extract the prostate region, a new 3D approach that is based on a MAP estimate of a new log-likelihood function that accounts for a priori shape, the spatial interactions between the prostate voxels, and the current appearance of the prostate tissues and its background is proposed. Following segmentation, a nonrigid registration approach is introduced. The proposed approach deforms the prostate object on iso-contours instead of a square lattice, which provides more degrees of freedom to obtain accurate deformation. The agent kinetic curves of the co-aligned prostate regions are constructed and the two features extracted from these curves undergo k_n-classification. Applications of the proposed framework yield promising results that would, in the near future, represent a supplement of the current technologies to determine the type of prostate cancer.

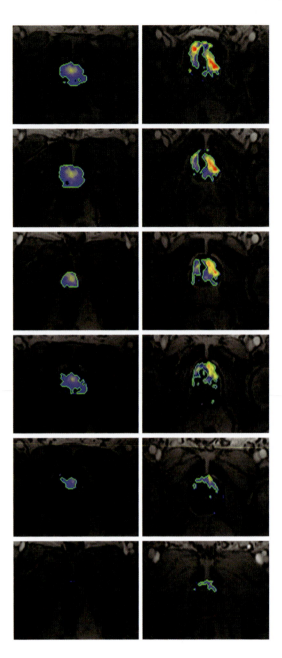

FIGURE 12.14 Color-coded maps of local tumor progression overlaid on anatomic DCE-MRI data for one benign (first column) and one malignant (second column) subject. The determined tumor contours are shown in green.

This work could also be applied to various other applications in medical imaging, such as the kidney, the heart, the lung, and the retina.

One application is renal transplant functional assessment. Chronic kidney disease (CKD) affects about 26 million people in the United States with 17,000 transplants being performed each year. In renal transplant patients, acute rejection is the leading cause of renal dysfunction. Given the limited number of donors, routine clinical post-transplantation evaluation is of immense importance to help clinicians initiate timely interventions with appropriate treatment and thus prevent graft loss.

Accurate assessment of renal transplant function is critically important for graft survival. Although transplantation can improve a patient wellbeing, there is a potential post-transplantation risk of kidney dysfunction that, if not treated in a timely manner, can lead to the loss of the entire graft, and even patient death. Thus, accurate assessment of renal transplant function is crucial for the identification of proper treatment. In recent years, an increased area of research has been dedicated to developing noninvasive image-based CAD systems for the assessment of renal transplant function utilizing different image modalities (e.g., ultrasound, CT, MRI, etc.). In particular, dynamic and diffusion MRI-based systems have been clinically used to assess transplanted kidneys with the advantage of providing information on each kidney separately. A variety of studies can be consulted for more details about renal transplant functional assessment [77–101].

The heart is also an important application for this work. The clinical assessment of myocardial perfusion plays a major role in the diagnosis, management, and prognosis of ischemic heart disease patients. Thus, there have been ongoing efforts to develop automated systems for accurate analysis of myocardial perfusion using first-pass images [102–118].

Another application for this work could be the detection of retinal abnormalities. The majority of ophthalmologists depend on visual interpretation for the identification of diseases types. However, inaccurate diagnosis will affect the treatment procedure which may lead to fatal results. Hence, there is a crucial need for computer automated diagnosis systems that yield highly accurate results. Optical coherence tomography (OCT) has become a powerful modality for noninvasive diagnosis of various retinal abnormalities such as glaucoma, diabetic macular edema, and macular degeneration. The problem with diabetic retinopathy (DR) is that the patient is not aware of the disease until the changes in the retina have progressed to a level at which treatment tends to be less effective. Therefore, automated early detection could limit the severity of the disease and assist ophthalmologists in investigating and treating it more efficiently [119,120].

Abnormalities of the lung could be another promising area of research and a related application for this work. Radiation-induced lung injury is the main side effect of radiation therapy for lung cancer patients. Although higher radiation doses increase the radiation therapy effectiveness for tumor control, this can lead to lung injury as a greater quantity of normal lung tissues is included in the treated area. Almost a third of patients who undergo radiation therapy develop lung injury following radiation treatment. The severity of radiation-induced lung injury ranges from ground-glass opacities and consolidation at the early phase to fibrosis and traction bronchiectasis in the late phase. Early detection of lung injury will thus help to improve treatment management [121–161].

This work can also be applied to other brain abnormalities, such as dyslexia and autism. Dyslexia is one of the most complicated developmental brain disorders that affect children's learning abilities. Dyslexia leads to the failure to develop age-appropriate reading skills in spite of a normal intelligence level and adequate reading instructions. Neuropathological studies have revealed an abnormal anatomy of some structures, such as the corpus callosum in dyslexic brains. There has been a lot of work in the literature that aims at developing CAD systems for diagnosing this disorder, along with other brain disorders [71,162–183].

This work could also be applied for the extraction of blood vessels from phase contrast (PC) magnetic resonance angiography (MRA). Accurate cerebrovascular segmentation using noninvasive MRA is crucial for the early diagnosis and timely treatment of intracranial vascular diseases [166,167,184,185].

REFERENCES

1. Gray, H. *Anatomy of the Human Body*. Lea & Febiger: Philadelphia, PA (2000).
2. HealthNews Texas. *PSA Test Reduces Prostate Cancer Deaths* [Online]. Available: http://healthnewstexas.com/5262/psa-test-reduces-prostate-cancer-deaths/
3. Shier, D., Butler, J., Lewis, R. *Human Anatomy and Physiology*. McGraw-Hill: New York (2001).
4. McNeal, J.E. The zonal anatomy of the prostate. *Prostate* **2**(1) (1981) 35–49.

5. SIU School of Medicine. *Enlarged Prostate* [Online]. Available: http://www.siumed.edu/surgery/urology/bph.html

6. Stevermer, J.J., Easley, S.K. Treatment of prostatitis. *Am. Fam. Physician* **61**(10) (2000) 3015–3034.

7. Meares, E., Stamey, T.A. Bacteriologic localization patterns in bacterial prostatitis and urethritis. *Invest. Urol.* **5**(5) (1968) 492.

8. Hedayati, T., Stehman, C. Prostatitis. emedicine from WebMD website (2011).

9. Piovesan, A.C., Freire, G.D.C., Torricelli, F.C.M., Cordeiro, P., Yamada, R., Srougi, M. Incidence of histological prostatitis and its correlation with PSA density. *Clinics* **64**(11) (2009) 1049–1051.

10. Urology Care Foundation. *BPH: Management* [Online]. Available: http://www.urologyhealth.org/urology/index.cfm?article=144

11. Lee, C.H., Akin-Olugbade, O., Kirschenbaum, A. Overview of prostate anatomy, histology, and pathology. *Endocrinol. Metab. Clin. N. Am.* **40**(3) (2011) 565–575.

12. Baade, P.D., Youlden, D.R., Krnjacki, L.J. International epidemiology of prostate cancer: Geographical distribution and secular trends. *Mol. Nutr. Food Res.* **53**(2) (2009) 171–184.

13. American Cancer Society. Cancer facts and figures (2013).

14. Hugosson, J., Carlsson, S., Aus, G., Bergdahl, S., Khatami, A., Lodding, P., Pihl, C.G., Stranne, J., Holmberg, E., Lilja, H. Mortality results from the göteborg randomised population-based prostate-cancer screening trial. *Lancet Oncol.* **11**(8) (2010) 725–732.

15. Hricak, H., Choyke, P.L., Eberhardt, S.C., Leibel, S.A., Scardino, P.T. Imaging prostate cancer: A multidisciplinary perspective. *Radiology* **243**(1) (2007) 28–53.

16. Applewhite, J.C., Matlaga, B., McCullough, D., Hall, M. Transrectal ultrasound and biopsy in the early diagnosis of prostate cancer. *Cancer Contr.* **8**(2) (2001) 141–150.

17. Ren, J., Huan, Y., Wang, H., Chang, Y.J., Zhao, H.T., Ge, Y.L., Liu, Y., Yang, Y. Dynamic contrast-enhanced MRI of benign prostatic hyperplasia and prostatic carcinoma: Correlation with angiogenesis. *Clin. Radiol.* **63**(2) (2008) 153–159.

18. Puech, P., Betrouni, N., Makni, N., Dewalle, A.S., Villers, A., Lemaitre, L. Computer-assisted diagnosis of prostate cancer using DCE-MRI data: Design, implementation and preliminary results. *Int. J. Comput. Assist. Radiol. Surg.* **4**(1) (2009) 1–10.

19. Haider, M.A., Chung, P., Sweet, J., Toi, A., Jhaveri, K., Ménard, C., Warde, P., Trachtenberg, J., Lockwood, G., Milosevic, M. Dynamic contrast-enhanced magnetic resonance imaging for localization of recurrent prostate cancer after external beam radiotherapy. *Int. J. Radiat. Oncol. Biol. Phys.* **70**(2) (2008) 425–430.

20. Casciani, E., Polettini, E., Carmenini, E., Floriani, I., Masselli, G., Bertini, L., Gualdi, G.F. Endorectal and dynamic contrast-enhanced MRI for detection of local recurrence after radical prostatectomy. *Am. J. Roentgenol.* **190**(5) (2008) 1187–1192.

21. Valerio, M., Panebianco, V., Sciarra, A., Osimani, M., Salsiccia, S., Casciani, L., Giuliani, A., Bizzarri, M., Di Silverio, F., Passariello, R., Filippo, C. Classification of prostatic diseases by means of multivariate analysis on in vivo proton MRSI and DCE-MRI data. *NMR Biomed.* **22**(10) (2009) 1036–1046.

22. Loiselle, C.R., Eby, P.R., DeMartini, W.B., Peacock, S., Bittner, N., Lehman, C.D., Kim, J.N. Dynamic contrast-enhanced MRI kinetics of invasive breast cancer: A potential prognostic marker for radiation therapy. *Int. J. Radiat. Oncol. Biol. Phys.* **76**(5) (2010) 1314–1319.

23. Isebaert, S., De Keyzer, F., Haustermans, K., Lerut, E., Roskams, T., Roebben, I., Van Poppel, H., Joniau, S., Oyen, R. Evaluation of semi-quantitative dynamic contrast-enhanced MRI parameters for prostate cancer in correlation to whole-mount histopathology. *Eur. J. Radiol.* **81**(3) (2012) 217–222.

24. Niaf, E., Rouvière, O., Mège-Lechevallier, F., Bratan, F., Lartizien, C. Computer-aided diagnosis of prostate cancer in the peripheral zone using multiparametric MRI. *Phys. Med. Biol.* **57**(12) (2012) 3833–3851.

25. Fütterer, J.J., Engelbrecht, M.R., Huisman, H.J., Jager, G.J., Hulsbergen-van De Kaa, C.A., Witjes, J.A., Barentsz, J.O. Staging prostate cancer with dynamic contrast-enhanced endorectal MR imaging prior to radical prostatectomy: Experienced versus less experienced readers. *Radiology* **237**(2) (2005) 541–549.

26. Fütterer, J.J., Heijmink, S.W.T.P.J., Scheenen, T.W.J., Veltman, J., Huisman, H.J., Vos, P., Hulsbergen-Van de Kaa, C.A., Witjes, J.A., Krabbe, P.F.M., Heerschap, A., Barentsz, J.O. Prostate cancer localization with dynamic contrast-enhanced MR imaging and proton MR spectroscopic imaging. *Radiology* **241**(2) (2006) 449–458.

27. Firjani, A., Khalifa, F., Elnakib, A., Gimelfarb, G., Abo El-Ghar, M., Elmaghraby, A., El-Baz, A. A novel image-based approach for early detection of prostate cancer using DCE-MRI. In: Suzuki, K. (Ed.) *Computational Intelligence in Biomedical Imaging*. Springer Science and Business Media: Berlin, Germany (2014) pp. 55–85.

28. Firjani, A., Elnakib, A., Khalifa, F., Gimelfarb, G., Abou El-Ghar, M., Elmaghraby, A., El-Baz, A. A diffusion-weighted imaging based diagnostic system for early detection of prostate cancer. *J. Biomed. Sci. Eng.* **6**(3A) (2013) 346–356.

29. Firjani, A., Khalifa, F., Elnakib, A., Gimelfarb, G., Abo El-Ghar, M., Elmaghraby, A., El-Baz, A. Noninvasive image-based approach for early detection of prostate cancer. In: *Proceedings of the International Conference On the Developments on eSystems Engineering (DeSE'11)* IEEE (2011) pp. 172–177.

30. Firjani, A., Khalifa, F., Elnakib, A., Gimelfarb, G., Elmaghraby, A., El-Baz, A. A novel image-based approach for early detection of prostate cancer. In: *Proceedings of IEEE International Conference on Image Processing (ICIP'12)* (2012) pp. 2849–2852.

31. Zwiggelaar, R., Zhu, Y., Williams, S. Semi-automatic segmentation of the prostate. In: *Proceedings of First Iberian Conference on Pattern Recognition and Image Analysis*, Springer, Berlin, Germany (2003) pp. 1108–1116.

32. Allen, P.D., Graham, J., Williamson, D.C., Hutchinson, C.E. Differential segmentation of the prostate in MR images using combined 3D shape modelling and voxel classification. In: *Proceedings of IEEE International Symposium on Biomedical Imaging: From Nano to Macro (ISBI'06)* (2006) pp. 410–413.

33. Zhu, Y., Williams, S., Zwiggelaar, R. A hybrid ASM approach for sparse volumetric data segmentation. *Pattern Recogn. Image Anal.* **17**(2) (2007) 252–258.

34. Klein, S., van der Heide, U.A., Raaymakers, B.W., Kotte, A.N., Staring, M., Pluim, J.P. Segmentation of the prostate in MR images by atlas matching. In: *Proceedings of IEEE International Symposium on Biomedical Imaging: From Nano to Macro (ISBI'07)* (2007) pp. 1300–1303.

35. Klein, S., van der Heide, U.A., Lips, I.M., van Vulpen, M., Staring, M., Pluim, J.P. Automatic segmentation of the prostate in 3D MR images by atlas matching using localized mutual information. *Med. Phys.* **35**(5) (2008) 1407–1417.

36. Flores-Tapia, D., Thomas, G., Venugopal, N., McCurdy, B., Pistorius, S. Semi automatic MRI prostate segmentation based on wavelet multiscale products. In: *Proceedings of the Annual IEEE Conference of the Engineering in Medicine and Biology Society (EMBS'08)* (2008) pp. 3020–3023.

37. Pesquet, J.C., Krim, H., Carfantan, H. Time-invariant orthonormal wavelet representations. *IEEE Trans. Image Process.* **44**(8) (1996) 1964–1970.

38. Toth, R., Tiwari, P., Rosen, M., Kalyanpur, A., Pungavkar, S., Madabhushi, A. A multimodal prostate segmentation scheme by combining spectral clustering and active shape models. In: *Proceedings of SPIE Medical Imaging: Image Processing*, SPIE, Bellingham, WA (2008) pp. 1–12.

39. Vikal, S., Haker, S., Tempany, C., Fichtinger, G. Prostate contouring in MRI guided biopsy. In: *Proceedings of SPIE Medical Imaging: Image Processing*, SPIE, Bellingham, WA (2009) pp. 1–11.

40. Liu, X., Langer, D., Haider, M., Van der Kwast, T., Evans, A., Wernick, M., Yetik, I. Unsupervised segmentation of the prostate using MR images based on level set with a shape prior. In: *Proceedings of the Annual IEEE Conference of the Engineering in Medicine and Biology Society (EMBS'09)* (2009) pp. 3613–3616.

41. Otsu, N. A threshold selection method from gray-level histograms. *IEEE Trans. Syst. Man Cybern.* **9**(1) (1979) 62–66.

42. Makni, N., Puech, P., Lopes, R., Dewalle, A.S., Colot, O., Betrouni, N. Combining a deformable model and a probabilistic framework for an automatic 3D segmentation of prostate on MRI. *Int. J. Comput. Assist. Radiol. Surg.* **4**(2) (2009) 181–188.

43. Liu, X., Langer, D.L., Haider, M.A., Yang, Y., Wernick, M.N., Yetik, I.S. Prostate cancer segmentation with simultaneous estimation of Markov random field parameters and class. *IEEE Trans. Med. Imaging* **28**(6) (2009) 906–915.

44. Artan, Y., Haider, M.A., Langer, D.L., van der Kwast, T.H., Evans, A.J., Yang, Y., Wernick, M.N., Trachtenberg, J., Yetik, I.S. Prostate cancer localization with multispectral MRI using cost-sensitive support vector machines and conditional random fields. *IEEE Trans. Image Process.* **19**(9) (2010) 2444–2455.

45. Ozer, S., Haider, M.A., Langer, D.L., van der Kwast, T.H., Evans, A.J., Wernick, M.N., Trachtenberg, J., Yetik, I.S. Prostate cancer localization with multispectral MRI based on relevance vector machines. In: *Proceedings of IEEE International Symposium on Biomedical Imaging: From Nano to Macro (ISBI'09)* (2009) pp. 73–76.

46. Tipping, M.E. Sparse Bayesian learning and the relevance vector machine. *J. Mach. Learning Res.* **1**(9) (2001) 211–244.

47. Gao, Y., Sandhu, R., Fichtinger, G., Tannenbaum, A.R. A coupled global registration and segmentation framework with application to magnetic resonance prostate imagery. *IEEE Trans. Med. Imaging* **29**(10) (2010) 1781–1794.

48. Martin, S., Troccaz, J., Daanen, V. Automated segmentation of the prostate in 3D MR images using a probabilistic atlas and a spatially constrained deformable model. *Med. Phys.* **37** (2010) 1579–1590.

49. Firjany, A., Elnakib, A., El-Baz, A., Gimelfarb, G., Abo El-Ghar, M., Elmagharby, A. Novel stochastic framework for accurate segmentation of prostate in dynamic contrast-enhanced MRI. In: *Proceedings of International Workshop Prostate Cancer Imaging: Computer-Aided Diagnosis, Prognosis, and Intervention*, Springer, Berlin, Germany (2010) pp. 121–130.

50. Firjani, A., Elnakib, A., Khalifa, F., Gimelfarb, G., Abo El-Ghar, M., Suri, J., Elmaghraby, A., El-Baz, A. A new 3D automatic segmentation framework for accurate extraction of prostate from DCE-MRI. In: *Proceedings of IEEE International Symposium on Biomedical Imaging: From Nano to Macro (ISBI'11)* (2011) pp. 1476–1479.

51. Dowling, J.A., Fripp, J., Chandra, S., Pluim, J.P.W., Lambert, J., Parker, J., Denham, J., Greer, P.B., Salvado, O. Fast automatic multi-atlas segmentation of the prostate from 3D MR images. In: *Proceedings of International Workshop on Prostate Cancer Imaging: Image Analysis and Image-guided Intervention*, Springer, Berlin, Germany (2011) pp. 10–21.

52. Langerak, T.R., van der Heide, U.A., Kotte, A.N., Viergever, M.A., van Vulpen, M., Pluim, J.P. Label fusion in atlas-based segmentation using a selective and iterative method for performance level estimation (SIMPLE). *IEEE Trans. Med. Imaging* **29**(12) (2010) 2000–2008.

53. Ghose, S., Mitra, J., Oliver, A., Marti, R., Llado, X., Freixenet, J., Vilanova, J.C., Sidibé, D., Mériaudeau, F. Graph cut energy minimization in a probabilistic learning framework for 3D prostate segmentation in MRI. In: *Proceedings of the IEEE International Conference on Pattern Recognition (ICPR'12)* (2012) pp. 125–128.

54. Ghose, S., Oliver, A., Mart, R., Lladó, X., Freixenet, J., Mitra, J., Vilanova, J.C., Meriaudeau, F. A hybrid framework of multiple active appearance models and global registration for 3D prostate segmentation in MRI. In: *Proceedings of the SPIE Medical Imaging: Image Process*, SPIE, Bellingham, WA (2012) pp. 83140S–83140S.

55. Chan, I., Wells III, W., Mulkern, R.V., Haker, S., Zhang, J., Zou, K.H., Maier, S.E., Tempany, C.M. Detection of prostate cancer by integration of line-scan diffusion, T2-mapping and T2-weighted magnetic resonance imaging; a multichannel statistical classifier. *Med. Phys.* **30**(9) (2003) 2390–2398.

56. Madabhushi, A., Feldman, M.D., Metaxas, D.N., Tomaszeweski, J., Chute, D. Automated detection of prostatic adenocarcinoma from high-resolution ex vivo MRI. *IEEE Trans. Med. Imaging* **24**(12) (2005) 1611–1625.

57. Engelbrecht, M.R., Huisman, H.J., Laheij, R.J., Jager, G.J., van Leenders, G.J., Hulsbergen-Van De Kaa, C.A., de la Rosette, J.J., Blickman, J.G., Barentsz, J.O. Discrimination of prostate cancer from normal peripheral zone and central gland tissue by using dynamic contrast-enhanced MR imaging. *Radiology* **229**(1) (2003) 248–254.

58. Kim, J.K., Hong, S.S., Choi, Y.J., Park, S.H., Ahn, H., Kim, C.S., Cho, K.S. Wash-in rate on the basis of dynamic contrast-enhanced MRI: Usefulness for prostate cancer detection and localization. *J. Magn. Reson. Imaging* **22**(5) (2005) 639–646.

59. Rouvière, O., Valette, O., Grivolat, S., Colin-Pangaud, C., Bouvier, R., Chapelon, J.Y., Gelet, A., Lyonnet, D. Recurrent prostate cancer after external beam radiotherapy: Value of contrast-enhanced dynamic MRI in localizing intraprostatic tumor correlation with biopsy findings. *Urology* **63**(5) (2004) 922–927.

60. Puech, P., Betrouni, N., Viard, R., Villers, A., Leroy, X., Lemaitre, L. Prostate cancer computer-assisted diagnosis software using dynamic contrast-enhanced MRI. In: *Proceedings of the Annual IEEE Conference on Engineering in Medicine and Biology Society (EMBS'07)* (2007) pp. 5567–5570.

61. Ocak, I., Bernardo, M., Metzger, G., Barrett, T., Pinto, P., Albert, P.S., Choyke, P.L. Dynamic contrast-enhanced MRI of prostate cancer at 3T: A study of pharmacokinetic parameters. *Am. J. Roentgenol.* **189**(4) (2007) W192–W201.

62. Viswanath, S., Bloch, B.N., Genega, E., Rofsky, N., Lenkinski, R., Chappelow, J., Toth, R., Madabhushi, A. A comprehensive segmentation, registration, and cancer detection scheme on 3 tesla in vivo prostate DCE-MRI. In: *Proceedings of the Medical Image Computing and Computer-Assisted Intervention (MICCAI'08)*, Springer, Berlin, Germany (2008) pp. 662–669.

63. Viswanath, S., Bloch, B.N., Rosen, M., Chappelow, J., Toth, R., Rofsky, N., Lenkinski, R., Genega, E., Kalyanpur, A., Madabhushi, A. Integrating structural and functional imaging for computer assisted detection of prostate cancer on multi-protocol in vivo 3 Tesla MRI. In: *Proceedings of the SPIE Medical Imaging: Image Process*, SPIE, Bellingham, WA (2009) pp. 72603I–72603I.

64. Vos, P.C., Hambrock, T., Hulsbergen-van de Kaa, C.A., Fütterer, J.J., Barentsz, J.O., Huisman, H.J. Computerized analysis of prostate lesions in the peripheral zone using dynamic contrast enhanced MRI. *Med. Phys.* **35**(3) (2008) 888–899.

65. Ampeliotis, D., Antonakoudi, A., Berberidis, K., Psarakis, E., Kounoudes, A. A computer-aided system for the detection of prostate cancer based on magnetic resonance image analysis. In: *Proceedings of the 3rd International Symposium on Communications, Control, and Signal Processing (ISCCSP'08)*, IEEE (2008) pp. 1372–1377.

66. Litjens, G., Vos, P., Barentsz, J., Karssemeijer, N., Huisman, H. Automatic computer aided detection of abnormalities in multi-parametric prostate MRI. In: *Proceedings of the SPIE Medical Imaging: Computer-Aided Diagnosis*, SPIE, Bellingham, WA (2011) pp. 79630T–79630T.

67. Vos, P.C., Barentsz, J.O., Karssemeijer, N., Huisman, H.J. Automatic computer-aided detection of prostate cancer based on multiparametric magnetic resonance image analysis. *Phys. Med. Biol.* **57**(6) (2012) 1527–1542.

68. Roweis, S.T., Saul, L.K. Nonlinear dimensionality reduction by locally linear embedding. *Science* **290**(5500) (2000) 2323–2326.

69. Peng, Y., Jiang, Y., Yang, C., Brown, J.B., Antic, T., Sethi, I., Schmid-Tannwald, C., Giger, M.L., Eggener, S.E., Oto, A. Quantitative analysis of multiparametric prostate MR images: Differentiation between prostate cancer and normal tissue and correlation with Gleason score. *Radiology* **267**(3) (2013) 787–796.

70. Farag, A., El-Baz, A., Gimelfarb, G. Precise segmentation of multimodal images. *IEEE Trans. Image Process.* **15**(4) (2006) 952–968.

71. El-Baz, A., Elnakib, A., Khalifa, F., Abou El-Ghar, M., McClure, P., Soliman, A., Gimelfarb, G. Precise segmentation of 3-D magnetic resonance angiography. *IEEE Trans. Biomed. Eng.* **59**(7) (2012) 2019–2029.

72. Viola, P.A., Wells III, W.M. Alignment by maximization of mutual information. *Int. J. Comput. Vis.* **24**(2) (1997) 137–154.

73. Besag, J. On the statistical analysis of dirty pictures. *J. Roy. Stat. Soc. Ser. B* **48**(3) (1986) 259–302.

74. Bouman, C., Sauer, K. A generalized Gaussian image model for edge-preserving MAP estimation. *IEEE Trans. Image Process.* **2**(3) (1993) 296–310.

75. Reda, I., Elmogy, M., Aboulfotouh, A., Ismail, M., El-Baz, A., Keynton, R. Prostate segmentation using deformable model-based methods. In: El-Baz, A., Jiang, X., Suri, J.S. (Eds.) *Biomedical Image Segmentation: Advances and Trends.* CRC Press: Boca Raton, FL (2016) pp. 293–308

76. Tsai, A., Yezzi, A.J., Wells III, W.M., Tempany, C.M., Tucker, D., Fan, A.C., Grimson, W.E.L., Willsky, A.S. A shape-based approach to the segmentation of medical imagery using level sets. *IEEE Trans. Med. Imaging* **22**(2) (2003) 137–154.

77. Ali, A.M., Farag, A.A., El-Baz, A. Graph cuts framework for kidney segmentation with prior shape constraints. In: *Proceedings of the Medical Image Computing and Computer-Assisted Intervention (MICCAI'07)*, Springer, Berlin, Germany, Vol. 1 (2007) pp. 384–392.

78. Chowdhury, A.S., Roy, R., Bose, S., Elnakib, F.K.A., El-Baz, A. Non-rigid biomedical image registration using graph cuts with a novel data term. In: *Proceedings of IEEE International Symposium on Biomedical Imaging: From Nano to Macro (ISBI'12)*, Barcelona, Spain, May 2–5 (2012) pp. 446–449.

79. El-Baz, A., Farag, A.A., Yuksel, S.E., El-Ghar, M.E.A., Eldiasty, T.A., Ghoneim, M.A. Application of deformable models for the detection of acute renal rejection. In: Farag, A.A., Suri, J.S. (Eds.) *Deformable Models*, Vol. 1 (2007) pp. 293–333.

80. El-Baz, A., Farag, A., Fahmi, R., Yuksel, S., El-Ghar, M.A., Eldiasty, T. Image analysis of renal DCE MRI for the detection of acute renal rejection. In: *Proceedings of IAPR International Conference on Pattern Recognition (ICPR'06)*, Hong Kong, August 20–24 (2006) pp. 822–825.

81. El-Baz, A., Farag, A., Fahmi, R., Yuksel, S., Miller, W., El-Ghar, M.A., El-Diasty, T., Ghoneim, M. A new CAD system for the evaluation of kidney diseases using DCE-MRI. In: *Proceedings of International Conference on Medical Image Computing and Computer-Assisted Intervention (MICCAI'08)*, Copenhagen, Denmark, October 1–6 (2006) pp. 446–453.

82. El-Baz, A., Gimelfarb, G., El-Ghar, M.A. A novel image analysis approach for accurate identification of acute renal rejection. In: *Proceedings of IEEE International Conference on Image Processing (ICIP'08)*, San Diego, CA, October 12–15 (2008) pp. 1812–1815.

83. El-Baz, A., Gimelfarb, G., El-Ghar, M.A. Image analysis approach for identification of renal transplant rejection. In: *Proceedings of IAPR International Conference on Pattern Recognition (ICPR'08)*, IEEE Tampa, FL, December 8–11 (2008) pp. 1–4.

84. El-Baz, A., Gimelfarb, G., El-Ghar, M.A. New motion correction models for automatic identification of renal transplant rejection. In: *Proceedings of International Conference on Medical Image Computing and Computer-Assisted Intervention (MICCAI'07)*, Brisbane, Australia, October 29–November 2 (2007) pp. 235–243.

85. Farag, A., El-Baz, A., Yuksel, S., El-Ghar, M.A., Eldiasty, T. A framework for the detection of acute rejection with Dynamic Contrast Enhanced Magnetic Resonance Imaging. In: *Proceedings of IEEE International Symposium on Biomedical Imaging: From Nano to Macro (ISBI'06)*, Arlington, VA, April 6–9 (2006) pp. 418–421.

86. Khalifa, F., Beache, G.M., Abou El-Ghar, M., El-Diasty, T., Gimelfarb, G., Kong, M., El-Baz, A. Dynamic contrast-enhanced MRI-based early detection of acute renal transplant rejection. *IEEE Trans. Med. Imaging* **32**(10) (2013) 1910–1927.

87. Khalifa, F., El-Baz, A., Gimelfarb, G., Abo El-Ghar, M. Non-invasive image-based approach for early detection of acute renal rejection. In: *Proceedings of the Medical Image Computing and Computer-Assisted Intervention (MICCAI'10)*, Springer, Berlin, Germany (2010) pp. 10–18.

88. Khalifa, F., El-Baz, A., Gimelfarb, G., Ouseph, R., El-Ghar, M.A. Shape-appearance guided level-set deformable model for image segmentation. In: *Proceedings of the International Conference on Pattern Recognition (ICPR'10)* IEEE (2010) pp. 4581–4584.

89. Khalifa, F., Abou El-Ghar, M., Abdollahi, B., Frieboes, H.B., El-Diasty, T., El-Baz, A. A comprehensive non-invasive framework for automated evaluation of acute renal transplant rejection using DCE-MRI. *NMR Biomed.* **26**(11) (2013) 1460–1470.

90. Khalifa, F., El-Ghar, M.A., Abdollahi, B., Frieboes, H.B., El-Diasty, T., El-Baz, A. Dynamic contrast-enhanced MRI-based early detection of acute renal transplant rejection. In: *2014 Annual Scientific Meeting and Educational Course Brochure of the Society of Abdominal Radiology (SAR'14)*, Boca Raton, FL, March 23–28 (2014) CID: 1855912.

91. Khalifa, F., Elnakib, A., Beache, G.M., Gimelfarb, G., El-Ghar, M.A., Sokhadze, G., Manning, S., McClure, P., El-Baz, A. 3D kidney segmentation from CT images using a level set approach guided by a novel stochastic speed function. In: *Proceedings of the Medical Image Computing and Computer-Assisted Intervention (MICCAI'11)*, Springer, Berlin, Germany (2011) pp. 587–594.

92. Khalifa, F., Gimelfarb, G., El-Ghar, M.A., Sokhadze, G., Manning, S., McClure, P., Ouseph, R., El-Baz, A. A new deformable model-based segmentation approach for accurate extraction of the kidney from abdominal CT images. In: *Proceedings of the IEEE International Conference on Image Processing (ICIP'11)* (2011) pp. 3393–3396.

93. Mostapha, M., Khalifa, F., Alansary, A., Soliman, A., Suri, J., El-Baz, A. Computer-aided diagnosis systems for acute renal transplant rejection: Challenges and methodologies. In: El-Baz, A., Saba, L., Suri, J. (Eds.) *Abdomen and Thoracic Imaging*. Springer: Berlin, Germany (2014) pp. 1–35.

94. Shehata, M., Khalifa, F., Hollis, E., Soliman, A., Hosseini-Asl, E., El-Ghar, M.A., El-Baz, M., Dwyer, A.C., El-Baz, A., Keynton, R. A new non-invasive approach for early classification of renal rejection types using diffusion-weighted MRI. In: *IEEE International Conference on Image Processing (ICIP)*, IEEE (2016) pp. 136–140.

95. Khalifa, F., Soliman, A., Takieldeen, A., Shehata, M., Mostapha, M., Shaffie, A., Ouseph, R., Elmaghraby, A., El-Baz, A. Kidney segmentation from CT images using a 3D NMF-guided active contour model. In: *IEEE 13th International Symposium on Biomedical Imaging (ISBI)*, IEEE (2016) pp. 432–435.

96. Shehata, M., Khalifa, F., Soliman, A., Takieldeen, A., El-Ghar, M.A., Shaffie, A., Dwyer, A.C., Ouseph, R., El-Baz, A., Keynton, R. 3D diffusion MRI-based CAD system for early diagnosis of acute renal rejection. In: *Biomedical Imaging (ISBI), 2016 IEEE 13th International Symposium on*, IEEE (2016) pp. 1177–1180.

97. Shehata, M., Khalifa, F., Soliman, A., Alrefai, R., El-Ghar, M.A., Dwyer, A.C., Ouseph, R., El-Baz, A. A level set-based framework for 3D kidney segmentation from diffusion MR images. In: *IEEE International Conference on Image Processing (ICIP)*, IEEE (2015) pp. 4441–4445.

98. Shehata, M., Khalifa, F., Soliman, A., El-Ghar, M.A., Dwyer, A.C., Gimelfarb, G., Keynton, R., El-Baz, A. A promising non-invasive CAD system for kidney function assessment. In: *International Conference on Medical Image Computing and Computer-Assisted Intervention*, Springer (2016) pp. 613–621.

99. Khalifa, F., Soliman, A., Elmaghraby, A., Gimelfarb, G., El-Baz, A. 3D kidney segmentation from abdominal images using spatial-appearance models. *Comput. Math. Methods Med.* **2017** (2017) 9818506.

100. Hollis, E., Shehata, M., Khalifa, F., El-Ghar, M.A., El-Diasty, T., El-Baz, A. Towards non-invasive diagnostic techniques for early detection of acute renal transplant rejection: A review. *Egyptian J. Radiol. Nucl. Med.* **48**(1) (2016) 257–269.

101. Shehata, M., Khalifa, F., Soliman, A., El-Ghar, M.A., Dwyer, A.C., El-Baz, A. Assessment of renal transplant using image and clinical-based biomarkers. In: *Proceedings of 13th Annual Scientific Meeting of American Society for Diagnostics and Interventional Nephrology (ASDIN'17)*, New Orleans, LA, February 10–12 (2017).

102. Shehata, M., Khalifa, F., Soliman, A., El-Ghar, M.A., Dwyer, A.C., El-Baz, A. Early assessment of acute renal rejection. In: *Proceedings of 12th Annual Scientific Meeting of American Society for Diagnostics and Interventional Nephrology (ASDIN'16)*, Pheonix, AZ, February 19–21, 2016 (2017).

103. Khalifa, F., Beache, G., El-Baz, A., Gimelfarb, G. Deformable model guided by stochastic speed with application in cine images segmentation. In: *Proceedings of the IEEE International Conference on Image Processing (ICIP'10)*, Hong Kong, September 26–29 (2010) pp. 1725–1728.
104. Khalifa, F., Beache, G.M., Elnakib, A., Sliman, H., Gimelfarb, G., Welch, K.C., El-Baz, A. A new shape-based framework for the left ventricle wall segmentation from cardiac first-pass perfusion MRI. In: *Proceedings of IEEE International Symposium on Biomedical Imaging: From Nano to Macro (ISBI'13)* (2013) pp. 41–44.
105. Khalifa, F., Beache, G.M., Elnakib, A., Sliman, H., Gimelfarb, G., Welch, K.C., El-Baz, A. A new non-rigid registration framework for improved visualization of transmural perfusion gradients on cardiac first-pass perfusion MRI. In: *Proceedings of IEEE International Symposium on Biomedical Imaging: From Nano to Macro (ISBI'12)* (2012) pp. 828–831.
106. Khalifa, F., Beache, G.M., Firjani, A., Welch, K.C., Gimelfarb, G., El-Baz, A. A new nonrigid registration approach for motion correction of cardiac first-pass perfusion MRI. In: *Proceedings of the IEEE International Conference on Image Processing (ICIP'12)* (2012) pp. 1665–1668.
107. Khalifa, F., Beache, G.M., Gimelfarb, G., El-Baz, A. A novel CAD system for analyzing cardiac first-pass MRI images. In: *Proceedings of the IEEE International Conference on Pattern Recognition (ICPR'12)* (2012) pp. 77–80.
108. Khalifa, F., Beache, G.M., Gimelfarb, G., El-Baz, A. A novel approach for accurate estimation of left ventricle global indexes from short-axis cine MRI. In: *Proceedings of the IEEE International Conference on Image Processing (ICIP'11)* (2011) pp. 2645–2649.
109. Khalifa, F., Beache, G.M., Gimelfarb, G., Giridharan, G.A., El-Baz, A. A new image-based framework for analyzing cine images. In: El-Baz, A., Acharya, U.R., Mirmehdi, M., Suri, J.S. (Eds.) *Handbook of Multi Modality State-of-the-Art Medical Image Segmentation and Registration Methodologies*, Vol. 2. Springer: New York (2011) pp. 69–98.
110. Khalifa, F., Beache, G.M., Gimelfarb, G., Giridharan, G.A., El-Baz, A. Accurate automatic analysis of cardiac cine images. *IEEE Trans. Biomed. Eng.* **59**(2) (2012) 445–455.
111. Khalifa, F., Beache, G.M., Nitzken, M., Gimelfarb, G., Giridharan, G.A., El-Baz, A. Automatic analysis of left ventricle wall thickness using short-axis cine CMR images. In: *Proceedings of IEEE International Symposium on Biomedical Imaging: From Nano to Macro (ISBI'11)* (2011) pp. 1306–1309.
112. Nitzken, M., Beache, G., Elnakib, A., Khalifa, F., Gimelfarb, G., El-Baz, A. Accurate modeling of tagged CMR 3D image appearance characteristics to improve cardiac cycle strain estimation. In: *Image Processing (ICIP), 2012 19th IEEE International Conference on*, Orlando, FL, IEEE, September (2012) pp. 521–524.
113. Nitzken, M., Beache, G., Elnakib, A., Khalifa, F., Gimelfarb, G., El-Baz, A. Improving full-cardiac cycle strain estimation from tagged CMR by accurate modeling of 3D image appearance characteristics. In: *Biomedical Imaging (ISBI), 2012 9th IEEE International Symposium on*, Barcelona, Spain, IEEE, May (2012) pp. 462–465 (Selected for oral presentation)..
114. Nitzken, M.J., El-Baz, A.S., Beache, G.M. Markov-Gibbs random field model for improved full-cardiac cycle strain estimation from tagged CMR. *J. Cardiovasc. Magn. Reson.* **14**(1) (2012) 1–2.
115. Sliman, H., Elnakib, A., Beache, G., Elmaghraby, A., El-Baz, A. Assessment of myocardial function from cine cardiac MRI using a novel 4D tracking approach. *J. Comput. Sci. Syst. Biol.* **7** (2014) 169–173.
116. Sliman, H., Elnakib, A., Beache, G.M., Soliman, A., Khalifa, F., Gimelfarb, G., Elmaghraby, A., El-Baz, A. A novel 4D PDE-based approach for accurate assessment of myocardium function using cine cardiac magnetic resonance images. In: *Proceedings of IEEE International Conference on Image Processing (ICIP'14)*, Paris, France, October 27–30 (2014) pp. 3537–3541.
117. Sliman, H., Khalifa, F., Elnakib, A., Beache, G.M., Elmaghraby, A., El-Baz, A. A new segmentation-based tracking framework for extracting the left ventricle cavity from cine cardiac MRI. In: *Proceedings of IEEE International Conference on Image Processing (ICIP'13)*, Melbourne, Australia, September 15–18 (2013) pp. 685–689.
118. Sliman, H., Khalifa, F., Elnakib, A., Soliman, A., Beache, G.M., Elmaghraby, A., Gimelfarb, G., El-Baz, A. Myocardial borders segmentation from cine MR images using bi-directional coupled parametric deformable models. *Med. Phys.* **40**(9) (2013) 1–13.
119. Sliman, H., Khalifa, F., Elnakib, A., Soliman, A., Beache, G.M., Gimelfarb, G., Emam, A., Elmaghraby, A., El-Baz, A. Accurate segmentation framework for the left ventricle wall from cardiac cine MRI. In: *Proceedings of the International Symposium on Computational Models for Life Sciences*, AIP, College Park, MD (*CMLS'13*), Vol. 1559 (2013) pp. 287–296.

120. Eladawi, N., Elmogy, M.M., Ghazal, M., Helmy, O., Aboelfetouh, A., Riad, A., Schaal, S., El-Baz, A. Classification of retinal diseases based on OCT images. *Front. Biosci. (Landmark Ed.)* **23**(2018) 247–264.

121. ElTanboly, A., Ismail, M., Shalaby, A., Switala, A., El-Baz, A., Schaal, S., Gimelfarb, G., El-Azab, M. A computer aided diagnostic system for detecting diabetic retinopathy in optical coherence tomography images. *Med. Phys.* **44**(2017) 914–923.

122. Abdollahi, B., Civelek, A.C., Li, X.F., Suri, J., El-Baz, A. PET/CT nodule segmentation and diagnosis: A survey. In: Saba, L., Suri, J.S. (Eds.) *Multi Detector CT Imaging.* Taylor & Francis Group: New York (2014) pp. 639–651.

123. Abdollahi, B., El-Baz, A., Amini, A.A. A multi-scale non-linear vessel enhancement technique. In: *Engineering in Medicine and Biology Society, EMBC, 2011 Annual International Conference of the IEEE*, IEEE (2011) pp. 3925–3929.

124. Abdollahi, B., Soliman, A., Civelek, A., Li, X.F., Gimelfarb, G., El-Baz, A. A novel 3D joint MGRF framework for precise lung segmentation. In: *Machine Learning in Medical Imaging.* Springer: Berlin, Germany (2012) pp. 86–93.

125. Ali, A.M., El-Baz, A.S., Farag, A.A. A novel framework for accurate lung segmentation using graph cuts. In: *Proceedings of IEEE International Symposium on Biomedical Imaging: From Nano to Macro (ISBI'07)* (2007) pp. 908–911.

126. El-Baz, A., Beache, G.M., Gimelfarb, G., Suzuki, K., Okada, K. Lung imaging data analysis. *Int. J. Biomed. Imaging* **2013** (2013) 618561.

127. El-Baz, A., Beache, G.M., Gimelfarb, G., Suzuki, K., Okada, K., Elnakib, A., Soliman, A., Abdollahi, B. Computer-aided diagnosis systems for lung cancer: Challenges and methodologies. *Int. J. Biomed. Imaging* **2013** (2013) 1–46.

128. El-Baz, A., Elnakib, A., Abou El-Ghar, M., Gimelfarb, G., Falk, R., Farag, A. Automatic detection of 2D and 3D lung nodules in chest spiral CT scans. *Int. J. Biomed. Imaging* **2013** (2013) 517632.

129. El-Baz, A., Farag, A.A., Falk, R., La Rocca, R. A unified approach for detection, visualization, and identification of lung abnormalities in chest spiral CT scans. In: *International Congress Series*, Vol. 1256 (2003) pp. 998–1004.

130. El-Baz, A., Farag, A.A., Falk, R., La Rocca, R. Detection, visualization and identification of lung abnormalities in chest spiral CT scan: Phase-I. In: *Proceedings of International conference on Biomedical Engineering*, Vol. 12, Cairo, Egypt (2002).

131. El-Baz, A., Farag, A., Gimelfarb, G., Falk, R., El-Ghar, M.A., Eldiasty, T. A framework for automatic segmentation of lung nodules from low dose chest CT scans. In: *Proceedings of International Conference on Pattern Recognition (ICPR'06)*, IEEE (2006) pp. 611–614.

132. El-Baz, A., Farag, A., Gimelfarb, G., Falk, R., El-Ghar, M.A. A novel level set-based computer-aided detection system for automatic detection of lung nodules in low dose chest computed tomography scans. *Lung Imaging Comput. Aided Diagno.* **10** (2011) 221–238.

133. El-Baz, A., Gimelfarb, G., Abou El-Ghar, M., Falk, R. Appearance-based diagnostic system for early assessment of malignant lung nodules. In: *Proceedings of IEEE International Conference on Image Processing (ICIP'12)* (2012) pp. 533–536.

134. El-Baz, A., Gimelfarb, G., Falk, R. A novel 3D framework for automatic lung segmentation from low dose CT images. In: El-Baz, A., Suri, J.S. (Eds.) *Lung Imaging and Computer Aided Diagnosis.* Taylor & Francis Group: Boca Raton, FL (2011) pp. 1–16.

135. El-Baz, A., Gimelfarb, G., Falk, R., El-Ghar, M. Appearance analysis for diagnosing malignant lung nodules. In: *Proceedings of IEEE International Symposium on Biomedical Imaging: From Nano to Macro (ISBI'10)* (2010) pp. 193–196.

136. El-Baz, A., Gimelfarb, G., Falk, R., El-Ghar, M.A. A novel level set-based CAD system for automatic detection of lung nodules in low dose chest CT scans. In: El-Baz, A., Suri, J.S. (Eds.) *Lung Imaging and Computer Aided Diagnosis*, Vol. 1. Taylor & Francis Group: Boca Raton, FL (2011) pp. 221–238.

137. El-Baz, A., Gimelfarb, G., Falk, R., El-Ghar, M.A. A new approach for automatic analysis of 3D low dose CT images for accurate monitoring the detected lung nodules. In: *Proceedings of IEEE International Conference on Pattern Recognition (ICPR'08)* (2008) pp. 1–4.

138. El-Baz, A., Gimelfarb, G., Falk, R., El-Ghar, M.A. A novel approach for automatic follow-up of detected lung nodules. In: *Proceedings of IEEE International Conference on Image Processing (ICIP'07)*, Vol. 5 (2007) pp. V–501.

139. El-Baz, A., Gimelfarb, G., Falk, R., El-Ghar, M.A. A new CAD system for early diagnosis of detected lung nodules. In: *Image Processing, 2007. ICIP 2007. IEEE International Conference on*, Vol. 2, IEEE (2007) pp. II–461.

140. El-Baz, A., Gimelfarb, G., Falk, R., El-Ghar, M.A., Refaie, H. Promising results for early diagnosis of lung cancer. In: *Proceedings of IEEE International Symposium on Biomedical Imaging: From Nano to Macro (ISBI'08)* (2008) pp. 1151–1154.

141. El-Baz, A., Gimelfarb, G.L., Falk, R., Abou El-Ghar, M., Holland, T., Shaffer, T. A new stochastic framework for accurate lung segmentation. In: *Proceedings of Medical Image Computing and Computer-Assisted Intervention (MICCAI'08)*, Springer, Berlin, Germany (2008) pp. 322–330.

142. El-Baz, A., Gimelfarb, G.L., Falk, R., Heredis, D., Abou El-Ghar, M. A novel approach for accurate estimation of the growth rate of the detected lung nodules. In: *Proceedings of the International Workshop Pulmonary Image Analysis*, IEEE (2008) pp. 33–42.

143. El-Baz, A., Gimelfarb, G.L., Falk, R., Holland, T., Shaffer, T. A framework for unsupervised segmentation of lung tissues from low dose computed tomography images. In: *Proceedings of the British Machine Vision (BMVC'08)* (2008) pp. 1–10.

144. El-Baz, A., Gimelfarb, G., Falk, R., El-Ghar, M.A. 3D MGRF-based appearance modeling for robust segmentation of pulmonary nodules in 3D LDCT chest images. In: *Lung Imaging and Computer Aided Diagnosis* (2011) pp. 51–63.

145. El-Baz, A., Gimelfarb, G., Falk, R., El-Ghar, M.A. Automatic analysis of 3D low dose CT images for early diagnosis of lung cancer. *Pattern Recognit.* **42**(6) (2009) 1041–1051.

146. El-Baz, A., Gimelfarb, G., Falk, R., El-Ghar, M.A., Rainey, S., Heredia, D., Shaffer, T. Toward early diagnosis of lung cancer. In: *Proceedings of Medical Image Computing and Computer-Assisted Intervention (MICCAI'09)*, Springer, Berlin, Germany (2009) pp. 682–689.

147. El-Baz, A., Gimelfarb, G., Falk, R., El-Ghar, M.A., Suri, J. Appearance analysis for the early assessment of detected lung nodules. In: *Lung Imaging and Computer Aided Diagnosis* (2011) pp. 395–404.

148. El-Baz, A., Khalifa, F., Elnakib, A., Nitkzen, M., Soliman, A., McClure, P., Gimelfarb, G., El-Ghar, M.A. A novel approach for global lung registration using 3D Markov Gibbs appearance model. In: *Proceedings of International Conference Medical Image Computing and Computer-Assisted Intervention (MICCAI'12)*, Nice, France, October 1–5 (2012) pp. 114–121.

149. El-Baz, A., Nitzken, M., Elnakib, A., Khalifa, F., Gimelfarb, G., Falk, R., El-Ghar, M.A. 3D shape analysis for early diagnosis of malignant lung nodules. In: *Proceedings of International Conference Medical Image Computing and Computer-Assisted Intervention (MICCAI'11)*, Toronto, Canada, September 18–22 (2011) pp. 175–182.

150. El-Baz, A., Nitzken, M., Gimelfarb, G., Van Bogaert, E., Falk, R., El-Ghar, M.A., Suri, J. Three-dimensional shape analysis using spherical harmonics for early assessment of detected lung nodules. In: *Lung Imaging and Computer Aided Diagnosis* (2011) pp. 421–438.

151. El-Baz, A., Nitzken, M., Khalifa, F., Elnakib, A., Gimelfarb, G., Falk, R., El-Ghar, M.A. 3D shape analysis for early diagnosis of malignant lung nodules. In: *Proceedings of International Conference on Information Processing in Medical Imaging (IPMI'11)*, Monastery Irsee, Germany, July 3–8 (2011) pp. 772–783.

152. El-Baz, A., Nitzken, M., Vanbogaert, E., Gimelfarb, G., Falk, R., Abo El-Ghar, M. A novel shape-based diagnostic approach for early diagnosis of lung nodules. In: *Biomedical Imaging: From Nano to Macro, 2011 IEEE International Symposium on*, IEEE (2011) pp. 137–140.

153. El-Baz, A., Sethu, P., Gimelfarb, G., Khalifa, F., Elnakib, A., Falk, R., El-Ghar, M.A. Elastic phantoms generated by microfluidics technology: Validation of an imaged-based approach for accurate measurement of the growth rate of lung nodules. *Biotech. J.* **6**(2) (2011) 195–203.

154. El-Baz, A., Sethu, P., Gimelfarb, G., Khalifa, F., Elnakib, A., Falk, R., El-Ghar, M.A. A new validation approach for the growth rate measurement using elastic phantoms generated by state-of-the-art microfluidics technology. In: *Proceedings of IEEE International Conference on Image Processing (ICIP'10)*, Hong Kong, September 26–29 (2010) pp. 4381–4383.

155. El-Baz, A., Sethu, P., Gimelfarb, G., Khalifa, F., Elnakib, A., Falk, R., Suri, M.A.E.G.J. Validation of a new imaged-based approach for the accurate estimating of the growth rate of detected lung nodules using real CT images and elastic phantoms generated by state-of-the-art microfluidics technology. In: El-Baz, A., Suri, J.S. (Eds.) *Handbook of Lung Imaging and Computer Aided Diagnosis*, Vol. 1. Taylor & Francis Group: New York (2011) pp. 405–420.

156. El-Baz, A., Soliman, A., McClure, P., Gimelfarb, G., El-Ghar, M.A., Falk, R. Early assessment of malignant lung nodules based on the spatial analysis of detected lung nodules. In: *Proceedings of IEEE International Symposium on Biomedical Imaging: From Nano to Macro, (ISBI'12)* (2012) pp. 1463–1466.

157. El-Baz, A., Yuksel, S.E., Elshazly, S., Farag, A.A. Non-rigid registration techniques for automatic follow-up of lung nodules. In: *Proceedings of Computer Assisted Radiology and Surgery (CARS'05)*, Berlin, Germany Vol. 1281 (2005) pp. 1115–1120.

158. El-Baz, A.S., Suri, J.S. *Lung Imaging and Computer Aided Diagnosis.* CRC Press: Boca Raton, FL (2011).

159. Oliman, A., Khalifa, F., Shaffie, A., Liu, N., Dunlap, N., Wang, B., Elmaghraby, A., Gimelfarb, G., El-Baz, A. Image-based CAD system for accurate identification of lung injury. In: *Proceedings of IEEE International Conference on Image Processing, (ICIP'16)* IEEE (2016) pp. 121–125.

160. Soliman, A., Khalifa, F., Dunlap, N., Wang, B., El-Ghar, M., El-Baz, A. An iso-surfaces based local deformation handling framework of lung tissues. In: *Biomedical Imaging (ISBI), 2016 IEEE 13th International Symposium on*, IEEE (2016) pp. 1253–1259.

161. Soliman, A., Khalifa, F., Shaffie, A., Dunlap, N., Wang, B., Elmaghraby, A., El-Baz, A. Detection of lung injury using 4D-CT chest images. In: *Biomedical Imaging (ISBI), 2016 IEEE 13th International Symposium on*, IEEE (2016) pp. 1274–1277.

162. Dombroski, B., Nitzken, M., Elnakib, A., Khalifa, F., El-Baz, A., Casanova, M.F. Cortical surface complexity in a population-based normative sample. *J. Transl. Neurosci.* **5**(1) (2014) 1–8.

163. El-Baz, A., Casanova, M., Gimelfarb, G., Mott, M., Switala, A. An MRI-based diagnostic framework for early diagnosis of dyslexia. *Int. J. Comput. Assist. Radiol. Surg.* **3**(3–4) (2008) 181–189.

164. El-Baz, A., Casanova, M., Gimelfarb, G., Mott, M., Switala, A., Vanbogaert, E., McCracken, R. A new CAD system for early diagnosis of dyslexic brains. In: *Proceedings of the International Conference on Image Processing (ICIP'2008)*, IEEE (2008) pp. 1820–1823.

165. El-Baz, A., Casanova, M.F., Gimelfarb, G., Mott, M., Switwala, A.E. A new image analysis approach for automatic classification of autistic brains. In: *Proceedings of IEEE International Symposium on Biomedical Imaging: From Nano to Macro (ISBI'2007)*, IEEE (2007) pp. 352–355.

166. El-Baz, A., Farag, A.A., Gimelfarb, G.L., El-Ghar, M.A., Eldiasty, T. Probabilistic modeling of blood vessels for segmenting MRA images. In: *ICPR* (2006) pp. 917–920.

167. El-Baz, A., Farag, A.A., Gimelfarb, G., El-Ghar, M.A., Eldiasty, T. A new adaptive probabilistic model of blood vessels for segmenting MRA images. In: *Medical Image Computing and Computer-Assisted Intervention–MICCAI 2006*, Vol. 4191, Springer (2006) pp. 799–806.

168. El-Baz, A., Farag, A.A., Gimelfarb, G., Hushek, S.G. Automatic cerebrovascular segmentation by accurate probabilistic modeling of TOF-MRA images. In: *Medical Image Computing and Computer-Assisted Intervention–MICCAI 2005*, Springer (2005) pp. 34–42.

169. El-Baz, A., Farag, A., Elnakib, A., Casanova, M.F., Gimelfarb, G., Switala, A.E., Jordan, D., Rainey, S. Accurate automated detection of autism related corpus callosum abnormalities. *J. Med. Syst.* **35**(5) (2011) 929–939.

170. El-Baz, A., Farag, A., Gimelfarb, G. Cerebrovascular segmentation by accurate probabilistic modeling of tof-mra images. In: *Image Analysis*, Vol. 3540, Springer (2005) pp. 1128–1137.

171. El-Baz, A., Gimelfarb, G., Falk, R., El-Ghar, M.A., Kumar, V., Heredia, D. A novel 3D joint Markov-Gibbs model for extracting blood vessels from PC–MRA images. In: *Medical Image Computing and Computer-Assisted Intervention–MICCAI 2009*, Vol. 5762, Springer (2009) pp. 943–950.

172. Elnakib, A., El-Baz, A., Casanova, M.F., Gimelfarb, G., Switala, A.E. Image-based detection of corpus callosum variability for more accurate discrimination between dyslexic and normal brains. In: *Proceedings of IEEE International Symposium on Biomedical Imaging: From Nano to Macro (ISBI'2010)*, IEEE (2010) pp. 109–112.

173. Elnakib, A., Casanova, M.F., Gimelfarb, G., Switala, A.E., El-Baz, A. Autism diagnostics by centerline-based shape analysis of the corpus callosum. In: *Proceedings of IEEE International Symposium on Biomedical Imaging: From Nano to Macro (ISBI'2011)*, IEEE (2011) pp. 1843–1846.

174. Elnakib, A., Nitzken, M., Casanova, M., Park, H., Gimelfarb, G., El-Baz, A. Quantification of age-related brain cortex change using 3D shape analysis. In: *Pattern Recognition (ICPR), 2012 21st International Conference on*, IEEE (2012) pp. 41–44.

175. Mostapha, M., Soliman, A., Khalifa, F., Elnakib, A., Alansary, A., Nitzken, M., Casanova, M.F., El-Baz, A. A statistical framework for the classification of infant DT images. In: *Image Processing (ICIP), 2014 IEEE International Conference on*, IEEE (2014) pp. 2222–2226.

176. Nitzken, M., Casanova, M., Gimelfarb, G., Elnakib, A., Khalifa, F., Switala, A., El-Baz, A. 3D shape analysis of the brain cortex with application to dyslexia. In: *Image Processing (ICIP), 2011 18th IEEE International Conference on*, IEEE: Brussels, Belgium, September (2011), pp. 2657–2660 (Selected for oral presentation. Oral acceptance rate is 10 percent and the overall acceptance rate is 35 percent).

177. El-Gamal, F.E.Z.A., Elmogy, M., Ghazal, M., Atwan, A., Barnes, G., Casanova, M., Keynton, R., El-Baz, A. A novel CAD system for local and global early diagnosis of Alzheimer's disease based on PIB-PET scans. In: *Image Processing (ICIP), 2017 IEEE International Conference on*, IEEE: Beijing, China (2017).

178. Ismail, M., Soliman, A., Ghazal, M., Switala, A.E., Gimelfarb, G., Barnes, G.N., Khalil, A., El-Baz, A. A fast stochastic framework for automatic mr brain images segmentation. *PLoS One* **12**(11) (2017) e0187391.

179. Ismail, M.M., Keynton, R.S., Mostapha, M.M., ElTanboly, A.H., Casanova, M.F., Gimelfarb, G.L., El-Baz, A. Studying autism spectrum disorder with structural and diffusion magnetic resonance imaging: A survey. *Front. Hum. Neurosci.* **10** (2016) 211.

180. Alansary, A., Ismail, M., Soliman, A., Khalifa, F., Nitzken, M., Elnakib, A., Mostapha, M. et al. Infant brain extraction in T1-weighted MR images using BET and refinement using LCDG and MRGF models. *IEEE J. Biomed. Health Inform.* **20**(3) (2016) 925–935.

181. Ismail, M., Barnes, G., Nitzken, M., Switala, A., Shalaby, A., Hosseini-Asl, E., Casanova, M., Keynton, R., Khalil, A., El-Baz, A.S. A new deep-learning CAD system for early diagnosis of autism using structural MR. In: *Proceedings of the IEEE Conference on Image Processing* (*ICIP 17*), Beijing, China (2017).

182. Ismail, M., Soliman, A., ElTanboly, A., Switala, A., Mahmoud, M., Khalifa, F., Gimelfarb, G., Casanova, M.F., Keynton, R., El-Baz, A. Detection of white matter abnormalities in MR brain images for diagnosis of autism in children. In: *2016 IEEE 13th International Symposium on Biomedical Imaging* (*ISBI*) (2016) pp. 6–9.

183. Ismail, M., Mostapha, M., Soliman, A., Nitzken, M., Khalifa, F., Elnakib, A., Gimelfarb, G., Casanova, M., El-Baz, A. Segmentation of infant brain MR images based on adaptive shape prior and higher-order MGRF. In: *2015 IEEE International Conference on Image Processing* (*ICIP*) (2015) pp. 4327–4331.

184. Shalaby, A., Taher, F., El-Baz, M., Ghazal, V., Abou El-Ghar, M., Takieldeen, A., El-Baz, A. Probabilistic modeling of blood vessels for segmenting magnetic resonance angiography images. In: *Medical Research Archive- MRA. KEI* (2017) pp. 34–42.

185. Chowdhury, A.S., Rudra, A.K., Sen, M., Elnakib, A., El-Baz, A. Cerebral white matter segmentation from MRI using probabilistic graph cuts and geometric shape priors. In: *ICIP* (2010) pp. 3649–3652.

13 Prostate Segmentation from DW-MRI Using Level-Set Guided by Nonnegative Matrix Factorization

Islam Reda, Patrick McClure, Ahmed Shalaby, Mohammed Elmogy, Ahmed Aboulfotouh, Mohamed Abou El-Ghar, Moumen El-Melegy, Jasjit S. Suri, and Ayman El-Baz

CONTENTS

INTRODUCTION

Prostate cancer is one of the leading causes of cancer-related deaths in American men. Fortunately, the survival rate is relatively high for patients who are diagnosed with the disease in its early stages. Currently, in vivo imaging modalities have a major role in both the diagnosis and treatment of prostate cancer. The most common types of imaging modalities used in clinical diagnosis and treatment of prostate cancer are ultrasound and magnetic resonance imaging (MRI) [1–6]. The main strength of MRI over ultrasound is that MRI provides improved soft tissue contrast. Accurate prostate localization is an important step in diagnosis and treatment, such as developing computer-aided diagnostic (CAD) systems, guiding biopsy [7], and radiotherapy [8]. This accurate segmentation of the prostate can be done in a manual or an automated manner. Manual segmentation of the prostate is time-consuming, tiresome, and suffers from intra- and inter-observer variability [9]. As a result, developing automated and reliable prostate segmentation techniques from MRI is a clinically required task. The challenges related to this task include the following: the border between the prostate and its surrounding background is generally weak, the intensity distributions of the voxels around the border of the prostate vary across different subjects, and the shape of the prostate differs both across the different slices of the same subject and across different subjects [10].

Several methods have been developed for segmenting the prostate from a variety of MRI modalities. Two deformable model (DM)-based methods have been widely used: active shape models (ASMs) [11] and level-sets [12]. For instance, Allen et al. [13] developed a DM-based technique for segmenting the prostate from three dimensional (3D) T2-MRI. In their technique, the evolution of the DM was guided by voxel intensity and a statistical shape model. Zhu et al. [14] developed a 2D/3D ASM-based technique for prostate segmentation from 3D MRI. Their idea was that combining 2D and 3D models can lead to a global optimum delineation of the prostate rather than a local optimum delineation at each individual slice. Moreover, Ghose et al. [15] proposed an active appearance model (AAM)-based methodology that utilized multiple statistical shape and intensity models to segment the prostate in 2D and a global registration scheme to impose shape constraint in 3D. In addition, Martin et al. [16] proposed an automated approach for prostate segmentation from 3D MRI that used an anatomical atlas to generate an initial probabilistic segmentation. This probabilistic segmentation introduced a spatial constraint to control the evolution of a deformable model for accurate segmentation. Gao et al. [17] proposed a global affine registration to align the MR images before segmenting the prostate using a level-set controlled by a learned shape prior and local image statistics. Also, Yang et al. [10] proposed a semi-automated approach for prostate segmentation from MRI using level-sets. In their approach, the evolution of the level-set was preceded by a background simplification process that involved a prostate landmark detection and a texture constraint. The formulation of the level-set was expanded with shape prior for accurate segmentation of the prostate border.

Statistical-based techniques have also been used for prostate segmentation from MRI data. For instance, Ghose et al. [18] proposed an automated prostate segmentation method from 3D T2-MRI. The proposed method first used a probabilistic atlas and a random forest classifier to obtain classification probabilities of the prostate voxels. The final prostate segmentation was based on energy minimization using 3D graph cut. Firjany et al. [19] introduced a Markov random field (MRF) image model [20] for segmenting the prostate from 2D dynamic contrast-enhanced (DCE)-MRI. Their technique integrated a graph cut approach with a prior shape model of the prostate and the visual appearance of the prostate image, modeled using a linear combination of discrete Gaussian (LCDG) [21]. Their technique was later extended in other studies [22,23] to allow for 3D prostate segmentation from DCE-MRI. Makni et al. [24] developed an automated approach for 3D prostate segmentation from MRI. In their approach, intensity levels were modeled using a Gaussian mixture and the final prostate segmentation was performed by a Bayesian maximum a posteriori (MAP) [25] classifier that used both Markov fields and statistical shape information. A semi-automated method for prostate segmentation from MRI was proposed by Tian et al. [26]. The proposed approach integrated 3D graph cut and 3D active contours in an iterative mode for accurate prostate segmentation by combining the advantages of both graph cut and active contours. The 3D graph cut was used to obtain an initial segmentation of the supervoxels which is smoothed in turn by the 3D active contours.

Atlas-based techniques have also been used to delineate the prostate from MRI. The atlas is composed of original images and their corresponding manual delineation. It is used as a reference to delineate the prostate of new subjects. For example, Klein et al. [27] proposed an automatic 3D prostate segmentation technique from MRI based on nonrigid registration of each pre-labeled atlas image with the target image. Then, the closest atlases to the target image are fused to obtain the segmentation of the target images. Another automatic method, presented by Dowling et al. [28], used an automated atlas approach to segment the prostate region from 3D MR scans based on a selective and iterative method for performance level estimation (SIMPLE)-based registration approach [29]. Litjens et al. [30] developed a similar segmentation technique to the one proposed in the PROMISE12 challenge [31]. Their technique was multi-atlas-based for prostate segmentation from multiparametric images. However, to obtain the final segmentation, the SIMPLE method was used instead in order to fuse labels after the alignment of the different atlases.

Besides the previously mentioned techniques, several other techniques have been proposed for prostate segmentation from MR images. For example, multiple edge-detection-based techniques have been developed for prostate segmentation. The basic idea of those techniques is to produce a set of edges using edge-detection operators. Then, the candidate edges are selected and connected to obtain the prostate border. For example, Zwiggelaar et al. [32] proposed a semi-automatic technique for prostate delineation from MR images. Their technique used the anatomical shape of the prostate when represented in a polar transform space. The prostate border was tracked using a non-maximum suppression method. Another semi-automatic edge-detection technique for MRI prostate segmentation was proposed by Flores-Tapia et al. [33]. Their technique exploited the behavioral variation between the signal and the noise after applying a wavelet transform [34] to detect the prostate boundary. In their semi-automatic method, Vikal et al. [35] exploited shape prior to detect the prostate boundary in each slice. Then, a 3D surface was generated after refining the detected boundaries. Moreover, random walk classification [36] was utilized to segment the prostate from MR images by Khurd et al. [37].

Most of the aforementioned techniques segment prostate from T2-MRI. Currently, diffusion-weighted (DW)-MRI has emerged as a promising imaging modality for diagnosing prostate cancer because of its ability to measure both structural and functional qualities. DW-MRI measures the sensitivity of tissues to the water molecule motion by applying pairs of opposing magnetic field gradients. Although the resolution of DW-MR images is lower than DCE-MR images, DW-MR images have distinct advantages over DCE-MR images as they can be acquired very quickly and without injecting a patient with a contrast agent that could be harmful to the patient's kidneys [38]. Specifically for prostate cancer, the apparent diffusion coefficient (ADC), a feature calculated using DW-MRI images acquired at different magnetic field strengths (or b-values), has been found capable of distinguishing between malignant and benign prostate tissues [39–46]. The reported accuracy of DW-MRI for diagnosing prostate cancer is better than T2-MRI and DCE-MRI [47].

As a consequence of the discriminative nature of DW-MRI-based features, prostate segmentation is an essential step in many DW-MRI-based CAD systems for diagnosing prostate cancer. Precise segmentation of the prostate can be challenging because of image noise, intra- and inter-patient differences, and the similar appearance of the prostate and neighboring tissues, such as the bladder. A small number of techniques for prostate localization from DW-MRI have been proposed to overcome those challenges. For instance, Firjani et al. [39,48,49] proposed the use of a MAP [25] approach that exploited intensity, shape, and spatial features for prostate segmentation from 3D DW-MRI data. The appearance was modeled using the LCDG model and the used spatial model was 3D Markov-Gibbs random field (MGRF). Liu et al. [50] developed a 2D level-set guided by intensity and shape information for prostate delineation from DW-MRI. The intensity of a pixel was found by taking the average of the pixel's intensity at a b-value of 0 s/mm^2 and the ADC value found using b-values of 0 and 100 s/mm^2. The shape model of the prostate was estimated by fitting an ellipse to an initial segmentation generated using Otsu intensity thresholding [51]. Similarly, Liu et al. [52] developed a 3D level-set method guided by intensity and shape information. The intensity of a voxel was the ADC value found using b-values of 0 and 600 s/mm^2. An initial segmentation was performed using a 3D level-set guided by this intensity information. The shape of the prostate was then approximated by fitting an ellipsoid and a series of ellipses to the initial segmentation. This intensity and shape information was then used to guide another 3D level-set for final segmentation. While these techniques have successfully performed DW-MRI prostate segmentation, they can be sensitive to similarities between the intensities of object and background voxels. To overcome this challenge, nonnegative matrix factorization (NMF) feature fusion is introduced to generate a more robust model for guiding the evolution of a 3D level-set for DW-MRI prostate segmentation.

METHODS

In this chapter, a DW-MRI-based prostate segmentation framework is developed, as shown in Figure 13.1. It utilizes an NMF-based feature fusion algorithm that includes three features, which are DW-MRI intensities, shape, and spatial interactions between voxels. The features resulted by applying NMF-based feature fusion are then used to guide the propagation of a geometric deformable model (3D level-set) to delineate the prostate from DW-MRI data. Geometric deformable models based on level-sets are widely utilized for object segmentation from different medical imaging modalities. Level-sets have been successfully applied to delineate several organs in the human body (e.g., kidney [53], heart [54], and prostate [17,50,52]).

According to the level-set definition, the propagating surface of the level-set at any time instant t is represented by the zero level, $\phi_{n+1}(x, y, z)=0$, of an implicit level-set function, that is a distance map of the signed minimum Euclidean distance from each voxel to the surface. This formulation results in points inside the surface having negative (or positive) values and voxels outside the surface having positive (or negative) values, respectively. Mathematically, the evolution of the level-set is defined by [12]:

$$\phi_{n+1}(x, y, z) = \phi_n(x, y, z) - \tau V_n(x, y, z) \,|\, \nabla \phi_n(x, y, z) \,| \tag{13.1}$$

where t is the discrete time instant $t = n\tau$ taken with a step τ, $\tau > 0$ and $\nabla = [(\partial/\partial x, \partial/\partial y, \partial/\partial z)]$ is the differential operator. This evolution is guided by the speed function $V_n(x, y, z)$ [55].

Previous speed functions that utilize image intensities, gradient vector flow, and object edges have had difficulty delineating noisy images and those with poor object-background contrast. More effective speed functions have been developed by using shape priors to incorporate shape information of the object of interest. Nevertheless, this has not completely overcome image inhomogeneities (e.g., large image noise and discontinuous object borders). In order to more precisely delineate the prostate from DW-MRI data, we introduce a speed function that considers the 3D appearance, shape prior, and spatial interactions between voxels of the DW-MRI data. These features are integrated using an NMF-based fusion approach to provide the voxelwise guidance of the deformable model.

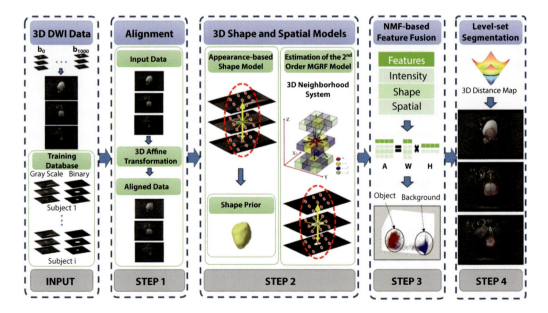

FIGURE 13.1 A schematic diagram of the proposed DW-MRI prostate segmentation framework.

3D Appearance, Shape, and Spatial Features

Basic Notation: Let $\mathbf{Q} = \{0, \ldots, Q-1$ and $\mathbf{L} = \{0, 1\}$ be the set of Q integer gray levels and a set of object (1) and background (0) labels, respectively. Also, let a 3D arithmetic lattice $\mathbf{R} = \{(x, y, z) : 0 \leq x \leq X-1; 0 \leq y \leq Y-1; 0 \leq z \leq Z-1\}$ support the grayscale DW-MRI data $\mathbf{g}: \mathbf{R} \to \mathbf{Q}$ and their binary region maps $\mathbf{m}: \mathbf{R} \to \mathbf{L}$. Each voxel (x, y, z) is associated with its neighbors, $\{(x + \xi, y + \eta, z + \zeta): (x + \xi, y + \eta, z + \zeta) \in \mathbf{R}; (\xi, \eta, \zeta) \in \mathbf{N}\}$ where $\mathbf{N}$ is the 26 neighborhood system (Figure 13.2) defined by $\xi \in \{-1, 0, 1\}$, $\eta \in \{-1, 0, 1\}$, and $\zeta \in \{-1, 0, 1\}$.

Appearance-Based Shape Model: Most prostates have a similar near-ellipsoidal shape [56]. As a consequence, the incorporation of a shape prior can significantly enhance the accuracy of prostate segmentation. In the developed framework, an appearance-based shape model is constructed to take into account not only voxels' intensities, but also their spatial interactions. A shape database was created from all available subjects except the one to be segmented (leave-one-out methodology). So in each experiment, the shape prior consists a total of 52 subjects. The training data sets were co-aligned to be in the reference domain using a 3D affine transformation with 12 degrees of freedom (3 for the 3D translation, 3 for the 3D rotation, 3 for the 3D scaling, and 3 for the 3D shearing) to decrease the variability and maximize the overlap by maximizing mutual information (MI) [57]. The obtained transformation matrix used to map each subject to the reference volume is applied to the manually delineated segmentation also to create the shape prior. In the case of any new subject, it can be tested directly using all the available 53 subjects as the shape prior. The superposition of training maps before (A) and after (B) registration at different slices (a–e) is illustrated in Figure 13.3. A shape prior is a spatially variant independent random field of region labels for the co-aligned data. Mathematically, this is defined as:

$$P_{\text{shape}}(\mathbf{m}) = \prod_{(x,y,z)\in R} P_{\text{shape}:x,y,z}(m_{x,y,z}) \tag{13.2}$$

where $P_{\text{shape}:x,y,z}(l)$ is the voxel-wise empirical probability for label $l \in \mathbf{L}$. For each input DW-MRI volume to be delineated, the shape prior is built by a process guided by the visual appearance features of the DW-MRI data. The appearance-based shape prior is then estimated using the methodology summarized in Algorithm 13.1.

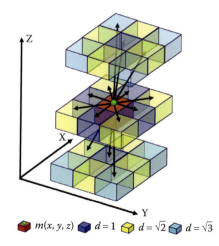

FIGURE 13.2   Illustration of a voxel's neighborhood.

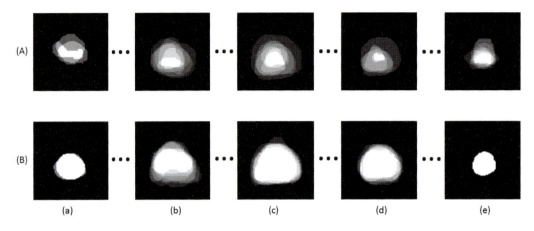

FIGURE 13.3 The superposition of training maps before (A) and after (B) registration at different slices (a–e).

Spatial Voxel Interaction Model: Besides the prostate shape prior, analyzing the interactions of a voxel and its neighbors can enhance segmentation [39,58]. In order to model these interactions, a second-order 3D MGRF model [59] is used. The MGRF model of the region map **m** is defined as:

Algorithm 13.1   Algorithm for Calculating an Appearance-Based Shape Model

Calculate the value of the shape prior probability at each voxel using the following steps:

1. Transform each test subject voxel to the shape database domain using the calculated 3D affine transformation matrix (T).
2. Initialize an $N_{1i} \times N_{2i} \times N_{3i}$ search space centered at the voxel.
3. Find voxels inside the search space with corresponding gray levels to the center voxel in all training data sets.
4. If no corresponding voxels are found, increase the search space size and repeat the previous step.
5. Calculate the label probabilities for each voxel based on the relative occurrence of each label in the search results.

$$P(\mathbf{m}) = \frac{1}{Z_N} \exp \sum_{(x,y,z) \in \mathbf{R}} \sum_{(\varepsilon,\upsilon,\varsigma) \in \mathbf{N}} V_{eq}(m_{x,y,z}, m_{x+\varepsilon,y+\upsilon,z+\varsigma}) \tag{13.3}$$

where $V_{eq}\left(m_{x,y,z}, m_{x+\varepsilon,y+\upsilon,z+\varsigma}\right)$ is the Gibbs potential and Z_N is the normalization factor which can be approximated as [60]:

$$Z_N \approx \exp \sum_{(x,y,z) \in \mathbf{R}} \sum_{(\varepsilon,\upsilon,\varsigma) \in \mathbf{N}} \sum_{l \in \mathbf{L}} V_{eq}(l, m_{x+\varepsilon,y+\upsilon,z+\varsigma}) \tag{13.4}$$

The MGRF used can be viewed as a 3D extension of the auto-binomial, or Potts, model with the exception that the Gibbs potential is estimated analytically. The maximum likelihood estimate of the potential is given as [61]:

$$V_{eq} = -V_{ne} = 2\left(f_{eq}(\mathbf{m}) - \frac{1}{2}\right) \tag{13.5}$$

where $f_{eq}(\mathbf{m})$ is the relative frequency of equal labels in the voxel pairs $\left((x,y,z),(x+\xi,y+\eta,z+\zeta)\right)$.

NMF-Based Feature Fusion

NMF is a method for extracting meaningful features from data sets for representing different classes in the data [62]. This is done by calculating a weight matrix W that transforms a vector from the input space into a new feature space (H-space) through factorizing the input matrix A so that $A \approx WH$. The input data matrix A contains the intensities for each voxel and its neighbors in addition to the shape and spatial probabilities of each voxel (Figure 13.4). NMF has been applied to various data analysis problems such as document clustering [63] and facial recognition [64]. In addition, it has been used in a few segmentation systems. Particularly, Xie et al. [65] used NMF to segment the spinal cord, corpus callosum, and hippocampus regions of rats from diffusion tensor imaging (DTI) by k-means clustering the column vectors of the produced H matrix. Also, Sandler et al. [66] proposed using NMF to factorize intensity histogram data for generic image segmentation.

In this chapter, an NMF-based technique is introduced to find the weights for each feature in order to create a feature space where object and background classes are better separated, dimensionality is reduced, and information from the training data set is encoded. NMF factorizes a k by n input matrix A into a k by r weight matrix W, which contains the basis vectors of the new space as columns, and an r by n output matrix H where k is the dimensionality of the input column vectors, n is the number of input and output column vectors, and r is the dimensionality of the output column vectors [62]. Mathematically, this is defined as

$$A \approx WH \tag{13.6}$$

W and H are calculated by minimizing the Euclidean distance between A and WH with the constraint that W and H contain only nonnegative values. This results in the following constrained optimization problem:

$$\underset{W,H}{\text{minimize}} \quad \frac{1}{2}\|A - WH\|^2 \tag{13.7}$$
$$\text{subject to} \quad W, H \geq 0$$

In the literature, several approaches have been used to optimize this function. The most prominent methods have been multiplicative gradient descent, alternating least square (ALS),

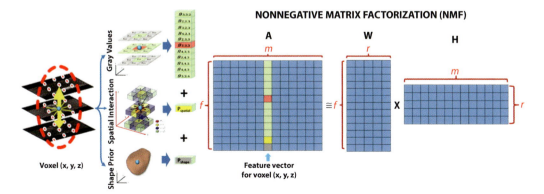

FIGURE 13.4 An illustration for the NMF-based fusion of input features (intensity, spatial, and shape) where f is the dimensionality of the feature vector, m is the total number of the input voxels, and r is the dimensionality of the output space.

and projected gradient descent (PGD) [67]. In this chapter, the multiplicative method [68] is used because of its ease of implementation. This method iteratively updates W and H until convergence using the following rules:

$$H_{\alpha\beta} \leftarrow H_{\alpha\beta} \frac{\left(W^T A\right)_{\alpha\beta}}{\left(W^T W H\right)_{\alpha\beta}} \tag{13.8}$$

$$W_{\gamma\alpha} \leftarrow W_{\gamma\alpha} \frac{\left(AH^T\right)_{\gamma\alpha}}{\left(W H H^T\right)_{\gamma\alpha}} \tag{13.9}$$

where $\alpha: 1 \rightarrow r$, $\beta: 1 \rightarrow n$, and $\gamma: 1 \rightarrow k$.

In the proposed framework, NMF is performed on a matrix that has a kth dimensional, one dimension for each calculated feature, column vector for each pixel in the training volumes. The resulting W is used as the basis vectors to transform new feature vectors into the new r-dimensional space (H-space). The resulting H is used to find the r-dimensional centroids corresponding to the object and background classes, C_{object} and $C_{background}$, respectively. For each voxel in a testing volume, a kth dimensional feature vector was calculated. This resulted in a k by n feature matrix B where n is the number of voxels in the volume. The new r dimensional vectors corresponding to the input voxels are calculated by multiplying B by the pseudo-inverse of W, which can be replaced by W^T assuming orthogonality of the columns of W [69]. Mathematically, this is described as

$$H_B = W^T B \tag{13.10}$$

ESTIMATION OF THE STOCHASTIC SPEED FUNCTION

In this chapter, a novel speed function to control the evolution of the level-set deformable model is proposed. This speed function is derived using the NMF-based fusion of DW-MRI features, $H_{B:x,y,z}$ for voxel (x, y, z). The proposed speed function $V_n(x, y, z)$ is defined as $V_n(x, y, z) = k\vartheta(x, y, z)$, where κ is the curvature and $\vartheta(x, y, z)$ is defined as

$$\vartheta(x, y, z) = \begin{cases} -E_{obj:x,y,z} & \text{if } E_{obj:x,y,z} > -E_{bg:x,y,z} \\ E_{bg:x,y,z} & \text{otherwise} \end{cases} \tag{13.11}$$

Here, $E_{obj:x,y,z} = P_{nmf:x,y,z}(1) + P_{shape:x,y,z}(1) + P_{spatial:x,y,z}(1)$, where $P_{shape:x,y,z}(1)$ is the object shape prior probability, and $P_{spatial:x,y,z}(1)$ is the object MGRF model probability. Similarly, $E_{bg:x,y,z} = P_{nmf:x,y,z}(0) + P_{shape:x,y,z}(0) + P_{spatial:x,y,z}(0)$, where $P_{shape:x,y,z}(0)$ is the background shape prior probability, and $P_{spatial:x,y,z}(0)$ is the background MGRF model probability. $P_{nmf:x,y,z}(1)$ and $P_{nmf:x,y,z}(0)$ are defined using the distances from the two class centroids produced by performing k-means clustering on the columns of H. The overall segmentation framework is summarized by Algorithm 13.2.

PERFORMANCE EVALUATION METRICS

The performance of the proposed segmentation framework was evaluated using three metrics: (1) Dice similarity coefficient (DSC), (2) Hausdorff distance (HD), and (3) absolute relative volume difference (ARVD). These metrics are detailed below.

Algorithm 13.2   Proposed Algorithm for DW-MRI Prostate Segmentation

Segment the prostate from a DW-MRI volume using the following steps:

1. Align the input DW-MRI volume with the training database using the MI-based affine transformation.
2. Calculate the appearance-based shape prior using Algorithm 13.1.
3. Calculate the 3D pairwise voxel interactions.
4. Perform NMF-based feature fusion.
5. Calculate the probabilities that each voxel is object or background using the NMF-based features.
6. Use these probabilities to guide the evolution of a level-set to segment the prostate.

DICE SIMILARITY COEFFICIENT (DSC)

Many segmentation and classification metrics are based on the determination of true positive (TP), false positive (FP), true negative (TN), and false negative (FN) values (see Figure 13.5). The TP is the number of correctly positively labeled samples; the FP is the number of incorrectly positively labeled samples; the TN is the number of correctly negatively labeled samples; and the FN is the number of incorrectly negatively labeled samples. These values can be used to calculate the DSC as shown by the following:

$$DSC = \frac{2TP}{2TP + FP + FN} \tag{13.12}$$

The value of the DSC ranges from 0 to 1, where 0 means that there is no similarity and 1 means that there is a perfect similarity.

HAUSDORFF DISTANCE (HD)

Distance measures are another type of performance metric used for evaluating segmentation methods. The Euclidean distance is often utilized, but another common measure is the HD. The HD from a set $\mathbf{A_1}$ to a set $\mathbf{A_2}$ is defined as the maximum distance of the set $\mathbf{A_1}$ to the nearest point in the set $\mathbf{A_2}$ [70] (Figure 13.6):

$$HD(\mathbf{A_1}, \mathbf{A_2}) = \max_{a_1 \in A_1} \left\{ \min_{a_2 \in A_2} \left\{ d(a_1, a_2) \right\} \right\} \tag{13.13}$$

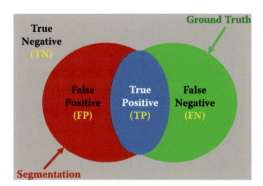

FIGURE 13.5   Diagram illustrating the meaning of TP, FP, TN, and FP.

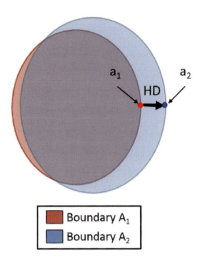

FIGURE 13.6   Diagram illustrating the 2D HD of boundaries A_1 and A_2 for points a_1 and a_2.

where a_1 and a_2 are points of sets A_1 and A_2, respectively, and $d(a_1, a_2)$ is Euclidean distance between these points. The bidirectional Hausdorff distance, denoted by $HD_{Bi}(GT, SR)$, between the segmented region (SR) and its ground truth (GT) is defined as

$$HD_{Bi}(GT, SR) = \max\{HD(GT, SR), HD(SR, GT)\} \tag{13.14}$$

The smaller the distance, the better the segmentation. The ideal case with perfect segmentation is when the bidirectional Hausdorff distance is equal to 0.

ABSOLUTE RELATIVE VOLUME DIFFERENCE (ARVD)

Besides the DSC and the HD, the ARVD has been used as an additional metric for evaluating the segmentation accuracy. The ARVD is the percentage volume difference between the segmented and the ground truth volumes. The lower the ARVD, the higher the segmentation accuracy.

EXPERIMENTAL RESULTS

MEDICAL IMAGES

The proposed system was tested on 53 DW-MRI volumes acquired using a body coil Signa Horizon GE scanner in axial plane with the following parameters:

- Magnetic field strength: 1.5 Tesla
- TE: 84.6 ms
- TR: 8000 ms
- Bandwidth: 142.86 kHz
- FOV: 34 cm
- Slice thickness: 3 mm
- Inter-slice gap: 0 mm
- Acquisition sequence: conventional EPI;
- Diffusion weighting directions: mono direction
- Used range of b-values from 0 to 700 s/mm²

On average, 26 slices were obtained in 120 seconds to cover the prostate in each patient with a voxel size of $1.25 \times 1.25 \times 3.00$ mm^3. The ground truth segmentation used in training and in verifying the segmentation results were verified by an MR expert for each subject.

SEGMENTATION RESULTS

The proposed NMF-based level set has been tested on DW-MRI dataset of 53 subjects at different b-values. Evaluation of the system was done using a leave-one-out methodology, where 52 subjects were used as training data and the remaining subject was used as test data. This was repeated so that each subject was tested once. In order to evaluate the proposed method, we compared the segmentation results of our method with the following approaches: (1) a level-set guided by the MAP model proposed by Firjani et. al. [39] and (2) the reported results for the 3D approach developed by Liu et al. [52]. Table 13.1 summarizes the average segmentation accuracy in terms of the DSC, ARVD, and HD for each method.

Tables 13.2 and 13.3 show the DSC results and the HD results, respectively, for nine subjects using the proposed segmentation approach and the MAP-guided level-set method [39].

As can be seen, the proposed method leads to superior results over the compared methods. The proposed method reaches 85.9% ± 4% overall DSC and 1.6% ± 3.2% ARVD. It reaches 5.84% ± 2.14 mm overall HD which reflects the high accuracy of the proposed

TABLE 13.1

A Comparison of the Average DSC and HD Values Over All Subjects for the Compared Segmentation Methods

Measures	NMF	MAP [39]	Liu et al. [52]
DSC (%)	85.9 ± 4	83.4 ± 7	81 ± 5
ARVD (%)	1.6 ± 3.2	1.8 ± 4.3	—
HD (mm)	5.8 ± 2.1	6.7 ± 2.0	9.1 ± 1.6

TABLE 13.2

The DSC Segmentation Performances of the NMF and MAP-Guided Level-Set Methods for Nine Subjects

Method	S_1	S_2	S_3	S_4	S_5	S_6	S_7	S_8	S_9
NMF	0.822	0.861	0.907	0.862	0.905	0.828	0.851	0.886	0.905
MAP	0.816	0.858	0.881	0.836	0.900	0.827	0.849	0.647	0.880

TABLE 13.3

The HD Segmentation Performances of the NMF and MAP-Guided Level-Set Methods for Nine Subjects

Method	S_1	S_2	S_3	S_4	S_5	S_6	S_7	S_8	S_9
NMF	5.30	3.00	6.00	6.00	5.96	8.72	9.75	3.49	3.25
MAP	5.30	3.00	6.34	6.00	6.93	8.75	9.08	9.27	6.00

segmentation approach. Figure 13.7 illustrates the evolution of the level-set for two different cases. Figure 13.8 shows that the NMF-based approach used in the proposed framework is more accurate than the MAP-based approach described in [39]. Figure 13.9a illustrates the 2D projection in the axial view at different cross sections of the final 3D level-set segmentation for 3 different subjects using the proposed method. The resultant 3D mesh (from 3 different views) of the prostate is shown in Figure 13.9b.

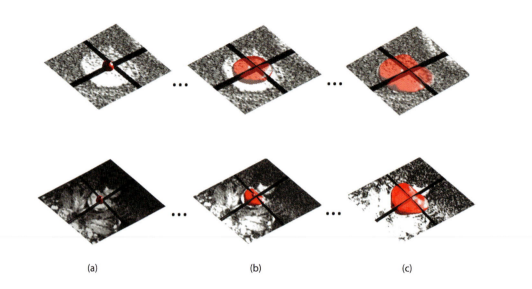

(a)   (b)   (c)

FIGURE 13.7 The propagation of the level set for two subjects (rows): initial surface (a), propagation after 20 iterations (b), and final surface (c).

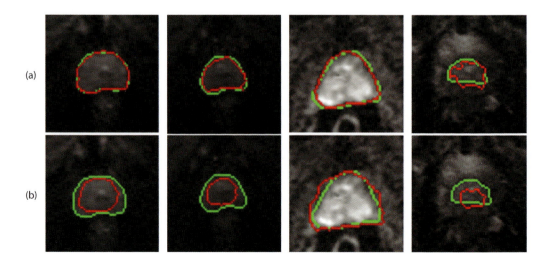

FIGURE 13.8 Visual comparison of the segmentation accuracy between (a) the NMF-based approach and (b) MAP-based approach at different cross sections. The green and red colors show the contour of the ground truth and segmented regions, respectively.

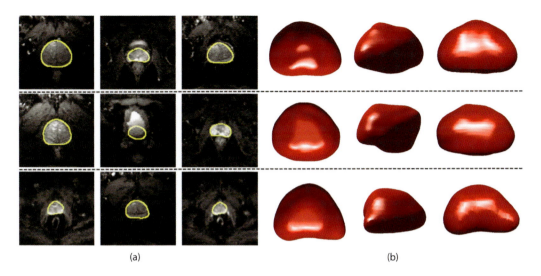

(a)   (b)

FIGURE 13.9 The final segmentation results for three different subjects (a) 2D axial projections at different cross sections and (b) the resultant 3D mesh at different views.

CONCLUSION

In this chapter, an NMF-based DW-MRI prostate delineation framework was introduced. The use of 3D intensity, shape, and spatial features combined with NMF-based feature fusion is significantly better at guiding a level-set for DW-MRI prostate delineation than either using MAP with the same input information or intensity and shape information alone. The addition of NMF-based feature fusion allows the proposed framework to perform robust prostate segmentation despite image noise, inter-patient anatomical differences, and the similar intensities of the prostate and surrounding tissues. In future work, this segmentation framework will be tested with a larger data set in order to verify its robustness. In addition, the effectiveness of using the proposed method to segment the prostate at varying b-values will be investigated. Since segmentation is a key step in developing CAD systems for diagnosing different disorders of various human organs, such as the brain [71–93], the lung [94–133], the retina [134,135], the heart [136–152], and the kidney [153–178], another future work could be the application of the developed framework in segmenting those organs to verify its effectiveness.

REFERENCES

1. Reda, I., Shalaby, A., Elmogy, M., Elfotouh, A.A., Khalifa, F., El-Ghar, M.A., Hosseini-Asl, E., Gimelfarb, G., Werghi, N., El-Baz, A. A comprehensive non-invasive framework for diagnosing prostate cancer. *Computers in Biology and Medicine* **81** (2017) 148–158.
2. Reda, I., Shalaby, A., Elmogy, M., Aboulfotouh, A., Khalifa, F., El-Ghar, M.A., Gimelfarb, G., El-Baz, A. Image-based computer-aided diagnostic system for early diagnosis of prostate cancer. In: *International Conference on Medical Image Computing and Computer-Assisted Intervention*, Athens, Greece, Springer (October 17–21, 2016) pp. 610–618.
3. Reda, I., Shalaby, A., El-Ghar, M.A., Khalifa, F., Elmogy, M., Aboulfotouh, A., Hosseini-Asl, E., El-Baz, A., Keynton, R. A new NMF-autoencoder based CAD system for early diagnosis of prostate cancer. In: *Biomedical Imaging (ISBI), 2016 IEEE 13th International Symposium on*, IEEE (2016) pp. 1237–1240.
4. Reda, I., Shalaby, A., Khalifa, F., Elmogy, M., Aboulfotouh, A., El-Ghar, M.A., Hosseini-Asl, E., Werghi, N., Keynton, R., El-Baz, A. Computer-aided diagnostic tool for early detection of prostate cancer. In: *Image Processing (ICIP), 2016 IEEE International Conference on*, IEEE (2016) pp. 2668–2672.

5. Reda, I., Elmogy, M., Aboulfotouh, A., Ismail, M., El-Baz, A., Keynton, R. Prostate segmentation using deformable model-based methods. In: EI-Baz, A., Jiang, X., Suri, J.S. (Eds.) *Biomedical Image Segmentation: Advances and Trends.* Boca Raton, FL, CRC Press (2016) pp. 293–308.

6. Reda, I., Shalaby, A., Elmogy, M., Aboulfotouh, A., Werghi, N., Elmaghraby, A., El-Baz, A. Prostate cancer diagnosis based on the fusion of imaging-markers with clinical-biomarkers. In: *Biomedical Engineering Society* (*BMES*), Phoenix, Arizona, USA (2017).

7. Pondman, K.M., Fütterer, J.J., ten Haken, B., Kool, L.J.S., Witjes, J.A., Hambrock, T., Macura, K.J., Barentsz, J.O. MR-guided biopsy of the prostate: An overview of techniques and a systematic review. *European Urology* **54**(3) (2008) 517–527.

8. Hricak, H., Wang, L., Wei, D.C., Coakley, F.V., Akin, O., Reuter, V.E., Gonen, M., Kattan, M.W., Onyebuchi, C.N., Scardino, P.T. The role of preoperative endorectal magnetic resonance imaging in the decision regarding whether to preserve or resect neurovascular bundles during radical retropubic prostatectomy. *Cancer* **100**(12) (2004) 2655–2663.

9. Guo, Y., Gao, Y., Shen, D. Deformable MR prostate segmentation via deep feature learning and sparse patch matching. *IEEE Transactions on Medical Imaging* **35**(4) (2016) 1077–1089.

10. Yang, X., Zhan, S., Xie, D. Landmark based prostate MRI segmentation via improved level set method. In: *Signal Processing (ICSP), 2016 IEEE 13th International Conference on*, IEEE (2016) pp. 29–34.

11. Cootes, T.F., Taylor, C.J. Active shape models: Smart snakes. In: *Proceedings of the British Machine Vision Conference (BMVC'92)*, Leeds, UK, Springer (September 1992) pp. 266–275.

12. Osher, S., Sethian, J.A. Fronts propagating with curvature-dependent speed: Algorithms based on Hamilton-Jacobi formulations. *Journal of Computational Physics* **79**(1) (1988) 12–49.

13. Allen, P.D., Graham, J., Williamson, D.C., Hutchinson, C.E. Differential segmentation of the prostate in MR images using combined 3D shape modelling and voxel classification. In: *Proceedings of the 3rd IEEE International Symposium on Biomedical Imaging: (ISBI'06)*, Arlington, VA, IEEE (April 6–9, 2006) pp. 410–413.

14. Zhu, Y., Williams, S., Zwiggelaar, R. A hybrid ASM approach for sparse volumetric data segmentation. *Pattern Recognition and Image Analysis* **17**(2) (2007) 252–258.

15. Ghose, S., Oliver, A., Martí, R., Lladó, X., Freixenet, J., Mitra, J., Vilanova, J.C., Meriaudeau, F. A hybrid framework of multiple active appearance models and global registration for 3D prostate segmentation in MRI. In: *Proceedings of the SPIE Conference on Medical Imaging 2012* (February 4–9, 2012) p. 83140S.

16. Martin, S., Troccaz, J., Daanen, V. Automated segmentation of the prostate in 3D MR images using a probabilistic atlas and a spatially constrained deformable model. *Medical Physics* **37** (2010) 1579.

17. Gao, Y., Sandhu, R., Fichtinger, G., Tannenbaum, A.R. A coupled global registration and segmentation framework with application to magnetic resonance prostate imagery. *IEEE Transactions on Medical Imaging* **29**(10) (2010) 1781–1794.

18. Ghose, S., Mitra, J., Oliver, A., Marti, R., Llado, X., Freixenet, J., Vilanova, J.C., Sidibé, D., Mériaudeau, F. Graph cut energy minimization in a probabilistic learning framework for 3D prostate segmentation in MRI. In: *Proceedings of the 21st International Conference on Pattern Recognition (ICPR'12)*, Tsukuba Science City, Japan, IEEE (November 11–15, 2012) pp. 125–128.

19. Firjany, A., Elnakib, A., El-Baz, A., Gimelfarb, G., El-Ghar, M., Elmagharby, A. Novel stochastic framework for accurate segmentation of prostate in dynamic contrast enhanced MRI. In: *Proceedings of the First International Workshop on Prostate Cancer Imaging: Computer-Aided Diagnosis, Prognosis, and Intervention*, Volume 1, Beijing, China (September 24, 2010) pp. 123–130.

20. Li, S.Z., Singh, S. *Markov Random Field Modeling in Image Analysis*, Vol. 3. Berlin, Germany, Springer (2009).

21. El-Baz, A. Novel stochastic models for medical image analysis. PhD thesis, University of Louisville, Louisville, KY (2006).

22. Firjani, A., Elnakib, A., Khalifa, F., Gimelfarb, G., Abo El-Ghar, M., Suri, J., Elmagharby, A., El-Baz, A. A new 3D automatic segmentation framework for accurate segmentation of prostate from DCE-MRI. In: *Proceedings of the IEEE International Conference on Image Processing (ICIP'11)*, Brussels, Belgium (September 11–14, 2011).

23. Firjani, A., Elnakib, A., Khalifa, F., Gimelfarb, G., Abo El-Ghar, M., Suri, J., Elmaghraby, A., El-Baz, A. A new 3D automatic segmentation framework for accurate segmentation of prostate from DCE-MRI. In: *Proceedings of the IEEE International Symposium on Biomedical Imaging (ISBI'11)*, Chicago, IL, IEEE (March 30–April 2, 2011) pp. 1476–1479.

24. Makni, N., Puech, P., Lopes, R., Dewalle, A.S., Colot, O., Betrouni, N. Combining a deformable model and a probabilistic framework for an automatic 3D segmentation of prostate on MRI. *International Journal on Computer Assisted Radiology Surgery* **4**(2) (2009) 181–188.

25. Mark, B.L., Turin, W. *Probability, Random Processes, and Statistical Analysis*. Cambridge, UK, Cambridge University Press Textbooks (2011).
26. Tian, Z., Liu, L., Zhang, Z., Fei, B. Superpixel-based segmentation for 3D prostate MR images. *IEEE Transactions on Medical Imaging* **35**(3) (2016) 791–801.
27. Klein, S., van der Heide, U.A., Lips, I.M., van Vulpen, M., Staring, M., Pluim, J.P. Automatic segmentation of the prostate in 3D MR images by atlas matching using localized mutual information. *Medical Physics* **35** (2008) 1407.
28. Dowling, J.A., Fripp, J., Chandra, S., Pluim, J.P.W., Lambert, J., Parker, J., Denham, J., Greer, P.B., Salvado, O. Fast automatic multi-atlas segmentation of the prostate from 3D MR images. In: *Prostate Cancer Imaging*. Berlin, Germany, Springer (2011) pp. 10–21.
29. Langerak, T.R., van der Heide, U.A., Kotte, A.N., Viergever, M.A., van Vulpen, M., Pluim, J.P. Label fusion in atlas-based segmentation using a selective and iterative method for performance level estimation (SIMPLE). *IEEE Transactions on Medical Imaging* **29**(12) (2010) 2000–2008.
30. Litjens, G., Debats, O., Barentsz, J., Karssemeijer, N., Huisman, H. Computer-aided detection of prostate cancer in MRI. *IEEE Transactions on Medical Imaging* **33**(5) (2014) 1083–1092.
31. Litjens, G., Toth, R., van de Ven, W. et al. Evaluation of prostate segmentation algorithms for MRI: The promise 12 challenge. *Medical Image Analysis* **18**(2) (2014) 359–373.
32. Zwiggelaar, R., Zhu, Y., Williams, S. Semi-automatic segmentation of the prostate. In: Perales, F.J., Campilho, A.J., de la Blanca, N.P., Sanfeliu, A. (Eds.), *Pattern Recognition and Image Analysis*. Berlin, Germany, Springer (2003) pp. 1108–1116.
33. Flores-Tapia, D., Thomas, G., Venugopal, N., McCurdy, B., Pistorius, S. Semi automatic MRI prostate segmentation based on wavelet multiscale products. In: *Proceedings of the 30th Annual International Conference of the IEEE Engineering in Medicine and Biology Society* (*EMBS'08*), Vancouver, Canada, IEEE (August 20–25, 2008) pp. 3020–3023.
34. Pesquet, J.C., Krim, H., Carfantan, H. Time-invariant orthonormal wavelet representations. *IEEE Transactions on Signal Processing* **44**(8) (1996) 1964–1970.
35. Vikal, S., Haker, S., Tempany, C., Fichtinger, G. Prostate contouring in MRI guided biopsy. In: *Proceedings of the SPIE Conference on Medical Imaging 2009*, Lake Buena Vista, FL (2009) pp. 1–11.
36. Grady, L. Random walks for image segmentation. *IEEE Transactions on Pattern Analysis and Machine Intelligence* **28**(11) (2006) 1768–1783.
37. Khurd, P., Grady, L., Gajera, K., Diallo, M., Gall, P., Requardt, M., Kiefer, B., Weiss, C., Kamen, A. Facilitating 3D spectroscopic imaging through automatic prostate localization in MR images using random walker segmentation initialized via boosted classifiers. In: *Prostate Cancer Imaging*. Berlin, Germany, Springer (2011) pp. 47–56.
38. Tan, C.H., Wang, J., Kundra, V. Diffusion weighted imaging in prostate cancer. *European Radiology* **21**(3) (2011) 593–603.
39. Firjani, A., Elnakib, A., Khalifa, F., Gimelfarb, G., El-Ghar, M.A., Elmaghraby, A., El-Baz, A. A diffusion-weighted imaging based diagnostic system for early detection of prostate cancer. *Journal of Biomedical Science and Engineering* **6** (2013) 346–356.
40. Litjens, G., Vos, P., Barentsz, J., Karssemeijer, N., Huisman, H. Automatic computer aided detection of abnormalities in multi-parametric prostate MRI. In: *SPIE Medical Imaging, International Society for Optics and Photonics* (2011) pp. 79630T–79630T.
41. Vos, P.C., Hambrock, T., Barenstz, J.O., Huisman, H.J. Computer-assisted analysis of peripheral zone prostate lesions using T2-weighted and dynamic contrast enhanced T1-weighted MRI. *Physics in Medicine and Biology* **55**(6) (2010) 1719.
42. Vos, P., Barentsz, J., Karssemeijer, N., Huisman, H. Automatic computer-aided detection of prostate cancer based on multiparametric magnetic resonance image analysis. *Physics in Medicine and Biology* **57**(6) (2012) 1527.
43. Ozer, S., Haider, M.A., Langer, D.L., van der Kwast, T.H., Evans, A.J., Wernick, M.N., Trachtenberg, J., Yetik, I.S. Prostate cancer localization with multispectral MRI based on relevance vector machines. In: *Proceedings of the IEEE International Symposium on Biomedical Imaging: From Nano to Macro* (*ISBI'09*), Boston, MA, IEEE (June 28–July 1, 2009) pp. 73–76.
44. Niaf, E., Rouvi`ere, O., M`ege-Lechevallier, F., Bratan, F., Lartizien, C. Computer-aided diagnosis of prostate cancer in the peripheral zone using multiparametric MRI. *Physics in Medicine and Biology* **57**(12) (2012) 3833.
45. Peng, Y., Jiang, Y., Yang, C., Brown, J.B., Antic, T., Sethi, I., Schmid-Tannwald, C., Giger, M.L., Eggener, S.E., Oto, A. Quantitative analysis of multiparametric prostate MR images: Differentiation between prostate cancer and normal tissue and correlation with Gleason score. *Radiology* **267**(3) (2013) 787–796.

46. Hambrock, T., Vos, P.C., Hulsbergen-van de Kaa, C.A., Barentsz, J.O., Huisman, H.J. Prostate cancer: Computer-aided diagnosis with multiparametric 3-T MR imaging– effect on observer performance. *Radiology* **266**(2) (2013) 521–530.

47. Tamada, T., Sone, T., Jo, Y., Yamamoto, A., Ito, K. Diffusion-weighted MRI and its role in prostate cancer. *NMR in Biomedicine* **27**(1) (2014) 25–38.

48. Firjani, A., Khalifa, F., Elnakib, A., Gimelfarb, G., Abo El-Ghar, M., El-magharby, A., El-Baz, A. 3D automatic approach for precise segmentation of the prostate from diffusion-weighted magnetic resonance imaging. In: *Proceedings of the IEEE International Conference on Image Processing (ICIP'11)*, Brussels, Belgium (September 11–14, 2011).

49. Firjani, A., Elnakib, A., Khalifa, F., Gimelfarb, G., Abo El-Ghar, M., El-maghraby, A., El-Baz, A. A new 3D automatic segmentation framework for accurate extraction of prostate from diffusion imaging. In: *Proceedings of the Biomedical Sciences and Engineering Conference (BSEC'11)*, Knoxville, TN (March 15–17, 2011) pp. 1–4.

50. Liu, X., Langer, D., Haider, M., Van der Kwast, T., Evans, A., Wernick, M., Yetik, I. Unsupervised segmentation of the prostate using MR images based on level set with a shape prior. In: *Proceedings of the Annual International Conference of the IEEE Engineering in Medicine and Biology Society (EMBC'09)*, Minneapolis, MN, IEEE (September 2–6, 2009) pp. 3613–3616.

51. Otsu, N. A threshold selection method from gray-level histograms. *Automatica* **11**(285–296) (1975) 23–27.

52. Liu, X., Haider, M.A., Yetik, I.S. Unsupervised 3D prostate segmentation based on diffusion-weighted imaging MRI using active contour models with a shape prior. *Journal of Electrical and Computer Engineering* **2011** (2011) 11.

53. Khalifa, F., Elnakib, A., Beache, G., Gimelfarb, G., El-Ghar, M., Ouseph, R., Sokhadze, G., Manning, S., McClure, P., El-Baz, A. 3D kidney segmentation from CT images using a level set approach guided by a novel stochastic speed function. In: Fichtinger, G., Martel, A., Peters, T. (Eds.), *Proceedings of the International Conference on Medical Image Computing and Computer-Assisted Intervention (MICCAI'11)*, Volume 6893 of Lecture Notes in Computer Science, Toronto, Canada. Berlin, Germany, Springer (September 18–22, 2011) pp. 587–594.

54. Khalifa, F., Beache, G., Elnakib, A., Sliman, H., Gimelfarb, G., Welch, K., El-Baz, A. A new shape-based framework for the left ventricle wall segmentation from cardiac first-pass perfusion MRI. In: *Proceedings of the International Symposium on Biomedical Imaging (ISBI'13)*, San Francisco, CA (April 7–11, 2013) pp. 41–44.

55. Osher, S., Fedkiw, R. *Level Set Methods and Dynamic Implicit Surfaces*. New York, Springer-Verlag (2006).

56. Shier, D., Butler, J., Lewis, R. *Hole's Essentials of Human Anatomy and Physiology*. New York, McGraw-Hill (2006).

57. Viola, P.A., Wells III, W.M. Alignment by maximization of mutual information. *International Journal on Computer Vision* **24**(2) (1997) 137–154.

58. Khalifa, F., El-Baz, A., Gimelfarb, G., Ouseph, R., El-Ghar, M. Shape-appearance guided level-set deformable model for image segmentation. In: *Proceedings of the 20th International Conference on Pattern Recognition (ICPR'10)*, Istanbul, Turkey (August 23–26, 2010).

59. El-Baz, A., Soliman, A., McClure, P., Gimelfarb, G., El-Ghar, M.A., Falk, R. Early assessment of malignant lung nodules based on the spatial analysis of detected lung nodules. In: *Proceedings of the IEEE International Symposium on Biomedical Imaging: From Nana to Macro (ISBI'12)*, IEEE (2012) pp. 1463–1466.

60. Besag, J. Spatial interaction and the statistical analysis of lattice systems. *Journal of the Royal Statistical Society. Series B (Methodological)* **36** (1974) 192–236.

61. Farag, A.A., El-Baz, A.S., Gimelfarb, G. Precise segmentation of multimodal images. *IEEE Transactions on Image Processing* **15**(4) (2006) 952–968.

62. Lee, D.D., Seung, H.S. Learning the parts of objects by non-negative matrix factorization. *Nature* **401**(6755) (1999) 788–791.

63. Shahnaz, F., Berry, M.W., Pauca, V.P., Plemmons, R.J. Document clustering using nonnegative matrix factorization. *Information Processing & Management* **42**(2) (2006) 373–386.

64. Zafeiriou, S., Tefas, A., Buciu, I., Pitas, I. Exploiting discriminant information in nonnegative matrix factorization with application to frontal face verification. *IEEE Transactions on Neural Netwoks*, **17**(3) (2006) 683–695.

65. Xie, Y., Ho, J., Vemuri, B.C. Nonnegative factorization of diffusion tensor images and its applications. In: Székely, G., Hahn, H.K. (Eds.), *Information Processing in Medical Imaging*. Berlin, Germany, Springer (2011) pp. 550–561.

66. Sandler, R., Lindenbaum, M. Nonnegative matrix factorization with earth mover's distance metric for image analysis. *IEEE Transactions on Pattern Analysis* **33**(8) (2011) 1590–1602.

67. Berry, M.W., Browne, M., Langville, A.N., Pauca, V.P., Plemmons, R.J. Algorithms and applications for approximate nonnegative matrix factorization. *Computational Statistics & Data Analysis* **52**(1) (2007) 155–173.

68. Lee, D.D., Seung, H.S. Algorithms for non-negative matrix factorization. *Advances in Neural Information Processing Systems* **13** (2000) 556–562.

69. Hyv¨arinen, A. Sparse code shrinkage: Denoising of nongaussian data by maximum likelihood estimation. *Neural Computation* **11**(7) (1999) 1739–1768.

70. Babalola, K.O., Patenaude, B., Aljabar, P., Schnabel, J., Kennedy, D., Crum, W., Smith, S., Cootes, T., Jenkinson, M., Rueckert, D. An evaluation of four automatic methods of segmenting the subcortical structures in the brain. *Neuroimage* **47**(4) (2009) 1435–1447.

71. Dombroski, B., Nitzken, M., Elnakib, A., Khalifa, F., El-Baz, A., Casanova, M.F. Cortical surface complexity in a population-based normative sample. *Translational Neuroscience* **5**(1) (2014) 17–24.

72. El-Baz, A., Casanova, M., Gimelfarb, G., Mott, M., Switala, A. An MRI-based diagnostic framework for early diagnosis of dyslexia. *International Journal of Computer Assisted Radiology and Surgery* **3**(3–4) (2008) 181–189.

73. El-Baz, A., Casanova, M., Gimelfarb, G., Mott, M., Switala, A., Vanbogaert, E., McCracken, R. A new CAD system for early diagnosis of dyslexic brains. In: *Proceedings of the International Conference on Image Processing (ICIP'2008)*, IEEE (2008) pp. 1820–1823.

74. El-Baz, A., Casanova, M.F., Gimelfarb, G., Mott, M., Switwala, A.E. A new image analysis approach for automatic classification of autistic brains. In: *Proceedings of the IEEE International Symposium on Biomedical Imaging: From Nano to Macro (ISBI'2007)*, IEEE (2007) pp. 352–355.

75. El-Baz, A., Elnakib, A., Khalifa, F., El-Ghar, M.A., McClure, P., Soliman, A., Gimelfarb, G. Precise segmentation of 3-D magnetic resonance angiography. *IEEE Transactions on Biomedical Engineering* **59**(7) (2012) 2019–2029.

76. El-Baz, A., Farag, A.A., Gimelfarb, G.L., El-Ghar, M.A., Eldiasty, T. Probabilistic modeling of blood vessels for segmenting MRA images. *ICPR* **3** (2006) 917–920.

77. El-Baz, A., Farag, A.A., Gimelfarb, G., El-Ghar, M.A., Eldiasty, T. A new adaptive probabilistic model of blood vessels for segmenting MRA images. In: *Medical Image Computing and Computer-Assisted Intervention–MICCAI 2006*, Volume 4191. Berlin, Germany, Springer (2006) pp. 799–806.

78. El-Baz, A., Farag, A.A., Gimelfarb, G., Hushek, S.G. Automatic cerebrovascular segmentation by accurate probabilistic modeling of TOF-MRA images. In: *Medical Image Computing and Computer-Assisted Intervention–MICCAI 2005*. Berlin, Germany, Springer (2005) pp. 34–42.

79. El-Baz, A., Farag, A., Elnakib, A., Casanova, M.F., Gimelfarb, G., Switala, A.E., Jordan, D., Rainey, S. Accurate automated detection of autism related corpus callosum abnormalities. *Journal of Medical Systems* **35**(5) (2011) 929–939.

80. El-Baz, A., Farag, A., Gimelfarb, G. Cerebrovascular segmentation by accurate probabilistic modeling of TOF-MRA images. In: *Image Analysis*, Volume 3540. Berlin, Germany, Springer (2005) pp. 1128–1137.

81. El-Baz, A., Gimelfarb, G., Falk, R., El-Ghar, M.A., Kumar, V., Heredia, D. A novel 3D joint Markov-Gibbs model for extracting blood vessels from PC–MRA images. In: *Medical Image Computing and Computer-Assisted Intervention– MICCAI 2009*, Volume 5762. Berlin, Germany, Springer (2009) pp. 943–950.

82. Elnakib, A., El-Baz, A., Casanova, M.F., Gimelfarb, G., Switala, A.E. Image-based detection of corpus callosum variability for more accurate discrimination between dyslexic and normal brains. In: *Proceeding of the IEEE International Symposium on Biomedical Imaging: From Nano to Macro (ISBI'2010)*, IEEE (2010) pp. 109–112.

83. Elnakib, A., Casanova, M.F., Gimelfarb, G., Switala, A.E., El-Baz, A. Autism diagnostics by centerline-based shape analysis of the corpus callosum. In: *Proceedings of the IEEE International Symposium on Biomedical Imaging: From Nano to Macro (ISBI'2011)*, IEEE (2011) pp. 1843–1846.

84. Elnakib, A., Nitzken, M., Casanova, M., Park, H., Gimelfarb, G., El-Baz, A. Quantification of age-related brain cortex change using 3D shape analysis. In: *Pattern Recognition (ICPR), 2012 21st International Conference on*, IEEE (2012) pp. 41–44.

85. Mostapha, M., Soliman, A., Khalifa, F., Elnakib, A., Alansary, A., Nitzken, M., Casanova, M.F., El-Baz, A. A statistical framework for the classification of infant DT images. In: *Image Processing (ICIP), 2014 IEEE International Conference on*, IEEE (2014) pp. 2222–2226.

86. Nitzken, M., Casanova, M., Gimelfarb, G., Elnakib, A., Khalifa, F., Switala, A., El-Baz, A. 3D shape analysis of the brain cortex with application to dyslexia. In: *Image Processing (ICIP), 2011 18th IEEE International Conference on*, Brussels, Belgium, IEEE (September 2011) pp. 2657–2660 (Selected for oral presentation. Oral acceptance rate is 10 percent and the overall acceptance rate is 35 percent).

87. El-Gamal, F.E.Z.A., Elmogy, M., Ghazal, M., Atwan, A., Barnes, G., Casanova, M., Keynton, R., El-Baz, A. A novel CAD system for local and global early diagnosis of Alzheimer's disease based on PIB-PET scans. In: *Image Processing (ICIP), 2017 IEEE International Conference on*, Beijing, China, IEEE (2017).

88. Ismail, M., Soliman, A., Ghazal, M., Switala, A. E., Gimelfarb, G., Barnes, G. N., Khalil, A., El-Baz, A. A fast stochastic framework for automatic MR brain images segmentation. *PLoS One* **12**(11) (2017) e0187391.

89. Ismail, M.M., Keynton, R.S., Mostapha, M.M., ElTanboly, A.H., Casanova, M.F., Gimelfarb, G.L., El-Baz, A. Studying autism spectrum disorder with structural and diffusion magnetic resonance imaging: A survey. *Frontiers in Human Neuroscience* **10** (2016) 211.

90. Alansary, A., Ismail, M., Soliman, A. et al. Infant brain extraction in T1-weighted MR images using bet and refinement using LCDG and MGRF models. *IEEE Journal of Biomedical and Health Informatics* **20**(3) (2016) 925–935.

91. Ismail, M., Barnes, G., Nitzken, M., Switala, A., Shalaby, A., Hosseini-Asl, E., Casanova, M., Keynton, R., Khalil, A., and El-Baz, A. A new deep-learning CAD system for early diagnosis of autism using structural MR. In: *Proceedings of the IEEE Conference on Image Processing (ICIP 17)*, Beijing, China (2017).

92. Ismail, M., Soliman, A., ElTanboly, A., Switala, A., Mahmoud, M., Khalifa, F., Gimelfarb, G., Casanova, M.F., Keynton, R., El-Baz, A. Detection of white matter abnormalities in MR brain images for diagnosis of autism in children. In: *2016 IEEE 13th International Symposium on Biomedical Imaging 2016 IEEE 13th International Symposium on Biomedical Imaging*, Prague, Czech Republic (2016) pp. 6–9.

93. Ismail, M., Mostapha, M., Soliman, A., Nitzken, M., Khalifa, F., Elnakib, A., Gimelfarb, G., Casanova, M., El-Baz, A. Segmentation of infant brain MR images based on adaptive shape prior and higher-order MGRF. In: *2015 IEEE International Conference on Image Processing (ICIP)*, Quebec City, Canada (2015) pp. 4327–4331.

94. Abdollahi, B., Civelek, A.C., Li, X.F., Suri, J., El-Baz, A. PET/CT nodule segmentation and diagnosis: A survey. In: Saba, L., Suri, J.S. (Eds.), *Multi Detector CT Imaging*. New York, Taylor & Francis Group (2014) pp. 639–651.

95. Abdollahi, B., El-Baz, A., Amini, A.A. A multi-scale non-linear vessel enhancement technique. In: *Engineering in Medicine and Biology Society, EMBC, 2011 Annual International Conference of the IEEE*, IEEE (2011) pp. 3925–3929.

96. Abdollahi, B., Soliman, A., Civelek, A., Li, X.F., Gimelfarb, G., El-Baz, A. A novel gaussian scale space-based joint MGRF framework for precise lung segmentation. In: *Proceedings of IEEE International Conference on Image Processing (ICIP'12)*, IEEE (2012) pp. 2029–2032.

97. Abdollahi, B., Soliman, A., Civelek, A., Li, X.F., Gimelfarb, G., El-Baz, A. A novel 3D joint MGRF framework for precise lung segmentation. In: *Machine Learning in Medical Imaging*. Berlin, Germany, Springer (2012) pp. 86–93.

98. Ali, A.M., El-Baz, A.S., Farag, A.A. A novel framework for accurate lung segmentation using graph cuts. In: *Proceedings of IEEE International Symposium on Biomedical Imaging: From Nano to Macro (ISBI'07)*, IEEE (2007) pp. 908–911.

99. El-Baz, A., Beache, G.M., Gimelfarb, G., Suzuki, K., Okada, K. Lung imaging data analysis. *International Journal of Biomedical Imaging* **2013** (2013) 1–2.

100. El-Baz, A., Beache, G.M., Gimelfarb, G., Suzuki, K., Okada, K., Elnakib, A., Soliman, A., Abdollahi, B. Computer-aided diagnosis systems for lung cancer: Challenges and methodologies. *International Journal of Biomedical Imaging* **2013** (2013) 1–46.

101. El-Baz, A., Elnakib, A., Abou El-Ghar, M., Gimelfarb, G., Falk, R., Farag, A. Automatic detection of 2D and 3D lung nodules in chest spiral CT scans. *International Journal of Biomedical Imaging* **2013** (2013) 1–11.

102. El-Baz, A., Farag, A.A., Falk, R., La Rocca, R. A unified approach for detection, visualization, and identification of lung abnormalities in chest spiral CT scans. In: *International Congress Series*, Volume 1256. Amsterdam, the Netherlands, Elsevier (2003) pp. 998–1004.

103. El-Baz, A., Farag, A.A., Falk, R., La Rocca, R. Detection, visualization and identification of lung abnormalities in chest spiral CT scan: Phase-I. In: *Proceedings of International conference on Biomedical Engineering*, Cairo, Egypt, Volume 12 (2002).

104. El-Baz, A., Farag, A., Gimelfarb, G., Falk, R., El-Ghar, M.A., Eldiasty, T. A framework for automatic segmentation of lung nodules from low dose chest CT scans. In: *Proceedings of International Conference on Pattern Recognition (ICPR'06)*, Volume 3, IEEE (2006) pp. 611–614.

105. El-Baz, A., Farag, A., Gimelfarb, G., Falk, R., El-Ghar, M.A. A novel level set-based computer-aided detection system for automatic detection of lung nodules in low dose chest computed tomography scans. *Lung Imaging and Computer Aided Diagnosis* **10** (2011) 221–238.

106. El-Baz, A., Gimelfarb, G., Abou El-Ghar, M., Falk, R. Appearance-based diagnostic system for early assessment of malignant lung nodules. In: *Proceedings of IEEE International Conference on Image Processing (ICIP'12)*, IEEE (2012) pp. 533–536.

107. El-Baz, A., Gimelfarb, G., Falk, R. A novel 3D framework for automatic lung segmentation from low dose CT images. In: El-Baz, A., Suri, J.S. (Eds.), *Lung Imaging and Computer Aided Diagnosis*. Boca Raton, FL, Taylor & Francis Group (2011) pp. 1–16.

108. El-Baz, A., Gimelfarb, G., Falk, R., El-Ghar, M. Appearance analysis for diagnosing malignant lung nodules. In: *Proceedings of IEEE International Symposium on Biomedical Imaging: From Nano to Macro (ISBI'10)*, IEEE (2010) pp. 193–196.

109. El-Baz, A., Gimelfarb, G., Falk, R., El-Ghar, M.A. A novel level set-based CAD system for automatic detection of lung nodules in low dose chest CT scans. In: El-Baz, A., Suri, J.S. (Eds.), *Lung Imaging and Computer Aided Diagnosis*, Volume 1. Boca Raton, FL, Taylor & Francis Group (2011) pp. 221–238.

110. El-Baz, A., Gimelfarb, G., Falk, R., El-Ghar, M.A. A new approach for automatic analysis of 3D low dose CT images for accurate monitoring the detected lung nodules. In: *Proceedings of International Conference on Pattern Recognition (ICPR'08)*, IEEE (2008) pp. 1–4.

111. El-Baz, A., Gimelfarb, G., Falk, R., El-Ghar, M.A. A novel approach for automatic follow-up of detected lung nodules. In: *Proceedings of IEEE International Conference on Image Processing (ICIP'07)*, Volume 5, IEEE (2007) pp. V–501.

112. El-Baz, A., Gimelfarb, G., Falk, R., El-Ghar, M.A. A new CAD system for early diagnosis of detected lung nodules. In: *Image Processing, 2007. ICIP 2007. IEEE International Conference on*, Volume 2, IEEE (2007) pp. II–461.

113. El-Baz, A., Gimelfarb, G., Falk, R., El-Ghar, M.A., Refaie, H. Promising results for early diagnosis of lung cancer. In: *Proceedings of IEEE International Symposium on Biomedical Imaging: From Nano to Macro (ISBI'08)*, IEEE (2008) pp. 1151–1154.

114. El-Baz, A., Gimelfarb, G.L., Falk, R., Abou El-Ghar, M., Holland, T., Shaffer, T. A new stochastic framework for accurate lung segmentation. In: *Proceedings of Medical Image Computing and Computer-Assisted Intervention (MICCAI'08)*, New York (2008) pp. 322–330.

115. El-Baz, A., Gimelfarb, G.L., Falk, R., Heredis, D., Abou El-Ghar, M. A novel approach for accurate estimation of the growth rate of the detected lung nodules. In: *Proceedings of International Workshop on Pulmonary Image Analysis*, New York (2008) pp. 33–42.

116. El-Baz, A., Gimelfarb, G.L., Falk, R., Holland, T., Shaffer, T. A framework for unsupervised segmentation of lung tissues from low dose computed tomography images. In: *Proceedings of British Machine Vision (BMVC'08)*, Leeds, UK (2008) pp. 1–10.

117. El-Baz, A., Gimelfarb, G., Falk, R., El-Ghar, M.A. 3D MGRF-based appearance modeling for robust segmentation of pulmonary nodules in 3D LDCT chest images. In: El-Baz, A., Suri, J.S. (Eds.), *Lung Imaging and Computer Aided Diagnosis*, Chapter 3. Boca Raton, FL, Taylor & Francis Group (2011) pp. 51–63.

118. El-Baz, A., Gimelfarb, G., Falk, R., El-Ghar, M.A. Automatic analysis of 3D low dose CT images for early diagnosis of lung cancer. *Pattern Recognition* **42**(6) (2009) 1041–1051.

119. El-Baz, A., Gimelfarb, G., Falk, R., El-Ghar, M.A., Rainey, S., Heredia, D., Shaffer, T. Toward early diagnosis of lung cancer. In: *Proceedings of Medical Image Computing and Computer-Assisted Intervention (MICCAI'09)*, London, UK, Springer (2009) pp. 682–689.

120. El-Baz, A., Gimelfarb, G., Falk, R., El-Ghar, M.A., Suri, J. Appearance analysis for the early assessment of detected lung nodules. In: El-Baz, A., Suri, J. (Eds.), *Lung Imaging and Computer Aided Diagnosis*, Chapter 17, Boca Raton, FL, Taylor & Francis Group (2011) pp. 395–404.

121. El-Baz, A., Khalifa, F., Elnakib, A., Nitkzen, M., Soliman, A., McClure, P., Gimelfarb, G., El-Ghar, M.A. A novel approach for global lung registration using 3D Markov Gibbs appearance model. In: *Proceedings of International Conference Medical Image Computing and Computer-Assisted Intervention (MICCAI'12)*, Nice, France (October 1–5, 2012) pp. 114–121.

122. El-Baz, A., Nitzken, M., Elnakib, A., Khalifa, F., Gimelfarb, G., Falk, R., El-Ghar, M.A. 3D shape analysis for early diagnosis of malignant lung nodules. In: *Proceedings of International Conference Medical Image Computing and Computer-Assisted Intervention (MICCAI'11)*, Toronto, Canada (September 18–22, 2011) pp. 175–182.

123. El-Baz, A., Nitzken, M., Gimelfarb, G., Van Bogaert, E., Falk, R., El-Ghar, M.A., Suri, J. Three-dimensional shape analysis using spherical harmonics for early assessment of detected lung nodules. In: El-Baz, A., Suri, J. (Eds.), *Lung Imaging and Computer Aided Diagnosis*, Chapter 19, Boca Raton, FL, Taylor & Francis Group (2011) pp. 421–438.

124. El-Baz, A., Nitzken, M., Khalifa, F., Elnakib, A., Gimelfarb, G., Falk, R., El-Ghar, M.A. 3D shape analysis for early diagnosis of malignant lung nodules. In: *Proceedings of International Conference on Information Processing in Medical Imaging (IPMI'11)*, Bavaria, Germany, Monastery Irsee (July 3–8, 2011) pp. 772–783.

125. El-Baz, A., Nitzken, M., Vanbogaert, E., Gimelfarb, G., Falk, R., Abo El-Ghar, M. A novel shape-based diagnostic approach for early diagnosis of lung nodules. In: *Biomedical Imaging: From Nano to Macro, 2011 IEEE International Symposium on*, IEEE (2011) pp. 137–140.

126. El-Baz, A., Sethu, P., Gimelfarb, G., Khalifa, F., Elnakib, A., Falk, R., El-Ghar, M.A. Elastic phantoms generated by microfluidics technology: Validation of an imaged-based approach for accurate measurement of the growth rate of lung nodules. *Biotechnology Journal* **6**(2) (2011) 195–203.

127. El-Baz, A., Sethu, P., Gimelfarb, G., Khalifa, F., Elnakib, A., Falk, R., El-Ghar, M.A. A new validation approach for the growth rate measurement using elastic phantoms generated by state-of-the-art microfluidics technology. In: *Proceedings of IEEE International Conference on Image Processing (ICIP'10)*, Hong Kong (September 26–29, 2010) pp. 4381–4383.

128. El-Baz, A., Sethu, P., Gimelfarb, G., Khalifa, F., Elnakib, A., Falk, R., Suri, M.A.E.G.J. Validation of a new imaged-based approach for the accurate estimating of the growth rate of detected lung nodules using real CT images and elastic phantoms generated by state-of-the-art microfluidics technology. In: El-Baz, A., Suri, J.S. (Eds.), *Handbook of Lung Imaging and Computer Aided Diagnosis*, Volume 1. New York, Taylor & Francis Group (2011) pp. 405–420.

129. El-Baz, A., Yuksel, S.E., Elshazly, S., Farag, A.A. Non-rigid registration techniques for automatic follow-up of lung nodules. In: *Proceedings of Computer Assisted Radiology and Surgery (CARS'05)*, Berlin, Germany, Volume 1281. Elsevier (2005) pp. 1115–1120.

130. El-Baz, A.S., Suri, J.S. *Lung Imaging and Computer Aided Diagnosis*. Boca Raton, FL, CRC Press (2011).

131. Soliman, A., Khalifa, F., Shaffie, A., Liu, N., Dunlap, N., Wang, B., Elmaghraby, A., Gimelfarb, G., El-Baz, A. Image-based CAD system for accurate identification of lung injury. In: *Proceedings of IEEE International Conference on Image Processing (ICIP'16)*, IEEE (2016) pp. 121–125.

132. Soliman, A., Khalifa, F., Dunlap, N., Wang, B., El-Ghar, M., El-Baz, A. An iso-surfaces based local deformation handling framework of lung tissues. In: *Biomedical Imaging (ISBI), 2016 IEEE 13th International Symposium on*, IEEE (2016) pp. 1253–1259.

133. Soliman, A., Khalifa, F., Shaffie, A., Dunlap, N., Wang, B., Elmaghraby, A., El-Baz, A. Detection of lung injury using 4D-CT chest images. In: *Biomedical Imaging (ISBI), 2016 IEEE 13th International Symposium on*, IEEE (2016) pp. 1274–1277.

134. Eladawi, N., Elmogy, M., Ghazal, M., Helmy, O., Aboelfetouh, A., Riad, A., Schaal, S., El-Baz, A. Classification of retinal diseases based on OCT images. *Frontiers in Bioscience Landmark Journal* **23** (2018) 247–264.

135. ElTanboly, A., Ismail, M., Shalaby, A., Switala, A., El-Baz, A., Schaal, S., Gimelfarb, G., El-Azab, M. A computer aided diagnostic system for detecting diabetic retinopathy in optical coherence tomography images. *Medical Physics* **44** (2017) 914–923.

136. Khalifa, F., Beache, G., El-Baz, A., Gimelfarb, G. Deformable model guided by stochastic speed with application in cine images segmentation. In: *Proceedings of IEEE International Conference on Image Processing (ICIP'10)*, Hong Kong (September 26–29, 2010) pp. 1725–1728.

137. Khalifa, F., Beache, G.M., Elnakib, A., Sliman, H., Gimelfarb, G., Welch, K.C., El-Baz, A. A new shape-based framework for the left ventricle wall segmentation from cardiac first-pass perfusion MRI. In: *Proceedings of IEEE International Symposium on Biomedical Imaging: From Nano to Macro (ISBI'13)*, San Francisco, CA (April 7–11, 2013) pp. 41–44.

138. Khalifa, F., Beache, G.M., Elnakib, A., Sliman, H., Gimelfarb, G., Welch, K.C., El-Baz, A. A new non-rigid registration framework for improved visualization of transmural perfusion gradients on cardiac first–pass perfusion MRI. In: *Proceedings of IEEE International Symposium on Biomedical Imaging: From Nano to Macro (ISBI'12)*, Barcelona, Spain (May 2–5, 2012) pp. 828–831.

139. Khalifa, F., Beache, G.M., Firjani, A., Welch, K.C., Gimelfarb, G., El-Baz, A. A new nonrigid registration approach for motion correction of cardiac first-pass perfusion MRI. In: *Proceedings of IEEE International Conference on Image Processing (ICIP'12)*, Lake Buena Vista, FL (September 30–October 3, 2012) pp. 1665–1668.

140. Khalifa, F., Beache, G.M., Gimelfarb, G., El-Baz, A. A novel CAD system for analyzing cardiac first-pass MR images. In: *Proceedings of IAPR International Conference on Pattern Recognition (ICPR'12)*, Tsukuba Science City, Japan (November 11–15, 2012) pp. 77–80.

141. Khalifa, F., Beache, G.M., Gimelfarb, G., El-Baz, A. A novel approach for accurate estimation of left ventricle global indexes from short-axis cine MRI. In: *Proceedings of IEEE International Conference on Image Processing (ICIP'11)*, Brussels, Belgium (September 11–14, 2011) pp. 2645–2649.

142. Khalifa, F., Beache, G.M., Gimelfarb, G., Giridharan, G.A., El-Baz, A. A new image-based framework for analyzing cine images. In El-Baz, A., Acharya, U.R., Mirmedhdi, M., Suri, J.S. (Eds.), *Handbook of Multi Modality State-of-the-Art Medical Image Segmentation and Registration Methodologies*, Volume 2. New York, Springer (2011) pp. 69–98.

143. Khalifa, F., Beache, G.M., Gimelfarb, G., Giridharan, G.A., El-Baz, A. Accurate automatic analysis of cardiac cine images. *IEEE Transactions on Biomedical Engineering* **59**(2) (2012) 445–455.

144. Khalifa, F., Beache, G.M., Nitzken, M., Gimelfarb, G., Giridharan, G.A., El-Baz, A. Automatic analysis of left ventricle wall thickness using short-axis cine CMR images. In: *Proceedings of IEEE International Symposium on Biomedical Imaging: From Nano to Macro (ISBI'11)*, Chicago, IL (March 30–April 2, 2011) pp. 1306–1309.

145. Nitzken, M., Beache, G., Elnakib, A., Khalifa, F., Gimelfarb, G., El-Baz, A. Accurate modeling of tagged CMR 3D image appearance characteristics to improve cardiac cycle strain estimation. In: *Image Processing (ICIP), 2012 19th IEEE International Conference on*, Orlando, FL, IEEE (September 2012) pp. 521–524.

146. Nitzken, M., Beache, G., Elnakib, A., Khalifa, F., Gimelfarb, G., El-Baz, A. Improving full-cardiac cycle strain estimation from tagged CMR by accurate modeling of 3D image appearance characteristics. In: *Biomedical Imaging (ISBI), 2012 9th IEEE International Symposium on*, Barcelona, Spain, IEEE (May 2012) pp. 462–465 (Selected for oral presentation).

147. Nitzken, M.J., El-Baz, A.S., Beache, G.M. Markov-Gibbs random field model for improved full-cardiac cycle strain estimation from tagged CMR. *Journal of Cardiovascular Magnetic Resonance* **14**(1) (2012) 1–2.

148. Sliman, H., Elnakib, A., Beache, G., Elmaghraby, A., El-Baz, A. Assessment of myocardial function from cine cardiac MRI using a novel 4D tracking approach. *Journal of Computer Science and Systems Biology* **7** (2014) 169–173.

149. Sliman, H., Elnakib, A., Beache, G.M., Soliman, A., Khalifa, F., Gimelfarb, G., Elmaghraby, A., El-Baz, A. A novel 4D PDE-based approach for accurate assessment of myocardium function using cine cardiac magnetic resonance images. In: *Proceedings of IEEE International Conference on Image Processing (ICIP'14)*, Paris, France (October 27–30, 2014) pp. 3537–3541.

150. Sliman, H., Khalifa, F., Elnakib, A., Beache, G.M., Elmaghraby, A., El-Baz, A. A new segmentation-based tracking framework for extracting the left ventricle cavity from cine cardiac MRI. In: *Proceedings of IEEE International Conference on Image Processing (ICIP'13)*, Melbourne, Australia (September 15–18, 2013) pp. 685–689.

151. Sliman, H., Khalifa, F., Elnakib, A., Soliman, A., Beache, G.M., Elmaghraby, A., Gimelfarb, G., El-Baz, A. Myocardial borders segmentation from cine MR images using bi-directional coupled parametric deformable models. *Medical Physics* **40**(9) (2013) 1–13.

152. Sliman, H., Khalifa, F., Elnakib, A., Soliman, A., Beache, G.M., Gimelfarb, G., Emam, A., Elmaghraby, A., El-Baz, A. Accurate segmentation framework for the left ventricle wall from cardiac cine MRI. In: *Proceedings of International Symposium on Computational Models for Life Science (CMLS'13)*, Volume 1559, Sydney, Australia (November 27–29, 2013) pp. 287–296.

153. Ali, A.M., Farag, A.A., El-Baz, A. Graph cuts framework for kidney segmentation with prior shape constraints. In: *Proceedings of International Conference on Medical Image Computing and Computer-Assisted Intervention (MICCAI'07)*, Volume 1, Brisbane, Australia (October 29–November 2, 2007) pp. 384–392.

154. Chowdhury, A.S., Roy, R., Bose, S., Elnakib, F.K.A., El-Baz, A. Non-rigid biomedical image registration using graph cuts with a novel data term. In: *Proceedings of IEEE International Symposium on Biomedical Imaging: From Nano to Macro (ISBI'12)*, Barcelona, Spain (May 2–5, 2012) pp. 446–449.

155. El-Baz, A., Farag, A.A., Yuksel, S.E., El-Ghar, M.E.A., Eldiasty, T.A., Ghoneim, M.A. Application of deformable models for the detection of acute renal rejection. In Farag, A.A., Suri, J.S. (Eds.), *Deformable Models*, Volume 1. New York, Springer (2007) pp. 293–333.

156. El-Baz, A., Farag, A., Fahmi, R., Yuksel, S., El-Ghar, M.A., Eldiasty, T. Image analysis of renal DCE MRI for the detection of acute renal rejection. In: *Proceedings of IAPR International Conference on Pattern Recognition (ICPR'06)*, Hong Kong (August 20–24, 2006) pp. 822–825.

157. El-Baz, A., Farag, A., Fahmi, R., Yuksel, S., Miller, W., El-Ghar, M.A., El-Diasty, T., Ghoneim, M. A new CAD system for the evaluation of kidney diseases using DCE-MRI. In: *Proceedings of International Conference on Medical Image Computing and Computer-Assisted Intervention (MICCAI'08)*, Copenhagen, Denmark (October 1–6, 2006) pp. 446–453.

158. El-Baz, A., Gimelfarb, G., El-Ghar, M.A. A novel image analysis approach for accurate identification of acute renal rejection. In: *Proceedings of IEEE International Conference on Image Processing (ICIP'08)*, San Diego, CA (October 12–15, 2008) pp. 1812–1815.

159. El-Baz, A., Gimelfarb, G., El-Ghar, M.A. Image analysis approach for identification of renal transplant rejection. In: *Proceedings of IAPR International Conference on Pattern Recognition (ICPR'08)*, Tampa, FL (December 8–11, 2008) pp. 1–4.

160. El-Baz, A., Gimelfarb, G., El-Ghar, M.A. New motion correction models for automatic identification of renal transplant rejection. In: *Proceedings of International Conference on Medical Image Computing and Computer-Assisted Intervention (MICCAI'07)*, Brisbane, Australia (October 29–November 2, 2007) pp. 235–243.

161. Farag, A., El-Baz, A., Yuksel, S., El-Ghar, M.A., Eldiasty, T. A framework for the detection of acute rejection with Dynamic Contrast Enhanced Magnetic Resonance Imaging. In: *Proceedings of IEEE International Symposium on Biomedical Imaging: From Nano to Macro (ISBI'06)*, Arlington, VA (April 6–9, 2006) pp. 418–421.

162. Khalifa, F., Beache, G.M., El-Ghar, M.A., El-Diasty, T., Gimelfarb, G., Kong, M., El-Baz, A. Dynamic contrast-enhanced MRI-based early detection of acute renal transplant rejection. *IEEE Transactions on Medical Imaging* **32**(10) (2013) 1910–1927.

163. Khalifa, F., El-Baz, A., Gimelfarb, G., El-Ghar, M.A. Non-invasive image-based approach for early detection of acute renal rejection. In: *Proceedings of International Conference Medical Image Computing and Computer-Assisted Intervention (MICCAI'10)*, Beijing, China (September 20–24, 2010) pp. 10–18.

164. Khalifa, F., El-Baz, A., Gimelfarb, G., Ouseph, R., El-Ghar, M.A. Shape-appearance guided level-set deformable model for image segmentation. In: *Proceedings of IAPR International Conference on Pattern Recognition (ICPR'10)*, Istanbul, Turkey (August 23–26, 2010) pp. 4581–4584.

165. Khalifa, F., El-Ghar, M.A., Abdollahi, B., Frieboes, H., El-Diasty, T., El-Baz, A. A comprehensive non-invasive framework for automated evaluation of acute renal transplant rejection using DCE-MRI. *NMR in Biomedicine* **26**(11) (2013) 1460–1470.

166. Khalifa, F., El-Ghar, M.A., Abdollahi, B., Frieboes, H.B., El-Diasty, T., El-Baz, A. Dynamic contrast-enhanced MRI-based early detection of acute renal transplant rejection. In: *2014 Annual Scientific Meeting and Educational Course Brochure of the Society of Abdominal Radiology (SAR'14)*, Boca Raton, FL (March 23–28, 2014) CID: 1855912.

167. Khalifa, F., Elnakib, A., Beache, G.M., Gimelfarb, G., El-Ghar, M.A., Sokhadze, G., Manning, S., McClure, P., El-Baz, A. 3D kidney segmentation from CT images using a level set approach guided by a novel stochastic speed function. In: *Proceedings of International Conference Medical Image Computing and Computer-Assisted Intervention (MICCAI'11)*, Toronto, Canada (September 18–22, 2011) pp. 587–594.

168. Khalifa, F., Gimelfarb, G., El-Ghar, M.A., Sokhadze, G., Manning, S., McClure, P., Ouseph, R., El-Baz, A. A new deformable model-based segmentation approach for accurate extraction of the kidney from abdominal CT images. In: *Proceedings of IEEE International Conference on Image Processing (ICIP'11)*, Brussels, Belgium (September 11–14, 2011) pp. 3393–3396.

169. Mostapha, M., Khalifa, F., Alansary, A., Soliman, A., Suri, J., El-Baz, A. Computer-aided diagnosis systems for acute renal transplant rejection: Challenges and methodologies. In: El-Baz, A., Saba, J. Suri, L. (Eds.), *Abdomen and Thoracic Imaging*. Berlin, Germany, Springer (2014) pp. 1–35.

170. Shehata, M., Khalifa, F., Hollis, E., Soliman, A., Hosseini-Asl, E., El-Ghar, M.A., El-Baz, M., Dwyer, A.C., El-Baz, A., Keynton, R. A new non-invasive approach for early classification of renal rejection types using diffusion-weighted MRI. In: *IEEE International Conference on Image Processing (ICIP)*, IEEE (2016) pp. 136–140.

171. Khalifa, F., Soliman, A., Takieldeen, A., Shehata, M., Mostapha, M., Shaffie, A., Ouseph, R., Elmaghraby, A., El-Baz, A. Kidney segmentation from CT images using a 3D NMF-guided active contour model. In: *IEEE 13th International Symposium on Biomedical Imaging (ISBI)*, IEEE (2016) pp. 432–435.

172. Shehata, M., Khalifa, F., Soliman, A., Takieldeen, A., El-Ghar, M.A., Shaffie, A., Dwyer, A.C., Ouseph, R., El-Baz, A., Keynton, R. 3D diffusion MRI-based CAD system for early diagnosis of acute renal rejection. In: *Biomedical Imaging (ISBI), 2016 IEEE 13th International Symposium on*, IEEE (2016) pp. 1177–1180.

173. Shehata, M., Khalifa, F., Soliman, A., Alrefai, R., El-Ghar, M.A., Dwyer, A.C., Ouseph, R., El-Baz, A. A level set-based framework for 3D kidney segmentation from diffusion MR images. In: *IEEE International Conference on Image Processing (ICIP)*, IEEE (2015) pp. 4441–4445.

174. Shehata, M., Khalifa, F., Soliman, A., El-Ghar, M.A., Dwyer, A.C., Gimelfarb, G., Keynton, R., El-Baz, A. A promising non-invasive CAD system for kidney function assessment. In: *International Conference on Medical Image Computing and Computer-Assisted Intervention*, Athens, Greece, Springer (2016) pp. 613–621.

175. Khalifa, F., Soliman, A., Elmaghraby, A., Gimelfarb, G., El-Baz, A. 3D kidney segmentation from abdominal images using spatial-appearance models. *Computational and Mathematical Methods in Medicine* **2017** (2017) 9818506.

176. Hollis, E., Shehata, M., Khalifa, F., El-Ghar, M.A., El-Diasty, T., El-Baz, A. Towards non-invasive diagnostic techniques for early detection of acute renal transplant rejection: A review. *The Egyptian Journal of Radiology and Nuclear Medicine* **48**(1) (2016) 257–269.

177. Shehata, M., Khalifa, F., Soliman, A., El-Ghar, M.A., Dwyer, A.C., El-Baz, A. Assessment of renal transplant using image and clinical-based biomarkers. In: *Proceedings of 13th Annual Scientific Meeting of American Society for Diagnostics and Interventional Nephrology* (*ASDIN'17*), New Orleans, LA (February 10–12, 2017).

178. Shehata, M., Khalifa, F., Soliman, A., El-Ghar, M.A., Dwyer, A.C., El-Baz, A. Early assessment of acute renal rejection. In: *Proceedings of 12th Annual Scientific Meeting of American Society for Diagnostics and Interventional Nephrology* (*ASDIN'16*), Phoenix, AZ (February 19–21, 2016).

14 Automated Prostate Image Recognition and Segmentation

Ke Yan, Xiuying Wang, Jinman Kim, Changyang Li, Dagan Feng, and Mohamed Khadra

CONTENTS

INTRODUCTION

Prostate diseases, such as prostate cancer, prostatitis, and enlarged prostate, are common in males [1]. In addition to its high incidence, prostate cancer also brings high mortality. According to the American Cancer Society [2], prostate cancer was the second leading cause of cancer death in American men in 2016 (approximately 26,120 deaths), behind only lung and bronchus cancers.

In clinical practice, when a patient is deemed at risk of prostate cancer after blood test or rectal examination, the patient is generally required to have a biopsy to confirm diagnosis. A urologist will perform biopsy of the patient to cut out small samples (typically 12 sites) of tissue from the prostate and a pathologist will identify whether the cells are malignant or benign [3]. However, prostate biopsy is an invasive, painful procedure, has a significant risk of infection, and is subject to false-negative results, in particular, when none of the samples are cut from the lesion areas [3]. Alternative noninvasive, biomedical imaging-based methods have recently been widely explored for prostate cancer assessment [4–7]. Imaging-based prostate cancer assessment, computer-aided diagnosis (CAD) systems can be employed to provide automated approaches to the recognition and segmentation of the prostate and this is a fundamental requirement in the analysis of prostate cancer; recognition is to identify the site of the prostate in the image volume and segmentation is used to quantify the volume of the prostate [8]. This approach has the potential to negate the subjectivity and reduce the time needed in manual segmentation and recognition of the prostate [1].

This chapter introduces and discusses a wide range of methods for prostate image recognition and segmentation. We will first present common imaging modalities used for prostate cancer diagnoses and treatments; in particular, the imaging properties of prostate T2-weighted (T2W) MRI for its capabilities toward prostate recognition and segmentation. Then, we will review various conventional methods for prostate image recognition and segmentation, including recent approaches using deep learning-based methods.

CHALLENGES OF PROSTATE IMAGE RECOGNITION AND SEGMENTATION

TYPES OF BIOMEDICAL IMAGES

MRI, computed tomography (CT), and transrectal ultrasound (TRUS) are the three primary imaging modalities for prostate cancer diagnoses and treatments. The inner-sights of prostate provided by each imaging modality significantly differ from each other, and the use of a particular method depends on the clinical aim. For examples, MRI is normally used in diagnostic and treatment planning for prostate cancer [9–11]; in prostate brachytherapy, CT is employed for the radioactive seeds localization after treatment [9]; TRUS could assist in determining prostate volume and prostate biopsy [9,12]. The characteristics [9] of each imaging modality are summarized in Table 14.1.

As MRI allows cancer detection and staging which are the sequent aims of prostate recognition and segmentation, this chapter will focus on the methods conducted on prostate MRI. We suggest readers refer to other references for potential usage of TRUS and CT for prostate recognition and processing [13–15]. With regard to MRI, there are multiple parametric types of image acquisition protocols such as T2W, diffusion-weighted imaging (DWI), dynamic contrast-enhanced imaging (DCE), and MR spectroscopy imaging (MRS). These multiple types are often used in combination, for example, multiparametric MRI (mpMRI), where different imaging types provide complementary information. T2W-MRI provides reliable anatomical visualization of the transitional and peripheral zones [16], which enables the recognition of prostate tumors. DWI quantitatively provides tumor apparent diffusion coefficient (ADC) values, which can be used in predicting the aggressiveness of tumors in clinical practice [16]. High b-value image (BVAL) from DWI could generate increased delineation between tumors and healthy tissues. DWI is also usually combined

TABLE 14.1

The Characteristics of Prostate MRI, CT, and TRUS

	MRI	CT	TRUS
Price	Expensive	Expensive	Inexpensive
Portable	χ	χ	✓
Real-time imaging	χ	χ	✓
Radiation involved	χ	✓	χ
Imaging contrast for prostate	High	Medium	Low
Cancer detection	✓	χ	χ
Cancer assessment	✓	χ	χ

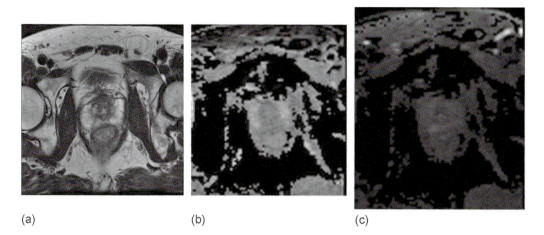

(a)   (b)   (c)

FIGURE 14.1   Example prostate MRI. (a) T2W, (b) ADC, and (c) BVAL.

with T2W-MRI to measure the prostate tumor volume. DCE can be used for the assessment of perfusion and vascular permeability of prostate tumor [16]. MRS can be used to assess the intracellular concentrations of choline and citrate, and thus can differentiate and grade prostate tumors in which the ratios of choline-to-citrate are higher. Since most prostate MRI recognition and segmentation methods work on T2W, we specify MRI to the certain type of T2W image in the rest of this chapter, unless otherwise specified (Figure 14.1).

IMAGING PROPERTIES OF PROSTATE MRI FOR RECOGNITION AND SEGMENTATION

MRI produces a set of tomographic slices of a prostate volume. As shown in Figure 14.2, in addition to prostate, other tissues and organs (i.e., bladder, hip, and rectum) are also scanned on the image.

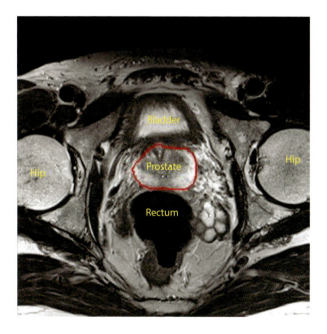

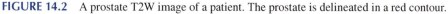

FIGURE 14.2   A prostate T2W image of a patient. The prostate is delineated in a red contour.

There are three major challenges to automated prostate MRI recognition and segmentation, which we define into three core categories:

1. *Image noise*: Circuit noise, transmission noise of imaging equipment [17], inappropriate imaging-testing position of patients, and other sources of noise inherently bring low quality to the MR images. Gaussian noise, salt-and-pepper noise, and speckle noise [18] are the major three types of image noises. The image noise distorts the one-channel pixels (image intensities) and makes them less informative, which increases the difficulty of prostate recognition.
2. *Intensity inhomogeneity*: Tumors' regions in the prostate are typically inhomogeneous. Such intensity inhomogeneity poses challenges to derive consistent image features to characterize the prostate, which are necessary for prostate recognition and segmentation.
3. *Blurred boundaries*: The blurred boundaries of prostate on MRI lead to the false positive predictions to recognition algorithms, and significantly impede segmentation algorithms delineating prostate.

PROSTATE IMAGE RECOGNITION

Many prostate image segmentation algorithms employ initial points or atlas mapping to localize prostate, thus we define two major categories for prostate image recognition.

SEMI-AUTOMATED APPROACHES

The prostate image segmentation algorithms [19–24] require one or more initial point(s) to trace the prostate boundary. The exact position of the initial point selected by a user depends on the particular algorithm, either inside the prostate [23,24] or around/on the boundary [19–22]. These user-intervened methods could be categorized into the semi-automated approach for prostate recognition and (or) segmentation which benefit by reliable point initialization but negate the possibility of developing fully-automated CAD.

ATLAS MAPPING

Atlas is a global probabilistic cloud, in which many human annotations corresponding to different prostate images are stacked and masked. The density of each pixel/voxel on the atlas indicates the corresponding likelihood the pixel/voxel being foreground. Many prostate image segmentation works [10,25–30] employ atlas mapping to obtain foreground seeds so that their algorithms could be fully automated. To serve for prostate image recognition, atlas is registered [31] with the testing image so that it is applicable to the particular image. Afterward, the foreground and background seeds could be selected by a pre-defined threshold as described in Li et al [25]. The atlas mapping based methods are robust to contrast differences and incorporate shape and intensity information; however, they are prone to registration errors as noted in Ghose et al. [9].

PROSTATE IMAGE SEGMENTATION

We categorize prostate image segmentation approaches into four major groups according to method models.

CONTOUR AND SHAPE-BASED APPROACHES

A set of works, including contour-based methods and deformable model-based methods, exploit the contours and shape information in prostate segmentation. Contour-based methods [19,22,23] usually extract edges and ridges in images via gradient filters, and recognize or trace the boundaries by their proposed schemes, for example, the longest curvilinear structure [23] and moving masks [19,22]. However, the edge detectors may not always be reliable due to the artifacts (blurred/broken boundaries) on biomedical images.

Since deformable model was first introduced by Terzopoulos [32], it has been widely applied in many prostate segmentation works [24,33–38] using contour and shape information. Deformable models are curves or surfaces and usually formed under the control of internal and external energies [39]. Internal energies preserve the smoothness of curves (surfaces) during deformation, and external energies force curves (surfaces) toward the anatomical structure boundaries [9]. By minimizing the joint internal and external energies, deformable models can be evolved to the desired positions. Active shape model (ASM) [40] is one of the most popular modalities used in deformable prostate models [37,41–46]. In ASM-based methods, a statistical shape model (SSM) [47] is constructed with shape variations using principle component analysis (PCA) on a set of landmarks, and then ASM is performed to delineate prostate. As ASM overlooks the interdependencies of shape and appearance [48], active appearance model (AAM) [49] thus is developed for the purpose of combination of shape and appearance. However, as noted in Toth et al. [48], conventional ASM and AAM based methods are hindered by the use of landmarks. To solve this issue, Toth et al. [48] proposed a novel landmark-free AAM-based method for more accurate and robust prostate segmentation on MRI. Other modalities applied in deformable models for prostate segmentation include level-set [50–55], active contour model [56–61], and so on.

GRAPH-BASED APPROACHES

Many prostate segmentation works [62–70] rebuild prostate images as (un)directed graphs, usually followed by a cost function. The atomic units (pixels, voxels, superpixels, or supervoxels) are the nodes of graph, and the edge weights are measured by the "distances" of pairs of nodes. The essential parts of these graph-based approaches are the design of edge weights on graphs and cost functions. Positions [62] and intensities [62,66,70] of pixels (voxels, superpixels, or supervoxels) are the two extensively used measurements for edge weights. As the utilization of position and intensity are usually limited by the biomedical image artifacts, some works employ other information, such as prior shape knowledge [67] and image gradients [69], to estimate edge weights. The cost functions are various across the graph-based methods, but most of them [63,64,66,68,70] are formulated based on graph-cut model [71]. In addition to graph-cut, Lagrange function [62], and other special designed functions (e.g., shape probability function and gradient profile model in [69]) can also be applied to energy minimization scheme. However, the fixed parameters for balancing cost function need carefully tuning so that may hinder the robustness of these methods across different datasets.

After the construction of graph model, some other works [72–74] formulate segmentation as labeling propagation problem, in which unlabeled nodes could be predicted by pre-defined labeled nodes. Random walker [75] could be an effective and efficient algorithm to solve the labelling propagation problem in prostate segmentation [72–74].

FEATURE EXTRACTION AND CLASSIFICATION APPROACHES

The classification-based approaches extract a set of image features as feature vectors, and tend to partition feature space (vector space associated with feature vectors [9]) into two or more groups. The classic classifiers, such as support vector machine [76] and random forest [77], have been extensively studied in the last decades and proved favorable capacity of feature space partition, thus can also be applied in prostate segmentation works. Gray level intensity and spatial coordinate are the simple but useful common features that are widely used in many works [78–81]. Other computer vision features, such as histogram of oriented gradients [82,83], Haar features [82,83], curvature [80], Haralick texture features [81], and Laws energy features [81], are also widely employed to differentiate prostate. Ghosh et al. [84] imposed prior knowledge on texture and shape features by genetic algorithm, which achieved better segmentation results compared to Laws energy features. Instead of classic classifiers, Li et al. [83] proposed a set of location-adaptive classifiers which enable effectively gathering of local information and propagation of them to other regions. Gao et al. [82] proposed an extended sparse representation based classification to address the issue of low contrast on prostate images.

HYBRID SEGMENTATION APPROACHES

As hybrid techniques are robust to noise and produce superior results in the presence of shape and texture variations of the prostate [9], most works combine two or even more methods for prostate segmentation.

As a common prostate segmentation approach, deformable models are usually combined with various techniques to boost performance. Graph-based methods and classification-based methods are usually employed to initialize deformable models in many works [33,36,52,85,86]. Zhan et al. [36] tentatively labeled voxels by proposed Gabor-SVM classifier to feed the later deformable surface model. Martin et al. [33] utilized atlas to map a specific prostate image before deformable model. For more reliable initialization of deformable model, Guo et al. [85] employed deep learning features to estimate rough prostate recognition map. Different from aforementioned works exploiting priors for deformable models, the results by deformable models in the work of [11,87] can also be treated as location and shape priors for other techniques (i.e., Bayesian classification).

Classification-based approaches are usually followed by a graph-cut based cost function in a set of works [63,66,80,88,89]. Such combination focuses on local features in patch classification phase; meanwhile, the correlations of neighboring patches/pixels can be attributed to smoothness in cost function. Other hybrid segmentation methods can be found in Martin et al. [10] (atlas and shape model combined), Lu et al. [90] (level-set and registration combined), Liao et al. [91] (representation learning and labeling propagation combined), and so on.

DEEP LEARNING FOR PROSTATE RECOGNITION AND SEGMENTATION

In computer vision, image features learned via deep neural networks (DNN) have proved to be more intrinsic and semantic encodings for image segmentation and classification. Many deep learning approaches are proposed to extract the high-level image features, such as with the stacked autoencoder (SAE) [92], convolutional neural network (CNN) [93], and deep Boltzmann machine [94]. To apply deep learning algorithms on prostate image recognition and segmentation, images are typically: either (1) partitioned into a set of superpixels and the deep learning algorithms then perform binary classification for each superpixel; (2) or directly fed into CNN and produce the corresponding pixelwise segmentation map. The first approach is a sparse segmentation as it predicts the segmentation map in superpixel scale, and the latter one is a dense segmentation. In this section, we first present two state-of-the-art deep learning-based methods for sparse prostate image recognition and segmentation, employing SAE and CNN, respectively. Then, we introduce two top-performing algorithms with CNN on dense prostate image segmentation. The prostate MR Image Segmentation 2012 (PROMISE12) dataset [95] is used to validate and evaluate the methods. This dataset contains 50 cases which are multicenter and multi-vendor and have different acquisition protocols [65]. Each case is composed of 15–54 prostate transverse T2W-MR images. Manual segmentation is available for each case and used as the ground truth.

COMPREHENSIVE AUTOENCODER FOR SUPERPIXEL CLASSIFICATION (PROSTATE IMAGE RECOGNITION)

The prostate recognition method [96] via SAE consists of four stages as shown in Figure 14.3.

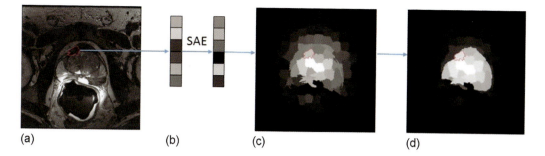

(a)   (b)   (c)   (d)

FIGURE 14.3 Pipeline of the SAE-based method [96] for prostate image recognition. (a) Early feature extraction. (b) Superpixel reconstruction. (c) Superpixel classification. (d) Refinement.

Early Feature Descriptors

Before feeding SAE, two early feature descriptors (i.e., the intensity descriptor and the position descriptor) should be gained. Denote a prostate image as I. SLIC algorithm [97] is applied on I to segment I into N superpixels $\{P\}$. Then, an early feature vector $f(P)$ could be gained for P with details as follows:

Intensity descriptor: Intensity histogram IH(P), with 20 bins in [96], is employed to describe P's intensity. Note that the number of pixels are variable among different superpixels; intensity histogram IH(P) should be normalized to have a uniform sum to address this issue.

Position descriptor: Generally, the prostate is approximately located at the center area of patient MR image. To use this spatial prior knowledge, the bounding box of P is extracted as

$$C(P) = \{c_v(\alpha_{v,1}, \alpha_{v,2}) : v = 1,2\} \tag{14.1}$$

where c_1 and c_2 are the top-left coordinate and bottom-right coordinate of $C(P)$ in image I, respectively. $\alpha_{v,1}$ and $\alpha_{v,2}$ are c_v's values corresponding to x-axis and y-axis, respectively. Then, the position information of P could be described by

$$POS(P) = \left\{ t(v,u) = \frac{\alpha_{v,u}}{(2-u)n + (u-1)m} : v = 1,2; u = 1,2 \right\} \tag{14.2}$$

Early feature vector: Given the intensity and position descriptors of P, a superpixel-wise feature vector $f(P)$ is generated as

$$f(P) = \{IH(P); POS(P)\} \tag{14.3}$$

Prostate Stacked Autoencoder Model

The obtained early feature vectors of prostate superpixels are input to a stacked autoencoder (SAE). SAE could extract high-level features and perform the reconstruction of input data. As shown in Figure 14.4, three autoencoders are stacked; hence a six-layer network, including three encoding layers and three decoding layers, is formed.

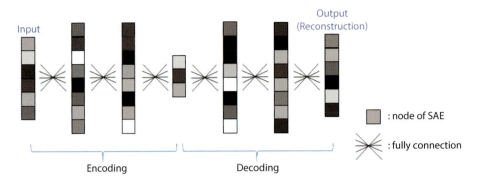

Input

Output
(Reconstruction)

: node of SAE

: fully connection

Encoding Decoding

FIGURE 14.4 Architecture of the SAE. The output of each layer is the input for its subsequent layer. The output of the last layer is a reconstruction for the input data.

Superpixel Classification

The output of the SAE is the reconstruction of the input superpixel, which could be used for classification. For a superpixel, set the reconstruction error as

$$\text{err}(P) = \sum_{\omega=1}^{W} \exp\left(\tau \| f(P)_\omega - y(P)_\omega \|^2\right) \tag{14.4}$$

where $f(P)_\omega$ and $y(P)_\omega$ are the ωth elements of $f(P)$ and the output of the SAE, respectively. W is the dimension of $f(P)$ and $y(P)$. τ controls the distance between different superpixels' reconstruction errors within an image and is set to 100 empirically. The reconstruction error is adopted to measure the probability of a superpixel being prostate tissue. This is because as the SAE model is learned from the set of prostate superpixels, the prostate superpixel should have a lower reconstruction error than the background superpixel does and vice versa [96].

Denote the probability map obtained from superpixels' reconstruction errors as D^{AE}. In the next subsection, a refined prostate detection map with better suppressed background, more smooth inner region, and clear boundary is generated based on D^{AE}.

Refinement

The refinement of D^{AE} is to assign a label $HO_p \in \{0,1\}$ to a pixel p to measure whether p belongs to foreground or not. For the set of pixels' labeling $O = \{O_p: p \in I\}$, this can be solved by minimizing the energy function [98]

$$E(O) = \sum_{p \in I} H(O_p) + \xi \sum_{(p,q) \in Y} \frac{1}{1 + \sqrt{3(I_p - I_q)^2}} \cdot T(O_p \neq O_q) \tag{14.5}$$

where Y is a set of all pairs of neighboring pixels. $H(O_p)$ is the cost for assigning a label O_p to a pixel p. D^{AE} is used to approximate the label cost of pixels. The second term in Equation 14.5 encourages intensity and spatial coherence by penalizing discontinuities [71] between neighboring pixels, with the parameter ξ controlling the scale of discontinuity penalty. $T(\cdot)$ is 1 if the condition inside the parentheses is true and 0 otherwise.

Minimum cut/maximum flow algorithms [71] can minimize Equation 14.5 and generate the corresponding prostate detection map D^{mf}. Then D^{AE} and D^{mf} are linearly combined as the final prostate detection map:

$$D = \frac{D^{AE} + D^{mf}}{2} \tag{14.6}$$

Results

Precision-recall (PR) curve and F-measure [98,99] are two major evaluation metrics in object recognition. The F-measure is calculated based on *Precision* and *Recall* by

$$F_\eta = \frac{(1+\eta^2)\cdot Precision\cdot Recall}{\eta^2\cdot Precision + Recall} \tag{14.7}$$

An atlas-based seeds-selection in segmentation approach (RW) [74] and three popular classifiers, that is, support vector machine (SVM) with radial basis function kernel, random forest (RF), and naïve Bayes (NB), were chosen as comparison methods. Precision and F-measure of the SAE-based method reported by Yan et al. [96] are 86.99% and 68.32%, respectively. SAE-based method [96] outperformed all the comparison methods by >4% precision and >5% F-measure (RW: 82.86% precision, 62.20% F-measure; SVM: 63.94% precision, 62.28% F-measure; RF: 55.06% precision, 57.66% F-measure; NB: 48.94% precision, 50.33% F- measure).

CONVOLUTIONAL NEURAL NETWORKS FOR SUPERPIXEL CLASSIFICATION (PROSTATE IMAGE SEGMENTATION)

This subsection will introduce a novel model [100] for prostate image segmentation via deep neural networks. A 3D prostate image volume P is composed of m transverses $\{T_1, T_2, ..., T_m\}$. The aim of the prostate segmentation of P is to generate m segmentation maps $\{S^{T1}, S^{T2}, ..., S^{Tm}\}$ corresponding to each transverse. The 3D prostate image segmentation method [100] via CNN consists of two stages. In the first stage, the algorithm performs binary classification for each superpixel and explores n prostate proposals $\{I_1^{T_j}, I_2^{T_j}, ..., I_n^{T_j}\}$ for each transverse T_j; In the second stage, the algorithm selects a typical prostate proposal from $\{I_k^{T_j}\}$, where $k \in \{1,2, ..., n\}$, as the segmentation map S^{T_j} for T_j. For simplification, we use T to denote T_j, that is, a specific transverse in the remaining parts of this subsection, unless otherwise specified.

Superpixel Classification and Prostate Proposal

A Geodesic Object Proposals (GOP) algorithm [101] is applied to find candidate objects $\{O^T\}$ over T. To improve efficiency of the algorithm, $\{O^T\}$ are trimmed by atlas probability map $\mathscr{A} \in [0,1]$ as follows.

For a specific O^T from $\{O^T\}$, the accuracy score $AS(O^T)$ and coverage score $CS(O^T)$ [102] compared to $\mathscr{A}$ can be calculated. The two scores are used to measure the confidence of prostate recognition by O^T [102]:

$$C\left(O^T\right) = \frac{(1+\beta)\times AS(O^T)\times CS(O^T)}{\beta \times AS(O^T) + CS(O^T)} \tag{14.8}$$

The global prostate proposals $\{I^{(g)T}\}$ for T can be formed by the candidate objects from $\{O^T\}$ with 25 top confidence values. Then, CNN is employed to refine each candidate object as follows.

For the transverse T, the local context $TL_{I(g)T}$ corresponding to the specific $I^{(g)T}$ is the subregion of T where the bounding box of the prostate proposal on $TL_{I(g)T}$ covers. In order to capture the context near the prostate boundary, $TL_{I(g)T}$ is expanded with 10 pixels on each side. The aim is to measure the likelihood of each superpixel on $TL_{I(g)T}$ being prostate. To achieve it, $TL_{I(g)T}$ is input to a deep convolutional network for classification of patches. As one of the most popular convolutional networks, the AlexNet [103] model is adopted and thus $TL_{I(g)T}$ is resized to 227×227 pixels to fit the input structure of AlexNet model. In addition to $TL_{I(g)T}$, a 227×227 size mask is also input to convolutional network together with $TL_{I(g)T}$ to indicate position of superpixel, in which the region of superpixel is set to 1 and the remaining is set to 0.

The final prostate proposal I^T can be obtained by

$$I^T = \alpha I^{(g)T} + (1-\alpha) I^{(l)T} \tag{14.9}$$

where α is set to 0.3 to emphasize the impact of local refinement and then binarized by the threshold of 0.5.

Graph Model for 3D Prostate Segmentation

In the previous stage, n prostate proposals as $L^T = \{I^T\}$ could be obtained for a specific transverse, corresponding to each $I^{(g)T}$ in $\{I^{(g)T}\}$. Then the features of each prostate proposal are calculated as edge weight of graph. The feature of I^T is composed of intensity histogram (intensity descriptor), Inner-Distance Shape Context [104] (shape descriptor), and $C(I^T)$ via (Equation 14.8) (position descriptor). Denote intensity descriptor and shape descriptor of I^T as ID_IT and SD_IT, respectively.

With the features of all I^T, that is, ID_IT, SD_IT, and $C(I^T)$, a directed graph $\mathcal{G} = (V, E)$ is constructed to indicate the differences among I^T. V is the set of nodes and $E \subseteq V \times V$ is the set of edges in $\mathcal{G}$. Inspired by Meng et al. [105], the construction of $\mathcal{G}$ is as follows:

1. $V = \{V_0, V_1, \ldots, V_m, V_{m+1}\}$; $V_0 = \mathcal{A}$; $V_{m+1} = \mathcal{A}$; and $V_j = L^{Tj}$
   where $j \in \{1, 2, \ldots, m\}$.
2. For $\forall (u, v) \in E$, if $u \in V_i$, then $v \in V_{i+1}$ where $i \in \{0, 1, \ldots m\}$.
3. The weight of edge $e = (u, v)$ is calculated by

$$w(u, v) = \left(1 - \sigma\left(ID_u, ID_v\right)\right) + \phi\left(SD_u, SD_v\right) + \| C(u) - C(v) \| \tag{14.10}$$

where $\sigma(\cdot)$ is the histogram intersection and $\phi(\cdot)$ is the Hausdorff distance.

Finally, the optimal prostate proposals for each transverse can be selected by searching the path on $\mathcal{G}$ with minimum weight cost from node V_0 to node V_{m+1}, which can be easily solved by any shortest path algorithm (such as Dijkstra's algorithm [106] and the Bellman-Ford algorithm [107,108]). The selected $\{I^{Tj}\}$ are adopted as the final segmentation maps $\{S^{Tj}\}$.

Results

Four state-of-the-art methods [34,41,79,109] are selected as the comparisons with the method. Following Kirschner et al. and Vincent et al. [34,109], dice similarity coefficient (*DSC*) and Hausdorff distance (*HD*) are used as the quantitative metrics for evaluation:

$$DSC = \frac{2|X \cap Y|}{|X| + |Y|} \tag{14.11}$$

$$HD_{asym}(X_s, Y_s) = \max\left(\min_{x \in X_s} \min_{y \in Y_s} \varphi(x, y)\right) \tag{14.12}$$

$$HD(X_s, Y_s) = \max\left(HD_{asym}(X_s, Y_s), HD_{asym}(X_s, Y_s)\right) \tag{14.13}$$

where X and Y are the algorithm segmentation and reference segmentation respectively; X_s and Y_s are the surface points of the algorithm segmentation and reference segmentation respectively; and $\varphi(\cdot)$ is the Euclidean distance. *DSC* of the CNN method [100], RF [79], PAS [34], MAC [41], and AAM [109] are 0.89, 0.73, 0.86, 0.85, and 0.88, respectively. *HD* of the CNN method [100], PAS [34], and AAM [109] are 3.8, 9.5, and 4.1, respectively. *HD* of RF [79] and MAC [41] are not available.

CONVOLUTIONAL NEURAL NETWORKS FOR DENSE PROSTATE IMAGE SEGMENTATION

The sparse segmentation (superpixel classification) methods are more likely to get trapped into the inherent limitations of superpixel pre-segmentation, in particular near the blurred prostate boundaries. To alleviate this problem and produce a dense segmentation map from CNN, Long et al. [110] proposed fully convolutional networks (FCN) for pixelwise semantic segmentation on general images. After that, some state-of-the-art CNN models were invented to segment 3D prostate image volume. V-Net [111] and Volumetric ConvNets [1] are the top two CNN-based 3D prostate image segmentation methods.

The structures of V-Net and Volumetric ConvNets are similar. They use the sequent convolution+pooling blocks to encode the images, producing compressed feature maps. To decompress the feature maps to gain the pixelwise segmentation maps, they then use deconvolution+convolution blocks to upsample the feature maps progressively. Convolutional layer is the essential component in CNN, which will filter the distracting information out of images so that the algorithm can focus on the intrinsic image structures. The convolutional layer in CNN can be illustrated as follows. A typical filter $F \in \mathbb{R}^{u \times v \times d}$ convolves the input data $X \in \mathbb{R}^{m \times h \times d}$ by [112]

$$Y_{ij} = b + \sum_{p=1}^{d} \sum_{k=1}^{u} \sum_{l=1}^{v} F_{klp} \times X_{i+k-1, j+l-1, p} \qquad (14.14)$$

where b is a bias attached with F. The filter F and the bias b are learnable during the training phase. The optimal F and b would urge CNN to produce ideal segmentation maps across different images. Deconvolution is the transpose of convolution, which supports input upsampling and output cropping [112]. Therefore, deconvolution is usually employed to predict dense segmentation maps from relatively small feature maps.

Both V-Net and Volumetric ConvNets participated in MICCAI Grand Challenge (Prostate MR Image Segmentation 2012). From the PROMISE12 leaderboard, V-Net and Volumetric ConvNets achieved scores of 82.39 and 86.65, respectively; particularly, Volumetric ConvNets ranked first among all participants.

SUMMARY

Prostate image recognition and segmentation are broadly categorized into DNN and non-DNN methods. In DNN models, sparse connectivity and shared weights allow features to be detected regardless of their position in visual field; pooling operation makes detected features less sensitive to input shift and distortion. Therefore, DNN methods are the state of the art in performance and could overcome some limitations in non-DNN methods. The future research direction on prostate imaging will move to prostate lesion detection and classification. By taking advantages of DNN features, deep learning-based approaches will be extensively explored in the field. The DNN methods introduced in this chapter on prostate image recognition and segmentation could be extended to lesion detection; however, huge variations among prostate lesions in terms of shape, size, and Gleason score make prostate lesion processing more difficult than prostate recognition and segmentation.

REFERENCES

1. L. Yu, X. Yang, H. Chen, J. Qin, and P.-A. Heng, "Volumetric ConvNets with mixed residual connections for automated prostate segmentation from 3D MR images," *AAAI*, 2017, pp. 66–72.
2. R. L. Siegel, K. D. Miller, and A. Jemal, "Cancer statistics, 2016," *CA: A Cancer Journal for Clinicians*, vol. 66, pp. 7–30, 2016.
3. Tests for Prostate Cancer. September, 2016. Available: https://www.cancer.org/cancer/prostate-cancer/detection-diagnosis-staging/how-diagnosed.html

4. G. P. Murphy, A. L. Boynton, E. H. Holmes, and R. J. Barren III, "Non-invasive methods to detect prostate cancer," ed: Google Patents, 2001.

5. P. Kozlowski, S. D. Chang, E. C. Jones, K. W. Berean, H. Chen, and S. L. Goldenberg, "Combined diffusion-weighted and dynamic contrast-enhanced MRI for prostate cancer diagnosis—Correlation with biopsy and histopathology," *Journal of Magnetic Resonance Imaging*, vol. 24, pp. 108–113, 2006.

6. S. A. Reinsberg, G. S. Payne, S. F. Riches, S. Ashley, J. M. Brewster, V. A. Morgan et al., "Combined use of diffusion-weighted MRI and 1H MR spectroscopy to increase accuracy in prostate cancer detection," *American Journal of Roentgenology*, vol. 188, pp. 91–98, 2007.

7. N. Hara, M. Okuizumi, H. Koike, M. Kawaguchi, and V. Bilim, "Dynamic contrast-enhanced magnetic resonance imaging (DCE-MRI) is a useful modality for the precise detection and staging of early prostate cancer," *The Prostate*, vol. 62, pp. 140–147, 2005.

8. G. Litjens, J. Barentsz, N. Karssemeijer, and H. Huisman, "Automated computer-aided detection of prostate cancer in MR images: From a whole-organ to a zone-based approach," in *SPIE Medical Imaging*, 2012, pp. 83150G.

9. S. Ghose, A. Oliver, R. Martí, X. Lladó, J. C. Vilanova, J. Freixenet et al., "A survey of prostate segmentation methodologies in ultrasound, magnetic resonance and computed tomography images," *Computer Methods and Programs in Biomedicine*, vol. 108, pp. 262–287, 2012.

10. S. Martin, V. Daanen, and J. Troccaz, "Atlas-based prostate segmentation using an hybrid registration," *International Journal of Computer Assisted Radiology and Surgery*, vol. 3, pp. 485–492, 2008.

11. N. Makni, P. Puech, R. Lopes, A.-S. Dewalle, O. Colot, and N. Betrouni, "Combining a deformable model and a probabilistic framework for an automatic 3D segmentation of prostate on MRI," *International Journal of Computer Assisted Radiology and Surgery*, vol. 4, pp. 181–188, 2009.

12. F. Shao, K. V. Ling, W. S. Ng, and R. Y. Wu, "Prostate boundary detection from ultrasonographic images," *Journal of Ultrasound in Medicine*, vol. 22, pp. 605–623, 2003.

13. Y. Liu, W. Ng, M. Teo, and H. Lim, "Computerised prostate boundary estimation of ultrasound images using radial bas-relief method," *Medical and Biological Engineering and Computing*, vol. 35, pp. 445–454, 1997.

14. Y. Yu, J. Cheng, J. Li, W. Chen, and B. Chiu, "Automatic prostate segmentation from transrectal ultrasound images," in *Biomedical Circuits and Systems Conference (BioCAS), 2014 IEEE*, 2014, pp. 117–120.

15. L. Ma, R. Guo, Z. Tian, R. Venkataraman, S. Sarkar, X. Liu et al., "Combining population and patient-specific characteristics for prostate segmentation on 3D CT images," in *SPIE Medical Imaging*, 2016, pp. 978427.

16. L. M. Johnson, B. Turkbey, W. D. Figg, and P. L. Choyke, "Multiparametric MRI in prostate cancer management," *Nature Reviews Clinical Oncology*, vol. 11, pp. 346–353, 2014.

17. A. Li, "Medical image segmentation based on Dirichlet energies and priors," 2014.

18. C. Y. Li, "Statistical analysis based segmentation for multimodality images," PhD, University of Sydney, 2012.

19. M. Samiee, G. Thomas, and R. Fazel-Rezai, "Semi-automatic prostate segmentation of MR images based on flow orientation," in *Signal Processing and Information Technology, 2006 IEEE International Symposium on*, 2006, pp. 203–207.

20. S. S. Mahdavi, N. Chng, I. Spadinger, W. J. Morris, and S. E. Salcudean, "Semi-automatic segmentation for prostate interventions," *Medical Image Analysis*, vol. 15, pp. 226–237, 2011.

21. J. Yuan, W. Qiu, E. Ukwatta, M. Rajchl, Y. Sun, and A. Fenster, "An efficient convex optimization approach to 3D prostate MRI segmentation with generic star shape prior," *Prostate MR Image Segmentation Challenge, MICCAI*, vol. 7512, pp. 82–89, 2012.

22. D. Flores-Tapia, G. Thomas, N. Venugopa, B. McCurdy, and S. Pistorius, "Semi automatic MRI prostate segmentation based on wavelet multiscale products," in *Engineering in Medicine and Biology Society, 2008. EMBS 2008. 30th Annual International Conference of the IEEE*, 2008, pp. 3020–3023.

23. R. Zwiggelaar, Y. Zhu, and S. Williams, "Semi-automatic segmentation of the prostate," in *Pattern Recognition and Image Analysis*, ed: Springer, Berlin, Heidelberg, 2003, pp. 1108–1116.

24. B. Maan and F. van der Heijden, "Prostate MR image segmentation using 3D active appearance models," in *MICCAI Grand Challenge: Prostate MR Image Segmentation*, 2012.

25. A. Li, C. Li, X. Wang, S. Eberl, D. Feng, and M. Fulham, "A combinatorial Bayesian and Dirichlet model for prostate MR image segmentation using probabilistic image features," *Physics in Medicine and Biology*, vol. 61, p. 6085, 2016.

26. S. Klein, U. A. van der Heide, I. M. Lips, M. van Vulpen, M. Staring, and J. P. Pluim, "Automatic segmentation of the prostate in 3D MR images by atlas matching using localized mutual information," *Medical Physics*, vol. 35, pp. 1407–1417, 2008.

27. J. A. Dowling, J. Fripp, S. Chandra, J. P. W. Pluim, J. Lambert, J. Parker et al., "Fast automatic multi-atlas segmentation of the prostate from 3D MR images," in *International Workshop on Prostate Cancer Imaging*, Springer, Berlin, Heidelberg, 2011, pp. 10–21.

28. T. R. Langerak, U. A. van der Heide, A. N. Kotte, M. A. Viergever, M. Van Vulpen, and J. P. Pluim, "Label fusion in atlas-based segmentation using a selective and iterative method for performance level estimation (SIMPLE)," *IEEE Transactions on Medical Imaging*, vol. 29, pp. 2000–2008, 2010.

29. O. Acosta, J. Dowling, G. Cazoulat, A. Simon, O. Salvado, R. De Crevoisier et al., "Atlas based segmentation and mapping of organs at risk from planning ct for the development of voxel-wise predictive models of toxicity in prostate radiotherapy," in *International Workshop on Prostate Cancer Imaging*, Springer, Berlin, Heidelberg, 2010, pp. 42–51.

30. O. Acosta, A. Simon, F. Monge, F. Commandeur, C. Bassirou, G. Cazoulat et al., "Evaluation of multi-atlas-based segmentation of CT scans in prostate cancer radiotherapy," in *Biomedical Imaging: From Nano to Macro, 2011 IEEE International Symposium on*, 2011, pp. 1966–1969.

31. D.-J. Kroon and C. H. Slump, "MRI modality transformation in demon registration," in *Biomedical Imaging: From Nano to Macro, 2009. ISBI'09. IEEE International Symposium on*, 2009, pp. 963–966.

32. D. Terzopoulos, "On matching deformable models to images," in *Topical Meeting on Machine Vision Technical Digest Series*, 1987, pp. 160–167.

33. S. Martin, J. Troccaz, and V. Daanen, "Automated segmentation of the prostate in 3D MR images using a probabilistic atlas and a spatially constrained deformable model," *Medical Physics*, vol. 37, pp. 1579–1590, 2010.

34. M. Kirschner, F. Jung, and S. Wesarg, "Automatic prostate segmentation in MR images with a probabilistic active shape model," *MICCAI Grand Challenge: Prostate MR Image Segmentation*, vol. 2012, 2012.

35. Y. Guo, Y. Gao, Y. Shao, T. Price, A. Oto, and D. Shen, "Deformable segmentation of 3D MR prostate images via distributed discriminative dictionary and ensemble learning," *Medical Physics*, vol. 41, p. 072303, 2014.

36. Y. Zhan and D. Shen, "Deformable segmentation of 3-D ultrasound prostate images using statistical texture matching method," *Medical Imaging, IEEE Transactions on*, vol. 25, pp. 256–272, 2006.

37. R. Toth, P. Tiwari, M. Rosen, G. Reed, J. Kurhanewicz, A. Kalyanpur et al., "A magnetic resonance spectroscopy driven initialization scheme for active shape model based prostate segmentation," *Medical Image Analysis*, vol. 15, pp. 214–225, 2011.

38. S. S. Chandra, J. A. Dowling, K.-K. Shen, P. Raniga, J. P. Pluim, P. B. Greer et al., "Patient specific prostate segmentation in 3-D magnetic resonance images," *Medical Imaging, IEEE Transactions on*, vol. 31, pp. 1955–1964, 2012.

39. C. Xu, D. L. Pham, and J. L. Prince, "Image segmentation using deformable models," *Handbook of Medical Imaging*, vol. 2, pp. 129–174, 2000.

40. T. F. Cootes, C. J. Taylor, D. H. Cooper, and J. Graham, "Active shape models-their training and application," *Computer Vision and Image Understanding*, vol. 61, pp. 38–59, 1995.

41. R. Toth, B. N. Bloch, E. M. Genega, N. M. Rofsky, R. E. Lenkinski, M. A. Rosen et al., "Accurate prostate volume estimation using multifeature active shape models on T2- weighted MRI," *Academic Radiology*, vol. 18, pp. 745–754, 2011.

42. X. Tang, Y. Jeong, R. J. Radke, and G. T. Chen, "Geometric- model-based segmentation of the prostate and surrounding structures for image-guided radiotherapy," in *Electronic Imaging 2004*, SPIE, Bellingham, Washington USA, 2004, pp. 168–176.

43. Y. Zhu, S. Williams, and R. Zwiggelaar, "A hybrid ASM approach for sparse volumetric data segmentation," *Pattern Recognition and Image Analysis*, vol. 17, pp. 252–258, 2007.

44. A. C. Hodge, A. Fenster, D. B. Downey, and H. M. Ladak, "Prostate boundary segmentation from ultrasound images using 2D active shape models: Optimisation and extension to 3D," *Computer Methods and Programs in Biomedicine*, vol. 84, pp. 99–113, 2006.

45. Q. Feng, M. Foskey, W. Chen, and D. Shen, "Segmenting CT prostate images using population and patient-specific statistics for radiotherapy," *Medical Physics*, vol. 37, pp. 4121–4132, 2010.

46. T. F. Cootes, A. Hill, C. J. Taylor, and J. Haslam, "The use of active shape models for locating structures in medical images," in *Information Processing in Medical Imaging*, Springer, Berlin, Heidelberg, 1993, pp. 33–47.

47. D. Shen, Y. Zhan, and C. Davatzikos, "Segmentation of prostate boundaries from ultrasound images using statistical shape model," *Medical Imaging, IEEE Transactions on*, vol. 22, pp. 539–551, 2003.

48. R. Toth and A. Madabhushi, "Multifeature landmark-free active appearance models: Application to prostate MRI segmentation," *Medical Imaging, IEEE Transactions on*, vol. 31, pp. 1638–1650, 2012.

49. T. F. Cootes, G. J. Edwards, and C. J. Taylor, "Active appearance models," *IEEE Transactions on Pattern Analysis & Machine Intelligence*, pp. 681–685, 2001.

50. S. Fan, L. K. Voon, and N. W. Sing, "3D prostate surface detection from ultrasound images based on level set method," in *Medical Image Computing and Computer-Assisted Intervention—MICCAI 2002*, ed: Springer, Berlin, Heidelberg, 2002, pp. 389–396.

51. K. Zhang, L. Zhang, H. Song, and W. Zhou, "Active contours with selective local or global segmentation: A new formulation and level set method," *Image and Vision Computing*, vol. 28, pp. 668–676, 2010.

52. W. Xiong, A. L. Li, S. H. Ong, and Y. Sun, "Automatic 3D prostate MR image segmentation using graph cuts and level sets with shape prior," in *Advances in Multimedia Information Processing–PCM 2013*, ed: Springer, Cham, 2013, pp. 211–220.

53. N. N. Kachouie, P. Fieguth, and S. Rahnamayan, "An elliptical level set method for automatic TRUS prostate image segmentation," in *Signal Processing and Information Technology, 2006 IEEE International Symposium on*, 2006, pp. 191–196.

54. C. Li, R. Huang, Z. Ding, J. C. Gatenby, D. N. Metaxas, and J. C. Gore, "A level set method for image segmentation in the presence of intensity inhomogeneities with application to MRI," *Image Processing, IEEE Transactions on*, vol. 20, pp. 2007–2016, 2011.

55. A. Tsai, A. Yezzi Jr, W. Wells, C. Tempany, D. Tucker, A. Fan et al., "A shape-based approach to the segmentation of medical imagery using level sets," *Medical Imaging, IEEE Transactions on*, vol. 22, pp. 137–154, 2003.

56. A. Zaim and J. Jankun, "An energy-based segmentation of prostate from ultrasound images using dot-pattern select cells," in *Acoustics, Speech and Signal Processing, 2007. ICASSP 2007. IEEE International Conference on*, 2007, pp. I-297.

57. C. Knoll, M. Alcañiz, V. Grau, C. Monserrat, and M. C. Juan, "Outlining of the prostate using snakes with shape restrictions based on the wavelet transform (Doctoral Thesis: Dissertation)," *Pattern Recognition*, vol. 32, pp. 1767–1781, 1999.

58. H. M. Ladak, F. Mao, Y. Wang, D. B. D. B. Downey, D. Steinman, and A. Fenster, "Prostate segmentation from 2D ultrasound images," in *Engineering in Medicine and Biology Society, 2000. Proceedings of the 22nd Annual International Conference of the IEEE*, 2000, pp. 3188–3191.

59. M. Ding, C. Chen, Y. Wang, I. Gyacskov, and A. Fenster, "Prostate segmentation in 3D US images using the cardinal- spline-based discrete dynamic contour," in *Medical Imaging 2003*, 2003, pp. 69–76.

60. A. Jendoubi, J. Zeng, and M. F. Chouikha, "Segmentation of prostate ultrasound images using an improved snakes model," in *Signal Processing, 2004. Proceedings. ICSP'04. 2004 7th International Conference on*, IEEE, Piscataway, New Jersey, US, 2004, pp. 2568–2571.

61. P. A. Yushkevich, J. Piven, H. C. Hazlett, R. G. Smith, S. Ho, J. C. Gee et al., "User-guided 3D active contour segmentation of anatomical structures: Significantly improved efficiency and reliability," *Neuroimage*, vol. 31, pp. 1116–1128, 2006.

62. W. Du, S. Wang, A. Oto, and Y. Peng, "Graph-based prostate extraction in T2-weighted images for prostate cancer detection," in *Fuzzy Systems and Knowledge Discovery (FSKD), 2015 12th International Conference on*, IEEE, Piscataway, New Jersey, US, 2015, pp. 1225–11229.

63. S. Ghose, J. Mitra, A. Oliver, R. Marti, X. Llado, J. Freixenet et al., "Graph cut energy minimization in a probabilistic learning framework for 3D prostate segmentation in MRI," in *Pattern Recognition (ICPR), 2012 21st International Conference on*, IEEE, Piscataway, New Jersey, US, 2012, pp. 125–128.

64. A. S. Korsager, V. Fortunati, F. van der Lijn, J. Carl, W. Niessen, L. R. Østergaard et al., "The use of atlas registration and graph cuts for prostate segmentation in magnetic resonance images," *Medical Physics*, vol. 42, pp. 1614–1624, 2015.

65. D. Mahapatra, "Graph cut based automatic prostate segmentation using learned semantic information," in *Biomedical Imaging (ISBI), 2013 IEEE 10th International Symposium on*, 2013, pp. 1316–1319.

66. D. Mahapatra and J. M. Buhmann, "Visual saliency based active learning for prostate MRI segmentation," in *Machine Learning in Medical Imaging*, ed: Springer, Cham, 2015, pp. 9–16.

67. Q. Song, X. Wu, Y. Liu, M. Smith, J. Buatti, and M. Sonka, "Optimal graph search segmentation using arc-weighted graph for simultaneous surface detection of bladder and prostate," in *Medical Image Computing and Computer-Assisted Intervention–MICCAI 2009*, ed: Springer, Berlin, Heidelberg, 2009, pp. 827–835.

68. Z. Tian, L. Liu, and B. Fei, "A supervoxel-based segmentation for prostate MR images," in *SPIE Medical Imaging*, 2015, pp. 941318.

69. K. Wu, C. Garnier, H. Shu, and J.-L. Dillenseger, "Prostate segmentation on T2 MRI using Optimal Surface Detection," *IRBM*, vol. 34, pp. 287–290, 2013.

70. M. Zouqi and J. Samarabandu, "Prostate segmentation from 2- D ultrasound images using graph cuts and domain knowledge," in *Computer and Robot Vision, 2008. CRV'08. Canadian Conference on*, IEEE, Piscataway, New Jersey, US, 2008, pp. 359–362.

71. Y. Boykov and V. Kolmogorov, "An experimental comparison of min-cut/max-flow algorithms for energy minimization in vision," *Pattern Analysis and Machine Intelligence, IEEE Transactions on*, vol. 26, pp. 1124–1137, 2004.

72. Y. Artan, M. A. Haider, and I. S. Yetik, "Prostate cancer segmentation using multispectral random walks," in *Prostate Cancer Imaging: Computer-Aided Diagnosis, Prognosis, and Intervention*, ed: Springer, Berlin, Heidelberg, 2010, pp. 15–24.

73. P. Khurd, L. Grady, K. Gajera, M. Diallo, P. Gall, M. Requardt et al., "Facilitating 3D spectroscopic imaging through automatic prostate localization in MR images using random walker segmentation initialized via boosted classifiers," in *Prostate Cancer Imaging. Image Analysis and Image-Guided Interventions*, ed: Springer, Berlin, Heidelberg, 2011, pp. 47–56.

74. A. Li, C. Li, X. Wang, S. Eberl, D. D. Feng, and M. Fulham, "Automated Segmentation of Prostate MR Images Using Prior Knowledge Enhanced Random Walker," in *Digital Image Computing: Techniques and Applications (DICTA), 2013 International Conference on*, IEEE, Piscataway, New Jersey, US, 2013, pp. 1–7.

75. L. Grady, "Random walks for image segmentation," *Pattern Analysis and Machine Intelligence, IEEE Transactions on*, vol. 28, pp. 1768–1783, 2006.

76. B. E. Boser, I. M. Guyon, and V. N. Vapnik, "A training algorithm for optimal margin classifiers," in *Proceedings of the Fifth Annual Workshop on Computational Learning Theory*, ACM, New York City, 1992, pp. 144–152.

77. T. K. Ho, "Random decision forests," in *Document Analysis and Recognition, 1995, Proceedings of the Third International Conference on*, 1995, pp. 278–282.

78. S. Ghose, A. Oliver, J. Mitra, R. Martí, X. Lladó, J. Freixenet et al., "A supervised learning framework of statistical shape and probability priors for automatic prostate segmentation in ultrasound images," *Medical Image Analysis*, vol. 17, pp. 587–600, 2013.

79. S. Ghose, J. Mitra, A. Oliver, R. Martí, X. Lladó, J. Freixenet et al., "A random forest based classification approach to prostate segmentation in MRI," *MICCAI Grand Challenge: Prostate MR Image Segmentation*, vol. 2012, pp. 125–128, 2012.

80. D. Mahapatra and J. M. Buhmann, "Prostate MRI segmentation using learned semantic knowledge and graph cuts," *Biomedical Engineering, IEEE Transactions on*, vol. 61, pp. 756–764, 2014.

81. E. Moschidis and J. Graham, "Automatic differential segmentation of the prostate in 3-D MRI using Random Forest classification and graph-cuts optimization," in *Biomedical Imaging (ISBI), 2012 9th IEEE International Symposium on*, 2012, pp. 1727–1730.

82. Y. Gao, S. Liao, and D. Shen, "Prostate segmentation by sparse representation based classification," *Medical Physics*, vol. 39, pp. 6372–6387, 2012.

83. W. Li, S. Liao, Q. Feng, W. Chen, and D. Shen, "Learning image context for segmentation of the prostate in CT-guided radiotherapy," *Physics in Medicine and Biology*, vol. 57, p. 1283, 2012.

84. P. Ghosh and M. Mitchell, "Segmentation of medical images using a genetic algorithm," in *Proceedings of the 8th Annual Conference on Genetic and Evolutionary Computation*, 2006, pp. 1171–1178.

85. Y. Guo, Y. Gao, and D. Shen, "Deformable MR prostate segmentation via deep feature learning and sparse patch matching," *IEEE Transactions on Medical Imaging*, vol. 35, pp. 1077–1089, 2015.

86. Z. Tian, L. Liu, Z. Zhang, and B. Fei, "Superpixel-based segmentation for 3D prostate MR images," *IEEE Transactions on Medical Imaging*, vol. 35, pp. 791–801, 2015.

87. L. Gong, S. D. Pathak, D. R. Haynor, P. S. Cho, and Y. Kim, "Parametric shape modeling using deformable superellipses for prostate segmentation," *Medical Imaging, IEEE Transactions on*, vol. 23, pp. 340–349, 2004.

88. Q. Gao, A. Asthana, T. Tong, Y. Hu, D. Rueckert, and P. Edwards, "Hybrid Decision Forests for Prostate Segmentation in Multi-channel MR Images," in *2014 22nd International Conference on Pattern Recognition (ICPR)*, IEEE, Piscataway, New Jersey, US, 2014, pp. 3298–3303.

89. P. Wu, Y. Liu, Y. Li, and B. Liu, "Robust Prostate Segmentation Using Intrinsic Properties of TRUS Images," *Medical Imaging, IEEE Transactions on*, vol. 34, pp. 1321–1335, 2015.

90. C. Lu, S. Chelikani, X. Papademetris, J. P. Knisely, M. F. Milosevic, Z. Chen et al., "An integrated approach to segmentation and nonrigid registration for application in image-guided pelvic radiotherapy," *Medical Image Analysis*, vol. 15, pp. 772–785, 2011.

91. S. Liao, Y. Gao, A. Oto, and D. Shen, "Representation learning: A unified deep learning framework for automatic prostate MR segmentation," in *Medical Image Computing and Computer-Assisted Intervention–MICCAI 2013*, ed: Springer, Berlin, Heidelberg, 2013, pp. 254–261.

92. S. Liu, S. Liu, W. Cai, S. Pujol, R. Kikinis, and D. Feng, "Early diagnosis of Alzheimer's disease with deep learning," in *Biomedical Imaging (ISBI), 2014 IEEE 11th International Symposium on*, 2014, pp. 1015–1018.

93. K. Simonyan and A. Zisserman, "Very deep convolutional networks for large-scale image recognition," *arXiv preprint arXiv:1409.1556*, 2014.

94. R. Salakhutdinov and G. E. Hinton, "Deep Boltzmann machines," in *AISTATS*, 2009, p. 3.

95. G. Litjens, R. Toth, W. van de Ven, C. Hoeks, S. Kerkstra, B. van Ginneken et al., "Evaluation of prostate segmentation algorithms for MRI: The PROMISE12 challenge," *Medical Image Analysis*, vol. 18, pp. 359–373, 2014.

96. K. Yan, C. Li, X. Wang, Y. Yuan, A. Li, J. Kim et al., "Comprehensive autoencoder for prostate recognition on MR images," in *2016 IEEE 13th International Symposium on Biomedical Imaging (ISBI)*, 2016, pp. 1190–1194.

97. R. Achanta, A. Shaji, K. Smith, A. Lucchi, P. Fua, and S. Susstrunk, "SLIC superpixels compared to state-of-the-art superpixel methods," *Pattern Analysis and Machine Intelligence, IEEE Transactions on*, vol. 34, pp. 2274–2282, 2012.

98. N. Tong, H. Lu, X. Ruan, and M.-H. Yang, "Salient Object Detection via Bootstrap Learning," in *Proceedings of the IEEE Conference on Computer Vision and Pattern Recognition*, 2015, pp. 1884–1892.

99. J. Xu, L. Xiang, Q. Liu, H. Gilmore, J. Wu, J. Tang et al., "Stacked Sparse Autoencoder (SSAE) for nuclei detection on breast cancer histopathology images," *IEEE Transactions on Medical Imaging*, vol. 35, pp. 119–130, 2015.

100. K. Yan, C. Li, X. Wang, A. Li, Y. Yuan, D. Feng et al., "Automatic prostate segmentation on MR images with deep network and graph model," in *Engineering in Medicine and Biology Society (EMBC), 2016 IEEE 38th Annual International Conference of the*, 2016, pp. 635–638.

101. P. Krähenbühl and V. Koltun, "Geodesic object proposals," in *Computer Vision–ECCV 2014*, ed: Springer, Cham, 2014, pp. 725–739.

102. L. Wang, H. Lu, X. Ruan, and M.-H. Yang, "Deep Networks for Saliency Detection via Local Estimation and Global Search," in *Proceedings of the IEEE Conference on Computer Vision and Pattern Recognition*, 2015, pp. 3183–3192.

103. A. Krizhevsky, I. Sutskever, and G. E. Hinton, "ImageNet classification with deep convolutional neural networks," in *Advances in Neural Information Processing Systems*, MIT, Cambridge, Massachusetts, 2012, pp. 1097–1105.

104. H. Ling and D. W. Jacobs, "Shape classification using the inner-distance," *Pattern Analysis and Machine Intelligence, IEEE Transactions on*, vol. 29, pp. 286–299, 2007.

105. F. Meng, H. Li, G. Liu, and K. N. Ngan, "Object co- segmentation based on shortest path algorithm and saliency model," *Multimedia, IEEE Transactions on*, vol. 14, pp. 1429–1441, 2012.

106. E. W. Dijkstra, "A note on two problems in connexion with graphs," *Numerische Mathematik*, vol. 1, pp. 269–271, 1959.

107. R. Bellman, "On a routing problem," Technical report, DTIC Document, 1956.

108. L. R. Ford, *Network Flow Theory*, Santa Monica, CA: Rand Corporation, 1956.

109. G. Vincent, G. Guillard, and M. Bowes, "Fully automatic segmentation of the prostate using active appearance models," *MICCAI Grand Challenge: Prostate MR Image Segmentation*, vol. 2012, pp. 359–373, 2012.

110. J. Long, E. Shelhamer, and T. Darrell, "Fully convolutional networks for semantic segmentation," in *Proceedings of the IEEE Conference on Computer Vision and Pattern Recognition*, 2015, pp. 3431–3440.

111. F. Milletari, N. Navab, and S.-A. Ahmadi, "V-Net: Fully Convolutional Neural Networks for Volumetric Medical Image Segmentation," *arXiv preprint arXiv:1606.04797*, 2016.

112. A. Vedaldi and K. Lenc, "MatConvNet: Convolutional neural networks for MATLAB," in *Proceedings of the 23rd Annual ACM Conference on Multimedia Conference*, ACM, New York City, 2015, pp. 689–692.

15 Precision Imaging of Prostate Cancer

Computer-Aided Detection and Their Clinical Applications

Baowei Fei

CONTENTS

INTRODUCTION

Prostate cancer (PCa) is currently the most common cancer in men and the second leading cause of cancer-related deaths among men in the United States [1]. In 2015, it was estimated that the number of new cases and deaths would be 220,800 and 27,540, respectively, accounting for 26.0% of new cancer cases and 8.8% of cancer deaths for American men [1].

The prostate is subdivided into the base, mid-gland, and apex from superior to inferior. The prostate also has four anatomic zones: the transition zone (TZ), which contains 5% of the glandular tissue and accounts for around 25% of PCa; the central zone (CZ), which contains 20% of the glandular tissue and accounts for around 5% of PCa; the peripheral zone (PZ), which contains 70%–80% of the glandular tissue and accounts for about 70% of PCa; and the non-glandular anterior fibromuscular stroma. Accurate localization of PCa within the TZ or the PZ is extremely important as TZ prostate cancer is associated with favorable pathologic features and better recurrence-free survival [2].

At present, the clinical standard for definitive diagnosis of prostate cancer is transrectal ultrasound (TRUS)-guided sextant or systematic biopsy. The prostate-specific antigen (PSA) blood test and digital rectal examination (DRE) results are considered to identify patients who need biopsy. The actual impact of MRI for prostate cancer management is through guided biopsies and improved cancer diagnosis and staging yield. In recent years, magnetic resonance imaging (MRI) targeted prostate biopsies have been showing better disease localization and more accurate sampling than conventional TRUS-guided biopsy in various studies [3–6]. Sophisticated MRI-based computer-assisted imaging for individual patients would offer such a significant role in defining an optimal targeted biopsy and interventional approach. Several approaches have been explored to improve the accuracy of image-guided targeted prostate biopsy, including in-bore MRI-guided, cognitive fusion, and MRI/TRUS fusion-guided biopsy [7].

MR imaging provides excellent soft-tissue contrast and has become an imaging modality of choice for localization of prostate tumors. Multiparametric MRI (mpMRI) includes high-resolution T2-weighted (T2W) MRI, diffusion-weighted imaging (DWI), dynamic contrast-enhanced imaging (DCE-MR), and MR spectroscopy (MRS). The mpMRI has proven to be an effective technique to localize high-risk prostate cancer [8,9]. The combined use of anatomic and functional information provided by the multiparametric approach increases the accuracy of MR imaging in detecting and staging prostate cancer [8,9]. It can also help guide biopsies to achieve a higher tumor detection rate and better reflect the true Gleason grade. The European Society of Urogenital Radiology (ESUR) in 2012 established the Prostate Imaging-Reporting and Data System (PI-RADS) scoring system for multiparametric MRI of the prostate [10]. The MR PI-RADS aims to enable consistent interpretation, communication, and reporting of prostate mpMRI findings [10,11]. A joint steering committee, formed by the American College of Radiology, ESUR, and the AdMeTech Foundation, has recently announced an updated version of the proposals of PI-RADS version 2 (v2) [12]. Prostate mpMRI at 3 T had been recommended in PI-RADS v2. Generally, CAD systems are classified into two categories: computer-aided detection (CADe) and computer-aided diagnosis (CADx) systems. Currently, most CAD systems in prostate MRI focus on local suspicious lesions and discrimination between benign and malignant lesions; most of them are computer-aided diagnosis systems. As the combination of various MR images creates large amounts of data, supportive techniques or tools, such as computer-aided diagnosis (CADx), are needed in order to make a clinical decision in a fast, effective, and reliable way.

In the past 10 years, computer-aided techniques have developed rapidly. Automated computer-aided detection and diagnosis may help improve diagnostic accuracy of PCa, and reduce interpretation variation between and within observers [13,14]. Prostate cancer diagnosis requires an experienced radiologist to read prostate MRI, and such expertise is not widely available. Addition of CADx may significantly improve the performance of less-experienced observers in prostate cancer diagnosis. When less-experienced observers used CADx, they reached similar performance as experienced observers [13]. In a more recent study, the use of CAD can also improve prostate mpMRI study interpretation in experienced readers [15]. For cases in which radiologists are less confident, they can get higher performance by using the computer output. A recent study showed a pattern recognition system enables radiologists to have a lower variability in diagnosis, decreases false negative rates, and reduces the time to recognize and delineate structures in the prostate [16]. The benefit of CADx also includes guiding biopsy using cancer location information from MRI [14]. Therefore, along with rapid development of MR technique, CADx of prostate cancer has become an active field of research in the last 5 years.

This chapter starts with the review of MR image acquisition technology and then focuses on a comprehensive review of the state-of-the-art image quantification methods. The part on validation and clinical applications is a reference of the literature available in the clinical management of the disease. The chapter closes with a discussion and future perspectives.

MR IMAGE ACQUISITIONS

Contemporary MR imaging of the prostate combines anatomic images from high-resolution T1W and T2W sequences and functional information obtained from DWI, DCE, and MRS. The combination of conventional anatomical and functional MRI is known as multiparametric MRI. The PI-RADS Prostate MR Guidelines published in 2012 suggest the use of T2W images plus 2 functional techniques [10]. The anatomy of the prostate gland is visualized with T2W images; DWI and MRS add specificity to lesion characterization, while DCE-MRI has a high sensitivity in cancer detection. In the PI-RADS v2, the essential components of the mpMRI prostate examination are T2W, DWI, and DCE [12]. For the PZ, DWI is the primary determining sequence. For the TZ, T2W is the primary determining sequence. In order to obtain high and stable accuracy, a combination of anatomical and functional imaging is necessary in clinical practice. Recent studies showed an increasing interest in developing CADx systems to detect and characterize prostate cancer on the basis of an mpMR imaging approach [14,15,17,18]. T2W MR images are frequently used in mpMRI CADx systems. T2W plus DWI and DCE-MRI are also commonly used among the combinations.

T2WI and T2 Mapping

The anatomy of the prostate gland is best visualized with T2W images. The acquisition of high-resolution T2W images of the prostate is the first and most important step in an mpMR imaging protocol. In T2W images, the peripheral zone of the prostate has hyperintense signal, whereas the central and transition zones have low signal, allowing the zonal anatomy of the prostate to be clearly delineated (Figure 15.1). In T2W images (Figure 15.2), PCa in the peripheral zone is usually depicted as a low-signal area. However, the growth pattern and the aggressiveness of the tumor can

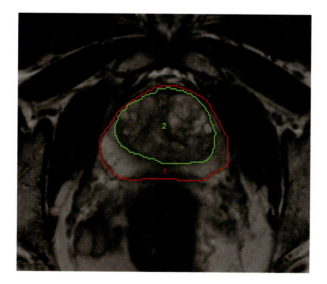

FIGURE 15.1 High-resolution T2-weighted MRI. T2-weighted MR images can differentiate the normal intermediate- to high-signal-intensity peripheral zone (Region 1) from the low-signal-intensity central and transition zones (Region 2).

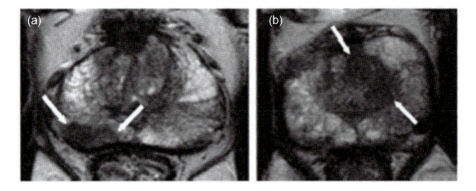

FIGURE 15.2 High-resolution T2-weighted MR images of prostate cancer. (a) There is a low-signal intensity lesion on the right peripheral zone (white arrows) at the mid-gland of the prostate. At prostatectomy, the lesion was classified as a Gleason grade 7 (4 + 3) prostate adenocarcinoma. (b) An ill-defined homogeneous low-signal intensity area at the left transition zone (white arrows) at mid-gland of the prostate in another patient. TRUS-guided biopsy showed a Gleason grade 8 (4 + 4) prostate adenocarcinoma on the corresponding position. (From Neto, J.A., and Parente, D.B., *Magn. Reson. Imaging Clin. N. Am.*, 21, 409–426, 2013.)

alter its appearance. T2W MR imaging has been advocated as an accurate technique in the detection of PCa in the transition zone [19,20]. The value of T2W MR images is also in predicting pathological stage and extracapsular extension of PCa [21].

Because T2W MR images play an important role in both location and staging of PCa, T2W MRI is the basis and important sequence in CADx systems for PCa. In T2W MR images, the tumor region of interest (ROI) has more dark pixels than bright pixels, whereas the normal tissue ROI has more bright pixels than dark pixels. Different features, including fractal features, textural features, and signal intensity can be used by CADx. Because prostate cancers at the central gland and peripheral zone usually have significantly different texture on T2W MR images [22], and because the use of mpMRI may have challenges for detecting cancer at the transition zone [23], a CADx system that can analyze features based on the lesion's location may be able to aid in the detection of suspicious lesions.

T2 maps offer quantitative T2 values. As the standard T2 mapping approach of performing multiple single spin-echo acquisitions with a range of TE settings requires excessive scan times, the T2 mapping is not include in most clinical applications. Recently, some new sequences can provide an effective approach to speed up T2 quantification [24,25]. T2 values of histologically proven malignant tumor areas were significantly lower than the suspicious lesions but nonmalignant lesions or normal areas [26]. The use of quantitative T2 measurement improves the specificity and/or sensitivity of prostate cancer detection [27] and aggressiveness assessment [28,29]. There is a potential benefit of incorporating quantitative T2 values into CADx systems.

DYNAMIC CONTRAST-ENHANCED MRI (DCE-MRI)

DCE-MRI, which enables visualization of vascular permeability and perfusion, is an important tool in oncology to define tumor. DCE-MRI is sensitive to alterations in vascular permeability, extracellular space, and blood flow. The clinical application of DCE-MRI for prostate cancer is based on data showing that malignant lesions show earlier and faster enhancement and earlier contrast agent washout compared with healthy prostate tissues (Figure 15.3) [30].

The DCE-MRI data can be analyzed with various semiquantitative or quantitative models to extract parameters related to vascular permeability, extracellular space, blood flow, and water exchange [31]. Semiquantitative DCE-MRI data are only relative to the patient; the baseline intensity is highly variable depending on the patient and the MRI protocol. It is necessary to use indicators relating to signal amplitude. The most commonly quantitative approach to analyzing DCE-MRI

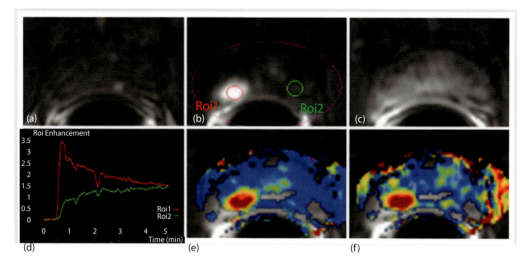

FIGURE 15.3 Dynamic contrast-enhanced MRI (DCE-MRI) of the prostate. (a) Axial T1 GRE unenhanced image. (b) After contrast agent administration, an area with early enhancement is seen on the right in the peripheral zone (ROI1) with significant washout in the late-phase image (c). (d) The curve (red) with early enhancement is a typical finding in the case of prostate cancer, while healthy prostate tissue is characterized by a steady slow enhancement (green). High transport constants K^{trans} (e) and k_{ep} (f) can confirm suspicion of prostate cancer. Prostate adenocarcinoma with a Gleason score of $4 + 5 = 9$ was diagnosed after prostatectomy. (From Durmus, T. et al., *Aktuelle Urol.*, 45, 119–126, 2014.)

involves two-compartment pharmacokinetic (PK) models that can be used to generate pharmacokinetic parameters such as K^{trans} (transfer of gadolinium contrast from the vasculature to the tumor, representing forward vascular perfusion and permeability) and K_{ep} (reverse transfer of contrast agent from the extracellular space back to the plasma, representing backward leakage) in order to quantify tumor enhancement and the contrast uptake and washout [32]. However, pharmacokinetic model implementation typically involves assuming some prior knowledge; and the arterial input function (AIF) estimation methodology can have significant effects on the parameters estimated by PK modeling [33]. The empirical approach based on phenomenological universalities (PUN) is able to reproduce experimental data from a DCE-MRI acquisition [34,35].

Different CADx systems have been developed to analyze the DCE-MRI data. Vos et al. developed a CADx system capable of discriminating PCa from nonmalignant disorders in the peripheral zone and achieved a diagnostic accuracy of 0.83 (0.75–0.92) [36]. They also developed an automated segmentation per patient calibration method to improve the diagnostic accuracy of CADx [37]. Puech et al. designed a prostate CADx software to provide a 5-level cancer suspicion score for suspicious foci detected in DCE-MRI and T1-weighted images [38,39].

DCE-MRI usually has lower spatial resolution than other sequences, especially when DCE-MRI is performed rapidly in a short period of time. Limitations in the interpretation of DCE-MRI data include overlap in enhancement properties between benign and malignant regions in the transition zone. Benign prostatic hyperplasia and other benign inflammatory conditions within the transition zone also exhibit substantial hypervascularity [40]. Diagnostic models containing contrast enhancement parameters have reduced performance when applied across zones, so zone-specific models can improve classification of prostate cancer on mpMRI [41].

Diffusion-Weighted MR Imaging (DWI)

The diffusion properties of tissue are related to the amount of interstitial free water and permeability. In general, cancer tends to have more restricted diffusion than normal tissue, because of the

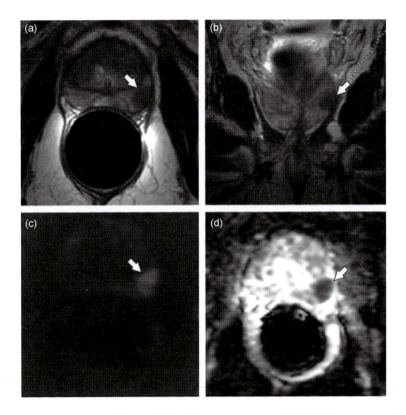

FIGURE 15.4 Multiparametric MRI (mpMRI) of the prostate. Axial T2 TSE (a) and coronal T2 TSE (b) images show a well-defined T2 hypointense lesion in the peripheral zone (arrow) with corresponding high signal on DWI (c) and low signal on the ADC map (d). Biopsy of this region was positive for Gleason 4 + 3 prostate cancer. (From Yacoub, J.H. et al., *Radiol. Clin. North Am.*, 52, 811–837, 2014.)

higher cell densities and abundance of intra- and intercellular membranes in cancer [42]. Diffusion-weighted MRI images can be used to detect prostate cancer from differences in the diffusion of water molecules of the normal and tumor tissues (Figure 15.4) [42]. The diffusion-weighted image is usually generated with different b-values that can be used to calculate the apparent diffusion coefficient (ADC), and the ADC for each pixel of the image is displayed as an ADC map. Diffusion of water molecules in tumor tissue is thought to reflect tissue architecture such as cell density and nucleus/cytoplasm ratio, and reductions in ADC values. For these reasons, ADC values have received attention as a predictor of Gleason score in prostate cancer [43,44]. Studies show that DWI findings may indicate tumor aggressiveness [27,45,46].

Technologic advances enable performance of DWI at high b- or ultrahigh b-values (greater than 1000 s/mm^2). High b-value images can be obtained in one of two ways: either directly by acquiring a high b-value DWI sequence or by calculating (synthesizing) the high b-value image by extrapolation from the acquired lower b-value data. Previous research has shown that high b-value DWI images allow for increased delineation between tumors and healthy tissue which makes the prostate cancer detection more robust [47,48]. Whereas contrast in ADC maps does not significantly change with different b-values, contrast ratios of DWI images are significantly higher at b-values of 1500 and 2000 s/mm^2 in comparison to b-values of 800 and 1000 s/mm^2 [49]. Wang et al. have reported that DWI images and ADC maps using $b = 1500$ s/mm^2 should be considered more effective than those at $b = 2000$ s/mm^2 or $b = 1000$ s/mm^2 for detecting prostate cancer at 3 T MRI [50].

DWI images and ADC maps are the key component of the prostate mpMRI exam. Several CADx systems adopting DWI images or ADC maps have been developed. DWI was mostly often combined with T2W in these CADx systems. Peng et al. demonstrated that the combination of 10th percentile ADC, average ADC, and T2-weighted skewness with CADx is promising in the differentiation of prostate cancer from normal tissue [27]. Niaf et al. presented a CADx system based on T2W, DWI, and DCE for assisting cancer identification in the PZ [18]. Stember et al. develop a software system that identifies suspicious regions at the prostate TZ using signal and textural features on T2W and ADC maps, free of user input [51]. Kwak et al. recently designed a prostate CADx combined T2W and high b-value ($b = 2000$ s/mm^2) DWI. They obtained an AUC of 0.89 [52].

MR Spectroscopy (MRS)

In MRS, the position of each metabolite peak in the output graph reflects the resonant frequencies or chemical shifts of its hydrogen protons, and the area of each peak reflects the relative concentration of that metabolite [53]. The dominant peaks observed in prostate MRS are from protons in citrate (2.60 ppm), creatine (3.04 ppm), and choline compounds (3.20 ppm) (Figure 15.5) [53].

As a metabolic biomarker for PCa, MRS has not gained wide acceptance in routine clinical practice due to a variety of factors including the length and complexity of data acquisition, zonal anatomy, processing, and analysis. Visual interpretation of the spectra by a trained spectroscopist is time-consuming and requires accurate knowledge of prostate anatomy. Therefore, a method for automated analysis of prostate MRS data is necessary.

Over the last decade, with a view to assisting radiologists in interpretation and analysis of MRS data, several researchers have begun to develop CADx schemes for PCa identification from spectroscopy. Tiwari et al. developed an approach that integrated a manifold learning scheme (spectral clustering) with an unsupervised hierarchical clustering algorithm to identify spectra corresponding to cancer on prostate MRS [54]. The scheme successfully identified MRS cancer voxels with a sensitivity of 77.8%, a false positive rate of 28.92%, and a false negative rate of 20.88% [54]. They also presented a CADx scheme that integrated nonlinear dimensionality reduction (NLDR) with an unsupervised hierarchical clustering algorithm to automatically identify suspicious regions on the prostate using MRS [55]. They introduced the use of wavelet embedding to map MRS and T2W texture features into a common space to identify the voxels that are affected by prostate cancer [56]. They recently presented a computerized decision support system called Semi Supervised Multi Kernel Graph Embedding (SeSMiK-GE) that may be developed into a powerful diagnostic and prognostic tool for distinguishing high- and low-grade PCa *in vivo*. Matulewicz et al. used an

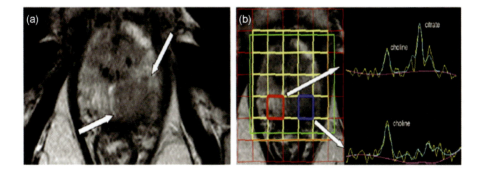

FIGURE 15.5 MR spectroscopy (MRS) of prostate cancer. (a) Axial T2-weighted MR images at the level of the prostate mid-gland to apex shows a large hypointense lesion on the left peripheral zone. (b) A 3D MRS shows a normal spectrum on the right peripheral zone (red box) with normal choline plus creatine-to-citrate ratio of 0.48. In the voxel placed over the lesion on the left peripheral zone (blue box), the curve shows an increased choline peak and the citrate peak is markedly reduced. Random systematic biopsy showed a Gleason grade 9 (4 + 5) prostate adenocarcinoma on the left apex. (From Neto, J.A., and Parente, D.B., *Magn. Reson. Imaging Clin. N. Am.*, 21, 409–426, 2013.)

artificial neural network (ANN) model to automatically detect cancerous voxels from prostate MRS datasets and found that the additional information concerning the prostate's zonal anatomy can improve the performance of the detection [57].

OTHER IMAGING METHODS

Although T2W, DWI, DCE-MRI, and MRS are more commonly used in mpMRI, some MRI methods, including diffusion tensor imaging (DTI), diffusion kurtosis imaging (DKI), and MR elastography (MRE), have been investigated for characterizing prostate cancer [58–61]. Other MRI methods, including proton density-weighted (PD-W) image [62] and T1 map [14], have also been added for feature calculation purposes in some CADx system.

DTI has been widely used in clinical applications, especially in neuro- and musculoskeletal imaging. Fractional anisotropy (FA) and apparent diffusion coefficient (ADC) values provided from DTI data reflect the degree of water diffusion restriction in different tissue. Pathological processes may cause change in normative FA values and disruption of fibers in tractography. The feasibility of performing DTI of the prostate had been demonstrated by some studies; and DTI tractography can successfully visualize fiber tracts around the prostate [58]. DTI tractography might be applicable to the estimation of structures of the prostate [59], the characterization of prostate cancer [60], and monitoring prostatic structural changes under radiotherapy [61].

The novel technique diffusion kurtosis imaging enables characterization of non-Gaussian water diffusion behavior. The DK model may add value in PCa detection and diagnosis, and DKI potentially offers a new metric for assessment of PCa [63]. A recent study demonstrated no significant benefit of DKI for detection and grading of PCa as compared with standard ADC in the peripheral zone determined from b-values of 0 and 800 s/mm [64]. The mechanical properties of the tissue of interest are calculated from the wave fields and displayed as an image, commonly referred as an elastogram. In MR elastography (MRE), an external mechanical excitation is applied to the tissue of interest to induce tissue vibrations [65]. MRE has been shown to be of clinical value in MRI for its ability to detect tissue abnormalities in organs such as the liver [66], brain [67], and breast [68–70]. More recently, researchers have also focused on the development of MRE methods to detect prostate cancer [71–73]. The resulting wave fields are imaged using a motion-sensitized MRI pulse sequence. Elastograms may add another dimension to current mpMRI techniques for diagnosing prostate cancer, and may further increase the sensitivity and specificity of such techniques.

T1 maps offer quantitative T1 values and can be produced by a variety of methods, such as multiple inversion or multiple repetition time acquisitions, typically requiring lengthy acquisition times. Another approach taken in the context of the prostate has been to employ spoiled gradient-echo (SPGR) sequences where it is possible to obtain T1 estimates in relatively short acquisition times by varying the radiofrequency (RF) flip angle [74]. The T1 mapping is not including in most CADx systems. Vos et al. [14] had presented a fully automatic CADx by combining a histogram analysis on mpMR images including T1, pharmacokinetic, T2, and ADC maps.

MR lymphography has been used for the investigation of the lymphatic channels and lymph glands. Different imaging techniques, including nanoparticle-enhanced [75,76] and non-contrast MR lymphography [77,78], had been developed for detection of nodal metastases. MR lymphography is a noninvasive technique that is well suited for the examination of regional (intrapelvic) lymph node metastases in PCa.

MR IMAGE QUANTIFICATION METHODS

GENERAL FRAMEWORK

Development of computer-aided detection systems includes several aspects: image pre-processing, algorithm development, methodology for assessing CADx performance, validation using appropriate cases to measure performance and robustness, observer performance studies, assessing

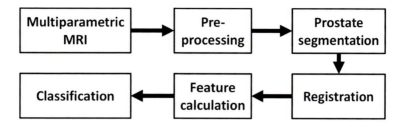

FIGURE 15.6 Flowchart for computer-aided detection of prostate cancer in mpMRI.

performance with a clinical trial, and ultimately commercialization. The development must confront several challenges. Computerized image procedure may cover different aspects of segmentation, registration, feature extraction, and classifiers. A computer algorithm should be developed based on the understanding of image reading by radiologists, such as how radiologists detect certain lesions, why they may miss some abnormalities, and how they can distinguish between benign and malignant lesions. It is important to develop CADx systems that extracts quantitative data in a more accurate and automated fashion.

Many different types of CADx systems are produced to locate/diagnose prostate cancer in MR imaging, including T2W, DWI, DCE-MRI, and MRS. Considering the particularity of prostate cancer in anatomy, pathology and clinic, the core of a CADx system for the detection of prostate cancer is associated with its computerized algorithms. In general, the pipeline of the CADx system for prostate cancer is visualized schematically in Figure 15.6. In the initial stage, lesion candidates are selected within a likelihood map that is generated by a voxel classification of one or more images. Hereafter, the lesion candidates are segmented into a region of interest from which region-based features are extracted. Finally, the extracted information is fused by a classifier into malignancy likelihood. The following sections describe each step in detail.

PRE-PROCESSING

The purpose of pre-processing is to normalize the MR data or to transform the MR data to a domain in which prostate lesions can be easily detected.

For T2W MRI, the image intensities can vary, even using the same protocol and the same scanner. The quality of images depends on the acquisition conditions such as temperature, calibration adjustment, B0 intensity, coil position, and the receiver gain value. In addition, the intensity variation will increase when different scanners are used. This relationship must be taken into account for MR image analysis. Collewet et al. [79] proposed four schemes for the intensity normalization. The most used method is that intensities are proportionally normalized by defining the median+2* (inter-quartile range).

ADC maps calculated from DWI are useful for detecting prostate cancer with a relatively high specificity. However, it has lower resolution than T2W MRI and is subject to magnetic susceptibility artifacts [17]. ADC represents a quantitative assessment of water diffusion. Lower ADC value is associated with higher rate of malignancy. Prostate cancer can be identified as a low signal region on ADC maps against a background of normal tissue with higher signal intensity [17].

Intensity inhomogeneity arises from the imperfections of the image acquisition, which can reduce the accuracy of segmentation, classification, and registration. The most intuitive method to correct intensity inhomogeneity is image smoothing or homomorphic filtering [80]. Vovk et al. [81] classify inhomogeneity correction methods into two categories, which are prospective and retrospective. Prospective methods aim at the calibration and improvement of image acquisition processes. Retrospective methods rely exclusively on the information of the acquired images or on a priori knowledge. Sled et al. [82] proposed a nonparametric nonuniform intensity normalization

(N3) method for inhomogeneity correction, which is independent of pulse sequence. Tustison et al. [83] proposed a variant of N3 for bias field correction. Similar to the N3, the source code, testing, and technical documentation are publicly available and the package is "N4ITK." This algorithm is available to the public through the Insight Toolkit of the National Institutes of Health.

SEGMENTATION

The segmentation aims to reduce the burden of the classifier in the later stages. Therefore, the classifiers only focus on the prostate region obtained by segmentation methods. T2W imaging provides the best resolution and contrast to show the anatomy of the prostate and has a very high sensitivity for prostate cancer. Therefore, T2W MRI is the most useful image sequence in determining the contours of prostate.

Extensive studies were developed to segment the prostate from MR images [62,84–90]. It can be a challenging task to obtain accurate prostate volume in T2W MRI. First, the contrast between the prostate and the surrounding tissues can be low. Therefore, it may be difficult to accurately segment the boundary of the prostate. Second, the prostate shapes of different patients can be significantly different. Even for the same patient, the prostate motion at different patient positions can be large, which results in a shape difference on MR images. Third, MR image appearance, quality, and the presence of artifacts can be affected by different scanners, which in turn can have a large influence on the performance of computerized algorithms. All these aspects need to be considered when developing a robust and accurate segmentation method for prostate MR images.

Contour- and shape-based methods [91–95] exploit edge and shape features to segment the prostate, which contains two categories. The first category is edge-based segmentation methods. The edge detection operators are used to produce edges on MR images. The candidate edges are picked up and then connected to obtain the prostate boundary. Zwiggelaar et al. [91] developed a semiautomatic method to segment the prostate in MRI data. Their method exploits the characteristics of the anatomical shape of the prostate when represented in a polar transform space. The edge detection and non-maximum suppression are used to track the boundary of the prostate.

The second category is deformable model-based segmentation methods. Kass et al. [96] proposed an active contour model and used the image gradient to evolve a curve. The internal spline force pushes the curve toward the salient image feature, while external force is responsible for putting the curve near the object. Chan and Vese [97] proposed a level-set algorithm of the piecewise constant variant of the Mumford-Shah model [98] for segmentation.

Atlas based methods are also used to segment the prostate in MR images [99]. An atlas consists of original image data and its corresponding manual segmentation. The atlas can be used as a reference to segment the prostate of a new patient. Klein et al. [99] proposed an automatic method for segmenting the prostate in 3D MR images. Their method is based on non-rigid registration of a set of pre-labeled atlas images. The label images of the deformed atlas are fused to yield a segmentation of images from a new patient.

Besides the above methods, a global optimization algorithm called graph cut [100,101] is becoming more and more popular due to its efficient global minimization. The segmentation problem can be formulated as a minimization of an energy minimization. Egger [102] proposed a graph-based approach to automatically segment prostate based on a spherical template. The minimal cost on the graph is optimized by a graph cut algorithm, which can get the segmentation of the prostate volume. Mahapatra and Buhmann [85] proposed a fully automatic method for prostate segmentation using random forest classifiers and graph cuts. The prostate probability map was generated based on a random forest classifier. The negative log-likelihood of the probability maps was used as the penalty cost in an energy function, which was minimized by graph cuts. Tian et al. [103] proposed a supervoxel-based segmentation method for the prostate. The prostate segmentation problem was considered as assigning labels to supervoxels. An energy function with both data and smoothness terms was used to model the labels, which was minimized using graph cuts. The segmentation

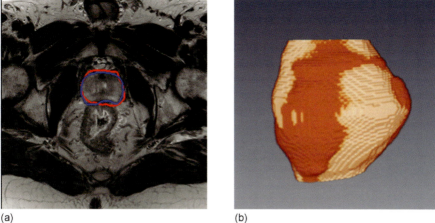

(a)   (b)

FIGURE 15.7 Prostate segmentation on MR images. (a) 2D MR image and segmentation results where the red curve represents the segmentation from a computer algorithm while the blue curve is the ground truth labeled by a radiologist. (b) 3D visualization after segmentation. The gold region is the prostate surface obtained by the computer algorithm while the red region is the ground truth.

results are shown in Figure 15.7. Other segmentation methods were also developed for the prostate [104,105]. Ghose et al. [105] reviewed segmentation methods for the prostate in TRUS, MR, and CT images. They studied the similarities and differences among the different methods, highlighting their advantages and disadvantages in order to assist in the choice of an appropriate segmentation method. They also provided a comprehensive description of the existing methods in all TRUS, MR, and CT images and highlighted their key points and features. They provided a strategy for choosing segmentation method for a given image modality.

A publicly available dataset called MICCAI Challenge Prostate MR Image Segmentation (PROMISE12) [104] can be used to evaluate the performances of the new proposed methods. This data set contains 50 cases with ground truths for training, and 30 cases without ground truths for test, which are 3D T2W MR transverse images of the prostate. The MR images were obtained from multicenter, multivendor, and different acquisition protocols (i.e., with/without endorectal coil, differences in slice thickness).

REGISTRATION

Image registration is a process of aligning two or more images, which aims to find the optimal transformation that best aligns the structures of interest in the input images. Image registration is needed in order to integrate the features from different images of mpMRI such as DCE-MRI and T2W MRI. The registration of images requires the selection of the feature space, a similarity measure, a transformation type, and a search strategy [106]. The DICOM header of MR images can provide coordination and orientation information that are useful for registering T2W, ADC, and K^{trans} maps. T2W-MRI is considered as the reference. Other modalities can be registered to T2W-MRI by aligning the coordinates of their origins, which are obtained from the DICOM header. If necessary, resolution adjustment is also performed after the alignment.

Registration is also used to validate *in vivo* MR imaging using *ex vivo* histologic images [107,108]. To obtain the reliable ground truth of the prostate cancer region, whole-mount histology is performed on *ex vivo* prostate. The pathologist labels the cancer region in the histology images. Based on the registration between the whole-mount histology and T2W MRI, the labeling of the cancer in histology can be mapped to T2W MRI for validation [107,108]. Kalavagunta et al. [108] proposed a method to register MRI and histology using local affine transformations guided by internal structures. First, the histologic and MR images are segmented, scaled, and translated. Second, the prostate capsule and internal structure masks are identified to constrain the pathology transformation. A transformation matrix is obtained by registering two images based on capsule and internal structure masks. Third, the pathology images are warped using a computed transformation matrix. Fourth, a transformation matrix is applied for each annotated cancer region. The warped cancer regions are superposed on registered pathology images. Last, the cancer regions in MRI can be obtained by mapping the cancer regions of pathologic images to MR images. In another study, Chappelow et al. [107] presented a new registration method that maximizes the combined mutual information shared by the intensity of the reference image and multiple representations of the floating images in multiple feature spaces. The method provides enhanced registration performance by combining the intensity information with transformed feature images from the images. These feature images are not as susceptible to intensity artifacts and provide additional similarity information regarding the reference image but not contained in the floating image. This method is particularly useful for registering MRI and histology.

FEATURE EXTRACTION

Feature extraction plays an important role in prostate MRI CADx systems. Classic features for medical images include intensity, shape, texture, and statistical features. For medical image classification, choosing the right features for a classifier is more important than choosing the classifier itself [62].

Litjens et al. classified the features into five types: intensity, pharmacokinetic, texture, blobness, and anatomical features [62]. For the intensity feature, a T2-estimate map is generated by using the MR signal equation, the proton density image, and a reference tissue [88]. Anatomical features include the relative distance to the prostate boundary and the relative position feature. Both the relative distance and relative position features are calculated with respect to the prostate surface obtained by segmentation methods. For the pharmacokinetic feature, the traditional analysis is incorporated in their CADx system by using a curve fitting technique to fit a bi-exponential curve to the time data, as presented in Huisman et al. [109]. For the texture feature, a Gaussian texture bank was used to capture the textural distortions [22]. For the blobness feature, it was found that prostate cancer tends to appear as a blob-like lesion in DWI and DCE-MRI. The blobness-filter presented by Li et al. was chosen as a blobness measure [110]. Blobness is calculated on the ADC, tau and LateWash images, and on the K^{trans} and K_{ep} images as well [110].

Shah et al. [17] created an mpMRI feature set for CADx systems (Figure 15.8). First, in order to reduce interpatient variability, normalized T2W maps were calculated from the transversal T2W intensities using the average fat signal adjacent to the prostate as a reference. Second, quantitative ADC maps were computed from the transversal DWI by fitting the dependence of the signal intensity in each pixel. Third, each dynamic curve was de-noised by using a wavelet filter for DCE-MRI. The pharmacokinetic parameters were extracted by using the generalized kinetic model (GKM) [111,112]. Then, the GKM was fitted to the measured concentration time curves, using the linear least squared method [112] to yield the volume transfer constant, K^{trans}, and the rate constant, k_{ep}. Finally, the normalized T2W and ADC maps were resized to have a pixel resolution equal to the T1 and K^{trans} and k_{ep} maps in order to form the final feature set for the CADx system.

Niaf et al. extracted about 140 kinds of features for a CADx system [18]. Most of these features were chosen based on their proven efficiency between cancer and non-cancer. Two categories of features were proposed: image features and functional features. For image features, there were three types: gray-level features, texture features, and gradient features. The image intensity values of T2, DCE, and ADC maps were used as gray-level features. First order texture measurements were

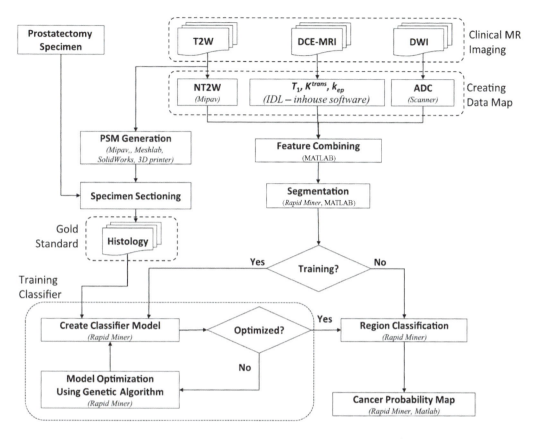

FIGURE 15.8 Flowchart for a CAD system based on a mpMRI. The cancer probability map is the final outcome of the algorithm. (From Shah, V. et al., *Med. Phys.*, 39, 4093–4103, 2012.)

computed for each pixel over a local window, which includes mean, median, standard deviation, and average deviation. Second order texture features were computed based on two neighboring pixels, which includes co-occurrence matrix. The Sobel and Kirsch filters and numerical gradient operators were used to compute gradient features (Figure 15.9).

Radiomics is an emerging field for the quantification of tumor phenotypes by applying a large number of quantitative image features [113,114]. Radiomics can provide complementary and interchangeable information to improve individualized treatment selection and monitoring. Since medical imaging technology is routinely used in clinical practice worldwide, radiomics may have a high clinical impact on future patient management. The workflow of radiomics consists of three steps [113]. The first step is the acquisition of standardized images for diagnostic or planning purposes. On the images, the tumor regions are extracted by an algorithm or an experienced radiologist. Second, quantitative imaging features are extracted from the tumor regions. These features involve tumor image intensity, texture, and shape and size of the tumor. Last, all the extracted features are analyzed and selected by a model. The most informative features are identified and incorporated into predictive models for treatment outcome. Radiomics, as a high-dimensional mineable feature space, can be used for prostate cancer. Cameron et al. constructed a comprehensive radiomics feature model to detect tumorous regions using mpMRI [115]. New radiomics-driven texture feature models have been developed for the detection of prostate cancer and for the classification of prostate cancer Gleason scores by utilizing mpMRI data [116–118].

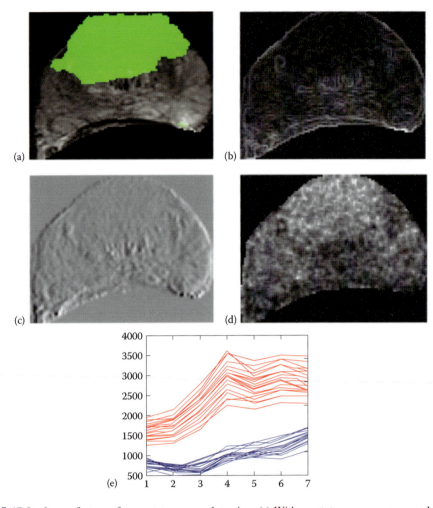

FIGURE 15.9 Image features for prostate cancer detection. (a) With prostate cancer superposed in green. (b) First order statistics (standard deviation). (c) Sobel-Kirsch feature. (d) Second order statistics (contrast inverse moment). (e) Corresponding time-intensity curves for PCa (red) and benign (blue) regions are shown based on DCE-MRI data. (From Viswanath, S. et al., *Proc. Soc. Photo. Opt. Instrum. Eng.*, 7260, 72603I, 2009.)

CLASSIFICATION

Image classification involves training and testing with features extracted from image data and its corresponding labels [62]. A classifier is usually trained by using the labeled image dataset and applied to unseen image datasets. Several classification techniques from the machine learning field have been developed for picking up discriminative features. Support vector machines (SVMs) and random forests could achieve good performance based on the positive and negative training samples [17,119]. A pixel classification provides a likelihood between 0 and 1 for each pixel, with 0 indicating no suspicion of prostate cancer and 1 indicating high suspicion of cancer.

Litjens et al. [62] experimented with three different classifiers: a linear discriminate classifier, a GentleBoost classifier [120], and a random forests classifier [119] with regression trees. Shah et al. used SVM to create a classifier model [17]. Because real data are not linearly separable, the SVM implementation was used to allow relaxed constraint for misclassified points. SVMs' "kernel trick" was also implemented to enable operations to be performed in the input space rather than the potentially high-dimensional feature space [121].

Chan et al. [122] investigated the use of a statistical classifier for detecting prostate cancer by combining information from MR images. SVM is used to predict the tumor likelihood in the peripheral zone using the derived features. For SVM training, they randomly sampled 10% of the PZ data and retained all the tumor data to confine the training dataset to a manageable size for SVM training convergence. The radial basis function kernel was used for SVM. These works indicate that the SVM classifiers and random forests work well on the problem of classifying prostate tumors on mpMRI.

VALIDATION

When developing a CADx system for prostate MRI, the accuracy of the "gold standard" is important. Histopathology, as the ground truth, usually includes findings from prostatectomy specimens or biopsy specimens. The validation of CADx systems is summarized in Table 15.1.

TABLE 15.1
Validation of CADx Systems

Reference	Ground Truth on the Histology	Candidate on MR Image	Image Registration
Chan et al. (2003) [122]	Biopsy	MO	NA
Puech et al. (2007) [39]	Needle biopsy or prostatectomy	MO	NA
Tiwari et al. (2007) [54]	Biopsy	Sextant location determined by radiologist	NA
Vos et al. (2008) [36]	WMHS + MO	MO	3D rendering mode
Viswanath et al. (2008) [140]	WMHS + MO	MANTRA	Multimodal image registration
Viswanath et al. (2009) [129]	WMHS	MANTRA	Multimodal image registration
Vos et al. (2009) [37]	WMHS	Not specified	Not specified
Liu et al. (2009) [141]	WMHS + MO	MO + *ex vivo* MRI	Manual
Tiwari et al. (2009) [55]	WMHS + sextant boundaries	A joint review session of trial imagers and pathologists	NA
Artan et al. (2010) [142]	WMHS + MO	Tumor location is transferred to the *in vivo* MRI from histologic images + *ex vivo* MRI	NA
Vos et al. (2010) [143]	WMHS + MO	MO	Mutual information registration
Viswanath et al. (2011) [144]	WMHS + MO	Registration from histologic images	MACMI
Lopes et al. (2011) [145]	WMHS + drawn by urologists	Drawn by urologists	Manual correspondence
Liu and Yetik (2011) [26]	WMHS + MO	MO + *ex vivo* MRI	Manual registration
Sung et al. (2011) [146]	Radical prostatectomy + MO	The radiologist matched the pathologic slices with corresponding MRI	NA
Tiwari et al. (2012) [56]	WMHS	MO + *ex vivo* MRI	Manual registration
Viswanath et al. (2012) [22]	WMHS + MO	Registration from histologic images	Multimodal elastic registration
Vos et al. (2012) [14]	Needle biopsy	Combining the findings with histopathology of MR-guided samples by radiologist	NA

(*Continued*)

TABLE 15.1 (*Continued*)

Validation of CADx Systems

Reference	Ground Truth on the Histology	Candidate on MR Image	Image Registration
Niaf et al. (2012) [18]	WMHS + MO	MO	Manual registration
Artan et al. (2012) [147]	WMHS + MO	MO + *ex vivo* MRI	Manual registration
Shah et al. (2012) [17]	WMHS + MO	Not specified	PSM
Matulewicz et al. (2013) [57]	WMHS + MO	MO	Manual registration
Hambrock et al. (2013) [13]	WMHS + MO	MO	Manual registration
Tiwari et al. (2013) [148]	WMHS + MO	MO	Manual registration
Peng et al. (2013) [27]	WMHS	MO	Manual registration
Ginsburg et al. (2014) [149]	WMHS + MO	Registration from histologic images	Nonlinear registration
Stember et al. (2014) [51]	Needle biopsy	Not specified	NA
Niaf et al. (2014) [150]	Prostatectomy + MO	MO	Manual registration
Garcia Molina et al. (2014) [16]	Prostatectomy + MO	MO	Manual registration
Litjens et al. (2014) [62]	Needle biopsy	Not specified	NA
Kwak et al. (2015) [52]	Needle biopsy	Determined by radiologists	NA
Zhao et al. (2015) [151]	Biopsy	MO	NA

Abbreviations: MO: manual outlined regions of lesions; MANTRA: multi-attribute, non-initializing, texture reconstruction-based ASM; MACMI: multi-attribute, higher-order mutual information-based elastic registration scheme; PSM: patient-specific molds; WMHS: whole-mount histological sections; NA: no registration was used.

In order to transfer the labels from pathology to MR images, MR images usually need to be registered with pathological sections of the prostate. An accurate registration of histologic and MR images serves as the bridge between *in vivo* anatomical information and *ex vivo* pathologic information, which is valuable in developing a CADx system.

Whole-mount sections are generated from tissue slices and microscopic slices are stained with hematoxylin-eosin staining after being embedded in paraffin [111,123]. Pathologists outline each lesion on the microscopic slices. Gleason scores of different regions may also be provided on the microscopic slices. For correlation between MR images and histopathologic images, the corresponding anatomical landmarks and cancerous regions are manually labeled by an expert. The urethra may serve as a guide for correlating the images. In order to improve the accuracy and efficiency of the correlation, some automatic methods have been developed [111,124].

There are several challenges in establishing automatic correlation between *in vivo* MR images and histopathologic images. The orientation of the specimen and its sections may be different from that of *in vivo* MR imaging. There are mismatches between MR imaging and histopathology, which make it difficult to assess the true accuracy of MRI. Once the anatomic orientation in the body is lost, it may be difficult to section the prostate in the same plane as that of *in vivo* MR images. The specimen can be marked with separate colors on the left, right, and anterior aspects for anatomic orientation [111]. Using image processing, computer-aided design, and rapid prototyping technology, a customized mold has been used to process prostatectomy specimens for each patient [124]. The customized mold holds the prostate in the same position and the same shape as those of *in vivo* MR images and guides the cutting knife to obtain tissue blocks that correspond to the image slices.

The prostate is an easily deformable organ, hence, the gland deforms during and after prostatectomy. Additionally, prostate MRI is often performed by using an endorectal coil, which further deforms the gland. Specimen formalin fixation and paraffin embedding also induce variable tissue shrinkage. Deformable image registration provides a high degree of flexibility for registration of histologic images with *in vivo/ex vivo* MR images, and can assist in more accurate evaluation of MRI findings. Boundary landmarks and internal landmarks of the same prostate have been used in a deformable registration algorithm. Mazaheri et al. describe a semiautomatic method by using a free-form deformation (FFD) algorithm based on B-splines [125]. This method enabled successful registration of anatomical prostate MR images to pathologic slices. Jacobs et al. [126] proposed a method for the registration and warping of MR images to histologic sections. This method consists of a modified surface-based registration algorithm followed by an automated warping approach using nonlinear thin plate splines to compensate for the distortions between the datasets.

There are two general approaches to map *ex vivo* histological PCa extent to preoperative MR images. The first method, perhaps the more intuitive approach, is to reconstruct the 3D histologic volume, and then register the 3D histologic volume with the 3D MR volume [127,128]. The second approach is to register each 2D histology slice to its corresponding 2D MRI slice separately [107,129]. In the first approach, one critical prerequisite was the accurate reconstruction of the histologic volume; while in the second approach, the prerequisite was to determine the histology-MRI slice correspondence. In some cases, the former prerequisite may not be achievable, hence the only solution is to take the second approach. There is an increasing interest in the registration of 3D histopathology with prostate MR imaging. Three-dimensional reconstruction of prostate histology facilitates these registration-based evaluations by reintroducing 3D spatial information lost during histology processing [130,131]. Patel et al. [132] presented a scheme for the registration of digitally reconstructed whole-mount histology to preoperative *in vivo* mpMRI using spatially weighted mutual information. McGrath et al. [133] used reference landmarks that are visible in both datasets to assist 3D histopathology reconstruction and thus can provide important information on the deformation effects of fixation, and hence improved registration accuracy. Histostitcher, a software system designed to create a pseudo whole-mount histology section from a stitching of four individual histology quadrant images, is another alternative for reconstructing pseudo whole-mount prostate images [134].

Registering pathologic information to mpMRI is a challenging problem in developing a CADx system for mpMRI (Figure 15.10). Chappelow et al. [135] described a method based on mutual information that registers T2W, DCE-MRI, and ADC. However, this method is based on 2D histology and requires considerable expertise to determine the correspondence between histologic and MR images. Orczyk et al. [136] described a method based on the present registration method and were the first to create a 3D counterpart within the same reference space

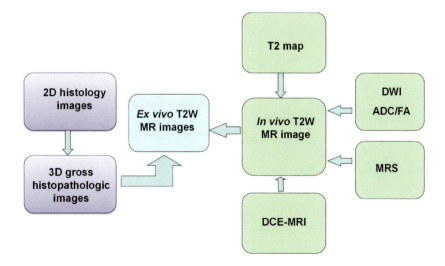

FIGURE 15.10 Registration between mpMRI and histology.

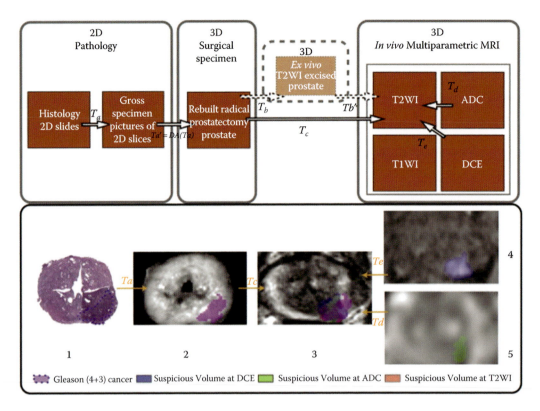

FIGURE 15.11 Registration between MRI and histology. Top: Workflow for pathology-mpMRI registration in a surgical 3D space. Bottom: 3D deformable registration of virtual whole-mount histology (1), fresh specimen (2), T2 weighted MRI (3), perfusion (4), and diffusion (5) sequences (ADC) applied to prostate cancer. (From Orczyk, C. et al., *Clin. Radiol.*, 68, e652–e658, 2013.)

between histology and both anatomical and functional sequences provided by prostate mpMRI (Figure 15.11). The method enables a true, deformable transformation and achieves an accuracy of 1–2 mm. The registration of different MR images is critical considering prostate motion, especially related to rectal peristalsis. Orczyk et al. [136] used rigid registration to correct motion between difference sequences.

Although whole-mount prostate histological analysis provides accurate label information for training a CADx system, whole-mount histology is expensive and registering whole-mount histologic slices with 3D mpMRI is a challenging problem. Therefore, histologic interpretations from biopsy specimens are used to determine the ground truth in some studies [14,62,122,137,138]. *In vivo* biopsy can only label the pathology of the core inside the prostate. Radiologists must manually define lesion boundaries on mpMRI retrospectively based on the biopsy results.

Meyer et al. [139] reviewed the registration methods of 3D medical images and histopathology of the prostate. They examined the registration process and techniques for registering MRI or PET with whole-mounted prostatectomy specimens.

CLINICAL APPLICATIONS

DIAGNOSIS

The functional MR imaging data, like DCE-MRI and MRS, are more complex and larger in amounts than anatomic MR imaging. There are clinical needs to develop fast, cost-effective, supportive techniques, such as computer-aided analysis tools, for easy and more reproducible diagnosis of prostate cancer. Researchers have focused on developing CADx methodology for automated prostate MRS classification and DCE-MRI analysis. Because all functional MR imaging techniques have their strengths and shortcomings, a single technique cannot adequately detect and characterize PCa. The combination of anatomic (T2W) images and functional techniques has been shown to increase the accuracy of MR imaging for diagnosis of PCa. Table 15.2 compares the performance of the major published prostate CADx systems [13,14,16–18,22,26,27,36,37,39,51,52,54–57,62,122,129,140–151]. Chan et al. were one of the first groups who implemented an mpMRI CADx system for the diagnosis of prostate cancer [122]. In their approach they used line-scan diffusion, T2, and T2-weighted images to identify predefined areas of the peripheral zone of the prostate for the presence of prostate cancer. Viswanath et al. [129] present an mpMRI CADx system for PCa detection by integrating functional and structural information obtained via DCE and T2W MRI. Liu et al. [141] present fuzzy MRF models for prostate cancer detection of multispectral MR prostate images. Tiwari et al. [55] investigated the use of MR spectroscopy in combination with T2W MRI to identify the voxels that are affected by prostate cancer. They also introduced the use of wavelet embedding to map MRS and T2W texture features into a common space. In a study by Peng et al. [27], the combination of 10th percentile ADC, average ADC, and T2-weighted skewness with CADx yielded an AUC value of 0.95 in differentiating prostate cancer from normal tissue. The combination achieved higher accuracy than any MR parameter alone. In a more recent study by Litjens et al. [62], they developed a fully automated computer-aided detection system which consists of two stages. The first (detection) stage consists of segmentation of the prostate on the transversal T2W MRI, extraction of voxel features from the image volumes, classification of the voxels, and candidate selection. The second (diagnosis) stage consists of candidate segmentation, candidate feature extraction, and candidate classification. The system was evaluated on a large consecutive cohort of 347 patients, and yielded an AUC value of 0.889.

AGGRESSIVENESS

Treatment choice for prostate cancer is based on initial PSA level, clinical stage of disease, and Gleason score, together with baseline urinary function, comorbidities, and patient age [152,153]. Therefore, there is an urgent clinical need to detect high-grade cancers and to differentiate them from the indolent, slow-growing tumors. The Gleason system, using a rating system to determine the grade of prostate cancer, remains one of the widely used prognostic factors in prostate cancer. The higher-grade tumors have a tendency to grow quickly and to spread faster than lower-grade tumors.

DWI, DCE-MRI, and MRS are noninvasive assessment methods of PCa aggressiveness. The Gleason grading system is a fundamental indicator of the aggressive nature of prostate cancer. Studies found that ADC image features correlate with Gleason scores [27,28,46,154–156]. A study by Yamamura et al. found a highly significant negative correlation between ADC-value and the Gleason score, while MRS did not show a significant correlation [157]. Recently, Zhang et al. found that TRUS-guided, MRI-directed biopsies improved the prediction of PCa aggressiveness in comparison with 12-core TRUS-guided biopsies. DWI-directed biopsies had a superior performance when compared with MRS directed biopsies in the peripheral zone [6]. Diffusion of water molecules in tumor tissue was thought to reflect tissue architecture such as cell density and nucleus/cytoplasm ratio, and reductions in ADC values in tumor tissue in fact correlates well with increases in cellular density [158–160]. For these reasons, ADC value has received more attention as a predictor of Gleason score in prostate cancer.

DCE-MRI is based on the permeability of blood vessels and extravasation of contrast agent into the surrounding tissue. Investigators have observed that quantitative parameters (K^{trans} and K_{ep}) and semiquantitative parameters (wash-in and washout) derived from DCE-MRI have the potential to assess the aggressiveness of PCa. Oto et al. found a moderate correlation between k_{ep} and microvessel density of prostate cancer [154]. Peng et al. found K^{trans} moderately correlate with Gleason scores [27].

In vivo MRS imaging has revealed a trend toward an increased (choline+ creatine)/citrate (CC/C) ratio with increased Gleason score [161,162]. This relationship has also been demonstrated by

TABLE 15.2

Summary of Representative Studies in the Literature

Reference	Modality	Validation	Region	Classifier	Data Size	Performance
Chan et al. (2003) [122]	T2WI, ADC, T2	Biopsy	PZ	SVM, FLD	15	FLD, AUC = 0.839; SVM, AUC = 0.761
Puech et al. (2007) [39]	DCE	Prostatectomy	PZ & TZ	Software titled "ProCAD"	100	PZ, Se/Sp = 100/49%; TZ, Se/Sp = 100/40%
Tiwari et al. (2007) [54]	MRS	Biopsy	WP	Spectral clustering	14	Se = 77.8%, FP = 28.92%, and FN = 20.88%
Vos et al. (2008) [36]	DCE	WMHS	PZ	SVM	34	AUC = 0.83
Viswanath et al. (2008) [140]	DCE	WMHS	WP	LLE and Consensus Clustering	6	Se = 60.72%, Sp = 83.24%
Viswanath et al. (2009) [129]	T2WI, DCE	WMHS	WP	Random forest	6	AUC = 0.815
Vos et al. (2009) [37]	DCE	WMHS	PZ	SVM	38	AUC = 0.80
Liu et al. (2009) [141]	T2W, T2, ADC, DCE	WMHS	PZ	Fuzzy MRF model	11	Se = 89.58%, Sp = 87.50%
Tiwari et al. (2009) [55]	MRS	Prostatectomy	WP	NLDR	18	Se = 89.33%, Sp = 79.79%
Artan et al. (2010) [142]	T2, ADC, DCE	Biopsy	PZ	Cost-sensitive CRF	21	AUC = 0.79
Vos et al. (2010) [143]	T2WI, DCE	WMHS	PZ	SVM	29	AUC = 0.89
Viswanath et al. (2011) [144]	T2W, DWI, DCE	WMHS	WP	EMPrAvISE	12	AUC = 0.77
Lopes et al. (2011) [145]	T2WI	WMHS	WP	SVM, AdaBoost	17	SVM, Se/Sp = 83/91%; AdaBoost, Se/Sp = 85/93%
Liu and Yetik (2011) [26]	T2W, DWI, DCE	WMHS	WP	SVM	20	AUC = 0.89
Sung et al. (2011) [146]	DCE	Prostatectomy	PZ & TZ	SVM	42	PZ, Se/Sp = 89/89%; TZ, Se/Sp = 91/64%
Tiwari et al. (2012) [56]	T2WI, MRS	WMHS	WP	Random forest	36	AUC = 0.89
Viswanath et al. (2012) [22]	T2WI	WMHS	PZ & CG	QDA	22	CG, AUC = 0.86; PZ, AUC = 0.73
Vos et al. (2012) [14]	T1, T2, ADC, DCE	Biopsy	WP	LDA	200	Se = 0.74, at a FP level of 5 per patient
Niaf et al. (2012) [18]	T2W, DWI, DCE	WMHS	PZ	SVM	30	AUC = 0.89
Artan et al. (2012) [147]	T2, ADC, T1-PC	WMHS	WP	SVM	15	Se = 76%, Sp = 86%
Shah et al. (2012) [17]	T2WI, ADC, DCE	WMHS	PZ	SVM	31	F-measure = 89%
Matulewicz et al. (2013) [57]	MRS	WMHS	WP	ANN	18	AUC = 0.968
Hambrock et al. (2013) [13]	T2WI, DWI, DCE	Prostatectomy	PZ & TZ	In-house–developed CAD system	34	Experienced observers, AUC = 0.91

(Continued)

TABLE 15.2 (*Continued*)

Summary of Representative Studies in the Literature

Reference	Modality	Validation	Region	Classifier	Data Size	Performance
Tiwari et al. (2013) [148]	T2WI, MRS	WMHS	WP	SeSMiK-GE	29	AUC = 0.89
Peng et al. (2013) [27]	T2WI, ADC, DCE	Prostatectomy	WP	LDA	48	AUC = 0.95
Ginsburg et al. (2014) [149]	T2WI, DWI, DCE	WMHS	PZ and CG	PCA-VIP	108	CG, AUC = 0.85; PZ, AUC = 0.79
Stember et al. (2014) [51]	T2WI, ADC	Biopsy	TZ	Naïve Bayes classifier	18	Predicted TZ tumor in all test patients
Niaf et al. (2014) [150]	T2WI, DWI, DCE	Prostatectomy	WP	P-SVM	48	AUC = 0.889
Garcia Molina et al. (2014) [16]	T2WI, ADC, DCE	Prostatectomy	PZ	Incremental learning ensemble SVM	12	Se = 84.4%, Sp = 78.0%
Litjens et al. (2014) [62]	T2WI, DWI, DCE, PDWI	Biopsy	WP	Random forest	347	AUC = 0.889
Kwak et al. (2015) [52]	T2WI, DWI	Biopsy	PZ & TZ	SVM	244	AUC of 0.89
Zhao et al. (2015) [151]	T2WI	Biopsy/follow-up	PZ & CG	ANN	71	CG, AUC = 0.821; PZ, AUC = 0.849

Abbreviations: T2W: T2-weighted; ADC: apparent diffusion coefficient; DCE: dynamic contrast-enhanced; MRS: magnetic resonance spectroscopy; DWI: diffusion-weighted imaging; T1-PC: principal component of T1-weighted dynamic series; T1: T1 mapping; T2: T2 mapping; SVM: support vector machine; P-SVM: probabilistic SVM; FLD: Fisher linear discriminant; MRF: Markov random field; NLDR: nonlinear dimensionality reduction; CRF: conditional random fields; EMPrAvISE: Enhanced Multi-Protocol Analysis via Intelligent Supervised Embedding; QDA: Quadratic Discriminant Analysis; ANN: artificial neural network; SeSMiK-GE: Semi Supervised Multi Kernel Graph Embedding; LDA: linear discriminant analysis; PCA: principal component analysis; PCA-VIP: variable importance on projection measure for PCA; LLE: locally linear embedding; AUC: area under a receiver operating characteristic curve; Se: sensitivity; Sp: specificity; FP: false positive; FN: false negative; TZ: transition zone; PZ: peripheral zone; CG: central gland; WP: whole prostate; WMHS: whole-mount histological sections.

ex vivo HR-MAS MRS [163]. However, other *in vivo* MRS imaging studies have found no correlation between metabolite ratios and aggressiveness [164,165].

On T2W MRI, changes in signal intensity for prostate cancer detection have been associated with its aggressiveness [166]. In a large retrospective study with 220 patients [166], T2W MRI and MRS imaging scores based on a 3-point scale for clinical prostate cancer aggressiveness were significantly correlated to biologic markers such as androgen receptor levels, which were associated with PCa progression. In that study, the combination of biomarkers with T2W MRI and MRS imaging results did discriminate clinically unimportant prostate cancer. If mpMRI can potentially aid in identifying low-grade disease *in vivo*, this might allow PCa patients to opt for active surveillance rather than immediately opting for aggressive therapy. Lee et al. demonstrated that the simple measurement of the diameter of suspicious tumor lesions on DWI could improve the prediction of insignificant prostate cancer in candidates for active surveillance therapy [167].

Although these MRI metrics are related to Gleason score, the power and threshold value of each metric are different and how to combine these anatomic and functional MRI information is still a problem. Developing a computerized decision support system may help in noninvasive assessment of PCa aggressiveness. Recently, the SeSMiK-GE system was developed to quantitatively combine T2WI and MRS data for distinguishing benign versus cancerous, and high- versus low-Gleason grade PCa regions *in vivo* [148].

BIOPSY GUIDANCE

TRUS-guided sextant or systematic prostate biopsy is the clinical standard for definitive diagnosis of prostate cancer. The Gleason score derived from biopsy specimens is important for appropriate treatment selection. However, PCa is often heterogeneous and multicentric [168]. In addition, the biopsy, which samples a small portion of the prostate, might not represent the whole gland efficiently. Traditionally, it is believed that Gleason score in systematic random TRUS-guided biopsy tends to downgrade the surgical specimen because a less differentiated pattern may not have been sampled in the biopsy [169,170]. Systematic random TRUS-guided biopsies often require repeated biopsy procedures, which are associated with discomfort and potential morbidity [171]. In order to reduce the overtreatment and the number of biopsies, lesions must be accurately detected, characterized, and targeted during biopsy. More effective imaging-guided targeted biopsy techniques are under investigation in order to improve the detection rate of prostate biopsies.

Optimization of prostate biopsy requires addressing the shortcomings of standard systematic TRUS-guided biopsy, including false negative rates, incorrect risk stratification, detection of clinically insignificant disease, and the need for repeat biopsy. MRI is an evolving noninvasive imaging modality that increases the accurate localization of prostate cancer at the time of biopsy, and thereby enhances clinical risk assessment and improves the ability to appropriately counsel patients regarding therapy.

Use of mpMRI for targeted prostate biopsies has the potential to reduce the sampling error associated with conventional biopsy by providing better disease localization and sampling, and also has a potential role in avoiding biopsy and reducing over detection/overtreatment. MRI-compatible biopsy systems were developed for this purpose [172]. More accurate risk stratification through improved cancer sampling may impact therapeutic decision making. Optimal clinical application of MRI-targeted biopsy remains under investigation.

There are three different manners in which an MRI-detected lesion can be targeted for biopsy: (1) direct targeting within the magnet using MR-compatible devices, also called in-bore MRI-guided biopsy; (2) use of fusion software to allow an MRI–defined lesion to be identified on ultrasound during a TRUS-guided biopsy procedure (Figure 15.12); or (3) cognitive targeting, in which the physician reviews the MRI data before the procedure and attempts to target the suspected area during the TRUS-guided biopsy using anatomic landmarks as reference [173]. An MRI-guided robotic prostate biopsy system, named APT-MRI robotic biopsy, has been reported with an accuracy within 2 mm [174]. A real-time phase-only cross correlation (POCC) algorithm-based sequence has been used

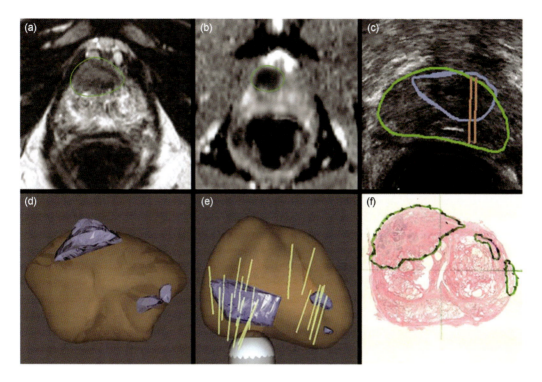

FIGURE 15.12 MRI and ultrasound fusion for targeted biopsy of the prostate. (a and b) Anterior lesion of the high suspicious lesion identified on mpMRI. (c) Real-time ultrasound targeting the corresponding lesion. (d and e) 3D models demonstrate the target (blue), prostate (brown), and biopsy cores (tan cylinders). (f) Radical prostatectomy pathology confirmed a 2.3 cm Gleason 8 (4 + 4) cancer centered in the right anterior prostate. (From Sonn, G.A. et al., *Urol. Oncol.*, 32, 903–911, 2014.)

in transrectal 3T in-bore MR-guided prostate biopsies [175]. Fusion of pre-biopsy MR images onto interventional TRUS images might increase the overall biopsy accuracy [176,177]. A novel method to identify the 2D axial MR slice from a pre-acquired MR prostate volume that closely corresponds to the 2D axial TRUS slice obtained during prostate biopsy has been reported by Mitra et al. [178].

TREATMENT PLANNING AND THERAPEUTIC RESPONSE ASSESSMENT

MRI-based techniques are used for computer-aided treatment procedures such as treatment planning of radiotherapy, MRI-guided radioactive seeds placement in prostate brachytherapy, and MRI-guided local ablation procedures [179–190].

The excellent soft-tissue contrast of MRI means that the technique is having an increasing role in contouring the gross tumor volume (GTV) and organs at risk (OAR) in radiation therapy treatment planning systems (TPS). MRI-planning scans from diagnostic MRI scanners are currently incorporated into the planning process by being registered to CT data. The soft-tissue data from the MRI provides target outline guidance and the CT provides a solid geometric and electron density map for accurate dose calculation on the TPS computer [191].

A number of minimally invasive, focal, organ-preserving methods have been used in recent years as further alternatives to the radical treatment of prostate cancer [170]. The focal therapy methods used to date for the prostate include cryotherapy, high-intensity focused ultrasound, laser-induced thermal ablation, and radioactive seed placement. MpMRI makes it possible to determine the exact location of tumor foci that are generally accessible for ablation or radioactive seed placement.

Moreover, mpMRI can also monitor treatment during and after minimally invasive therapy. A CADx system for the prostate may have potential value in helping clinicians to target tumor foci during treatment.

MpMRI can also be used as an imaging biomarker for monitoring therapeutic response, including radiotherapy of localized prostate cancer [191] and systemic therapy for metastatic disease. Successful treatment response to therapy is usually depicted by reductions in signal intensity accompanied by ADC increases [192–194]. There are clinical needs to develop mpMRI-based CADx systems for monitoring therapeutic response of the prostate in the future.

DISCUSSION AND FUTURE DIRECTIONS

Unlike breast and lung cancer, prostate cancer CADx systems for MR images have not been widely used in daily clinical work for detection or diagnosis. The majority of the prostate CADx systems reported the AUC in the range from 0.80 to 0.89 [179], while one reported AUCs of 0.96 [46], which represented a high performance. However, most systems generated lesion candidates based on manually selected ROIs, which may be dataset dependent, and employed a relatively small dataset. Validation on a large-scale dataset with several hundred patients is required. A prostate CADx system should be tested in multicenter trials to make the systems widely usable in clinical work.

One challenge of prostate CAD is related to mpMRI protocols. Both 3T protocols and endorectal coils have the advantage of increasing the signal-to-noise ratio (SNR). At 3T without the use of an endorectal coil (ERC), image quality can be comparable with that obtained at 1.5T with an endorectal coils [195]. Turkbey et al. found that dual-coil prostate MRI detected more cancer foci than non-endorectal coil MRI at 3T on T2W and DWI [196]. At 3T MRI, DWI images and ADC maps using $b = 1500$ s/mm^2 should be considered more effective than those at $b = 2000$ s/mm^2 or $b = 1000$ s/mm^2 for detecting prostate cancer [50]. Most members of the PI-RADS steering committee recommend 3T for prostate MRI. There is no consensus among experts concerning the potential benefits of the use of endorectal coils [12]. The impact of the mpMRI protocol on CADx systems should be considered and researched in the future. The combination of T2W, DWI, and DCE-MRI is the most commonly used set of parameters for the detection or diagnosis of prostate cancer. MRS with other parameters is also used in some research. The introduction of new imaging modalities or new modality combinations for mpMRI may lead to better CADx systems. Combining CAD prediction and PI-RADS into a combination score has the potential to improve diagnostic accuracy [197]. The MR PI-RADS system may provide a platform for CAD system development in the future.

The diagnostic value of these parameters for discrimination between benign and malignant tissue depend on the lesion's location. The parameter values of PCa are in the range of those of non-malignant diseases or conditions such as prostatitis, fibromuscular benign prostatic hyperplasia (BPH), post-biopsy hemorrhagic change, making for poor diagnostic value, especially in the transition zone. TZ and PZ cancer possess distinct quantitative imaging features on MRI. Computer-extracted parameters may be useful for cancer detection in the PZ, but are not suited in the TZ. In recent years, research focus has shifted from PZ prostate cancer to whole prostate cancer. There are more challenges in developing a CADx system for both PZ and TZ lesions than for PZ lesions only. Applications of anatomical segmentation from MRI as an additional input to ANN improve the accuracy of detecting cancerous voxels from MRS imaging [198]. A CAD system, utilizing two MRI sequences, such as T2-MRI and high b-value ($b = 2000$ s/mm^2) DWI, and texture features based on local binary patterns, is able to detect the discriminative texture features for cancer detection and localization, and the performance of the CADx system was not dependent on the specific regions of the prostate [52]. Future direction should also include whether zonal segmentation of the prostate is necessary when some new imaging sequences being used.

Ex vivo whole-mount prostate histological analysis provides more accurate label information for training a CADx system. However, whole-mount histology is expensive, and registering whole-mount histological slices with 3D mpMRI is a challenging problem. This is especially true during the preparation of the prostate histological data for training a CADx system. Pathologists must collect a large amount of training data from many patients, apply reliable biomarkers for each patient, prepare blocks, scan a large number of histological slices, and manually define lesion boundaries on histological slices. However, these are laborious and time-consuming procedures. Therefore, the histological image preparation procedures need to be performed by some automatic methods to improve efficacy. A software system has been designed to create a pseudo whole-mount histology section [134]. A computer-aided system to automatically grade pathological images according to the Gleason grading system has also been investigated [199]. A scheme, including automatic diagnosis from histologic images, 3D histologic reconstruction, and registration, should be developed for ground truth definition in the future.

Image quantification methods, such as accurate image registration for motion correction, compartment modeling for functional parameters estimation, feature extraction in high-dimensional data, automatic image classification for differentiating cancer from normal tissue, and correlation analyses among radiological data and genomic information, will play key roles in the future development of intelligent CAD systems.

Radiomics, as a high-dimensional extraction of large amounts of image features with high throughput from radiographic images, can provide valuable diagnostic, prognostic, or predictive information. Cameron et al. developed a quantitative radiomics feature model for performing prostate cancer detection using mpMRI [115].

Khalvati et al. [118] present new texture feature models for radiomics-driven detection of prostate cancer utilizing mpMRI data. Radiomics are emerging as a useful tool for prostate cancer detection. Further work is needed to build radiomics-based CAD systems for prostate cancer diagnosis, treatment planning, treatment prediction, and treatment response evaluation.

The Gleason grade of PCa is the most widely used prognostic factor for prostate cancer. MR metrics on T2W, DWI, DCE-MRI, and MRS imaging relate to microenvironment and microstructure. Therefore these MR metrics can predict the Gleason grade of the caner. Building a CAD system based on mpMRI and Gleason score is feasible. It can play a significant role in prognostic prediction, guiding biopsy, identifying suitable patients under active surveillance, and making a decision of appropriate treatment. CAD systems for prediction of Gleason score should be developed in the future.

As anatomic information is important when analyzing functional data, T2W images are frequently used in mpMRI CADx systems. T2W plus DWI and DCE-MRI are commonly used as the combinations. Chan et al. constructed a summary statistical map of the peripheral zone based on the utility of multichannel statistical classifiers by combining textural and anatomical features in PCa areas from T2W, DWI, proton density maps, and T2 maps [122]. Langer et al. included DCE-MRI and pharmacokinetic parameter maps as extra features to a CADx system for detecting prostate cancer at the peripheral zone [111]. They evaluated their system in predefined regions of interest, but on a per voxel basis. Vos et al. implemented a two-stage CADx system for prostate cancer using an initial blob detection approach combined with a candidate segmentation and classification using statistical region features [14]. Litjens et al. recently investigated a fully automated computer-aided detection system including a novel combination of segmentation, voxel classification, candidate extraction, and classification [62].

Promising preliminary results have been obtained with CADx systems that combine the analysis of statistical, structural, and functional MR imaging features and the use of an adapted classification scheme. Likelihood maps have been obtained by combining information from mpMRI using mathematical descriptors. These studies showed the discrimination between benign and malignant tissues is feasible with good performances [62,111].

CONCLUSION

In this chapter, we comprehensively reviewed mpMRI-based computer-aided technology for prostate cancer detection. Prostate CADx systems are a complicated composition of pre-processing, segmentation, registration, feature extraction, and classification modules. There are some challenges in accurate registration of MRI and histopathology, which is important for ground truth definition. Clinical applications of computer-aided systems include localization, diagnosis, staging, aggressiveness assessment, guiding biopsy, treatment planning, and therapeutic response assessment. Although the performance of some CADx systems is good, there is no such a system that has been wildly used in clinic. It is likely that more improvements in quantitative image analysis and computer-aided methods would need to be made in order to meet the clinical needs in near future work.

ACKNOWLEDGMENTS

This work was partially supported by NIH grants CA156775, CA176684, and CA204254. With permission, this chapter was reprinted from Liu L, Tian Z, Zhang Z, Fei B. Computer-aided Detection of Prostate Cancer with MRI: Technology and Applications. *Academic Radiology*. 2016 Aug; 23(8):1024-46.

REFERENCES

1. Siegel RL, Miller KD, Jemal A: Cancer statistics, 2015. *CA Cancer J Clin* 2015, 65:5–29.
2. Lee JJ, Thomas IC, Nolley R, Ferrari M, Brooks JD, Leppert JT: Biologic differences between peripheral and transition zone prostate cancer. *Prostate* 2015, 75:183–190.
3. Siddiqui MM, Rais-Bahrami S, Turkbey B, George AK, Rothwax J, Shakir N, Okoro C, Raskolnikov D, Parnes HL, Linehan WM et al.: Comparison of MR/ultrasound fusion-guided biopsy with ultrasound-guided biopsy for the diagnosis of prostate cancer. *JAMA* 2015, 313:390–397.
4. Pokorny MR, de Rooij M, Duncan E, Schroder FH, Parkinson R, Barentsz JO, Thompson LC: Prospective study of diagnostic accuracy comparing prostate cancer detection by transrectal ultrasound-guided biopsy versus magnetic resonance (MR) imaging with subsequent MR-guided biopsy in men without previous prostate biopsies. *Eur Urol* 2014, 66:22–29.
5. Schoots IG, Roobol MJ, Nieboer D, Bangma CH, Steyerberg EW, Hunink MG: Magnetic resonance imaging-targeted biopsy may enhance the diagnostic accuracy of significant prostate cancer detection compared to standard transrectal ultrasound-guided biopsy: A systematic review and meta-analysis. *Eur Urol* 2014, 68: 438–450.
6. Zhang J, Xiu J, Dong Y, Wang M, Han X, Qin Y, Huang Z, Cai S, Yuan X, Liu Q: Magnetic resonance imaging-directed biopsy improves the prediction of prostate cancer aggressiveness compared with a 12-core transrectal ultrasound-guided prostate biopsy. *Mol Med Rep* 2014, 9:1989–1997.
7. Brown AM, Elbuluk O, Mertan F, Sankineni S, Margolis DJ, Wood BJ, Pinto PA, Choyke PL, Turkbey B: Recent advances in image-guided targeted prostate biopsy. *Abdom Imaging* 2015, 40:1788–1799.
8. Puech P, Rouviere O, Renard-Penna R, Villers A, Devos P, Colombel M, Bitker MO, Leroy X, Mege-Lechevallier F, Comperat E et al.: Prostate cancer diagnosis: multiparametric MR-targeted biopsy with cognitive and transrectal US-MR fusion guidance versus systematic biopsy—Prospective multicenter study. *Radiology* 2013, 268:461–469.
9. Lawrence EM, Tang SY, Barrett T, Koo B, Goldman DA, Warren AY, Axell RG, Doble A, Gallagher FA, Gnanapragasam VJ et al.: Prostate cancer: Performance characteristics of combined T(2)W and DW-MRI scoring in the setting of template transperineal re-biopsy using MR-TRUS fusion. *Eur Radiol* 2014, 24:1497–1505.
10. Barentsz JO, Richenberg J, Clements R, Choyke P, Verma S, Villeirs G, Rouviere O, Logager V, Futterer JJ: ESUR prostate MR guidelines 2012. *Eur Radiol* 2012, 22:746–757.
11. Dickinson L, Ahmed HU, Allen C, Barentsz JO, Carey B, Futterer JJ, Heijmink SW, Hoskin PJ, Kirkham A, Padhani AR et al.: Magnetic resonance imaging for the detection, localisation, and characterisation of prostate cancer: Recommendations from a European consensus meeting. *Eur Urol* 2011, 59:477–494.

12. Weinreb JC, Barentsz JO, Choyke PL, Cornud F, Haider MA, Macura KJ, Margolis D, Schnall MD, Shtern F, Tempany CM et al.: PI-RADS Prostate Imaging-Reporting and Data System: 2015, Version 2. *Eur Urol* 2015, 69:16–40.

13. Hambrock T, Vos PC, Hulsbergen-van de Kaa CA, Barentsz JO, Huisman HJ: Prostate cancer: computer-aided diagnosis with multiparametric 3-T MR imaging—Effect on observer performance. *Radiology* 2013, 266:521–530.

14. Vos PC, Barentsz JO, Karssemeijer N, Huisman HJ: Automatic computer-aided detection of prostate cancer based on multiparametric magnetic resonance image analysis. *Phys Med Biol* 2012, 57:1527–1542.

15. Niaf E, Lartizien C, Bratan F, Roche L, Rabilloud M, Mege-Lechevallier F, Rouviere O: Prostate focal peripheral zone lesions: characterization at multiparametric MR imaging—Influence of a computer-aided diagnosis system. *Radiology* 2014, 271:761–769.

16. Garcia Molina JF, Zheng L, Sertdemir M, Dinter DJ, Schonberg S, Radle M: Incremental learning with SVM for multimodal classification of prostatic adenocarcinoma. *PLOS One* 2014, 9:e93600.

17. Shah V, Turkbey B, Mani H, Pang Y, Pohida T, Merino MJ, Pinto PA, Choyke PL, Bernardo M: Decision support system for localizing prostate cancer based on multiparametric magnetic resonance imaging. *Med Phys* 2012, 39:4093–4103.

18. Niaf E, Rouviere O, Mege-Lechevallier F, Bratan F, Lartizien C: Computer-aided diagnosis of prostate cancer in the peripheral zone using multiparametric MRI. *Phys Med Biol* 2012, 57:3833–3851.

19. Akin O, Sala E, Moskowitz CS, Kuroiwa K, Ishill NM, Pucar D, Scardino PT, Hricak H: Transition zone prostate cancers: Features, detection, localization, and staging at endorectal MR imaging. *Radiology* 2006, 239:784–792.

20. Li H, Sugimura K, Kaji Y, Kitamura Y, Fujii M, Hara I, Tachibana M: Conventional MRI capabilities in the diagnosis of prostate cancer in the transition zone. *AJR Am J Roentgenol* 2006, 186:729–742.

21. Cornud F, Rouanne M, Beuvon F, Eiss D, Flam T, Liberatore M, Zerbib M, Delongchamps NB: Endorectal 3D T2-weighted 1mm-slice thickness MRI for prostate cancer staging at 1.5 Tesla: Should we reconsider the indirect signs of extracapsular extension according to the D'Amico tumor risk criteria? *Eur J Radiol* 2012, 81:e591–e597.

22. Viswanath SE, Bloch NB, Chappelow JC, Toth R, Rofsky NM, Genega EM, Lenkinski RE, Madabhushi A: Central gland and peripheral zone prostate tumors have significantly different quantitative imaging signatures on 3 Tesla endorectal, in vivo T2-weighted MR imagery. *J Magn Reson Imaging* 2012, 36:213–224.

23. Hoeks CM, Hambrock T, Yakar D, Hulsbergen-van de Kaa CA, Feuth T, Witjes JA, Futterer JJ, Barentsz JO: Transition zone prostate cancer: Detection and localization with 3-T multiparametric MR imaging. *Radiology* 2013, 266:207–217.

24. Liu W, Turkbey B, Senegas J, Remmele S, Xu S, Kruecker J, Bernardo M, Wood BJ, Pinto PA, Choyke PL: Accelerated T2 mapping for characterization of prostate cancer. *Magn Reson Med* 2011, 65:1400–1406.

25. Yamauchi FI, Penzkofer T, Fedorov A, Fennessy FM, Chu R, Maier SE, Tempany CM, Mulkern RV, Panych LP: Prostate cancer discrimination in the peripheral zone with a reduced field-of-view T(2)-mapping MRI sequence. *Magn Reson Imaging* 2015, 33:525–530.

26. Liu X, Yetik IS: Automated prostate cancer localization without the need for peripheral zone extraction using multiparametric MRI. *Med Phys* 2011, 38:2986–2994.

27. Peng Y, Jiang Y, Yang C, Brown JB, Antic T, Sethi I, Schmid-Tannwald C, Giger ML, Eggener SE, Oto A: Quantitative analysis of multiparametric prostate MR images: Differentiation between prostate cancer and normal tissue and correlation with Gleason score—a computer-aided diagnosis development study. *Radiology* 2013, 267:787–796.

28. Nowak J, Malzahn U, Baur AD, Reichelt U, Franiel T, Hamm B, Durmus T: The value of ADC, T2 signal intensity, and a combination of both parameters to assess Gleason score and primary Gleason grades in patients with known prostate cancer. *Acta Radiol* 2014, 57:107–114.

29. Hoang Dinh A, Souchon R, Melodelima C, Bratan F, Mege-Lechevallier F, Colombel M, Rouviere O: Characterization of prostate cancer using T2 mapping at 3T: A multi-scanner study. *Diagn Interv Imaging* 2015, 96:365–372.

30. Durmus T, Baur A, Hamm B: Multiparametric magnetic resonance imaging in the detection of prostate cancer. *Aktuelle Urol* 2014, 45:119–126.

31. Ewing JR, Bagher-Ebadian H: Model selection in measures of vascular parameters using dynamic contrast-enhanced MRI: experimental and clinical applications. *NMR Biomed* 2013, 26:1028–1041.

32. Tofts PS, Brix G, Buckley DL, Evelhoch JL, Henderson E, Knopp MV, Larsson HB, Lee TY, Mayr NA, Parker GJ et al.: Estimating kinetic parameters from dynamic contrast-enhanced T(1)-weighted MRI of a diffusable tracer: Standardized quantities and symbols. *J Magn Reson Imaging* 1999, 10:223–232.

33. Fedorov A, Fluckiger J, Ayers GD, Li X, Gupta SN, Tempany C, Mulkern R, Yankeelov TE, Fennessy FM: A comparison of two methods for estimating DCE-MRI parameters via individual and cohort based AIFs in prostate cancer: A step towards practical implementation. *Magn Reson Imaging* 2014, 32:321–329.

34. Gliozzi AS, Mazzetti S, Delsanto PP, Regge D, Stasi M: Phenomenological universalities: A novel tool for the analysis of dynamic contrast enhancement in magnetic resonance imaging. *Phys Med Biol* 2011, 56:573–586.

35. Mazzetti S, Gliozzi AS, Bracco C, Russo F, Regge D, Stasi M: Comparison between PUN and Tofts models in the quantification of dynamic contrast-enhanced MR imaging. *Phys Med Biol* 2012, 57:8443–8453.

36. Vos PC, Hambrock T, Hulsbergen-van de Kaa CA, Futterer JJ, Barentsz JO, Huisman HJ: Computerized analysis of prostate lesions in the peripheral zone using dynamic contrast enhanced MRI. *Med Phys* 2008, 35:888–899.

37. Vos PC, Hambrock T, Barentsz JO, Huisman HJ: Automated calibration for computerized analysis of prostate lesions using pharmacokinetic magnetic resonance images. *Med Image Comput Comput Assist Interv* 2009, 12:836–843.

38. Puech P, Betrouni N, Makni N, Dewalle AS, Villers A, Lemaitre L: Computer-assisted diagnosis of prostate cancer using DCE-MRI data: Design, implementation and preliminary results. *Int J Comput Assist Radiol Surg* 2009, 4:1–10.

39. Puech P, Betrouni N, Viard R, Villers A, Leroy X, Lemaitre L: Prostate cancer computer-assisted diagnosis software using dynamic contrast-enhanced MRI. *Conf Proc IEEE Eng Med Biol Soc* 2007, 2007:5567–5570.

40. Padhani AR, Gapinski CJ, Macvicar DA, Parker GJ, Suckling J, Revell PB, Leach MO, Dearnaley DP, Husband JE: Dynamic contrast enhanced MRI of prostate cancer: Correlation with morphology and tumour stage, histological grade and PSA. *Clin Radiol* 2000, 55:99–109.

41. Dikaios N, Alkalbani J, Abd-Alazeez M, Sidhu HS, Kirkham A, Ahmed HU, Emberton M, Freeman A, Halligan S, Taylor S et al.: Zone-specific logistic regression models improve classification of prostate cancer on multi-parametric MRI. *Eur Radiol* 2015, 25:2727–2737.

42. Joseph H. Yacoub M, Aytekin Oto, Frank H. Miller: MR imaging of the prostate. *Radiol Clin N Am* 2014, 52:811–837.

43. Toivonen J, Merisaari H, Pesola M, Taimen P, Bostrom PJ, Pahikkala T, Aronen HJ, Jambor I: Mathematical models for diffusion-weighted imaging of prostate cancer using b values up to 2000 s/mm(2): Correlation with Gleason score and repeatability of region of interest analysis. *Magn Reson Med* 2015, 74:1116–1124.

44. Boesen L, Chabanova E, Logager V, Balslev I, Thomsen HS: Apparent diffusion coefficient ratio correlates significantly with prostate cancer Gleason score at final pathology. *J Magn Reson Imaging* 2015, 42:446–453.

45. Mazaheri Y, Shukla-Dave A, Hricak H, Fine SW, Zhang J, Inurrigarro G, Moskowitz CS, Ishill NM, Reuter VE, Touijer K et al.: Prostate cancer: Identification with combined diffusion-weighted MR imaging and 3D 1H MR spectroscopic imaging—Correlation with pathologic findings. *Radiology* 2008, 246:480–488.

46. Peng Y, Jiang Y, Antic T, Giger ML, Eggener SE, Oto A: Validation of quantitative analysis of multiparametric prostate MR images for prostate cancer detection and aggressiveness assessment: A cross-imager study. *Radiology* 2014, 271:461–471.

47. Kitajima K, Takahashi S, Ueno Y, Yoshikawa T, Ohno Y, Obara M, Miyake H, Fujisawa M, Sugimura K: Clinical utility of apparent diffusion coefficient values obtained using high b-value when diagnosing prostate cancer using 3 tesla MRI: Comparison between ultra-high b-value (2000 s/mm(2)) and standard high b-value (1000 s/mm(2)). *J Magn Reson Imaging* 2012, 36:198–205.

48. Kim CK, Park BK, Kim B: High-b-value diffusion-weighted imaging at 3 T to detect prostate cancer: Comparisons between b values of 1,000 and 2,000 s/mm^2. *AJR Am J Roentgenol* 2010, 194:W33–W37.

49. Wetter A, Nensa F, Lipponer C, Guberina N, Olbricht T, Schenck M, Schlosser TW, Gratz M, Lauenstein TC: High and ultra-high b-value diffusion-weighted imaging in prostate cancer: A quantitative analysis. *Acta Radiol* 2015, 56:1009–1015.

50. Wang X, Qian Y, Liu B, Cao L, Fan Y, Zhang JJ, Yu Y: High-b-value diffusion-weighted MRI for the detection of prostate cancer at 3 T. *Clin Radiol* 2014, 69:1165–1170.

51. Stember JN, Deng FM, Taneja SS, Rosenkrantz AB: Pilot study of a novel tool for input-free automated identification of transition zone prostate tumors using T2- and diffusion-weighted signal and textural features. *J Magn Reson Imaging* 2014, 40:301–305.

52. Kwak JT, Xu S, Wood BJ, Turkbey B, Choyke PL, Pinto PA, Wang S, Summers RM: Automated prostate cancer detection using T2-weighted and high-b-value diffusion-weighted magnetic resonance imaging. *Med Phys* 2015, 42:2368–2378.

53. Neto JA, Parente DB: Multiparametric magnetic resonance imaging of the prostate. *Magn Reson Imaging Clin N Am* 2013, 21:409–426.

54. Tiwari P, Madabhushi A, Rosen M: A hierarchical unsupervised spectral clustering scheme for detection of prostate cancer from magnetic resonance spectroscopy (MRS). *Med Image Comput Comput Assist Interv* 2007, 10:278–286.

55. Tiwari P, Rosen M, Madabhushi A: A hierarchical spectral clustering and nonlinear dimensionality reduction scheme for detection of prostate cancer from magnetic resonance spectroscopy (MRS). *Med Phys* 2009, 36:3927–3939.

56. Tiwari P, Viswanath S, Kurhanewicz J, Sridhar A, Madabhushi A: Multimodal wavelet embedding representation for data combination (MaWERiC): Integrating magnetic resonance imaging and spectroscopy for prostate cancer detection. *NMR Biomed* 2012, 25:607–619.

57. Matulewicz L, Jansen JF, Bokacheva L, Vargas HA, Akin O, Fine SW, Shukla-Dave A, Eastham JA, Hricak H, Koutcher JA, Zakian KL: Anatomic segmentation improves prostate cancer detection with artificial neural networks analysis of H magnetic resonance spectroscopic imaging. *J Magn Reson Imaging* 2013, 40:1414–1421.

58. Panebianco V, Barchetti F, Sciarra A, Marcantonio A, Zini C, Salciccia S, Collettini F, Gentile V, Hamm B, Catalano C: In vivo 3D neuroanatomical evaluation of periprostatic nerve plexus with 3T-MR Diffusion Tensor Imaging. *Eur J Radiol* 2013, 82:1677–1682.

59. Sinha S, Sinha U: In vivo diffusion tensor imaging of the human prostate. *Magn Reson Med* 2004, 52:530–537.

60. Xu J, Humphrey PA, Kibel AS, Snyder AZ, Narra VR, Ackerman JJ, Song SK: Magnetic resonance diffusion characteristics of histologically defined prostate cancer in humans. *Magn Reson Med* 2009, 61:842–850.

61. Takayama Y, Kishimoto R, Hanaoka S, Nonaka H, Kandatsu S, Tsuji H, Tsujii H, Ikehira H, Obata T: ADC value and diffusion tensor imaging of prostate cancer: Changes in carbon-ion radiotherapy. *J Magn Reson Imaging* 2008, 27:1331–1335.

62. Litjens G, Debats O, Barentsz J, Karssemeijer N, Huisman H: Computer-aided detection of prostate cancer in MRI. *IEEE Trans Med Imaging* 2014, 33:1083–1092.

63. Suo S, Chen X, Wu L, Zhang X, Yao Q, Fan Y, Wang H, Xu J: Non-Gaussian water diffusion kurtosis imaging of prostate cancer. *Magn Reson Imaging* 2014, 32:421–427.

64. Roethke MC, Kuder TA, Kuru TH, Fenchel M, Hadaschik BA, Laun FB, Schlemmer HP, Stieltjes B: Evaluation of Diffusion Kurtosis Imaging Versus Standard Diffusion Imaging for Detection and Grading of Peripheral Zone Prostate Cancer. *Invest Radiol* 2015, 50:483–489.

65. Suga M, Aga T, Minato K: Development of a magnetic resonance elastic microscope system. *Conf Proc IEEE Eng Med Biol Soc* 2004, 2:1025–1027.

66. Venkatesh SK, Yin M, Glockner JF, Takahashi N, Araoz PA, Talwalkar JA, Ehman RL: MR elastography of liver tumors: Preliminary results. *AJR Am J Roentgenol* 2008, 190:1534–1540.

67. Hamhaber U, Klatt D, Papazoglou S, Hollmann M, Stadler J, Sack I, Bernarding J, Braun J: In vivo magnetic resonance elastography of human brain at 7 T and 1.5 T. *J Magn Reson Imaging* 2010, 32:577–583.

68. Sinkus R, Tanter M, Xydeas T, Catheline S, Bercoff J, Fink M: Viscoelastic shear properties of in vivo breast lesions measured by MR elastography. *Magn Reson Imaging* 2005, 23:159–165.

69. McKnight AL, Kugel JL, Rossman PJ, Manduca A, Hartmann LC, Ehman RL: MR elastography of breast cancer: Preliminary results. *AJR Am J Roentgenol* 2002, 178:1411–1417.

70. Sinkus R, Lorenzen J, Schrader D, Lorenzen M, Dargatz M, Holz D: High-resolution tensor MR elastography for breast tumour detection. *Phys Med Biol* 2000, 45:1649–1664.

71. Arani A, Da Rosa M, Ramsay E, Plewes DB, Haider MA, Chopra R: Incorporating endorectal MR elastography into multi-parametric MRI for prostate cancer imaging: Initial feasibility in volunteers. *J Magn Reson Imaging* 2013, 38:1251–1260.

72. Li S, Chen M, Wang W, Zhao W, Wang J, Zhao X, Zhou C: A feasibility study of MR elastography in the diagnosis of prostate cancer at 3.0T. *Acta Radiol* 2011, 52:354–358.

73. Arani A, Plewes D, Krieger A, Chopra R: The feasibility of endorectal MR elastography for prostate cancer localization. *Magn Reson Med* 2011, 66:1649–1657.

74. Fennessy FM, Fedorov A, Gupta SN, Schmidt EJ, Tempany CM, Mulkern RV: Practical considerations in T1 mapping of prostate for dynamic contrast enhancement pharmacokinetic analyses. *Magn Reson Imaging* 2012, 30:1224–1233.

75. Fortuin AS, Smeenk RJ, Meijer HJ, Witjes AJ, Barentsz JO: Lymphotropic nanoparticle-enhanced MRI in prostate cancer: Value and therapeutic potential. *Curr Urol Rep* 2014, 15:389.

76. Thoeny HC, Triantafyllou M, Birkhaeuser FD, Froehlich JM, Tshering DW, Binser T, Fleischmann A, Vermathen P, Studer UE: Combined ultrasmall superparamagnetic particles of iron oxide-enhanced and diffusion-weighted magnetic resonance imaging reliably detect pelvic lymph node metastases in normal-sized nodes of bladder and prostate cancer patients. *Eur Urol* 2009, 55:761-769.

77. Derhy S, El Mouhadi S, Ruiz A, Azizi L, Menu Y, Arrive L: Non-contrast 3D MR lymphography of retroperitoneal lymphatic aneurysmal dilatation: A continuous spectrum of change from normal variants to cystic lymphangioma. *Insights Imaging* 2013, 4:753–758.

78. Arrive L, Derhy S, El Mouhadi S, Monnier-Cholley L, Menu Y, Becker C: Noncontrast magnetic resonance lymphography. *J Reconstr Microsurg* 2015, 32:80–86.

79. Collewet G, Strzelecki M, Mariette F: Influence of MRI acquisition protocols and image intensity normalization methods on texture classification. *Magn Reson Imaging* 2004, 22:81–91.

80. Vovk U, Pernuš F, Likar B: MRI intensity inhomogeneity correction by combining intensity and spatial information. *Phys Med Biol* 2004, 49:4119.

81. Vovk U, Pernuš F, Likar B: A review of methods for correction of intensity inhomogeneity in MRI. *IEEE Trans Med Imaging* 2007, 26:405–421.

82. Sled JG, Zijdenbos AP, Evans AC: A nonparametric method for automatic correction of intensity non-uniformity in MRI data. *IEEE Trans Med Imaging* 1998, 17:87–97.

83. Tustison NJ, Avants BB, Cook PA, Zheng Y, Egan A, Yushkevich PA, Gee JC: N4ITK: improved N3 bias correction. *IEEE Trans Med Imaging* 2010, 29:1310–1320.

84. Qiu W, Yuan J, Ukwatta E, Sun Y, Rajchl M, Fenster A: Dual optimization based prostate zonal segmentation in 3D MR images. *Med Image Anal* 2014, 18:660–673.

85. Mahapatra D, Buhmann JM: Prostate MRI segmentation using learned semantic knowledge and graph cuts. *IEEE Trans Biomed Eng* 2014, 61:756–764.

86. Liao S, Gao Y, Oto A, Shen D: Representation learning: A unified deep learning framework for automatic prostate MR segmentation. *Med Image Comput Comput Assist Interv* 2013, 16:254–261.

87. Toth R, Madabhushi A: Multifeature landmark-free active appearance models: Application to prostate MRI segmentation. *IEEE Trans Med Imaging* 2012, 31:1638–1650.

88. Litjens G, Debats O, van de Ven W, Karssemeijer N, Huisman H: A pattern recognition approach to zonal segmentation of the prostate on MRI. *Med Image Comput Comput Assist Interv* 2012, 15:413–420.

89. Qiu W, Yuan J, Ukwatta E, Sun Y, Rajchl M, and Fenster A: Prostate segmentation: An efficient convex optimization approach with axial symmetry using 3-D TRUS and MR images. *IEEE Trans Med Imaging* 2014, 33:947–960.

90. Yang M, Li X, Turkbey B, Choyke PL, Yan P: Prostate segmentation in MR images using discriminant boundary features. *Biomed Eng IEEE Trans* 2013, 60:479–488.

91. Zwiggelaar R, Zhu Y, Williams S: Semi-automatic segmentation of the prostate. In *Pattern Recognition and Image Analysis*. Springer; 2003: 1108–1116

92. Flores-Tapia D, Thomas G, Venugopa N, McCurdy B, Pistorius S: Semi automatic MRI prostate segmentation based on wavelet multiscale products. In *Engineering in Medicine and Biology Society, 2008 EMBS 2008 30th Annual International Conference of the IEEE*. IEEE; 2008: 3020–3023.

93. Samiee M, Thomas G, Fazel-Rezai R: Semi-automatic prostate segmentation of MR images based on flow orientation. In *Signal Processing and Information Technology, 2006 IEEE International Symposium on*. IEEE; 2006: 203–207.

94. Cootes TF, Hill A, Taylor CJ, Haslam J: The use of active shape models for locating structures in medical images. In *Information Processing in Medical Imaging*. Springer; 1993: 33–47.

95. Zhu Y, Williams S, Zwiggelaar R: A hybrid ASM approach for sparse volumetric data segmentation. *Pattern Recognition and Image Analysis* 2007, 17:252–258.

96. Kass M, Witkin A, Terzopoulos D: Snakes: Active contour models. *Int J Comput Vis* 1988, 1:321–331.

97. Chan TF, Vese LA: Active contours without edges. *IEEE Trans Image Process* 2001, 10:266–277.

98. Mumford D, Shah J: Optimal approximations by piecewise smooth functions and associated variational problems. *Commun Pure Appl Math* 1989, 42:577–685.

99. Klein S, van der Heide UA, Lips IM, van Vulpen M, Staring M, Pluim JPW: Automatic segmentation of the prostate in 3D MR images by atlas matching using localized mutual information. *Med Phys* 2008, 35:1407–1417.

100. Boykov Y, Veksler O, Zabih R: Fast approximate energy minimization via graph cuts. *IEEE Trans Pattern Anal Mach Intell* 2001, 23:1222–1239.

101. Boykov YY, Jolly M-P: Interactive graph cuts for optimal boundary & region segmentation of objects in ND images. In *Computer Vision, 2001 ICCV 2001 Proceedings Eighth IEEE International Conference on*. IEEE; 2001: 105–112.

102. Egger J: PCG-cut: Graph driven segmentation of the prostate central gland. *PLOS One* 2013, 8:6.

103. Tian Z, Liu L, Fei B: A supervoxel-based segmentation for prostate MR images. In SPIE Medical Imaging. *International Society for Optics and Photonics*; 2015: 941318-941318-941317.

104. Litjens G, Toth R, van de Ven W, Hoeks C, Kerkstra S, van Ginneken B, Vincent G, Guillard G, Birbeck N, Zhang J: Evaluation of prostate segmentation algorithms for MRI: The PROMISE12 challenge. *Med Image Anal* 2014, 18:359–373.

105. Ghose S, Oliver A, Marti R, Llado X, Vilanova JC, Freixenet J, Mitra J, Sidibe D, Meriaudeau F: A survey of prostate segmentation methodologies in ultrasound, magnetic resonance and computed tomography images. *Comput Methods Programs Biomed* 2012, 108:262–287.

106. Oliveira FP, Tavares JMR: Medical image registration: A review. *Comput Methods Biomech Biomed Eng* 2014, 17:73–93.

107. Chappelow J, Madabhushi A, Rosen M, Tomaszeweski J, Feldman M: Multimodal image registration of ex vivo 4 Tesla MRI with whole mount histology for prostate cancer detection. In Medical Imaging. *International Society for Optics and Photonics*; 2007: 65121S-65121S-65112.

108. Kalavagunta C, Zhou X, Schmechel SC, Metzger GJ: Registration of in vivo prostate MRI and pseudo-whole mount histology using Local Affine Transformations guided by Internal Structures (LATIS). *J Magn Reson Imaging* 2014, 41:1104–1114.

109. Huisman HJ, Engelbrecht MR, Barentsz JO: Accurate estimation of pharmacokinetic contrast-enhanced dynamic MRI parameters of the prostate. *J Magn Reson Imaging* 2001, 13:607–614.

110. Li Q, Sone S, Doi K: Selective enhancement filters for nodules, vessels, and airway walls in two- and three-dimensional CT scans. *Med Phys* 2003, 30:2040–2051.

111. Langer DL, van der Kwast TH, Evans AJ, Trachtenberg J, Wilson BC, Haider MA: Prostate cancer detection with multi-parametric MRI: Logistic regression analysis of quantitative T2, diffusion-weighted imaging, and dynamic contrast-enhanced MRI. *J Magn Reson Imaging* 2009, 30:327–334.

112. Murase K: Efficient method for calculating kinetic parameters using T1-weighted dynamic contrast-enhanced magnetic resonance imaging. *Magn Reson Med* 2004, 51:858–862.

113. Lambin P, Rios-Velazquez E, Leijenaar R, Carvalho S, van Stiphout RG, Granton P, Zegers CM, Gillies R, Boellard R, Dekker A: Radiomics: Extracting more information from medical images using advanced feature analysis. *Eur J Cancer* 2012, 48:441–446.

114. Kumar V, Gu Y, Basu S, Berglund A, Eschrich SA, Schabath MB, Forster K, Aerts HJ, Dekker A, Fenstermacher D: Radiomics: The process and the challenges. *Magn Reson Imaging* 2012, 30:1234–1248.

115. Cameron A, Khalvati F, Haider M, Wong A: MAPS: A quantitative radiomics approach for prostate cancer detection. *IEEE Trans Biomed Eng* 2015, 63:1145–1156.

116. Wibmer A, Hricak H, Gondo T, Matsumoto K, Veeraraghavan H, Fehr D, Zheng J, Goldman D, Moskowitz C, Fine SW et al.: Haralick texture analysis of prostate MRI: Utility for differentiating non-cancerous prostate from prostate cancer and differentiating prostate cancers with different Gleason scores. *Eur Radiol* 2015, 25:2840–2850.

117. Fehr D, Veeraraghavan H: Automatic classification of prostate cancer Gleason scores from multiparametric magnetic resonance images. *Proc Nat Acad Sci* 2015, 112:E6265–E6273.

118. Khalvati F, Wong A, Haider MA: Automated prostate cancer detection via comprehensive multi-parametric magnetic resonance imaging texture feature models. *BMC Med Imaging* 2015, 15:27.

119. Breiman L: Random forests. *Mach Lear* 2001, 45:5–32.

120. Friedman J, Hastie T, Tibshirani R: Additive logistic regression: A statistical view of boosting (with discussion and a rejoinder by the authors). *Ann Stat* 2000, 28:337–407.

121. Baeza-Yates R, Ribeiro-Neto B: *Modern Information Retrieval*. ACM Press, New York; 1999.

122. Chan I, Wells W, 3rd, Mulkern RV, Haker S, Zhang J, Zou KH, Maier SE, Tempany CM: Detection of prostate cancer by integration of line-scan diffusion, T2-mapping and T2-weighted magnetic resonance imaging; a multichannel statistical classifier. *Med Phys* 2003, 30:2390–2398.

123. Donati OF, Mazaheri Y, Afaq A, Vargas HA, Zheng J, Moskowitz CS, Hricak H, Akin O: Prostate cancer aggressiveness: Assessment with whole-lesion histogram analysis of the apparent diffusion coefficient. *Radiology* 2014, 271:143–152.

124. Shah V, Pohida T, Turkbey B, Mani H, Merino M, Pinto PA, Choyke P, Bernardo M: A method for correlating in vivo prostate magnetic resonance imaging and histopathology using individualized magnetic resonance-based molds. *Rev Sci Instrum* 2009, 80:104301.

125. Mazaheri Y, Bokacheva L, Kroon DJ, Akin O, Hricak H, Chamudot D, Fine S, Koutcher JA: Semiautomatic deformable registration of prostate MR images to pathological slices. *J Magn Reson Imaging* 2010, 32:1149–1157.

126. Jacobs MA, Windham JP, Soltanian-Zadeh H, Peck DJ, Knight RA: Registration and warping of magnetic resonance images to histological sections. *Med Phys* 1999, 26:1568–1578.

127. Park H, Piert MR, Khan A, Shah R, Hussain H, Siddiqui J, Chenevert TL, Meyer CR: Registration methodology for histological sections and in vivo imaging of human prostate. *Acad Radiol* 2008, 15:1027–1039.

128. Meyer CR, Moffat BA, Kuszpit KK, Bland PL, McKeever PE, Johnson TD, Chenevert TL, Rehemtulla A, Ross BD: A methodology for registration of a histological slide and in vivo MRI volume based on optimizing mutual information. *Mol Imaging* 2006, 5:16–23.

129. Viswanath S, Bloch BN, Rosen M, Chappelow J, Toth R, Rofsky N, Lenkinski R, Genega E, Kalyanpur A, Madabhushi A: Integrating Structural and Functional Imaging for Computer Assisted Detection of Prostate Cancer on Multi-Protocol 3 Tesla MRI. *Proc Soc Photo Opt Instrum Eng* 2009, 7260:72603I.

130. Gibson E, Gaed M, Gomez JA, Moussa M, Pautler S, Chin JL, Crukley C, Bauman GS, Fenster A, Ward AD: 3D prostate histology image reconstruction: Quantifying the impact of tissue deformation and histology section location. *J Pathol Inform* 2013, 4:31.

131. Gibson E, Gaed M, Gomez JA, Moussa M, Romagnoli C, Pautler S, Chin JL, Crukley C, Bauman GS, Fenster A, Ward AD: 3D prostate histology reconstruction: An evaluation of image-based and fiducial-based algorithms. *Med Phys* 2013, 40:093501.

132. Patel P, Chappelow J, Tomaszewski J, Feldman MD, Rosen M, Shih N, Madabhushi A: Spatially weighted mutual information (SWMI) for registration of digitally reconstructed ex vivo whole mount histology and in vivo prostate MRI. *Conf Proc IEEE Eng Med Biol Soc* 2011, 2011:6269–6272.

133. McGrath DM, Vlad RM, Foltz WD, Brock KK: Technical note: Fiducial markers for correlation of whole-specimen histopathology with MR imaging at 7 tesla. *Med Phys* 2010, 37:2321–2328.

134. Toth RJ, Shih N, Tomaszewski JE, Feldman MD, Kutter O, Yu DN, Paulus JC, Jr., Paladini G, Madabhushi A: Histostitcher: An informatics software platform for reconstructing whole-mount prostate histology using the extensible imaging platform framework. *J Pathol Inform* 2014, 5:8.

135. Chappelow J, Bloch BN, Rofsky N, Genega E, Lenkinski R, DeWolf W, Madabhushi A: Elastic registration of multimodal prostate MRI and histology via multiattribute combined mutual information. *Med Phys* 2011, 38:2005–2018.

136. Orczyk C, Rusinek H, Rosenkrantz AB, Mikheev A, Deng FM, Melamed J, Taneja SS: Preliminary experience with a novel method of three-dimensional co-registration of prostate cancer digital histology and in vivo multiparametric MRI. *Clin Radiol* 2013, 68:e652–e658.

137. Lv D, Guo X, Wang X, Zhang J, Fang J: Computerized characterization of prostate cancer by fractal analysis in MR images. *J Magn Reson Imaging* 2009, 30:161–168.

138. Rouviere O, Papillard M, Girouin N, Boutier R, Rabilloud M, Riche B, Mege-Lechevallier F, Colombel M, Gelet A: Is it possible to model the risk of malignancy of focal abnormalities found at prostate multiparametric MRI? *Eur Radiol* 2012, 22:1149–1157.

139. Meyer C, Ma B, Kunju LP, Davenport M, Piert M: Challenges in accurate registration of 3-D medical imaging and histopathology in primary prostate cancer. *Eur J Nucl Med Mol Imaging* 2013, 40:72–78.

140. Viswanath S, Bloch BN, Genega E, Rofsky N, Lenkinski R, Chappelow J, Toth R, Madabhushi A: A comprehensive segmentation, registration, and cancer detection scheme on 3 Tesla in vivo prostate DCE-MRI. *Med Image Comput Comput Assist Interv* 2008, 11:662–669.

141. Liu X, Langer DL, Haider MA, Yang Y, Wernick MN, Yetik IS: Prostate cancer segmentation with simultaneous estimation of Markov random field parameters and class. *IEEE Trans Med Imaging* 2009, 28:906–915.

142. Artan Y, Haider MA, Langer DL, van der Kwast TH, Evans AJ, Yang Y, Wernick MN, Trachtenberg J, Yetik IS: Prostate cancer localization with multispectral MRI using cost-sensitive support vector machines and conditional random fields. *IEEE Trans Image Process* 2010, 19:2444–2455.

143. Vos PC, Hambrock T, Barenstz JO, Huisman HJ: Computer-assisted analysis of peripheral zone prostate lesions using T2-weighted and dynamic contrast enhanced T1-weighted MRI. *Phys Med Biol* 2010, 55:1719–1734.

144. Viswanath S, Bloch BN, Chappelow J, Patel P, Rofsky N, Lenkinski R, Genega E, Madabhushi A: Enhanced multi-protocol analysis via intelligent supervised embedding (EMPrAvISE): Detecting prostate cancer on multi-parametric MRI. *Proc SPIE Int Soc Opt Eng* 2011, 7963:79630u.

145. Lopes R, Ayache A, Makni N, Puech P, Villers A, Mordon S, Betrouni N: Prostate cancer characterization on MR images using fractal features. *Med Phys* 2011, 38:83–95.

146. Sung YS, Kwon HJ, Park BW, Cho G, Lee CK, Cho KS, Kim JK: Prostate cancer detection on dynamic contrast-enhanced MRI: Computer-aided diagnosis versus single perfusion parameter maps. *AJR Am J Roentgenol* 2011, 197:1122–1129.

147. Artan Y, Yetik IS: Prostate cancer localization using multiparametric MRI based on semi-supervised techniques with automated seed initialization. *IEEE Trans Inf Technol Biomed* 2012, 16:1313–1323.

148. Tiwari P, Kurhanewicz J, Madabhushi A: Multi-kernel graph embedding for detection, Gleason grading of prostate cancer via MRI/MRS. *Med Image Anal* 2013, 17:219–235.

149. Ginsburg SB, Viswanath SE, Bloch BN, Rofsky NM, Genega EM, Lenkinski RE, Madabhushi A: Novel PCA-VIP scheme for ranking MRI protocols and identifying computer-extracted MRI measurements associated with central gland and peripheral zone prostate tumors. *J Magn Reson Imaging* 2014, 41: 1383–1393.

150. Niaf E, Flamary R, Rouviere O, Lartizien C, Canu S: Kernel-based learning from both qualitative and quantitative labels: Application to prostate cancer diagnosis based on multiparametric MR imaging. *IEEE Trans Image Process* 2014, 23:979–991.

151. Zhao K, Wang C, Hu J, Yang X, Wang H, Li F, Zhang X, Zhang J, Wang X: Prostate cancer identification: Quantitative analysis of T2-weighted MR images based on a back propagation artificial neural network model. *Sci China Life Sci* 2015, 58:666–673.

152. Saman DM, Lemieux AM, Nawal Lutfiyya M, Lipsky MS: A review of the current epidemiology and treatment options for prostate cancer. *Dis Mon* 2014, 60:150–154.

153. Keyes M, Crook J, Morton G, Vigneault E, Usmani N, Morris WJ: Treatment options for localized prostate cancer. *Can Fam Physician* 2013, 59:1269–1274.

154. Oto A, Yang C, Kayhan A, Tretiakova M, Antic T, Schmid-Tannwald C, Eggener S, Karczmar GS, Stadler WM: Diffusion-weighted and dynamic contrast-enhanced MRI of prostate cancer: Correlation of quantitative MR parameters with Gleason score and tumor angiogenesis. *AJR Am J Roentgenol* 2011, 197:1382–1390.

155. Anwar SS, Anwar Khan Z, Shoaib Hamid R, Haroon F, Sayani R, Beg M: Assessment of apparent diffusion coefficient values as predictor of aggressiveness in peripheral zone prostate cancer: Comparison with Gleason score. *ISRN Radiol* 2014, 2014:263417.

156. Hambrock T, Somford DM, Huisman HJ, van Oort IM, Witjes JA, Hulsbergen-van de Kaa CA, Scheenen T, Barentsz JO: Relationship between apparent diffusion coefficients at 3.0-T MR imaging and Gleason grade in peripheral zone prostate cancer. *Radiology* 2011, 259:453–461.

157. Yamamura J, Salomon G, Buchert R, Hohenstein A, Graessner J, Huland H, Graefen M, Adam G, Wedegaetner U: MR imaging of prostate cancer: Diffusion weighted imaging and (3D) Hydrogen 1 (H) MR spectroscopy in comparison with histology. *Radiol Res Pract* 2011, 2011:616852.

158. Gibbs P, Liney GP, Pickles MD, Zelhof B, Rodrigues G, Turnbull LW: Correlation of ADC and T2 measurements with cell density in prostate cancer at 3.0 Tesla. *Invest Radiol* 2009, 44:572–576.

159. Anderson AW, Xie J, Pizzonia J, Bronen RA, Spencer DD, Gore JC: Effects of cell volume fraction changes on apparent diffusion in human cells. *Magn Reson Imaging* 2000, 18:689–695.

160. Tanimoto K, Yoshikawa K, Obata T, Ikehira H, Shiraishi T, Watanabe K, Saga T, Mizoe J, Kamada T, Kato A, Miyazaki M: Role of glucose metabolism and cellularity for tumor malignancy evaluation using FDG-PET/CT and MRI. *Nucl Med Commun* 2010, 31:604–609.

161. Kobus T, Hambrock T, Hulsbergen-van de Kaa CA, Wright AJ, Barentsz JO, Heerschap A, Scheenen TW: In vivo assessment of prostate cancer aggressiveness using magnetic resonance spectroscopic imaging at 3 T with an endorectal coil. *Eur Urol* 2011, 60:1074–1080.

162. Zakian KL, Sircar K, Hricak H, Chen HN, Shukla-Dave A, Eberhardt S, Muruganandham M, Ebora L, Kattan MW, Reuter VE et al.: Correlation of proton MR spectroscopic imaging with gleason score based on step-section pathologic analysis after radical prostatectomy. *Radiology* 2005, 234:804–814.

163. van Asten JJ, Cuijpers V, Hulsbergen-van de Kaa C, Soede-Huijbregts C, Witjes JA, Verhofstad A, Heerschap A: High resolution magic angle spinning NMR spectroscopy for metabolic assessment of cancer presence and Gleason score in human prostate needle biopsies. *Magma* 2008, 21:435–442.

164. Garcia-Martin ML, Adrados M, Ortega MP, Fernandez Gonzalez I, Lopez-Larrubia P, Viano J, Garcia-Segura JM: Quantitative (1) H MR spectroscopic imaging of the prostate gland using LCModel and a dedicated basis-set: Correlation with histologic findings. *Magn Reson Med* 2011, 65:329–339.

165. Scheenen TW, Heijmink SW, Roell SA, Hulsbergen-Van de Kaa CA, Knipscheer BC, Witjes JA, Barentsz JO, Heerschap A: Three-dimensional proton MR spectroscopy of human prostate at 3 T without endorectal coil: feasibility. *Radiology* 2007, 245:507–516.

166. Shukla-Dave A, Hricak H, Ishill NM, Moskowitz CS, Drobnjak M, Reuter VE, Zakian KL, Scardino PT, Cordon-Cardo C: Correlation of MR imaging and MR spectroscopic imaging findings with Ki-67, phospho-Akt, and androgen receptor expression in prostate cancer. *Radiology* 2009, 250:803–812.

167. Lee DH, Koo KC, Lee SH, Rha KH, Choi YD, Hong SJ, Chung BH: Tumor lesion diameter on diffusion weighted magnetic resonance imaging could help predict insignificant prostate cancer in patients eligible for active surveillance: Preliminary analysis. *J Urol* 2013, 190:1213–1217.

168. Epstein JI, Allsbrook WC, Jr., Amin MB, Egevad LL: The 2005 International Society of Urological Pathology (ISUP) Consensus Conference on Gleason Grading of Prostatic Carcinoma. *Am J Surg Pathol* 2005, 29:1228–1242.

169. Cam K, Yucel S, Turkeri L, Akdas A: Accuracy of transrectal ultrasound guided prostate biopsy: Histopathological correlation to matched prostatectomy specimens. *Int J Urol* 2002, 9:257–260.

170. Quann P, Jarrard DF, Huang W: Current prostate biopsy protocols cannot reliably identify patients for focal therapy: Correlation of low-risk prostate cancer on biopsy with radical prostatectomy findings. *Int J Clin Exp Pathol* 2010, 3:401–407.

171. Djavan B, Ravery V, Zlotta A, Dobronski P, Dobrovits M, Fakhari M, Seitz C, Susani M, Borkowski A, Boccon-Gibod L et al.: Prospective evaluation of prostate cancer detected on biopsies 1, 2, 3 and 4: when should we stop? *J Urol* 2001, 166:1679–1683.

172. Futterer JJ, Barentsz JO: MRI-guided and robotic-assisted prostate biopsy. *Curr Opin Urol* 2012, 22:316–319.

173. Moore CM, Robertson NL, Arsanious N, Middleton T, Villers A, Klotz L, Taneja SS, Emberton M: Image-guided prostate biopsy using magnetic resonance imaging-derived targets: A systematic review. *Eur Urol* 2013, 63:125–140.

174. Xu H, Lasso A, Guion P, Krieger A, Kaushal A, Singh AK, Pinto PA, Coleman J, Grubb RL, 3rd, Lattouf JB et al.: Accuracy analysis in MRI-guided robotic prostate biopsy. *Int J Comput Assist Radiol Surg* 2013, 8:937–944.

175. Zamecnik P, Schouten MG, Krafft AJ, Maier F, Schlemmer HP, Barentsz JO, Bock M, Futterer JJ: Automated real-time needle-guide tracking for fast 3-T MR-guided transrectal prostate biopsy: A feasibility study. *Radiology* 2014, 273:879–886.

176. Fiard G, Hohn N, Descotes JL, Rambeaud JJ, Troccaz J, Long JA: Targeted MRI-guided prostate biopsies for the detection of prostate cancer: Initial clinical experience with real-time 3-dimensional transrectal ultrasound guidance and magnetic resonance/transrectal ultrasound image fusion. *Urology* 2013, 81:1372–1378.

177. Xu S, Kruecker J, Turkbey B, Glossop N, Singh AK, Choyke P, Pinto P, Wood BJ: Real-time MRI-TRUS fusion for guidance of targeted prostate biopsies. *Comput Aided Surg* 2008, 13:255–264.

178. Mitra J, Ghose S, Sidibe D, Marti R, Oliver A, Llado X, Vilanova JC, Comet J, Meriaudeau F: Joint probability of shape and image similarities to retrieve 2D TRUS-MR slice correspondence for prostate biopsy. *Conf Proc IEEE Eng Med Biol Soc* 2012, 2012:5416–5419.

179. Wang S, Burtt K, Turkbey B, Choyke P, Summers RM: Computer aided-diagnosis of prostate cancer on multiparametric MRI: A technical review of current research. *Biomed Res Int* 2014, 2014:789561.

180. Fei BW, Lee ZH, Boll DT, Duerk JL, Lewin JS, Wilson DL: Image registration and fusion for interventional MRI guided thermal ablation of the prostate cancer. In *Medical Image Computing and Computer-Assisted Intervention - Miccai 2003*, Pt 2. Vol. 2879. Edited by Ellis RE, Peters TM; 2003: 364–372: Lecture Notes in Computer Science.

181. Akbari H, Fei BW: 3D ultrasound image segmentation using wavelet support vector machines. *Med Phys* 2012, 39:2972–2984.

182. Fei BW, Lee ZH, Boll DT, Duerk JL, Sodee DB, Lewin JS, Wilson DL: Registration and fusion of SPECT, high-resolution MRI, and interventional MRI for thermal ablation of prostate cancer. *IEEE Trans Nucl Sci* 2004, 51:177–183.

183. Fei BW, Lee ZH, Duerk JL, Wilson DL: Image registration for interventional MRI guided procedures: Interpolation methods, similarity measurements, and applications to the prostate. In *Biomedical Image Registration*. Vol. 2717. Edited by Gee JC, Maintz JBA, Vannier MW; 2003: 321–329: Lecture Notes in Computer Science.

184. Fei BW, Ng WS, Chauhan S, Kwoh CK: The safety issues of medical robotics. *Reliab Eng Syst Safe* 2001, 73:183–192.

185. Fei BW, Wang H, Meyers JD, Feyes DK, Oleinick NL, Duerk JL: High-field magnetic resonance imaging of the response of human prostate cancer to pc 4-based photodynamic therapy in an animal model. *Lasers Surg Med* 2007, 39:723–730.

186. Fei BW, Wang HS, Wu CY, Chiu SM: Choline PET for monitoring early tumor response to photodynamic therapy. *J Nucl Med* 2010, 51:130–138.

187. Fei BW, Yang XF, Nye JA, Aarsvold JN, Raghunath N, Cervo M, Stark R, Meltzer CC, Votaw JR: MR/PET quantification tools: Registration, segmentation, classification, and MR-based attenuation correction. *Med Phys* 2012, 39:6443–6454.

188. Wang HS, Fei BW: Diffusion-weighted MRI for monitoring tumor response to photodynamic therapy. *J Magn Reson Imaging* 2010, 32:409–417.

189. Wang HS, Fei BW: An MR image-guided, voxel-based partial volume correction method for PET images. *Med Phys* 2012, 39:179–194.

190. Wang HS, Fei BW: Nonrigid point registration for 2D curves and 3D surfaces and its various applications. *Phys Med Biol* 2013, 58:4315–4330.

191. Song I, Kim CK, Park BK, Park W: Assessment of response to radiotherapy for prostate cancer: Value of diffusion-weighted MRI at 3 T. *AJR Am J Roentgenol* 2010, 194:W477–W482.

192. Padhani AR, Makris A, Gall P, Collins DJ, Tunariu N, de Bono JS: Therapy monitoring of skeletal metastases with whole-body diffusion MRI. *J Magn Reson Imaging* 2014, 39:1049–1078.

193. Graham TJ, Box G, Tunariu N, Crespo M, Spinks TJ, Miranda S, Attard G, de Bono J, Eccles SA, Davies FE, Robinson SP: Preclinical evaluation of imaging biomarkers for prostate cancer bone metastasis and response to cabozantinib. *J Natl Cancer Inst* 2014, 106:dju033.

194. Lee KC, Bradley DA, Hussain M, Meyer CR, Chenevert TL, Jacobson JA, Johnson TD, Galban CJ, Rehemtulla A, Pienta KJ, Ross BD: A feasibility study evaluating the functional diffusion map as a predictive imaging biomarker for detection of treatment response in a patient with metastatic prostate cancer to the bone. *Neoplasia* 2007, 9:1003–1011.

195. Sosna J, Pedrosa I, Dewolf WC, Mahallati H, Lenkinski RE, Rofsky NM: MR imaging of the prostate at 3 Tesla: Comparison of an external phased-array coil to imaging with an endorectal coil at 1.5 Tesla. *Acad Radiol* 2004, 11:857–862.

196. Turkbey B, Merino MJ, Gallardo EC, Shah V, Aras O, Bernardo M, Mena E, Daar D, Rastinehad AR, Linehan WM et al.: Comparison of endorectal coil and nonendorectal coil T2W and diffusion-weighted MRI at 3 Tesla for localizing prostate cancer: Correlation with whole-mount histopathology. *J Magn Reson Imaging* 2014, 39:1443–1448.

197. Litjens GJ, Barentsz JO, Karssemeijer N, Huisman HJ: Clinical evaluation of a computer-aided diagnosis system for determining cancer aggressiveness in prostate MRI. *Eur Radiol* 2015, 25:3187–3199.

198. Matulewicz L, Jansen JF, Bokacheva L, Vargas HA, Akin O, Fine SW, Shukla-Dave A, Eastham JA, Hricak H, Koutcher JA, Zakian KL: Anatomic segmentation improves prostate cancer detection with artificial neural networks analysis of 1H magnetic resonance spectroscopic imaging. *J Magn Reson Imaging* 2014, 40:1414–1421.

199. Huang PW, Lee CH: Automatic classification for pathological prostate images based on fractal analysis. *IEEE Trans Med Imaging* 2009, 28:1037–1050.

16 Computer-Aided Diagnosis of Prostate Magnetic Resonance Imaging
From Bench to Bedside

Valentina Giannini, Simone Mazzetti,
Filippo Russo, and Daniele Regge

CONTENTS

INTRODUCTION

Every 2 minutes, someone is diagnosed with prostate cancer (PCa) and every 6 minutes a person dies from PCa in Europe [1]. PCa represents the most common solid neoplasm in men, with an incidence rate of 214 cases per 1000, outnumbering lung and colorectal cancer [1]. Because of the increase in size of the population and aging, the number of cases is projected to increase, even if the age-specific incidence rate is projected to decrease [2]. This will have major economic implications for the future: in 2009 expenditures on PCa diagnosis, treatment, and follow-up were €8.43 billion in Europe [3], and they are projected to increase by 70% in 2030 [2]. Treatment affects costs significantly. Indeed, with the current diagnostic workflow the vast majority of men with PCa undergo radical treatment, such as radical prostatectomy (RP) or radiotherapy, including a large portion that, if left untreated, would not compromise either quality or quantity of life [4].

A major breakthrough could be accomplished by improving the diagnostic pipeline of PCa. Currently PCa diagnosis is obtained by performing multiple ultrasound-guided prostate biopsies in patients with high circulating levels of prostate-specific antigen (PSA) and/or a suspicious digital rectal examination (DRE). Pathological evaluation is performed by defining the Gleason score (GS), a histopathological score that correlates with biologic activity and prognosis [5]. According to GS and tumor size, patients can be classified as high or low risk. Some authors now argue that PCa lesions with a low Gleason pattern (i.e., 3, or GS 6 [3 + 3]), should not even be considered malignant and therefore should not be treated [6]. Hence, ruling out clinically insignificant cancer would limit the number of patients undergoing radical treatments with their related complications, reduce patient anxiety for having cancer, and limit the costs derived from overtreatment.

Unfortunately, since biopsy sampling is performed randomly, even when adopting extended biopsy schemes, up to 30% of transrectal ultrasonography (TRUS)-guided biopsies give false negative results [7]. As a consequence, these cases require clinical and/or pathological follow-up to ensure that PCa was not missed, or that any suspected premalignant lesion will not progress to a frank adenocarcinoma [8,9]. In an additional 12% biopsy GS overstages disease, which may lead to substantial overtreatment and consequent problems in terms of quality of life and socio-economic costs [10]. The magnitude of overdiagnosis is a critical issue if we compare a man's current lifetime risk of PCa, equal to 17%, with his approximate 3% risk of PCa mortality, providing one measure of the magnitude of wrong diagnosis of the disease (incidence-to-mortality ratio of 6:1) [11].

For these reasons, alternative modalities for imaging the prostate have been investigated. In the last decade, magnetic resonance imaging (MRI) has shown promise in the detection and staging of PCa because of its intrinsic high soft-tissue resolution [12]. T2-weighted (T2W) images allow clear visualization of the prostate anatomy: the central lobe can be easily distinguished from the periphery of the gland, and the capsule is clearly discernible as a thin dark linear structure. Dynamic contrast-enhanced MRI (DCE-MRI) captures T1-weighted (T1W) images while a dose of contrast agent is injected, and tumors can be detected since they usually show a distinctive early signal enhancement followed by a washout in the delayed phases. Diffusion-weighted imaging (DWI) can measure the diffusion of water molecules in tissues and hence provides information on the structural organization of a tissue. However, each MR approach has some drawbacks, which can be implied from the large range of sensitivity and specificity reported in the literature, only partially explained by the different diagnostic criteria used in the various studies [12,13]. To overcome these limitations, a multiparametric (mp) approach has been introduced, in which anatomical and functional information derived from different MRI sequences are combined to improve detection of PCas. MpMRI has been demonstrated to be very accurate in detecting clinically significant PCa, with a positive predictive value of 82% and a negative predictive value in excluding high-risk PCa greater than 95% [14,15]. As a consequence, the European Association of Urology (EAU) Guidelines have recently introduced mpMRI as strongly recommended examination before repeating biopsy when clinical suspicion of PCa persists [16]. Introducing mpMRI before prostate biopsy has the potential to improve selection of patients, and to make PCa sampling more efficient, since targeted cores contain a more complete pathological representation of the entire tumor, resulting in more personalized treatments for patients [17–19], and, perhaps, changing the way we think about initially approaching patients who present with an elevated PSA [9].

However, mpMRI has also some drawbacks: reporting is labor-intensive and time-consuming, requiring a steep learning curve. Indeed, interpretation requires experienced radiologists capable of analyzing data extracted from different MR sequences [20]. As for other consolidated applications [21–23], it has been hypothesized that computer-aided diagnosis (CAD) systems could increase the accuracy and efficiency of prostate MRI [24,25], by indicating suspicious regions and reducing oversight and perception errors [26], and, under certain conditions, also lower reading time [27]. The implementation of a fully automatic CAD system is not a trivial problem. In 2003, Chan et al. first implemented a CAD system for the diagnosis of peripheral zone (PZ) PCa, using a support vector machine (SVM) classifier [28]. In 2012, Vos et al. [25] developed a CAD scheme using multiple sequential steps, including an initial blob detection on apparent diffusion coefficient (ADC) maps followed by a local feature analysis by a supervised classifier. Similarly, Niaf et al. [29] used a SVM classifier combined with a *t* test feature-selection method, and achieved an area under the ROC curve (AUROC) equal to 0.82. Finally, Litjens et al. [30] included different stages in their CAD system, investigating a novel voxel classification step in combination with a candidate classification stage. More recently, Lemaitre et al. [31] assessed the stand-alone performance of more than 40 prostate CAD systems and reported sensitivities in the detection of PCa between 74% and 100%, and specificities between 43% and 93% when imaging was performed at 1.5T. However, there are a few studies in literature that evaluate the impact of CAD systems for PCa detection on the radiologists' performance, in particular in a condition where radiologists are not aware of disease prevalence, as it commonly happens in the daily clinical workflow.

In this chapter, we will describe a CAD for PCa detection using mpMRI and we will evaluate its application into clinical practice.

COMPUTER-AIDED DIAGNOSIS SYSTEM

STUDY POPULATION

The study population is composed of two different datasets: a training set used to develop and validate the CAD system, and a testing set on which the CAD performance was evaluated. Patients in the training set were enrolled at our Institute between April 2010 and November 2012. The following inclusion criteria were applied: (a) biopsy-proven PCa, (b) mpMRI examination including axial T2W, DW, and DCE-MR sequences, (c) radical prostatectomy (RP) within 3 months of mpMRI, and (d) a clinically significant PZ lesion (tumor volume ≥0.5 cc) [32] at the whole-mount histopathologic analysis.

Patients in the testing set were selected from a group of subjects with PSA≥4 ng/mL and/or a positive DRE, consecutively enrolled in a clinical trial where mpMRI was performed to triage patients for either in-bore prostate biopsy (maximum of 3 cores withdrawn from each lesion) or TRUS-guided saturation biopsy (at least 28 cores withdrawn from each patient) (ClinicalTrials.gov identifier: NCT02678481). The selection process is detailed in Figure 16.1. Exclusion criteria were age <18 years, history of PCa, contraindication to MRI, or a positive finding at a previous prostate biopsy.

The local Ethics Committee approved the study design, and all participants signed informed consent forms. This study was in accordance with the Helsinki Declaration.

MRI PROTOCOL

Patients of the training set were acquired with a 1.5T scanner (Signa Excite HD, GE Healthcare, Milwaukee, WI) using a four-channel phased-array coil combined with an endorectal coil (Medrad, Indianola, PA). The testing set was composed of patients acquired with a 1.5T scanner (Optima

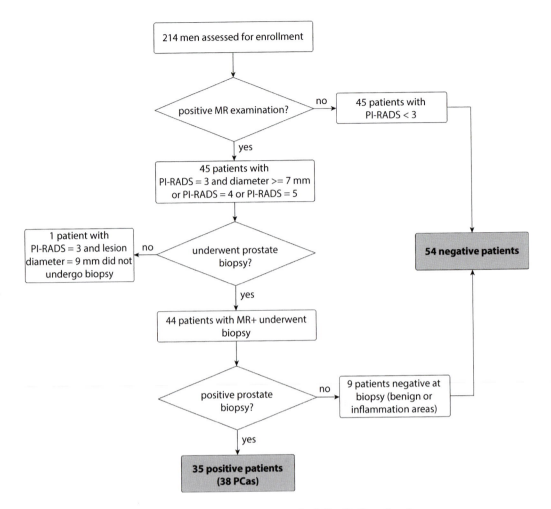

FIGURE 16.1 Flowchart showing case selection and the final distribution of study cases.

MR450w, GE Healthcare, Milwaukee, IL) using both 32-channel phased-array and endorectal coils (Medrad, Indianola, PA). Axial T2W, DW, and DCE sequences were obtained as detailed in Table 16.1. The DCE sequence was triggered to start simultaneously with the power injection of 0.1 mmol/kg gadobutrol (Gadovist, Bayer Schering, Berlin, Germany) through a peripheral line at 0.7 mL/s, followed by infusion of 20 cc normal saline at same rate. The average time to complete the whole MRI exam, including two additional T2W scans in the sagittal and coronal plane and an additional DW sequence with a higher b-value (i.e., 1400 or 2000 s/mm²), was 40 minutes. Imaging parameters satisfied the minimum scanning requirements for prostate imaging [33].

REFERENCE STANDARD

All patients belonging to the training set underwent RP within 3 months of mpMRI and the reference standard was created following the subsequent procedure. Each prostate specimen was step-sectioned at 3 mm intervals perpendicular to the long axis (apical-basal) of the gland [34]. This confidently reproduces the inclination of axial T2W images, which were acquired perpendicular to the rear gland surface. The bases and the apexes were cut parasagittally. Five μm sections were then obtained and colored with hematoxylin eosin. An experienced pathologist (with 24 years of

TABLE 16.1

MRI Sequence Details for the Different Types of Acquisitions

Sequence	ST (mm)	FOV (cm)	NEX	AM	RM	TR/TE/FA	Additional Information
T2W (fast spin echo—FSE)	3	16 × 16	2	384 × 288	512 × 512	3020/85/160°	
DW (echo planar imaging—EPI)[a]	3	16 × 16	6	128 × 128	256 × 256	7000/101/90°	b-values: 0–1000 s/mm^2
DW (single shot echo planar imaging—FOCUS)[b]	3	16 × 16	16	140 × 70	256 × 256	3200/73/90°	b-values: 0–800 s/mm^2; %FOV = 50
DCE (3D spoiled gradient echo—[SPGR])	3	20 × 20	0.5	224 × 192	512 × 512	3.6/1.3/20°	Temporal resolution = 13 s; 26 time points

[a] For acquisitions with Signa Excite HD (training set).

[b] For acquisitions with Optima MR450W (testing set).

Abbreviations: ST = slice thickness; FOV = field of view; NEX = number of executions; NEX = number of excitations; AM = acquisition matrix; RM = reconstruction matrix; TR/TE/FA = repetition time/echo time/flip angle.

experience in pathology, 20 attending uropathology) outlined each clinically significant PZ tumor on microscopic slices and assigned a pathological GS (pGS). The radiologist (F.R., with an experience of more than 500 prostate mpMRI studies interpreted per year for 7 years) in consensus with the pathologist, established the reference standard for PCa on T2W images drawing freehand regions of interest (ROIs) on cancer foci, following the outlines drawn by the pathologist on digital images of the pathologic slices. When pathological microslices and axial T2W images were not perfectly overlapped, usually due to modified prostate shape soaked by formaldehyde, the radiologist and the pathologist established the locations of tumors with respect to identifiable anatomic landmarks (e.g., adenoma nodule, urethra, ejaculatory ducts, and benign prostatic hyperplasia). If a lesion extended into more than one histopathologic slice, a ROI was drawn on each corresponding MR slice. For each patient, a ROI with extension similar to the tumoral one was also drawn on normal gland located in the contralateral PZ. This procedure is illustrated in Figure 16.2.

Conversely, the reference standard for the testing set was created following a slightly different approach, due to the fact that some patients did not undergo RP, but were treated with more conservative approaches (i.e., radiotherapy, hormonotherapy). Therefore, when the RP was not available, tumors were mapped to axial T2W images using the information gathered from biopsies. When the in-bore biopsy was performed the exact match between CAD findings and tumors was guaranteed by the fact that the experienced radiologist who performed all the in-bore biopsies was the same one who retrospectively reviewed all MR positive cases. Therefore, he was able to perfectly map biopsy findings to the MR images, by tracing the position of the needle tip on MRI images. Conversely, when the saturation biopsy was performed, at least 28 cores were obtained and a detailed report was provided by the uropathologist in which core location, presence of tumor, and the corresponding GS were reported for each core. Therefore, the experienced radiologist was able to map the biopsy results to MRI according to this information.

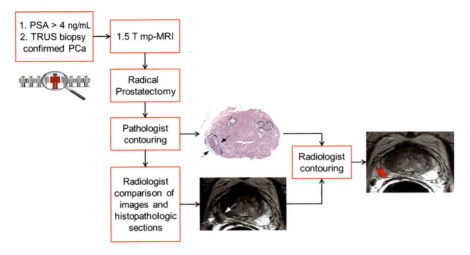

FIGURE 16.2 Flowchart illustrating the procedure used to create the reference standard.

CAD DEVELOPMENT

The CAD was conceived as a two-stage process. First, a parametric color-coded map of the prostate gland is created; colors are assigned to the map based on the likelihood of each voxel to be cancerous. Then, a candidate segmentation step is performed to highlight suspected areas. Different fully automatic steps, thoroughly described in the following subsections, compose each of these stages. All methods were implemented using C++ and the ITK libraries [35].

Image Registration

The first step to develop a CAD system which produces a voxelwise malignancy likelihood map of the prostate is image registration. This step aims to align all MRI sequences to the reference one, ensuring that different features, referring to the same voxel, may be correctly extracted. In our method, the reference image was the T2W sequence, therefore image registration algorithms were applied to both DWI and DCE sequences. The whole method was previously described [36], however, we will briefly report the main steps here. Before applying the registration methods, both DCE volumes and DW images were upsampled to the T2W image resolution. In addition, DCE volumes were automatically cropped to match the same field of view of the T2W image.

To register each DCE volume to the T2W image, a multiresolution strategy was applied to avoid local minima and to decrease the computational time. This approach uses image pyramids, which consist in a sequence of copies of an original image in which both sample density and resolution are decreased in regular steps. In the developed method, spatial resolution is halved from one level to another, and both the moving and the fixed image pyramids are composed by three levels, that is, subsampling scale factor = 444 222 111. In this case, the registration is solved as an optimization problem with the goal of finding the optimal transformation $T:(x,y,z) \rightarrow (x',y',z')$ which maps any point in the moving DCE dynamic image sequence $I(x,y,z,t)$ at time t into its corresponding point in the reference image $I(x,y,z,t0)$, that is, the T2W image. Since DCE sequences are not subjected to large elastic deformations, and it has been demonstrated that rigid-body registration of the prostate yields satisfactory results when images are acquired in the same position [37], a rigid-body registration, which is parametrized by 6 degrees of freedom, was preferred for its low computational costs [38]. The mutual information, which is a measure of statistical dependency between two datasets, was used as similarity metric and the regular step gradient descent algorithm was used as optimizer.

To register the DWI to the T2W image, a different approach was used, since in this case the algorithm needs to cope with distortions introduced by the echo planar imaging (EPI)-DWI sequence, which manifest as either local stretching or compression in the acquired image. Therefore, a non-rigid registration step was applied. To this scope, the endorectal coil was first automatically segmented in both DWI and T2W images by a region growing algorithm, which starts from a seed point inside the coil, automatically found by a circular Hough transform. Then, for each slice where the coil is visible, two spline smoothing curves were fitted on the coil border points on the DWI and T2W images, and used to estimate the initial distance (d_i) between the two coil surfaces, which is the difference between the upper points of these spline curves. Afterward, a deformation field T was modeled as a linear decay field along the vertical direction (Equation 16.1):

$$T(y) = \begin{cases} d_i - k * y & 0 < y < \dfrac{d_i}{k} \\ 0 & y > \dfrac{d_i}{k} \end{cases} \tag{16.1}$$

Prostate Segmentation

Prostate segmentation is of key importance to reduce the computational burden of the CAD system. In our method, we first automatically identify on each slice a rectangular region of fixed size (i.e., width = 7 cm, height = 6 cm). The rectangle is automatically generated in such a way that its posterior border is in contact with the anterior profile of the coil, which is segmented using the Hough transform on the T2W image, as detailed in the previous section. It may confidently enclose both a normal (size = $4 \times 2 \times 3$ cm^3) and an enlarged prostate [39]. Then, we extract the ADC map on this rectangular region and we apply, the multilevel Otsu threshold [40], that is, three levels. This method is able to select different threshold values by maximizing the between-class variance in a gray level image, thus separating the prostate from the darker background and the brighter coil. Once the thresholding has been applied, a 3-value map is provided, representing the three different classes of gray levels. Finally, we select all voxels belonging to the second class, which represents the prostate, and we apply some morphological operations to fill holes, that is, the darker voxels within the prostate, without enlarging the segmented prostate.

Feature Extraction and Classification

Once the prostate was segmented some quantitative features were extracted for each voxel belonging to the prostate region from each MRI sequence, as following detailed.

1. Normalized T2W signal intensities. Before extracting these parameters, some preprocessing steps were applied. First, image inhomogeneities introduced by the endorectal coil were corrected by using a variant of the popular nonparametric nonuniform intensity normalization (N3) algorithm, introduced by Tustison et al. [41], with the following parameters: FWHM = 0.5, Wiener = 0.1, convergence threshold = 0.001. Then, T2W images were normalized to reduce the differences between different patients. The normalization was performed by dividing the signal intensities of each voxel with the signal intensity of the obturator muscle, automatically segmented by our system, as previously described [42].
2. Image intensities from ADC maps. ADC maps, which give more standardized measurements with respect to DWI sequences, were computed using a monoexponential model [43].
3. Quantitative parameters from DCE-MRI sequences. First, we computed the signal intensity curves $S(t)$ of the DCE sequences normalized as following detailed:

$$\frac{\left(S(i) - S(0)\right)}{S(0)} \tag{16.2}$$

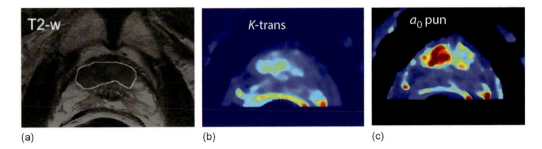

FIGURE 16.3 Example of kinetic features extracted using Tofts and PUN models. (a) T2W image of the prostate. The tumor in the transiton zone has been outlined by the radiologist. (b) k_{trans} derived from the Tofts model. In this case, the tumor does not show high values of k_{trans} in the malignant region. (c) a_0 parameter obtained from the PUN model. The tumor in the transition zone shows a suspected behavior in this map.

where $S(i)$ is the signal intensity at time i-th and $S(0)$ is the signal intensity at time 0, i.e., the first DCE frame. Then, kinetic features were extracted using the Phenomenological Universalities (PUN) approach [44,45]. This approach was preferred to the Tofts pharmacokinetic model because it was demonstrated to achieve similar results in the discrimination between malignant and benign regions of the prostate [46], while overcoming some limitations. Indeed, Tofts pharmacokinetic model suffers from complexity, because of the required conversion of MR signal intensities into contrast agent concentration. Moreover, the PUN model showed good discrimination performance also in detecting tumors in the transition zone (Figure 16.3).

The PUN model is characterized by three fitting parameters, a_0, β, and r, and the model equation is as follows:

$$y_{(PUN)} = \exp r\left[t + \frac{2}{3}\left(a\% - r\right)\exp\left(\beta t\right) - 1\right] \tag{16.3}$$

in which a_0 controls the steepness of the curve at $t = 0$ and, together with β, it primarily affects the growth rate of the curve in its first part; β is in inverse proportion to the time the system takes to reach the knee of the curve, and r determines the behavior of the second part of the curve where one can observe a further enhancement of the signal intensity or a washout phase [44]. Since a_0 and β were highly correlated (Spearman's correlation coefficient = −0.76), we decided to discard one of them to reduce overfitting problems. Therefore β, which had the lowest area under the ROC curve (0.57 vs. 0.65), was discarded.

Once these features were extracted, a four-dimensional vector of features was obtained for each voxel and it was fed into a SVM classifier, which uses the radial basis kernel and having the following parameters ($C = 2$ and $\gamma = 0.002$). Finally, a map was obtained, in which each voxel is represented by a likelihood between 0 and 1, 0 indicating no suspicion of PCa and 1 indicating very high suspicion of PCa.

Candidate Segmentation

On the likelihood map obtained during the previous step, we applied the second stage of the CAD pipeline to extract 3D candidates highly suspected to be cancers and reduce the number of false positive (FP) voxels. First, voxels having likelihood higher than 60% to be malignant were extracted from the voxelwise malignancy likelihood map, and connected regions with size <100 mm² were discarded. Then, for each of the remaining voxels we computed the time-intensity curves from the DCE-MR dataset, and voxels having maximum contrast uptake within the first minute <1 were discarded.

CAD Validation and Testing

The CAD system was first validated on the training set using the leave-one-out (LOO) method, which involves training on all but one case, estimating the likelihood of malignancy of the voxels belonging to the left-out patient, and repeating the procedure until each case has been tested individually. Both the voxel classification and the candidate selection steps were evaluated. The ROC analysis was used to assess the ability of the CAD system in discriminating between normal and malignant tissue. Since the LOO strategy was used, the median value of the AUROC, the median sensitivity, and the median specificity were provided. The ROC analysis, however, misses information about the number of FP candidates since it is evaluated on predetermined ROIs and does not consider the whole prostate. Therefore, for the candidate selection step, we provided the per-lesion and per-patient sensitivity, and the number of FP in both the PZ and the whole prostate for each patient. A 3D connected region was considered a true positive (TP) if the Dice overlap between the segmentation and the ROI drawn by the radiologist was higher than 0.10, vice versa it was considered a FP. We evaluated the system both for the detection of all tumors and for the detection of high-grade tumors ($pGS \geq 7$).

Similarly, the performance of the CAD system was evaluated on the testing set.

Clinical Application

Results obtained in the testing set were used to evaluate the potential of a fully automatic CAD scheme to improve reader performance in the detection of PCa at mpMRI. The aim of this step was to compare the per-patient sensitivity and specificity of experienced readers in the detection of PCa, using a color-coded map generated by a CAD scheme with that of unassisted interpretation of mpMRI. To this scope, three experienced radiologists in prostate MRI (reader 1, 2 years' experience and 200 reports/year; reader 2, 4 years' experience and 120 reports/year; reader 3, 4 years' experience and 200 reports/year), blinded to disease prevalence in this cohort, reported all examinations twice, more than 6 weeks apart to minimize recall bias. During the *CAD reading phase*, they were shown a 3D color-coded map of the prostate gland and were asked to classify as positive all CAD marks they considered suspicious for cancer. To discard findings outside the prostate gland or image artifacts, T2W images were transparently over-laid to the CAD map, and readers were allowed to modify the transparency, using a dedicated software (MIPAV, http://mipav.cit.nih.gov). However, they were not allowed to discard any suspicious finding based on T2W signal intensities other than the above-mentioned. In order to evaluate the CAD system, the reader could not include any tumors that were not detected by the CAD system. In the second session, cases were re-ordered randomly and readers reported without the support of the CAD system. During the unassisted interpretation, radiologists used the same workstation (Advantage Workstation 4.6, GE Healthcare, Milwaukee, IL) and were allowed to review using their favorite reading protocol. For both reading sessions, radiologists characterized each abnormality, annotating lesion coordinates, lesion size, Prostate Imaging-Reporting and Data System (PI-RADS) (only in the unassisted reading) and suggested a 5-point confidence score representing the subjective self-confidence that their finding was a tumor (1: absolutely not sure; 5: absolutely sure). Reader interpretation time was also recorded for both assisted and unassisted reading.

To assess the impact of CAD system in the clinical practice, per-patient sensitivity, specificity, positive predictive value (PPV), and negative predictive value (NPV) of *CAD interpretation* with that of *unassisted reading* were compared. For unassisted reporting, patients were considered positive for PCa when at least one lesion with a score of PI-RADS 3 and maximum lesion diameter ≥ 7 mm, or any PI-RADS lesion 4–5 was detected; all others were classified negative. In the CAD-assisted mode, patients were classified as positive when the readers marked as PCa at least one CAD prompt. This determination was deemed either true positive, false positive, true negative, or false negative depending on whether or not the lesion detected by the radiologist or the CAD system matched the exact location of a biopsy confirmed PCa. Sensitivity was stratified according to GS (GS ≤ 6 vs. GS > 6) and lesion size (<10 mm vs. ≥10 mm). Per-lesion analysis was similarly obtained.

Per-patient and per-lesion assessments were compared using McNemar test; other comparisons were performed with Mann-Whitney test. The AUROC was generated for each reader using the confidence scores and pathology results. Statistically significance was set at $p \leq 0.05$. Inter-observer agreement between reviewers was evaluated using Fleiss Kappa statistics on StatsToDo© [https://www.statstodo.com/CohenKappa_Pgm.php]. All other tests were conducted using MedCalc version 15.6.1.

RESULTS

The training set was composed of 58 patients, including 51 men (88%) with one clinically significant PZ tumor focus, and 7 patients (12%) with two clinically significant PZ tumor foci, for a total of 65 clinically significant peripheral PCas. Patients and lesion characteristics are summarized in Table 16.2.

The testing set comprised 89 patients, including 35 patients with at least one clinically significant tumor confirmed either by an in-bore biopsy ($n = 16$) or a TRUS-guided biopsy ($n = 19$). The total number of malignant lesions was 39. Patient and lesion characteristics are described in Table 16.3.

CAD VALIDATION

During the LOO validation of the CAD system using the training set, a median AUROC of 0.92 (1st–3rd quartile; 0.85–0.97), a median sensitivity of 0.85 (1st–3rd quartile; 0.71–0.92), and a median specificity of 0.88 (1st–3rd quartile; 0.58–0.97) were reached in the voxel classification stage. In the candidate segmentation step, the system was able to detect at least one lesion in 56 out of 58 patients, reaching a per-patient sensitivity of 0.97 (95%CI: 0.88–0.99). Besides, the CAD system detected 59 out of 65 lesions, leading to a per-lesion sensitivity of 0.91 (95% CI: 0.81–0.97), with a median

---

TABLE 16.2

Patient Demographics, Clinical Characteristics, and Lesion Characteristics

Parameter	Value
No. of patients included in the study	58
Patients median age [y] (1st–3rd quartile)	64 (60–69)
Median PSA at diagnosis [ng/mL] (1st–3rd quartile)	5.8 (4.8–8.6)
Median no. of days between biopsy and MR examination [d] (1st–3rd quartile)	92 (61–112)
Median time between MR imaging and prostatectomy [d] (1st–3rd quartile)	26 (13–47)
Median prostate volume [cc] (1st–3rd quartile)	44.8 (37.3–59.5)
No. of lesions with tumor volume ≥0.5 cc	65
Median volume (cc) (1st–3rd quartile)	1.6 (1.0–2.6)
Distribution of pathologic Gleason scores [no. of lesions]	
3 + 3	6 (9%)
3 + 4	31 (48%)
4 + 3	16 (24.5%)
4 + 4	9 (14%)
4 + 5	3 (4.5%)

TABLE 16.3

Patient and Lesion Characteristics. Two-Tailed *p*-Values Are Obtained Using Mann-Whitney Test

Patients	All	Positive (*n* = 35)	Negative (*n* = 54)	*p*
Age (y)	66.8 (63.0–73.0)[a]	68.5 (65.3–74.8)[a]	66.1 (61.4–72.9)[a]	0.0622
PSA (ng/mL)	7.50 (6.18–10.95)[a]	6.88 (5.89–12.29)[a]	7.77 (6.60–10.69)[a]	0.3801
Prostate volume (cc)	54.4 (38.1–82.2)[a]	40.2 (29.1–56.0)[a]	66.3 (47.5–88.9)[a]	**<0.0001**
No. of previous negative biopsy	1 (1–2)[a]	1 (0–1)[a]	1 (1–2)[a]	**0.0012**
No. patients with previous negative biopsies				
0	19	16	3	
1	41	11	30	
2	25	6	19	
3	3	2	1	
4	1	—	1	
No. patients with PI-RADS score				
1	23	—	23	
2	22	—	22	
3	8	3	5	
4	20	16	4	
5	16	16	—	

Lesions	All (*n* = 39)	Peripheral Zone (*n* = 30)	Transition Zone (*n* = 9)
No. lesions with GS			
3 + 3	13 (33%)	12 (40%)	1 (11%)
3 + 4	11 (28%)	7 (23%)	4 (44%)
4 + 3	9 (23%)	7 (23%)	2 (22%)
4 + 4	4 (10%)	2 (7%)	2 (22%)
4 + 5	1 (3%)	1 (3.5%)	0
5 + 5	1 (3%)	1 (3.5%)	0
Size (mm)	10 (4–30)[a]	8 (4–25)[a]	18 (10–30)[a]
≤7 mm	13 (33.5%)	13 (43%)	—
8–9 mm	6 (15%)	6 (20%)	—
≥10 mm	20 (51.5%)	11 (37%)	9 (100%)

[a] Measurements are given as median (range).

Abbreviation: GS = Gleason score.

number of FP per patient equal to 1 (1st–3rd quartile; 0–2), and 3 (1st–3rd quartile; 1–4) in the PZ and in the whole prostate, respectively. The per-lesion sensitivity increased to 0.95, if we consider only the high-grade tumors (pGS ≥ 7). Three of the 6 false negative (FN) lesions were pGS = 3 + 3 tumors, having volume equal to 0.59, 0.75, and 1.55 cc, respectively. Three of the six missed lesions were secondary tumors in patients in which the primary lesion was correctly detected by the system; one FN belonged to a patient with only one clinically significant tumor, while in one case the CAD missed both lesions belonging to a single patient.

Figure 16.4 shows the CAD output of a patient with two PCas. The index lesion (pGS = 3 + 4) was correctly detected by the system, while the secondary less aggressive tumor (pGS = 3 + 3) was missed.

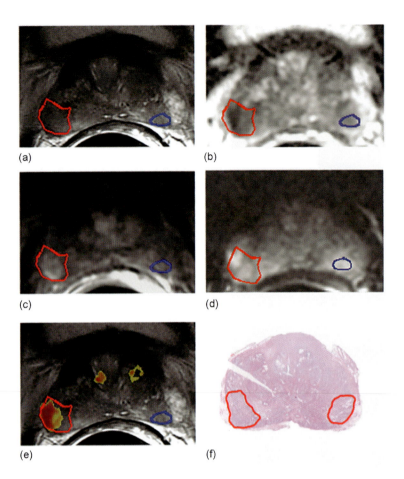

FIGURE 16.4 Example of CAD result of a patient harboring two PCas. The index tumor had pGS = 3 + 4 and volume = 1.55 cc (on the left), while the secondary had pGS = 3 + 3 and volume of 1.17 cc (on the right). The figure shows the manual masks of the tumors superimposed to (a) T2W image, (b) the ADC map, (c) the fourth enhanced frame of the DCE sequence, and (d) the DWI image. In (e), output of the CAD is superimposed to the T2W image. Reddish colors represent likelihood >80% to be cancerous. And (f) is the histopathological section of the prostate showing the ROIs drawn by the uropathologist.

CAD TESTING

When the CAD was applied on the testing set, at least one lesion was correctly detected in 33 of 35 positive patients, leading to a per-patient sensitivity of 94.3% (95% CI: 80.8%–99.3%). One FN patient had a sole lesion in the PZ with maximum diameter of 6 mm and pGS = 3 + 3, while the other one had a single lesion in the transition zone (TZ) with maximum diameter of 18 mm and biopsy GS = 3 + 4 (Figure 16.5). The latter patient underwent hormonotherapy rather than RP. In addition, CAD missed four other lesions, all of them smaller than 10 mm (range 5–8 mm), leading to a per-lesion sensitivity of 84.6% (95% CI: 69.5%–94.1%). Table 16.4 shows per-lesion and per-patient sensitivity of the CAD system stratified by lesion size and GS. Stratifying by lesion location, the CAD missed 5 out of 30 lesions in the PZ (sensitivity = 83.5%, 95% CI: 65.28%–94.36%) and 1

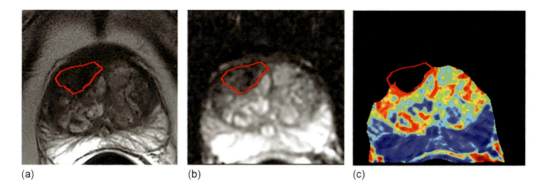

(a) (b) (c)

FIGURE 16.5 Example of a false negative case obtained in the testing set. The tumor was located in the TZ and had maximum diameter of 18 mm and biopsy GS = 3 + 4. It was discarded since it lied outside the segmentation of the prostate. The manual mask drawn by the radiologist is superimposed to the (a) T2W image, (b) the ADC map, and (c) the likelihood map obtained by the CAD.

TABLE 16.4

Per-Lesion and Per-Patient Sensitivity of the CAD System for All Cases and Stratified by Lesion Size and GS

	Per-Patient	Per-Lesion
Sensitivity	33/35 (94.3%) [80.8%–99.3%]	33/39 (84.6%) [69.5%–94.1%]
Sensitivity for GS = 6	11/12 (91.7%) [61.5%–99.8%]	12/13 (92.3%) [64.0%–99.8%]
Sensitivity for GS >6	22/23 (95.6%) [78.1%–99.9%]	21/26 (80.8%) [60.7%–93.4%]
Sensitivity for max diameter 4–9 mm	14/15 (93.3%) [68.1%–99.8%]	14/19 (73.7%) [48.8%–90.9%]
Sensitivity for max diameter ≥10 mm	19/20 (95.0%) [75.1%–99.9%]	19/20 (95.0%) [75.1%–99.9%]

Note: Sensitivity is expressed as number of patient/lesions over the total number of patients/lesions, with percentages in parentheses and corresponding 95% CIs in brackets.

---

out of 9 lesions in the TZ (sensitivity = 87.5%, 95% CI: 47.4%–99.7%). There was no statistical difference between sensitivity in the PZ and in the TZ (p-value of the Chi-squared test = 0.78).

IMPACT OF THE CAD SYSTEM IN CLINICAL PRACTICE

Per-Patient Analysis

Per-patient analysis is summarized in Table 16.5. Across all readers, sensitivity of unassisted and CAD-assisted interpretation was 80.9% (95% CI: 72.1%–88.0%) and 87.6% (95% CI: 79.8%–93.2%; $p = 0.105$), respectively. In general, readers rejected a few TP marks (reader 1, $n = 4$; reader 2, $n = 2$; reader 3, $n = 1$). Figure 16.6 shows an example of a PCa correctly identified by all readers with the CAD and missed by all readers in the unassisted reading. Across all readers, sensitivity was higher using the CAD-assisted interpretation in patients with at least one GS > 6 lesion (81.2% vs. 91.3%, $p = 0.046$) and in those with at least one lesion ≥10 mm (80.0% vs. 95.0%, $p = 0.006$). The reader with the lowest sensitivity when reporting unassisted improved the most by using the CAD

TABLE 16.5

Per-Patient Specificity and Sensitivity for All Lesions and Stratified by Lesion Size and GS for Unassisted and Assisted Reading

	Unassisted Reading	Assisted Reading	p-Value
Sensitivity			
Reader 1	28/35 (80.0) [63.1,91.6]	29/35 (82.9) [66.3,93.4]	0.5000
Reader 2	25/35 (71.4) [53.7,85.4]	31/35 (88.6) [73.3,95.8]	**0.0155**
Reader 3	32/35 (91.4) [76.9,98.2]	32/35 (91.4) [76.9,98.2]	0.5000
Average	85/105 (80.9) [72.1,88.0]	92/105 (87.6) [79.8–93.2]	0.1050
Sensitivity for GS = 6			
Reader 1	11/12 (91.7) [61.5,99.8]	8/12 (66.7) [34.9,90.1]	0.1875
Reader 2	6/12 (50.0) [21.1,78.98]	10/12 (83.3) [51.6,97.9]	0.0625
Reader 3	12/12 (100.0) [73.5,100.0]	11/12 (91.7) [61.5,99.8]	Not estimable
Average	29/36 (80.6) [64.0,91.8]	29/36 (80.6) [64.0,91.8]	0.5000
Sensitivity for GS > 6			
Reader 1	17/23 (73.9) [51.6,89.8]	21/23 (91.3) [72.0,98.9]	0.1095
Reader 2	19/23 (82.6) [61.2,95.1]	21/23 (91.3) [72.0,98.9]	0.2500
Reader 3	20/23 (87.0) [66.4,97.2]	21/23 (91.3) [72.0,98.9]	0.5000
Average	56/69 (81.2) [69.9,89.6]	63/69 (91.3) [82.0,96.7]	**0.0460**
Sensitivity for max. diameter 4–9 mm			
Reader 1	13/15 (86.7) [59.5,98.3]	10/15 (66.7) [38.4,88.2]	0.2265
Reader 2	10/15 (66.7) [38.4,88.2]	12/15 (80.0) [51.9,95.7]	0.2500
Reader 3	14/15 (93.3) [68.1,99.8]	13/15 (86.7) [59.5,98.3]	0.5000
Average	35/45 (77.8) [62.9,88.8]	37/45 (82.2) [67.9,92.0]	0.3870
Sensitivity for max. diameter ≥10 mm			
Reader 1	15/20 (75.0) [50.9,91.3]	19/20 (95.0) [75.1,99.9]	0.0625
Reader 2	15/20 (75.0) [50.9,91.3]	19/20 (95.0) [75.1,99.9]	0.0625
Reader 3	18/20 (90.0) [68.3,98.8]	19/20 (95.0) [75.1,99.9]	0.5000
Average	48/60 (80.0) [67.7,89.2]	57/60 (95.0) [86.1,-99.0]	**0.006**
Specificity			
Reader 1	41/54 (75.9) [62.3,86.5]	44/54 (81.5) [68.6,90.8]	0.2745
Reader 2	49/54 (90.7) [79.7,96.9]	48/54 (88.9) [77.4,95.8]	0.5000
Reader 3	32/54 (59.3) [45.0,72.4]	35/54 (64.8) [50.6,77.3]	0.3145
Average	122/162 (75.3) [67.9,91.7]	127/162 (78.4) [71.3,84.5]	0.2500

Note: Expressed as number of patient/total number of patients, with percentages in parentheses and corresponding 95% CIs in brackets. One-tailed *p*-value was obtained with the McNemar Chi-Squared test.

(71.4% vs. 88.6%, *p* = 0.0155). Overall mean NPV for unassisted and CAD-assisted reading was 85.9% (95% CI: 79.1%–91.2%) and 90.7% (95% CI: 84.6%–95.0%; *p* = 0.1055), respectively; mean PPV was 68.0% (95% CI: 59.1%–76.1%) and 72.4% (95% CI: 63.8%–80.0%; one-tailed *p* = 0.223), respectively. AUROC significantly increased with CAD for reader 2 (0.82 vs. 0.91; *p* = 0.012); no difference was observed for the other two readers (reader 1, 0.84 vs. 0.85, *p* = 0.8329; reader 3, 0.84 vs. 0.88, *p* = 0.3328).

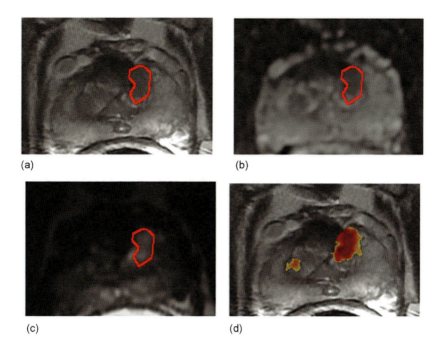

FIGURE 16.6 Example of a PCa with pGS = 4 + 4 and maximum diameter of 10 mm (red outline) that was correctly detected by all readers using the CAD and that was missed by all of them during the unassisted reading. (a) T2W image, (b) ADC map, (c) 4th enhanced frame of the DCE sequence, and (d) output of the CAD superimposed to the T2W image.

Per-Lesion Analysis

Per-lesion analysis is summarized in Table 16.6. With unassisted read, 21 PCa lesions were detected by all three readers, 7 lesions by two, 6 by one, and 5 by none. With CAD, 23 lesions were detected by all three readers, 8 by two, 1 by one, and 7 by none. Across all readers, we observed a marginal increase in the number of detected lesions when using CAD with respect to unassisted read (70.9% vs. 74.4%, $p = 0.309$). Two of the 6 CAD-missed lesions (33%), both with a GS = 3 + 4 and a diameter of 5 and 7 mm respectively, were picked up by at least two radiologists in the unassisted mode. Conversely, in the unassisted mode all three readers missed 5 PCa lesions detected by the CAD; two of the lesions had a diameter $\geq$10 mm (Figure 16.2). Across all readers, a sensitivity difference was observed in favor of CAD-assisted interpretation if only lesions $\geq$10 mm were considered (76.7% vs. 90%, $p = 0.019$). In the unassisted reading mode, readers 1, 2, and 3 reported 19, 9, and 42 FPs respectively, while using CAD first read FP were 15, 13 and 35, respectively.

Reading Time and Inter-reader Agreement

Reading times are summarized in Table 16.7. Overall, the average reading time of the unassisted and CAD first read mode was respectively 220 s (1st–3rd quartile, 147–359 s) and 60 s (1st–3rd quartile, 35–110 s). When using the CAD-assisted modality, a marginal increase of inter-reader agreement was observed in both per-patient (0.55 vs. 0.63; $p = 0.161$) and per-lesion (0.46 vs. 0.57; $p = 0.380$) analysis (Table 16.8).

TABLE 16.6
Per-Lesion Specificity and Sensitivity for All Lesions and Stratified by Lesion Size and GS for Unassisted and Assisted Reading

	Unassisted Reading	Assisted Reading	p-Value
Sensitivity			
Reader 1	25/39 (64.1) [47.2–78.8]	28/39 (71.8) [55.1–85.0]	0.2905
Reader 2	26/39 (66.7) [49.8–80.9]	30/39 (76.9) [60.7–88.9]	0.1940
Reader 3	32/39 (82.1) [66.5–92.5]	29/39 (74.4) [57.9–87.0]	0.2745
Average	83/117 (70.9) [61.8–79.0]	87/117 (74.4) [65.5–82.0]	0.3090
Sensitivity for GS = 6			
Reader 1	10/13 (76.9) [46.2,95.0]	9/13 (69.2) [38.6,90.9]	0.5000
Reader 2	6/13 (46.2) [19.2,74.9]	10/13 (76.9) [46.2,95.0]	0.1095
Reader 3	11/13 (84.6) [54.5,98.1]	9/13 (69.2) [38.6,90.9]	0.2500
Average	27/39 (69.2) [52.4–83.0]	28/39 (71.8) [55.1–85.0]	0.5000
Sensitivity for GS > 6			
Reader 1	15/26 (57.7) [36.9–76.7]	19/26 (73.1) [52.2–88.4]	0.1445
Reader 2	20/26 (76.9) [56.3–91.0]	20/26 (76.9) [56.3–91.0]	0.5000
Reader 3	21/26 (80.8) [60.6–93.4]	20/26 (76.9) [56.3–91.0]	0.5000
Average	56/78 (71.8) [60.5–81.4]	59/78 (75.6) [64.6–84.6]	0.3390
Sensitivity for max. diameter 4–9 mm			
Reader 1	11/19 (57.9) [33.5,79.7]	11/19 (57.9) [33.5,79.7]	0.5000
Reader 2	11/19 (57.9) [33.5,79.7]	12/19 (63.2) [38.4–83.7]	0.5000
Reader 3	15/19 (78.9) [54.4,93.9]	10/19 (52.6) [28.9,75.5]	0.0900
Average	37/57 (64.9) [51.1,77.1]	33/57 (57.9) [44.1–70.9]	0.2705
Sensitivity for max. diameter ≥10 mm			
Reader 1	14/20 (70.0) [45.7–88.1]	17/20 (85.0) [62.1–96.8]	0.1875
Reader 2	15/20 (75.0) [50.9–91.3]	18/20 (90.0) [68.3–98.8]	0.1875
Reader 3	17/20 (85.0) [62.1–96.8]	19/20 (95.0) [75.1–99.9]	0.2500
Average	46/60 (76.7) [64.0–86.7]	54/60 (90.0) [79.5–96.2]	**0.01950**

Note: Expressed as number of patient/total number of patients, with percentages in parentheses and corresponding 95% CIs in brackets. One-tailed p-value was obtained with the McNemar Chi-Squared test.

TABLE 16.7
Interpretation Times for Unassisted and Assisted Reading

	Unassisted Reading	p-Value	Assisted Reading		p-Value
Reader 1	410 (308–574)		85 (48–129)		**<0.0001**
Reader 2	124 (74–184)		60 (40–101)		**<0.0001**
Reader 3	210 (168–260)		48 (30–76)		**<0.0001**
Average	220 (147–359)		60 (35–110)		**<0.0001**
	Biopsy +	Biopsy −		Biopsy +	Biopsy −	
Reader 1	405 (331–540)	420 (273–600)	0.4547	117 (91–155)	60 (31–110)	**0.0002**
Reader 2	157 (125–220)	95 (71–147)	**0.0009**	95 (71–126)	43 (33–69)	**<0.0001**
Reader 3	225 (184–278)	200 (160–240)	**0.0376**	75 (40–128)	37 (20–59)	**<0.0001**
Average	235 (172–360)	203 (122–345)	**0.0187**	100 (63–132)	44 (30–74)	**<0.0001**

Note: Two-tailed p-value obtained with Mann-Whitney test was reported.

TABLE 16.8

Inter-observer Agreement between Reviewers Evaluated Using Fleiss Kappa Statistics. 95% CIs Are Reported in Brackets

CAD Paradigm	Per-Patient Analysis		Per-Lesion Analysis	
	Reader 1	Reader 3	Reader 1	Reader 3
Reader 2	0.561 (0.400–0.723)	0.679 (0.525–0.833)	0.494 (0.328–0.659)	0.655 (0.501–0.809)
Reader 3	0.647 (0.496–0.798)	—	0.575 (0.417–0.732)	
Fleiss Kappa	**0.625 (0.505–0.745)**		**0.570 (0.456–0.684)**	
Unassisted Reader	**Reader 1**	**Reader 3**	**Reader 1**	**Reader 3**
Reader 2	0.454 (0.301–0.607)	0.654 (0.500–0.808)	0.392 (0.240–0.544)	0.589 (0.427–0.751)
Reader 3	0.580 (0.420–0.741)		0.436 (0.272–0.600)	—
Fleiss Kappa	**0.549 (0.429–0.669)**		**0.455 (0.342–0.568)**	

DISCUSSION

In this chapter, we presented a two-stage CAD system providing both a voxelwise malignancy likelihood map of the entire prostate gland and segmentation of PCa candidates, with a possible application in a clinical scenario. The CAD system reached good performance both in the validation and in the testing phases. Using the training set composed of 58 patients, the AUROC of our CAD system was 0.92, while in the candidate segmentation step the per-patient sensitivity was 97%—that is, at least one PCa lesion was detected in 56 of the 58 patients—and the median number of FP per exam was 3 (1st–3rd quartile; 1–4). Other CAD systems relying on mpMRI for PCa detection showed slightly lower AUROC values (0.89 vs. 0.92) [25,29,30]. Recently, many CAD systems have been developed, showing different accuracies; however, comparison might be difficult for many reasons. First, CAD scheme accuracy may be influenced by the method used for drawing ROIs. Previously, only Langer et al. [47] computed the AUROC on ROIs drawn by an experienced radiologist using histopathology as the ground truth, obtaining an AUROC of 0.71, which is lower than our results. Conversely, authors who obtained AUROC similar to ours either adopted the overall lesion detection method [29,48] or considered only voxels belonging to an area with a predefined size, around the radiologist annotations [30]. The latter approaches tend to improve the apparent performance, since they do not take into consideration tumor heterogeneity and the overlying image noise; therefore, the ability to determine a strict threshold between tumor and normal values is increased [47]. The method implemented by our group, which relies on the analysis of every voxel belonging to the ROIs, may potentially extend the role of the CAD system to the evaluation of tumor aggressiveness, which might not be uniform within the lesion. The CAD system detected 59 of the 65 PZ PCas (per-lesion sensitivity of 91%). Three out of the six FNs lesions were tumors with a pGS of 3 + 3; 2 of the 3 patients had a second more aggressive tumor that was correctly detected by the CAD system. Two cases had very high ADC values (>1.6 × 10^{-3} mm^2/s) and one lesion had no contrast-uptake. Recently, it has been argued that low GS lesions—that is, ≤6—should not be defined as cancers, due to their *nihil* propensity to metastatization [49] and therefore should not be treated with surgery. Indeed, missing such indolent lesions at imaging could be beneficial, as it may reduce overtreatment which, in the conventional diagnostic pipeline, is estimated to occur in approximately 20% to 60% of cases [50].

Our CAD system has important strengths. First, the reference standard was established by using whole-mount pathological slices obtained from the prostate specimen, rather than relying on the radiologist's annotations, even if confirmed by biopsy [25,30]. The latter approach has an important limitation as no information is available on regions annotated as normal by the radiologist that could actually harbor PCa. Indeed, in a recent paper, Le et al. [51] showed that radiologists can miss up to 40% of clinically significant PCas. Conversely, using the whole-mount sections as histologic reference standard provides more accurate label information for training a CAD system [52], as it assesses the ground truth for PCa extent, grade, and disease infiltration [53]. Previously, other authors used the whole-mount histology as gold standard [47,54], however our method includes an automatic registration method. Second, we introduced a registration step to align both the DCE and the DW images to the reference T2W image [36]. This step is of key importance to correct misalignment due to both patient movements and image distortions that occur especially during DW images acquisition [52,55]. Most of the recent works describing the development of a CAD system did not apply a registration algorithm before feature extraction [29,30]. Previously, only Vos et al. [48] and Viswanath et al. [56] embedded a fully automatic registration algorithm into a CAD system for PCa on mpMRI. Vos et al. [48] aligned T2W and proton density (PD)-T1W images, from which they extracted pharmacokinetics maps, while Viswanath et al. [56] performed an affine registration between the T2W image and the fifth contrast-enhanced frame of the DCE acquisition. The latter approach does not consider that registration errors could occur due to patients' movements [30]. Conversely, our method is able to align each contrast-enhanced frame to the T2W image. Moreover, neither Vos et al. [48] nor Viswanath [56] assessed a specific framework to correct for image distortion and patients' movements during EPI-DW imaging acquisitions.

Indeed, although the mpMRI is implicitly registered (all sequences are acquired in one go, without the patient leaving the scanner), image deformation on DW images and registration errors between the different DCE volumes could occur due to patient movement [30]. The latter may strongly influence parameter estimation and cause apparently extreme changes in enhancement [57]. The registration step, together with the features selection method, may account for the lower number of FPs obtained by our CAD system.

Third, a novel empirical approach has been used to describe DCE-MRI curves, which could overcome some limitations of Tofts model. First, the empirical model implemented does not require any conversion of the MRI signal into contrast agent concentration, since it directly fits signal-intensity curves. Avoiding signal conversion to contrast agent concentration could reduce dramatically acquisition times and patient discomfort. Second, the arterial input function (AIF) is not required. It is known that wrong estimation of the AIF could potentially lead to large errors in parameters estimation, with clear implications for clinical utility of the model [58]. Third, empirical mathematical models were demonstrated able to fit DCE-MRI curves over long periods of time, differentiating benign from malignant lesions of the spine, prostate, and brain [44,46,59]. Finally, since the introduction of CAD systems in clinical settings aims to automatically highlight cancer-suspicious regions to the radiologist [29,30,48,60,61], it is not necessary anymore to implement biological-based models which produce as output tissue-related information. Indeed, all useful data are summarized in a likelihood map of malignancy.

One of the major strengths of the presented CAD is the fact that it was also tested on a different dataset, which was not used to train the system and which included also tumors located in the TZ. Using the testing set, the CAD obtained high per-patient sensitivity (94.3%), since it detected at least one lesion in 33 of 35 positive patients. Moreover, the CAD system detected 33 of 39 lesions (per-lesion sensitivity of 84.6%), and it was demonstrated that the sensitivity in the PZ was not statistically different from the sensitivity in the TZ. Most of FNs were secondary lesions smaller than 10 mm, while only a primary lesion with GS > 6 and diameter >10 mm was missed by the CAD, because of an error in the prostate segmentation step. These results showed that our CAD was able to deal with an independent dataset reaching high performance in discriminating between malignant from healthy voxels.

In addition, in this chapter, we demonstrated that the system could be integrated in the clinical practice, since we have shown that interpretation with CAD can significantly improve the sensitivity of MRI in detecting PCa in patients with at least one lesion with a diameter of 10 mm or more and for those with a GS > 6, while specificity is not altered.

The use of CAD reduced the average operator reading time from 220 to 60 seconds. Surprisingly, each one of the three experienced operators in this study had a different reading behavior. Reader 2 had the highest sensitivity gain by using CAD and retained the highest specificity; reader 3 reported with the highest sensitivity unassisted and no gain was observed by using CAD, but specificity was very low; reader 1 has a somewhat intermediate behavior, but took longer to report cases. We have hypothesized that reader 2 was trustier and leaned more on CAD, while reader 3 relied more on his personal experience and privileged sensitivity over specificity. The case that some TP CAD marks ($n = 7$) were rejected by readers is further evidence that operators where somewhat uncomfortable when using CAD. The above reported behavior patterns may have been determined by two reasons: (a) operators not being accustomed to interpreting with CAD, being that only 10 cases were reviewed with CAD prior to entering the study, as part of the preliminary training; and (b) interpreting prostate MRI on color-coded maps is something radiologists simply don't do when reading MRI examinations. As for other CAD applications, the next step will be to test CAD/reader interactions using different reading paradigms—that is, second reader, concurrent, or first reader—in order to establish which yields the best performances. Regardless of which CAD system is used, ultimately the reader will make the decision on whether or not disease is present.

From a general standpoint, there is a strong rationale in developing CAD systems for PCa detection at MRI. First, MRI is now on the front end of PCa diagnosis. In Europe, the number of yearly prostate MRI studies is increasing at a very fast rate (source: Millennium Research Group [62]) and this will inevitably lead to an increase of the individual reporting throughput. Second, since readers have to analyze data from several MRI sequences in parallel, each one yielding different information, reporting is time consuming and complex, requiring dedicated radiologists [24,25,63].

Further research should be conducted to validate these results and overcome some limitations. First, other readings protocol should be tested to avoid that readers rely only on CAD marks for diagnosis. Indeed, using only CAD findings, lesions missed by CAD were obviously ignored by operators. While planning the study we were aware that its design would limit the clinical usability of the CAD scheme. However, before testing other CAD paradigms we wanted to be confident that the CAD likelihood maps, which summarize the relevant information provided by mpMRI, could support radiologists in detecting PCa lesions. Therefore, in general our results add to the understanding of how radiologists interact with likelihood maps. Second, it would be useful to evaluate how the CAD impact on the performance of readers with less experience, that is, less than 5 years.

CONCLUSION

In conclusion, in this first study assessing interaction between CAD and experienced human operators reporting prostate MRI we have demonstrated that a CAD system, which reach high performance in detecting PCas, can allow the detection of more patients with GS > 6 and/or diameter ≥10 mm PCa lesions, additionally reducing overall reporting time. Since MRI will likely gain a leading role in PCa diagnosis, this finding may have a positive impact on clinical workflow. Multicenter studies involving a larger number of readers with different expertise will be necessary to deepen the knowledge of CAD/human interaction in this specific setting.

REFERENCES

1. Ferlay J, Steliarova-Foucher E, Lortet-Tieulent J, Rosso S, Coebergh J WW, Comber H, Forman D, Bray F. Cancer incidence and mortality patterns in Europe: Estimates for 40 countries in 2012. *Eur J Cancer* 2013;49:1374–1403. doi:10.1016/j.ejca.2012.12.027.
2. Mistry M, Parkin DM, Ahmad AS, Sasieni P. Cancer incidence in the United Kingdom: Projections to the year 2030. *Br J Cancer* 2011;105:1795–1803. doi:10.1038/bjc.2011.430.
3. Luengo-Fernandez R, Leal J, Gray A, Sullivan R. Economic burden of cancer across the European Union: A population-based cost analysis. *Lancet Oncol* 2013;14:1165–1174. doi:10.1016/S1470-2045(13)70442-X.

4. Ahmed HU, Arya M, Freeman A, Emberton M. Do low-grade and low-volume prostate cancers bear the hallmarks of malignancy? *Lancet Oncol* 2012;13:e509–e517. doi:10.1016/S1470-2045(12)70388-1.

5. Heidenreich A, Bastian PJ, Bellmunt J et al. EAU guidelines on prostate cancer. Part 1: Screening, diagnosis, and local treatment with curative intent-update 2013. *Eur Urol* 2014;65:124–137. doi:10.1016/j.eururo.2013.09.046.

6. Carter HB, Partin AW, Walsh PC, Trock BJ, Veltri RW, Nelson WG, Coffey DS, Singer EA, Epstein JI. Gleason score 6 adenocarcinoma: Should it be labeled as cancer? *J Clin Oncol* 2012;30:4294–4296. doi:10.1200/JCO.2012.44.0586.

7. Jones JS, Patel A, Schoenfield L, Rabets JC, Zippe CD, Magi-Galluzzi C. Saturation technique does not improve cancer detection as an initial prostate biopsy strategy. *J Urol* 2006;175(2):485–488.

8. Resnick MJ, Guzzo TJ. Patient selection essential in optimizing the benefit of radical prostatectomy for patients with organ-confined prostate cancer. *Asian J Androl* 2011;13:789–790. doi:10.1038/aja.2011.124.

9. Rothwax JT, George AK, Wood BJ. Multiparametric MRI in biopsy guidance for prostate cancer: Fusion-guided. *Biomed Res Int* 2014;2014:439171. doi:10.1155/2014/439171.

10. Epstein JI, Feng Z, Trock BJ et al. Upgrading and downgrading of prostate cancer from biopsy to radical prostatectomy: Incidence and predictive factors using the modified Gleason grading system and factoring in tertiary grades. *Eur Urol* 2012;61:1019–1024. doi:10.1016/j.eururo.2012.01.050.

11. Sandhu GS, Andriole GL. Overdiagnosis of prostate cancer. *J Natl Cancer Inst Monogr* 2012;2012:146–151. doi:10.1093/jncimonographs/lgs031.

12. Turkbey B, Pinto PA, Choyke PL. Imaging techniques for prostate cancer: Implications for focal therapy. *Nat Rev Urol* 2009;6(4):191–203. doi:10.1038/nrurol.2009.27.

13. Candefjord S, Ramser K, Lindahl OA. Technologies for localization and diagnosis of prostate cancer. *J Med Eng Technol* 2009;33(8):585–603. doi:10.3109/03091900903111966.

14. Russo F, Regge D, Armando E, Giannini V, Vignati A, Mazzetti S, Manfredi M, Bollito E, Correale L, Porpiglia F. Detection of prostate cancer index lesions with multiparametric magnetic resonance imaging (mp-MRI) using whole-mount histological sections as the reference standard. *BJU Int* 2016;118(1):84–94. doi:10.1111/bju.13234.

15. Arumainayagam N, Ahmed HU, Moore CM, Freeman A, Allen C, Sohaib SA, Kirkham A, van der Meulen J, Emberton M. Multiparametric MR imaging for detection of clinically significant prostate cancer: A validation cohort study with transperineal template prostate mapping as the reference standard. *Radiology* 2013;268(3):761–769. doi:10.1148/radiol.13120641.

16. Mottet N, Bellmunt J, Briers E et al. *Guidelines on Prostate Cancer.* European Association of Urology, 2015.

17. Porpiglia F, Manfredi M, Mele F et al. Diagnostic pathway with multiparametric magnetic resonance imaging versus standard pathway: Results from a randomized prospective study in biopsy-naïve patients with suspected prostate cancer. *Eur Urol* 2016. doi:10.1016/j.eururo.2016.08.041.

18. Wegelin O, van Melick HH, Hooft L, Bosch JL, Reitsma HB, Barentsz JO, Somford DM. Comparing three different techniques for magnetic resonance imaging-targeted prostate biopsies: A systematic review of in-bore versus magnetic resonance imaging-transrectal ultrasound fusion versus cognitive registration. Is there a preferred technique? *Eur Urol* 2017;71(4):517–531. doi:10.1016/j.eururo.2016.07.041.

19. Pokorny MR, de Rooij M, Duncan E, Schröder FH, Parkinson R, Barentsz JO, Thompson LC. Prospective study of diagnostic accuracy comparing prostate cancer detection by transrectal ultrasound-guided biopsy versus magnetic resonance (MR) imaging with subsequent MR-guided biopsy in men without previous prostate biopsies. *Eur Urol* 2014;66(1):22–29. doi:10.1016/j.eururo.2014.03.002.

20. Dickinson L, Ahmed HU, Allen C et al. Magnetic resonance imaging for the detection, localisation, and characterisation of prostate cancer: Recommendations from a European consensus meeting. *Eur Urol* 2011;59(4):477–494. doi:10.1016/j.eururo.2010.12.009.

21. Regge D, Della Monica P, Galatola G et al. Efficacy of computer-aided detection as a second reader for 6-9-mm lesions at CT colonography: Multicenter prospective trial. *Radiology* 2013;266(1):168–176. doi:10.1148/radiol.12120376.

22. Iussich G, Correale L, Senore C et al. CT colonography: Preliminary assessment of a double-read paradigm that uses computer-aided detection as the first reader. *Radiology* 2013;268(3):743–751. doi:10.1148/radiol.13121192.

23. Valente IR, Cortez PC, Neto EC, Soares JM, de Albuquerque VH, Tavares JM. Automatic 3D pulmonary nodule detection in CT images: A survey. *Comput Methods Programs Biomed* 2016;124:91–107. doi:10.1016/j.cmpb.2015.10.006.

24. Litjens GJ, Barentsz JO, Karssemeijer N, Huisman HJ. Clinical evaluation of a computer-aided diagnosis system for determining cancer aggressiveness in prostate MRI. *Eur Radiol* 2015;25(11):3187–3199. doi:10.1007/s00330-015-3743-y.

25. Vos PC, Barentsz JO, Karssemeijer N, Huisman HJ. Automatic computer-aided detection of prostate cancer based on multiparametric magnetic resonance image analysis. *Phys Med Biol* 2012;57(6):1527–1542. doi:10.1088/0031-9155/57/6/1527.

26. Litjens GJ, Vos PC, Barentsz JO, Karssemeijer N, Huisman HJ. Automatic computer aided detection of abnormalities in multi-parametric prostate MRI. *Proceedings of the SPIE 7963, Medical Imaging 2011: Computer-Aided Diagnosis*, 79630T, March 4, 2011. doi:10.1117/12.877844.

27. Iussich G, Correale L, Senore C, Hassan C, Segnan N, Campanella D, Bert A, Galatola G, Laudi C, Regge D. Computer-aided detection for computed tomographic colonography screening: A prospective comparison of a double-reading paradigm with first-reader computer-aided detection against second-reader computer-aided detection. *Invest Radiol* 2014;49(3):173–182. doi:10.1097/RLI.0000000000000009.

28. Chan I, Wells W 3rd, Mulkern RV, Haker S, Zhang J, Zou KH, Maier SE, Tempany CM. Detection of prostate cancer by integration of line-scan diffusion, T2-mapping and T2-weighted magnetic resonance imaging; a multichannel statistical classifier. *Med Phys* 2003;30(9):2390–2398.

29. Niaf E, Rouvière O, Mège-Lechevallier F, Bratan F, Lartizien C. Computer-aided diagnosis of prostate cancer in the peripheral zone using multiparametric MRI. *Phys Med Biol* 2012;57(12):3833–3851. doi:10.1088/0031-9155/57/12/3833.

30. Litjens G, Debats O, Barentsz J, Karssemeijer N, Huisman H. Computer-aided detection of prostate cancer in MRI. *IEEE Trans Med Imaging* 2014;33(5):1083–1092. doi:10.1109/TMI.2014.2303821.

31. Lemaître G, Martí R, Freixenet J, Vilanova JC, Walker PM, Meriaudeau F. Computer-aided detection and diagnosis for prostate cancer based on mono and multi-parametric MRI: A review. *Comput Biol Med* 2015;60:8–31. doi:10.1016/j.compbiomed.2015.02.009.

32. Stamey TA, Freiha FS, McNeal JE, Redwine EA, Whittemore AS, Schmid HP. Localized prostate cancer. Relationship of tumor volume to clinical significance for treatment of prostate cancer. *Cancer* 1993;71(suppl 3):933–938.

33. Barentsz JO, Weinreb JC, Verma S et al. Synopsis of the PI-RADS v2 guidelines for multiparametric prostate magnetic resonance imaging and recommendations for use. *Eur Urol* 2016;69(1):41–49. doi:10.1016/j.eururo.2015.08.038.

34. Montironi R, Lopez-Beltran A, Mazzucchelli R, Scarpelli M, Bollito E. Assessment of radical prostatectomy specimens and diagnostic reporting of pathological findings. *Pathologica* 2001;93(3):226–232.

35. Johnson HJ, McCormick M, Ibañez L. *The ITK Software Guide*. Kitware, Inc. 3rd ed., 2013. http://www.itk.org/ItkSoftwareGuide.pdf.

36. Giannini V, Vignati A, De Luca M, Mazzetti S, Russo F, Armando E, Stasi M, Bollito E, Porpiglia F, Regge D. A novel and fully automated registration method for prostate cancer detection using multiparametric magnetic resonance imaging. *J Med Imaging Health Inform* 2015;5(6):1171–1182. doi:10.1166/jmihi.2015.1518.

37. Khalifa F, Soliman A, El-Baz A, Abou El-Ghar M, El-Diasty T, Gimelfarb G, Ouseph R, Dwyer AC. Models and methods for analyzing DCE-MRI: A review. *Med Phys* 2014;41(12):124301. doi:10.1118/1.4898202.

38. Fan X, Medved M, Karczmar GS, Yang C, Foxley S, Arkani S, Recant W, Zamora MA, Abe H, Newstead GM. Diagnosis of suspicious breast lesions using an empirical mathematical model for dynamic contrast-enhanced MRI. *Magn Reson Imaging* 2007;25(5):593–603.

39. McVary KT. Clinical evaluation of benign prostatic hyperplasia. *Rev Urol* 2003;5(Suppl 4):S3–S11.

40. Otsu N. A threshold selection method from gray-level histogram. *IEEE Trans Syst Man Cybern* 1979;9(1):62–66.

41. Tustison NJ, Avants BB, Cook PA, Zheng Y, Egan A, Yushkevich PA, Gee JC. N4ITK: Improved N3 bias correction. *IEEE Trans Med Imaging* 2010;29(6):1310–1320. doi:10.1109/TMI.2010.2046908.

42. Giannini V, Vignati A, Mirasole S et al. MR-T2-weighted signal intensity: A new imaging biomarker of prostate cancer aggressiveness. *Comput Methods Biomech Biomed Eng Imaging Vis* 2016;4(3–4):130–134.

43. Peng Y, Jiang Y, Antic T, Giger ML, Eggener SE, Oto A. Validation of quantitative analysis of multiparametric prostate MR images for prostate cancer detection and aggressiveness assessment: A cross-imager study. *Radiology* 2014;271(2):461–471. doi:10.1148/radiol.14131320.

44. Gliozzi AS, Mazzetti S, Delsanto PP, Regge D, Stasi M. Phenomenological universalities: A novel tool for the analysis of dynamic contrast enhancement in magnetic resonance imaging. *Phys Med Biol* 2011;56(3):573–586. doi:10.1088/0031-9155/56/3/004.

45. Castorina P, Delsanto PP, Guiot C. Classification scheme for phenomenological universalities in growth problems in physics and other sciences. *Phys Rev Lett* 2006;96:188701.

46. Mazzetti S, Gliozzi AS, Bracco C, Russo F, Regge D, Stasi M. Comparison between PUN and Tofts models in the quantification of dynamic contrast-enhanced MR imaging. *Phys Med Biol* 2012;57(24):8443–8453. doi:10.1088/0031-9155/57/24/8443.

47. Langer DL, van der Kwast TH, Evans AJ, Trachtenberg J, Wilson BC, Haider MA. Prostate cancer detection with multi-parametric MRI: Logistic regression analysis of quantitative T2, diffusion weighted imaging, and dynamic contrast-enhanced MRI. *J Magn Reson Imaging* 2009;30(2):327–334.

48. Vos PC, Hambrock T, Barentsz JO, Huisman HJ. Computer-assisted analysis of peripheral zone prostate lesions using T2-weighted and dynamic contrast enhanced T1-weighted MRI. *Phys Med Biol* 2010;55(6):1719–1734.

49. Ross HM, Kryvenko ON, Cowan JE, Simko JP, Wheeler TM, Epstein JI. Do adenocarcinomas of the prostate with Gleason score (GS) ≤6 have the potential to metastasize to lymph nodes? *Am J Surg Pathol* 2012;36(9):1346–1352.

50. Loeb S, Bjurlin MA, Nicholson J et al. Overdiagnosis and overtreatment of prostate cancer. *Eur Urol* 2014;65(6):1046–1055.

51. Le JD, Tan N, Shkolyar E et al. Multifocality and prostate cancer detection by multiparametric magnetic resonance imaging: Correlation with whole-mount histopathology. *Eur Urol* 2015;67(3):569–576. doi:10.1016/j.eururo.2014.08.079.

52. Wang S, Burtt K, Turkbey B, Choyke P, Summers RM. Computer aided-diagnosis of prostate cancer on multiparametric MRI: A technical review of current research. *Biomed Res Int* 2014;2014:789561. doi:10.1155/2014/789561.

53. Chappelow J, Viswanath S, Monaco J et al. Improving supervised classification accuracy using non-rigid multimodal image registration: Detecting prostate cancer. In: *Proceedings of the SPIE 6915, Medical Imaging 2008: Computer-Aided Diagnosis*, 69150V, 2008. doi:10.1117/12.770703.

54. Shah V, Turkbey B, Mani H et al. Decision support system for localizing prostate cancer based on multi-parametric magnetic resonance imaging. *Med Phys* 2012;39(7):4093–4103. doi:10.1118/1.4722753.

55. De Luca M, Giannini V, Vignati A et al. A fully automatic method to register the prostate gland on T2-weighted and EPI-DWI images. *Conf Proc IEEE Eng Med Biol Soc* 2011;2011:8029–8032. doi:10.1109/IEMBS.2011.6091980.

56. Viswanath S, Bloch BN, Rosen M et al. Integrating structural. Functional imaging for computer assisted detection of prostate cancer on multi-protocol in vivo 3 Tesla MRI. *Proc Soc Photo Opt Instrum Eng* 2009;7260:72603I.

57. Melbourne A, Hipwell J, Modat M et al. The effect of motion correction on pharmacokinetic parameter estimation indynamic-contrast-enhanced MRI. *Phys Med Biol* 2011;56:7693–7708.

58. Orton MR, Collins DJ, Walker-Samuel S, d'Arcy JA, Hawkes DJ, Atkinson D, Leach MO. Bayesian estimation of pharmacokinetic parameters for DCE-MRI with a robust treatment of enhancement onset time. *Phys Med Biol* 2007;52(9):2393–2408. doi:10.1088/0031-9155/52/9/005.

59. Bergamino M, Barletta L, Castellan L, Mancardi G, Roccatagliata L. Dynamic contrast-enhanced MRI in the study of brain tumors. Comparison between the extended Tofts-Kety model and a Phenomenological Universalities (PUN) algorithm. *J Digit Imaging* 2015;28(6):748–754. doi:10.1007/s10278-015-9788-2.

60. Sung YS, Kwon HJ, Park BW, Cho G, Lee CK, Cho KS, Kim JK. Prostate cancer detection on dynamic contrast-enhanced MRI: Computer-aided diagnosis versus single perfusion parameter maps. *AJR Am J Roentgenol* 2011;197(5):1122–1129. doi:10.2214/AJR.10.6062.

61. Giannini V, Mazzetti S, Vignati A, Russo F, Bollito E, Porpiglia F, Stasi M, Regge D. A fully automatic computer aided diagnosis system for peripheral zone prostate cancer detection using multi-parametric magnetic resonance imaging. *Comput Med Imaging Graph* 2015;46(Pt 2):219–226. doi:10.1016/j.compmedimag.2015.09.001.

62. Millennium Research Group. DRG Medtech: Research quickly. Analyze thoroughly. Plan confidently. 2012. https://decisionresourcesgroup.com/solutions/medtech-solutions/.

63. Ruprecht O, Weisser P, Bodelle B, Ackermann H, Vogl TJ. MRI of the prostate: Interobserver agreement compared with histopathologic outcome after radical prostatectomy. *Eur J Radiol* 2012;81(3):456–460. doi:10.1016/j.ejrad.2010.12.076.

17 Magnetic Resonance Imaging in the Detection of Prostate Cancer

Timothy D. McClure, Daniel Margolis, and Peter N. Schlegel

CONTENTS

INTRODUCTION

Prostate cancer (PCa) is the most common noncutaneous malignancy in the United States with an estimated 161,360 cases and 26,370 deaths in 2017.[1] The choice of imaging modality for prostate cancer, including computed tomography (CT), magnetic resonance imaging (MRI), and ultrasound (US), depends on the clinical stage and specific component of prostate cancer being investigated. The role of CT is predominately focused on nodal and metastatic staging of prostate cancer and US is predominately used to assist in prostate biopsy. Accuracy of US in the diagnosis of prostate cancer is poor with specificity and sensitivity of approximately 66% and 46%.[2] MRI can be used for staging, surgical planning, radiation therapy planning, observation of patients on active surveillance, and the detection of local recurrence after treatment. Some recent studies have suggested that multiparametric MRI of the prostate can even be used in place of prostate biopsy in some clinical scenarios. The focus of this chapter is to discuss the ability of MRI to detect prostate cancer.

Dooms and Hricak first described MRI prostate imaging in 1986 but stated, "One cannot distinguish benign from malignant processes."[3] This perception has changed significantly and MRI is now used to diagnosis prostate cancer and assist in surgical planning.[4,5] In fact, the American Urologic Association and the Society of Abdominal Radiology in an joint consensus white paper recommend its use in men with elevated prostate-specific antigen (PSA) and a prior negative prostate biopsy.[6] Prostate multiparametric magnetic resonance imaging (mpMRI) includes multiple imaging sequences, at 1.5 or 3.0 Tesla, with or without the use of an endorectal coil. The "workhorse" pulse sequences are T1- and T2-weighted imaging, diffusion-weighted imaging (DWI) with the apparent diffusion coefficient (ADC) map, and dynamic contrast-enhanced (DCE) imaging.

T2-WEIGHTED IMAGING

T2-weighted imaging (T2WI) defines anatomy, assists in the detection of clinically significant cancer, and helps determine staging. Spin-echo T2WI has poor signal-to-noise and long imaging duration resulting in poor accuracy.[2] The advent of turbo spin echo (TSE) and fast spin echo (FSE), however, improved the accuracy of T2WI by reducing scan time and increasing signal-to-noise.[7] T2WI imaging includes the external urinary sphincter to the seminal vesicles and is obtained in axial (perpendicular to the axis of the prostate), coronal, and sagittal planes. Three-dimensional T2WI, known by the vendor designations of VISTA, SPACE, XETA, and CUBE, allows for reformatted planes and may potentially save time by avoiding three separate planar sequences, but is more sensitive to motion. The use of 3D T2WI has been shown to have similar sensitivity and specificity of 84% and 89%.[8]

The image slice thickness should be no greater than 3 mm. An antiperistaltic agent, such as hyoscine butylbromide or glucagon, can be used to limit movement of bowel during scanning. The use of an endorectal coil (ERC) is controversial, however, it may improve image quality, prostate cancer detection, and the accuracy of staging with T2WI in magnets of lower field strength.[9] Prostate Imaging Reporting and Data System (PI-RADS) v2 recommends the use of an ERC with a 1.5T magnet if a 3T magnet is not available.[10] The use of an ERC must be weighed against both the increased cost and patient discomfort with its use.

The prostate has no true fascial plane, however it does have a fibrous "capsule" which appears as a T2WI hypointensity encompassing the prostate posterior-laterally. Anteriorly the prostate cancer is covered by fibromuscular tissue which appears hypointense on T2WI.[11] The neurovascular bundles appear on T2WI as hypointense structures at the posterolateral "5 and 7 o'clock" positions.[12] The peripheral, central, and transition zones are easily characterized on T2WI. The healthy peripheral zone should be homogenously T2 hyperintense; the central zone, T2 hypointense; and the transition zone commonly of T2 hyperintensity owing to changes of prostatic hyperplasia. Axial T2WI is the primary diagnostic sequence; however, the coronal view is helpful to characterize tumors at the prostate base and seminal vesicles.

Prostate cancer characteristically appears as a distinct T2 hypointensity on MRI.[13]

This finding is not exclusive to prostate cancer with the differential diagnosis including hemorrhage, inflammation, calcification, or scar. In a meta-analysis evaluating the accuracy of T2WI in detecting prostate cancer, the sensitivity was in the range of 57%–67%, whereas the specificity was 74%–78%.[14] The use of mpMRI is important, however, with the accuracy of prostate cancer detection increasing when more than one sequence is used.[15] Location of prostate cancer also will determine the weight of what sequence predominates the PI-RADS v2 score. Transition zone lesions are best characterized by T2WI, whereas peripheral zone lesions are better characterized by DWI and the ADC map.[10]

DIFFUSION-WEIGHTED IMAGING

Diffusion-weighted imaging (DWI) evaluates the Brownian motion of water molecules in the prostate. This sequence does little to delineate the anatomy of the prostate, and it is the workhorse for prostate cancer detection within the peripheral zone.[10] When obtaining DWI, high b-values images and an apparent diffusion coefficient (ADC) map must be included. DWI sequences should be a free-breathing spin echo EPI with fat saturation.

The TE should be less than or equal to 90 msec and TR should be greater than 3000 msec. The slice thickness should be at most 4 mm. The FOV should be the same as that used in the T2WI and DCE, generally 12–20 cm. The reason for a similar FOV is to ensure an accurate comparison of a finding on each sequence in the prostate mpMRI. There should be at least 2 b-values for calculation of the ADC, the highest at 800–1000 sec/mm^2 and the lowest at 50–100 sec/mm^2. Additional b-values between these values improves the accuracy of the ADC calculations.[10] A high b-value image, at least 1400 s/mm^2, is also necessary for evaluation and can be natively acquired but is often more effectively calculated, which exploits the higher signal-to-noise ratio and shorter echo times of lower b-values. This sequence is highly susceptible to motion artifact and signal disturbance from orthopedic hardware within the prostate.

The appearance of prostate cancer will be hyperintense on a high b-value DWI and hypointense on the corresponding area on the ADC map on MRI. The differential diagnosis of these findings includes benign prostatic hyperplasia (BPH), in part due to diffusion restriction correlating with glandular and cell density, irrespective of the presence of hyperplasia or prostate cancer.[16] However, when specifically evaluating the peripheral zone, DWI and ADC maps strongly correlate with the presence of prostate cancer.

Verma et al. found that the ADC value was negatively correlated with the Gleason score. In 197 tumors detected in 110 men who underwent radical prostatectomy, ADC values less than 750–900 μm^2/sec correlated with greater aggressiveness of prostate cancer. This observation is only seen in prostate cancer within the peripheral zone and not the central/transition zone.[17] This observation is likely secondary to the confounding mp MRI appearance of nonmalignant nodules of BPH. This is an important point to highlight as well-circumscribed, capsulated lesions that are hyperintense on DWI and hypointense on the corresponding ADC map are presumed to be BPH nodules and do not warrant biopsy.

DWI and ADC maps are an integral component of prostate mpMRI and lesions identified on DWI must be compared to findings seen on T1WI, T2WI, and DCE. DWI has excellent accuracy in the detection of prostate cancer, particularly in the peripheral zone.

Standardized prostate mpMRI reporting with PI-RADS v2 uses the DWI and ADC maps as the primary determinate of the overall PI-RADS score in the peripheral zone.[10]

DYNAMIC CONTRAST-ENHANCED PERFUSION IMAGING

Unenhanced T1-weighted imaging is predominately used to evaluate hemorrhage within the prostate as it can confound the detection of prostate cancer. It is not otherwise useful in the detection of prostate cancer. Dynamic contrast-enhanced (DCE) T1-weighted MRI evaluates the prostate gland before and after the intravenous administration of a gadolinium-based contrast agent. The specific technical considerations are as follows: 3D T1 gradient echo (GRE) sequences should be obtained for several minutes to determine enhancement pattern of the prostate. Prostate cancer usually demonstrates early enhancement, hence temporal resolution is important. Subtracted imaging and fat supersession is helpful and advisable. The TR/TE should be less than 100/5 msec. A slice thickness of 3 mm with no gap is recommended with similar spatial parameters used for both T2 and DWI to allow for accurate comparisons.

The FOV should include the prostate and seminal vesicles. The duration of scanning needs to be greater than 2 minutes and the temporal resolution should be less than 10 seconds, preferably less than 7 seconds. The in-plane dimension should be $\leq 2 \times \leq 2$ mm. The dose of gadolinium contrast is generally 0.1 mmol/kg with an injection rate of 2–3 cc/sec.

Prostate cancer will demonstrate early enhancement when compared to surrounding tissue. Ocak et al. demonstrated the sensitivity, specificity, PPV, and NPV of DCE to be 73%, 88%, 75%, and 75%, respectively.[18] Dynamic enhancement curves are frequently used when assessing cancers and consist of three curve types. Type I is progressive enhancement, with an increase in signal as time progresses. There is no plateau or washout in a Type I curve and generally this pattern is seen with benign tissue. Type II and type III curves are more concerning for potential cancer. A type II enhancement curve will have an initial increase in signal intensity and then plateau with no continued enhancement or washout. A type III enhancement curve demonstrates this same initial enhancement but instead of a plateau will have washout. Enhancement curves have been shown to add value in breast cancer diagnosis with breast imaging.[19] The first version of PI-RADS recommended reporting enhancement curves as it was initially believed to be helpful in diagnosis and localization of prostate cancer sites. However, prostate cancer has very heterogeneous enhancement patterns and there is a lack of sufficient data demonstrating a benefit of curve analysis in prostate cancer diagnosis. Pharmacokinetic assessment with contrast wash-in (K^{trans}) and washout (k_{ep}) may provide utility for curve analysis in the future. Currently, no curve analysis is recommended to be used with prostate mpMRI.[10]

The specific suspicious finding on DCE MRI is a focal region of early enhancement with a correlating finding on either T2WI or DWI/ADC map. Color maps can be used for assistance with DCE MRI evaluation, however the authors find assessment with fat sat T1 post contrast is sufficient for accurate analysis. DCE MRI is useful in assessing indeterminate findings found on either T2WI or DWI/ADC map, especially in the central zone, apex, and anterior fibromuscular stroma.[20] False positives of DCE can be diffuse enhancement that is suggestive of prostatitis or marked enhancement within the central zone which can be seen with BPH nodules. The corresponding T2WI and DWI/ADC will, however, correctly characterize these false DCE findings, which highlights the need for multiple sequences to accurately perform prostate mpMRI.

DCE improves the accuracy of prostate mpMRI for prostate cancer localization but must be interpreted with other sequences. A recent meta-analysis demonstrated this by showing combined DCE-MRI, DWI, and T2WI had a notably better AUC of 0.110, 0.103–0.117 than DCE with an AUC of 0.075, 0.069–0.081; than T2WI with an AUC of 0.078, 0.073–0.083; or than DWI alone that had an AUC of 0.088, 0.079–0.095.[21] DCE MRI is an integral component of prostate mpMRI, but adds the least to suspicion characterization. Current PI-RADS v2 reporting uses DCE for suspicion assessment only for peripheral gland lesions of intermediate DWI suspicion.[10]

SPECTROSCOPY

Magnetic resonance spectroscopic imaging (MRSI) showed great promise in the detection of prostate cancer.[22] However due to the complexity of the technique and difficulty in applying this technique to the general population MRSI is not a required component of the current PI-RADS version.[23] The specifics of MRSI will not be discussed in this chapter as it is not currently being used clinically to detect prostate cancer in prostate mpMRI.

PROSTATE CANCER STAGING

The American Joint Committee on Cancer stages prostate cancer according to the tumor (T), regional lymph node status (N), and evidence of distant metastasis (M). T stage may be defined either clinically or pathologically. Clinical T1 disease is nonpalpable disease, clinical T2 disease is palpable disease on digital rectal exam, clinical T3 disease means disease extends beyond the capsule, and clinical T4 disease means the tumor has invaded surrounding structures such as the pelvic side wall. There is no pathologic T1 disease. Pathologic T2 disease is organ-confined and subcategorized into pT2a, pT2b, and pT2c depending on the extent to which the tumor involves the prostate. Pathologic T3 disease means there is extraprostatic extension with pT3a classification denoting tumor invasion into the surrounding fascia and pT3b into the seminal vesicles. N staging assesses the presence of regional lymph nodes. M staging assesses the presence of nonregional lymph nodes (M1a), bones (M1b), or other sites (M1c). Prostate mpMRI has improved accuracy in T staging when compared to DRE and transrectal ultrasound (TRUS) biopsy.[24]

Rooij et al. performed a meta-analysis of prostate MRI in the local staging of prostate cancer.[15] They reviewed a total of 75 studies that involved 9797 patients and assessed prostate MRI's ability to determine overall stage T3 disease, extracapsular extension (T3a), and seminal vesicle invasion (SVI). For overall stage T3 disease the sensitivity was 0.61 (95% CI 0.54–0.67) and the specificity was 0.88 (95% CI 0.85–0.91). For T3a disease the sensitivity was 0.57 (95% CI 0.49–0.65) and the specificity was 0.91 (95% CI 0.88–0.93). For T3b disease the sensitivity was 0.58 (95% CI 0.47–0.68) and the specificity was 0.97(95% CI 0.95–0.98). When assessing field strength, they noted improved sensitivity for T3a and overall T3 disease with 3.0 T when compared to 1.0 T or 1.5 T. This meta-analysis found the use of an endorectal coil (ERC) was only beneficial in patients being scanned in 1.5 T magnets. In summary, both mpMRI with 3.0 T or 1.5 T imaging with an ERC appear to have comparable and effective accuracy in prostate cancer staging.

Overall this meta-analysis noticed improved sensitivity when using more than one MRI sequence, highlighting the necessity of multiparametric prostate MRI. This is in accordance with PI-RADS v2 guidelines that suggest the use of T2WI, DWI with ADC map, and DCE imaging.

PROSTATE CANCER DETECTION

Prostate mpMRI is accurate in the staging of prostate cancer and is now increasingly being used to detect clinically significant prostate cancer. Prostate cancer outcome is largely determined by the overall risk that is determined by PSA, clinical stage, and Gleason score. Clinically significant cancer is now generally defined as a Gleason score greater than 6, as the majority of men with low-volume Gleason score 6 prostate cancers can be safely observed.

Clinically significant disease, which is generally viewed as when treatment for prostate cancer should occur, is commonly defined by prostate cancer of greater than Gleason score 6 or a tumor volume more than 1 cm. Prostate mpMRI is of particular value since it can help identify the majority of clinically significant prostate cancers and misses the majority of clinically insignificant disease.

Turkbey et al. evaluated 45 patients who underwent prostate mpMRI prior to prostatectomy.[25] These patients had a total of 342 prostate cancer foci and as expected 82% were found in the peripheral zone and 18% where found in the central gland. When assessing the sensitivity and specificity of T2WI, DCE, MRS, and DWI they found that the both the sensitivity and specificity of the MRI improved if the prostate cancer focus was greater than 5 mm in size and if the Gleason grade was greater than 7. Prostate cancer foci of Gleason score 6 which were less than 5 mm in size had the worst accuracy in all MRI sequences evaluated. This was one of the first papers to suggest that MRI is less likely to detect clinically insignificant disease.

Rosenkrantz et al. evaluated 49 patients who underwent prostate mpMRI prior to prostatectomy to provide pathological characterization of MRI-visible lesions.[26] Prostate mpMRI was done on at 1.5 T and included T1WI, T2WI, DWI, and DCE sequences. Lesions that were seen on MRI were then compared to lesions that were missed. This group found that size, Gleason score, and loose stroma were significant predictors of lesion detection on prostate mpMRI. The pathologist identified 87 tumors in 49 patients; 53 lesions were found on MRI of which 45 represented true foci of prostate cancer. These 45 tumors seen on MRI had a median size of 13 m (5–40 mm) and median Gleason score of 7 (6–9). A total of 42 prostate cancer lesions were missed on mpMRI. These lesions were, on average, smaller (5 mm; 2–17 mm) and were more likely to have a Gleason score of 6. On univariate analysis, MRI visible tumors were more likely to be at least 1 cm (OR 15.7), have a Gleason score greater than 6 (OR 9.8), have solid tumor growth (OR 37.6), have desmoplastic stroma, have a high ratio of malignant epithelium-to-stroma (OR 12.2), lack loose stroma (OR 0.078), and have an absence of intermixed benign epithelium (OR 0.14). Multivariate analysis demonstrated independent predictors of MRI-visible tumors were more likely to have a Gleason score greater than 6, be at least 1 cm in size, and have solid tumor growth pattern on histology.[26]

Tan et al. assessed 122 men who had prostate mpMRI and underwent a radical prostatectomy. This confirmed previous studies of what the histologic findings are of MRI-visible lesions.[27] In these 122 patients, 285 prostate cancer foci were identified, of which the majority were missed (53.3%). The large majority of these missed lesions were Gleason score 6 (75%) with only 4% of Gleason score greater than 8 being missed. When specifically looking at Gleason score equal to or great than 7, only 73% of these lesions where detected. Of lesions that were 1 cm or larger, 70% were detected. Interestingly, this study also suggested that apical lesions are harder to diagnose, with only 22% of apical lesions being detected, versus 52% in the midgland. As Turkbey et al. showed, as the lesion size and Gleason score increased, so too did the sensitivity and specificity of mpMRI for detection of these prostate cancers.

Le et al. evaluated the same patient population as Tan et al. but used the primary outcome of MRI's ability to detect the index lesion. The index lesion theory, presumes, that despite the multifocality of prostate cancer, the single, most advanced lesion determines the patient's overall prognosis from prostate cancer. This assumption is based on studies suggesting that tumors size predicts biochemical recurrence,[28] and that in multifocal disease, the dominant, index lesion (as determined by size or Gleason score) may predict overall oncologic outcome.[29–31] When only assessing mean prostate cancer focus size, MRI-visible cancers had a mean size of 1.8 cm, whereas MRI-missed cancers were 0.8 cm, nearly a centimeter difference in size. Prostate cancer foci greater than 3 cm were all detected and 72% where detected if greater than 1 cm, however, only 14% of tumors 0.5 cm in size were detected. "Index lesions," defined as a size greater than 1 cm and a Gleason score of 7 or above, were identified on mpMRI 80% of the time.

When specifically evaluating the identification of an index lesion in multifocal disease, 77% were identified. Of those lesions missed, the majority were less than 1 cm (83%) and of Gleason score 6 (79%). This study also showed that the presence of post biopsy hemorrhage and an increased prostate weight resulted in lower prostate mpMRI accuracy.

The PROMIS study group evaluated the role of prostate mpMRI in detecting clinically significant prostate cancer.[32] Clinically significant prostate cancer was defined as any focus of cancer equal to or greater than Gleason 4 + 3 or a maximum cancer core length greater than 6 mm. They assessed 576 men who underwent prostate mpMRI and then had both a TRUS biopsy and transperineal mapping (TPM) biopsy. The reason for the TPM biopsy is that it samples the entire prostate in 5 mm increments. Prostate cancer was diagnosed in 71% (408/576) of men in which 40% (230/576) had clinically significant cancer. Prostate mpMRI was statistically more sensitive (93%) than TRUS biopsy (48%, $p < 0.0001$) in detecting clinically significant cancer. Prostate mpMRI was less specific (41%) than TRUS biopsy (96% $p < 0.0001$). The authors suggested that prostate mpMRI could be used to triage men who needed prostate biopsy for an elevated PSA and prevent about 25% of men from undergoing a TRUS biopsy.

MRI lesions that are visible are clearly histologically distinct from those that are not. These MRI lesions tend to be greater than 1 cm and have a higher Gleason score (greater than 6). However, it is important to note and stress that despite this improved accuracy in detecting clinically significant, larger, higher-grade prostate cancer, up to 20% of cancers will be missed.

MRI FUSION BIOPSY

Prostate mpMRI has been a game changer in the detection of prostate cancer by improving our ability to noninvasively identify sites at high risk of having prostate cancer present, as well as providing the opportunity for fusion images, combining TRUS with MRI. The standard TRUS systematic biopsy samples the base, mid, and apex of the prostate.

Although, in theory, such sampling reflects the entire prostate, over 30% of significant prostate cancers are missed.[33] In-bore MRI-guided biopsy can be done but is costly and not available at many centers. MRI fusion biopsy brings the specificity of MRI to the office, allowing for accurate sampling of MRI lesions with a TRUS biopsy, which now reflects the standard of care for men being evaluated for prostate cancer. MRI fusion biopsy improves the accuracy of TRUS biopsy.[34] MRI fusion biopsy can be done cognitively or with fusion software/hardware.

Cognitive fusion was the first application of MRI fusion biopsy, and it has been reported in studies at multiple institutions to be better than standard biopsies.[35,36] Choyke and Pinto first reported on the utility of prostate mpMRI and fusion biopsy. They prospectively evaluated 583 patients who under mpMRI and then subsequent MR/US fusion-guided prostate biopsy. The mpMRI included T2WI, DWI, spectroscopy, and DCE. MRI findings were graded as either low, moderate, or high suspicion. The patient demographics were a mean age of 61.3 years, and a mean PSA of 9.9 ng/mL.

Univariate analysis demonstrated that age, PSA, prostate volume, and mpMRI suspicion were associated with the diagnosis of prostate cancer. When assessing Gleason score they found that mpMRI had a sensitivity of 98% for detection of sites with Gleason score 8 and 94% for Gleason score 7 detection. ROC analysis of mpMRI demonstrated an AUC of 0.64 for all prostate cancer, 0.69 for Gleason score greater or equal to 7, and 0.72 for Gleason score greater than or equal to 8.[37] The report by Pinto's group was one of the first published manuscripts to show that mpMRI of the prostate has improved performance in detecting clinically significant disease.

Wegelin et al. performed a meta-analysis that evaluated the difference between MRI-guided biopsy (in-bore MRI biopsy, fusion biopsy, cognitive biopsy) and the standard TRUS- guided biopsy. They found no significant difference between MRI-guided biopsy and standard TRUS biopsy overall in detection of any cancer. However, when looking specifically at detection of clinically significant prostate cancer, MRI-guided biopsy was significantly more likely to diagnose those clinically important prostate cancers.[38] The finding is of a clear advantage to fusion software in the ability to target small lesions within larger prostates, an approach that could fail with cognitive fusion.

MRI-guided fusion biopsy leads to improved detection of clinically significant prostate cancer. The specific approach (cognitive, US fusion, or in-bore) for the biopsy doesn't appear to be as important as the use of MRI-ultrasound fusion in the detection of clinically significant prostate cancer. MRI-guided prostate biopsy provides a safe, accurate approach to diagnose clinically significant prostate cancer.

REFERENCES

1. Siegel RL, Miller KD, Jemal A. Cancer statistics, 2017. *CA Cancer J Clin* 2017; 67: 7–30.
2. Rifkin MD, Zerhouni EA, Gatsonis CA et al. Comparison of magnetic resonance imaging and ultrasonography in staging early prostate cancer: Results of a multi-institutional cooperative trial. *N Engl J Med* 1990; 323: 621–6.
3. Dooms GC, Hricak H. Magnetic resonance imaging of the pelvis: Prostate and urinary bladder. *Urol Radiol* 1986; 8: 156–65.
4. McClure TD, Margolis DJA, Reiter RE et al. Use of MR imaging to determine preservation of the neurovascular bundles at robotic-assisted laparoscopic prostatectomy. *Radiology* 2012; 262: 874–83.
5. Le JD, Tan N, Shkolyar E et al. Multifocality and prostate cancer detection by multiparametric magnetic resonance imaging: Correlation with whole-mount histopathology. *Eur Urol* 2015; 67: 569–76.
6. Rosenkrantz AB, Verma S, Choyke P et al. Prostate magnetic resonance imaging and magnetic resonance imaging targeted biopsy in patients with a prior negative biopsy: A consensus statement by AUA and SAR. *J Urol* 2016; 196: 1613–18.
7. Gupta RT, Spilseth B, Patel N, Brown AF, Yu J. Multiparametric prostate MRI: Focus on T2-weighted imaging and role in staging of prostate cancer. *Abdom Radiol (NY)* 2016; 41: 831–43.
8. Cornud F, Rouanne M, Beuvon F et al. Endorectal 3D T2-weighted 1 mm-slice thickness MRI for prostate cancer staging at 1.5Tesla: should we reconsider the indirects signs of extracapsular extension according to the D'Amico tumor risk criteria? *Eur J Radiol* 2012; 81(4): e591–7.
9. Heijmink SWTPJ, Fütterer JJ, Hambrock T et al. Prostate cancer: Body-array versus endorectal coil MR imaging at 3 T—comparison of image quality, localization, and staging performance. *Radiology* 2007; 244: 184–95.
10. Weinreb JC, Barentsz JO, Choyke PL et al. PI-RADS prostate imaging—Reporting and data system: 2015, Version 2. *Eur Urol* 2016; 69: 16–40.
11. Hricak H, Dooms GC, McNeal JE et al. MR imaging of the prostate gland: Normal anatomy. *AJR Am J Roentgenol* 1987; 148: 51–8.
12. Rosenkrantz AB, Taneja SS. Radiologist, be aware: Ten pitfalls that confound the interpretation of multiparametric prostate MRI. *AJR Am J Roentgenol* 2014; 202: 109–20.
13. Turkbey B, Albert PS, Kurdziel K, Choyke PL. Imaging localized prostate cancer: Current approaches and new developments. *AJR Am J Roentgenol* 2009; 192: 1471–80.
14. Tan CH, Wei W, Johnson V, Kundra V. Diffusion-weighted MRI in the detection of prostate cancer: Meta-analysis. *AJR Am J Roentgenol* 2012; 199: 822–9.
15. de Rooij M, Hamoen EHJ, Witjes JA, Barentsz JO, Rovers MM. Accuracy of magnetic resonance imaging for local staging of prostate cancer: A diagnostic meta-analysis. *Eur Urol* 2016; 70: 233–45.

16. Borren A, Moman MR, Groenendaal G et al. Why prostate tumour delineation based on apparent diffusion coefficient is challenging: An exploration of the tissue microanatomy. *Acta Oncol* 2013; 52: 1629–36.

17. Verma S, Rajesh A, Morales H et al. Assessment of aggressiveness of prostate cancer: Correlation of apparent diffusion coefficient with histologic grade after radical prostatectomy. *AJR Am J Roentgenol* 2011; 196: 374–81.

18. Ocak I, Bernardo M, Metzger G et al. Dynamic contrast-enhanced MRI of prostate cancer at 3 T: A study of pharmacokinetic parameters. *AJR Am J Roentgenol* 2007; 189: 849.

19. Macura KJ, Ouwerkerk R, Jacobs MA, Bluemke DA. Patterns of enhancement on breast MR images: interpretation and imaging pitfalls. *Radiographics* 2006; 26: 1719–34; quiz 1719.

20. Hansford BG, Karademir I, Peng Y et al. Dynamic contrast-enhanced MR imaging features of the normal central zone of the prostate. *Acad Radiol* 2014; 21: 569–77.

21. Tan CH, Hobbs BP, Wei W, Kundra V. Dynamic contrast-enhanced MRI for the detection of prostate cancer: Meta-analysis. *AJR Am J Roentgenol* 2015; 204: W439–48.

22. Fuchsjäger M, Akin O, Shukla-Dave A, Pucar D, Hricak H. The role of MRI and MRSI in diagnosis, treatment selection, and post-treatment follow-up for prostate cancer. *Clin Adv Hematol Oncol* 2009; 7: 193–202.

23. Barentsz JO, Weinreb JC, Verma S et al. Synopsis of the PI-RADS v2 Guidelines for Multiparametric Prostate Magnetic Resonance Imaging and Recommendations for Use. *Eur Urol* 2016; 69: 41–9.

24. Mullerad M, Hricak H, Kuroiwa K et al. Comparison of endorectal magnetic resonance imaging, guided prostate biopsy and digital rectal examination in the preoperative anatomical localization of prostate cancer. *J Urol* 2005; 174: 2158–63.

25. Turkbey B, Mani H, Shah V et al. Multiparametric 3T prostate magnetic resonance imaging to detect cancer: Histopathological correlation using prostatectomy specimens processed in customized magnetic resonance imaging based molds. *J Urol* 2011; 186: 1818–24.

26. Rosenkrantz AB, Mendrinos S, Babb JS, Taneja SS. Prostate cancer foci detected on multiparametric magnetic resonance imaging are histologically distinct from those not detected. *J Urol* 2012; 187: 2032–8.

27. Tan N, Margolis DJ, Lu DY et al. Characteristics of detected and missed prostate cancer foci on 3-T multiparametric MRI using an endorectal coil correlated with whole-mount thin-section histopathology. *AJR Am J Roentgenol* 2015; 205: W87–92.

28. Stamey TA, McNeal JE, Yemoto CM, Sigal BM, Johnstone IM. Biological determinants of cancer progression in men with prostate cancer. *JAMA* 1999; 281: 1395–1400.

29. Noguchi M, Stamey TA, McNeal JE, Nolley R. Prognostic factors for multifocal prostate cancer in radical prostatectomy specimens: Lack of significance of secondary cancers. *J Urol* 2003; 170: 459–63.

30. Wise AM, Stamey TA, McNeal JE, Clayton JL. Morphologic and clinical significance of multifocal prostate cancers in radical prostatectomy specimens. *Urology* 2002; 60: 264–9.

31. Karavitakis M, Winkler M, Abel P, Livni N, Beckley I, Ahmed HU. Histological characteristics of the index lesion in whole-mount radical prostatectomy specimens: Implications for focal therapy. *Prostate Cancer Prostatic Dis* 2011; 14: 46–52.

32. Ahmed HU, El-Shater Bosaily A, Brown LC et al. Diagnostic accuracy of multi-parametric MRI and TRUS biopsy in prostate cancer (PROMIS): A paired validating confirmatory study. *The Lancet* 2017; 389: 815–22.

33. Hodge KK, McNeal JE, Stamey TA. Ultrasound guided transrectal core biopsies of the palpably abnormal prostate. *J Urol* 1989; 142: 66–70.

34. Le JD, Stephenson S, Brugger M et al. Magnetic resonance imaging-ultrasound fusion biopsy for prediction of final prostate pathology. *J Urol* 2014; 192: 1367–73.

35. Perrotti M, Han KR, Epstein RE et al. Prospective evaluation of endorectal magnetic resonance imaging to detect tumor foci in men with prior negative prostatic biopsy: A pilot study. *J Urol* 1999; 162: 1314–17.

36. Puech P, Rouvière O, Renard-Penna R et al. Prostate cancer diagnosis: Multiparametric MR-targeted biopsy with cognitive and transrectal US-MR fusion guidance versus systematic biopsy—prospective multicenter study. *Radiology* 2013; 268: 461–9.

37. Rais-Bahrami S, Siddiqui MM, Turkbey B et al. Utility of multiparametric magnetic resonance imaging suspicion levels for detecting prostate cancer. *J Urol* 2013; 190: 1721–7.

38. Wegelin O, van Melick HHE, Hooft L et al. Comparing three different techniques for magnetic resonance imaging-targeted prostate biopsies: A systematic review of in-bore versus magnetic resonance imaging-transrectal ultrasound fusion versus cognitive registration. Is there a preferred technique? *Eur Urol* 2017; 71: 517–31.

18 Diagnosing Prostate Cancer Based on Deep Learning with a Stacked Nonnegativity Constraint Autoencoder

*Islam Reda, Ahmed Shalaby, Mohammed Elmogy,
Ahmed Aboulfotouh, Mohamed Abou El-Ghar,
Adel Elmagharaby, and Ayman El-Baz*

CONTENTS

INTRODUCTION

Prostate cancer is the second most frequently diagnosed malignancy in men, and is the sixth most common cause of cancer-related male death worldwide [1]. Prostate cancer is also the most frequently diagnosed malignancy after skin cancer, and is the second primary reason of cancer-related death in American men after lung cancer. More than 180,000 new cases were diagnosed and about 26,120 deaths among Americans were attributed to prostate cancer in 2016 [2]. By 2030, it is estimated that the number of diagnosed prostate cancer cases will increase globally to 1.7 million, and this type of cancer will be the reason for up to 0.5 million male deaths per year [3]. Fortunately, the introduction and spread of different screening tests, and improvements in treatment procedures have been resulted in declining mortality rates, especially, if prostate cancer is diagnosed in its early stages.

Although many researchers have investigated the different causes of prostate cancer, only an indistinct list of risk factors has been recognized. Those risk factors include, for example, family history, genetic factors, race, and body mass index (BMI) [4]. The likelihood of developing prostate cancer for a man with a first-degree relative who suffered from prostate cancer was found to be twice that of a man with no affected relatives [5]. Moreover, this likelihood increases as the number of affected relatives increases; for example, a man with two affected first-degree family members has more risk of developing prostate cancer than a man with one affected relative [6].

The incidence of prostate cancer is also affected by race and ethnicity. For example, the incidence rate of prostate cancer for African Americans is 1.6 higher than for European Americans. The mortality rate due to prostate cancer for African Americans is 2.4 higher than for European Americans. Additionally, African Americans have twice the risk of non-Hispanic whites for developing aggressive prostate cancer [7].

Genetic factors are also correlated with the incidence of prostate cancer. According to the research conducted by Agalliu et al. [8] on 979 cases of prostate cancer, protein-truncating mutations BRCA2 genes have been associated with high Gleason score prostate cancer. Giovannucci et al. [9], examined 10 possible risk factors for prostate cancer using multivariate Cox regression. They found a statistically significant correlation between the incidence of prostate cancer and the African American race and the positive family history. Regarding aggressive prostate cancer, a statistically significant positive correlation was found with recent smoking history, higher BMI, and family history; while a negative correlation was found with vigorous exercise.

Rodriguez et al. [10] investigated the association between BMI and weight change with the incidence of prostate cancer. They found that there was a positive correlation between BMI with the risk of aggressive prostate cancer and they also found weight loss decreases the risk of prostate cancer. Therefore, diet has been proposed as a noninvasive and cost-effective technique for decreasing the jeopardy of prostate cancer as well as its treatment [11].

CURRENT SCREENING TECHNIQUES

Currently, the well-established techniques used for diagnosing prostate cancer are digital rectal exam (DRE) [12], prostate-specific antigen (PSA) [13], and transrectal ultrasound (TRUS)-guided needle biopsy [14]. In the DRE screening, a physician manually examines the prostate through the rectum to find out any anomalies in its size or hardness. Through this screening, some peripheral zone tumors can be detected. However, tumors that are not large enough to be palpated, in addition to most central zone and transitional zone tumors, cannot be detected through the DRE. As a consequence, the experience and the skills of the physician have a significant effect on the accuracy of the DRE.

PSA screening is a blood-based screening that measures the PSA level in the blood. An increased value of PSA indicates a higher probability for prostate cancer. However, elevated levels of PSA may also signify other conditions, such as prostatitis or benign prostatic hyperplasia. If the blood PSA levels exceed four nanograms per millimeter (4 ng/mL), patients undergo further screening, such as biopsy, to confirm the presence or absence of the prostate cancer. Generally, the sensitivity and specificity of PSA screening are higher than the DRE screening [12].

In a TRUS-guided biopsy, small tissue specimens are acquired from the prostate gland to be examined by a pathologist. To analyze the sample, a number of scoring systems have been developed, including the Gleason [15], the modified Gleason and Mellinger [16] and the International Society of Urological Pathology (ISUP) modified Gleason system [17,18]. The ISUP modified Gleason system involves pathologists assigning a score between 1 and 5 based on the degree of each of the two tumor patterns, that is, architectural and neoplasm patterns. A score of 5 for the architectural pattern indicates that the tissue is the least differentiated typical of cancerous tissue; while a neoplasm score of 5 signifies that the tumor resembles the most prevalent neoplasm pattern. Summation of these two scores indicates the severity of the neoplasm where a score between 6 and 10 means the tumor is cancerous [19]. TRUS-guided biopsy is an accurate technique for detecting cancer and determining its aggressiveness.

However, it is an expensive, highly invasive, and painful procedure. Moreover, as a result of the random strategy for acquiring the tissue samples, there is a possibility of missing some aggressive tumors. Thus, it is imperative that an accurate noninvasive method with high selectivity and specificity be developed.

Some of the major drawbacks with current prostate cancer screening are over diagnosis and overtreatment [20]. For instance, in an investigation that extended for 11 years of follow-up to determine the role of PSA and TRUS-guided biopsy in decreasing the mortality rate caused by prostate cancer, Schröder et al. [21] found that to obviate one death from prostate cancer, more than 1000 men would need to be examined and 37 would need to be treated. These problems of overdiagnosis and overtreatment motivated research toward developing techniques to visualize such structures and their associated abnormalities.

IMAGING TECHNIQUES

The field of medical imaging technology has provided excellent tools for visualizing different body structures and their correlated anomalies. Particularly, ultrasound and magnetic resonance imaging (MRI) have been used extensively to visualize the prostate to determine the severity of the disorders. As a consequence of the drawbacks associated with the current screening techniques previously described, *in vivo* image-based computer-aided diagnosis (CAD) systems have been utilized to identify and localize the size and extent of prostate cancer. In the following paragraphs, the uses and the advantages of both ultrasound and MRI are briefly described.

Transrectal ultrasound (TRUS) is the most commonly used prostate imaging technique since it is used primarily in guiding needle biopsies and identifying the prostate volume [22,23]. The fundamental advantages of TRUS are its portability, low cost compared to other imaging modalities, its ability to generate real-time imaging data, and absence of any type of radiation. On the other hand, it has some drawbacks: it produces low-contrast images that contain speckles, has low signal-to-noise (SNR) ratio, and generates shadow artifacts [24]. Consequently, it is hard to detect tumors with a high level of accuracy and/or identify the stage of cancer using TRUS imaging techniques.

MRI offers the best soft-tissue contrast compared to other image modalities, such as computed tomography (CT) and TRUS. MRI does not involve radiation and is useful for determining the stage of cancer. However, MRI is not portable, is sensitive to noise and image artifacts, has difficulties to implement real-time imaging due to its relatively long and complex acquisition, and has a relatively high cost [22,25].

Several different MRI techniques have been extensively used in the prostate cancer CAD systems, such as T2-MRI, dynamic contrast-enhanced (DCE)-MRI, and diffusion-weighted (DW)-MRI. Even though T2-MRI provides good contrast between soft tissues, it lacks functional information. DCE-MRI is a technique that provides detailed information on the anatomy and function of different tissues. It has gained wide attention due to the increased spatial resolution, the ability to yield information about the hemodynamics (i.e., perfusion), microvascular permeability, and extracellular leakage space [26]. DCE-MRI has been extensively used in many clinical applications [27–34] in addition to the detection of prostate cancer [35–41]. In DCE-MRI, a series of MR images are taken prior to and after administering a contrast agent into the bloodstream. Contrast agents significantly enhance the contrast between the different tissue types and ease visualization of the anatomical structures which have alternating magnetic properties in their vicinity. The acquired signal intensity is proportional to the concentration of contrast agent in each voxel. Several types of MRI contrast agents can be used depending on the application, such as paramagnetic agents, superparamagnetic agents, extracellular fluid space (ECF) agents, and tissue (organ)-specific agents.

DW-MRI is another MRI modality, which unlike DCE-MRI, does not involve the use of contrast agents and has been attracting researchers recently. DW-MRI is based on the measurement of micro-movements of water molecules inside the body [37–39,42]. It can be acquired in a short time and, as mentioned before, does not depend on any contrast agents. It can be classified into three major categories: diffusion-weighted imaging (DWI) [43,44], diffusion tensor imaging (DTI) [44–46], and diffusion spectrum imaging (DSI) [47,48].

Developing CAD systems for detecting prostate cancer is an ongoing research area [49]. Those CAD systems vary in their accuracy, speed, and level of automation. There are some common processing steps shared by CAD systems used for diagnosing prostate cancer, such as segmentation, feature extraction, and classification. Several classification techniques can be utilized, including neural networks [50,51], decision trees [52], support vector machines (SVM) [53,54], linear discriminant analysis (LDA) [55], *k-nearest neighbor* (*k*-NN) [56], and others.

Several studies have targeted early detection of prostate cancer through building CAD systems that would aid physicians in its early diagnosis. For example, Firjani et al. [42] developed a DW-MRI-based CAD system for prostate cancer diagnosis. In their system, the prostate segmentation was based on a maximum a posteriori (MAP) estimation that utilizes shape, spatial, and appearance information. A *k*-NN-based classifier used three intensity features to classify the prostate as benign or malignant. The first multiparametric CAD system was proposed by Chan et al. [57] using T2-MRI, T2-mapping, and line scan diffusion imaging (LSDI). In their system, the region of interest (ROI) was manually segmented by a radiologist, then intensity-based and textural features were extracted from those regions, finally, a SVM-based classifier and a Fisher linear discriminant (FLD)-based classifier utilized the extracted features to detect potential peripheral zone (PZ) tumors. The results showed that the area under curve (AUC) was 0.761 ± 0.043 for the SVM-based classifier and 0.839 ± 0.064 for the FLD-based classifier. Litjens et al. [58] developed a multiparametric CAD system that used a combination of T_2-MRI, DCE-MRI, and DWI-MRI. Prostate segmentation was based on appearance and anatomy models. A SVM-based classifier used ADC and pharmacokinetic parameters to classify the segmented prostate as malignant or benign. The system performance was 74.7% and 83.4% sensitivity at 7 and 9 false positives per patient, respectively. A CAD system was developed by Niaf et al. [56] to detect prostate cancer in the peripheral zone. Four types of classifiers were trained and their performance was evaluated using a database of 30 sets of multiparametric MRI. The AUC was 0.89. A fully automated multiparametric CAD system for detecting prostate cancer was presented by Vos et al. [59]. The prostate segmentation was performed using the technique developed by Litjens et al. [58]. A combination of features (e.g., texture-based, ADC maps) was used by a LDA classifier to determine malignant and benign regions; 74% of all tumors at a FP level of 5 per patient were detected.

The main focus of this chapter is on developing a CAD system for diagnosing prostate cancer from DW-MRI using a deep learning technique. The chapter is organized as follows: "Method" describes the proposed framework focusing on the stage of extracting discriminatory features (subsection "Extracting Discriminatory Features") and the classification stage (subsection "Stacked Nonnegatively Constrained Autoencoders (SNCAE)-based Classification"). Then, "Experimental Results" reports the experimental results. Finally, "Conclusions and Future Trends" provides conclusions and future trends.

METHOD

The proposed CAD system summarized in Figure 18.1 sequentially performs three steps. First, the prostate is segmented using our previously developed geometric deformable model (level-sets) as in McClure et al. [60]. The precise segmentation of the prostate is an essential step in diagnosing

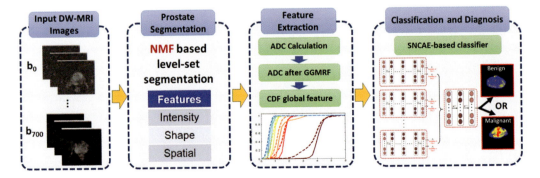

FIGURE 18.1 Schematic overview of a DW-MRI-based CAD system for diagnosing prostate cancer.

prostate cancer. This accurate segmentation can be achieved if it is done manually by an experienced radiologist. Nevertheless, manual segmentation is time-consuming, especially in the case of 3D volumes of MRI data, and also suffers from intra- and inter-observer variation. Therefore, an automatic segmentation model is used in the proposed CAD system. This model is guided by a stochastic speed function that is derived using nonnegative matrix factorization (NMF). The NMF attributes are calculated using information from the MRI intensity, a probabilistic shape model, and the spatial interactions between prostate voxels. The proposed approach reaches 86.89% overall Dice similarity coefficient and an average Hausdorff distance of 5.72 mm, indicating high segmentation accuracy. Details of this approach and comparisons with other segmentation approaches can be found in [60]. Afterward, global features describing the water diffusion inside the prostate tissue are extracted based on apparent diffusion coefficient cumulative distribution functions (ADC-CDFs). Finally, a two-stage structure of stacked nonnegativity constraint autoencoder (SNCAE) is trained to classify the prostate tumor as benign or malignant based on the cumulative distribution functions (CDFs) constructed in the previous step. The latter two steps of the proposed CAD system are discussed in the following sections.

EXTRACTING DISCRIMINATORY FEATURES

After the prostate is segmented, discriminatory features are estimated from the segmented DW-MRI data, which are used to distinguish between benign and malignant cases. In the proposed CAD system, ADCs were used as discriminatory features to assess the tumor status, where the malignant tissues show a lower ADC at different b-values compared with benign and normal tissue due to the replacement of normal tissue [61]. According to a published study [62], the DW-MRI features result in superior accuracy in diagnosing prostate cancer that is comparable to a combination of features from T_2-weighted MRI, DW-MRI, and DCE-MRI. The voxelwise ADC is computed according to Equation 18.1 to generate the ADC map at each b-value.

$$\text{ADC}(x,y,z) = \frac{\ln \dfrac{S_0(x,y,z)}{S_1(x,y,z)}}{b_1 - b_0} \tag{18.1}$$

where S_0 and S_1 are the signal intensity acquired at the b_0 and b_1 b-values, respectively. Then, all ADC maps at a certain b-value for all subjects are normalized with respect to the maximum value of all of these maps to make all calculated ADC maps in the same range (between 0 and 1) in order to use a unique color coding for all of them. The calculated ADC values are refined using a generalized Gauss-Markov random field (GGMRF) image model with a 26-voxel neighborhood to remove any data inconsistency and preserve continuity. Continuity of the constructed 3D volume is amplified by using their MAP estimates. The CDFs of the normalized ADCs of each subject are constructed. These CDFs are considered as global features distinguishing between benign and malignant cases. Instead of using the whole ADC volume, the resultant CDFs are used to train an SNCAE classifier using the deep learning approach. In our system, the CDFs for a training set of the DW-MR images are used for deep learning of a classifier with an SNCAE.

Experimental validation was performed using 53 (27 benign and 26 malignant) cases. The average training CDFs for the benign and malignant cases at six b-values, 100, 200, 300, 400, 500, and 700 s/mm^2, are shown in Figure 18.2. Figure 18.2 shows the maximum difference and best separation between these subjects are for the b-value of 700 s/mm^2. Therefore, the most accurate classification can be expected with the CDF at this b-value. The section titled "Diagnostic Results of the Single SNCAE Structure" will address this issue in more detail and present additional experiments.

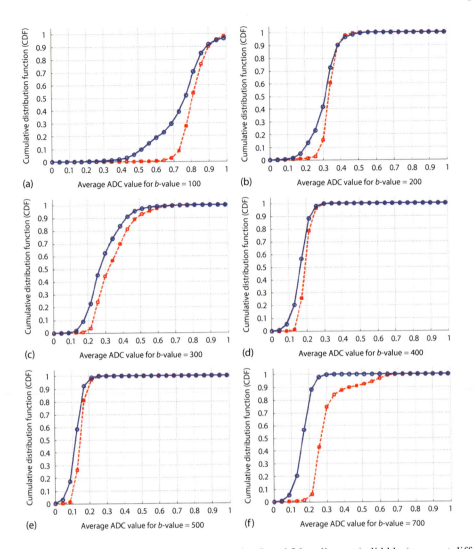

FIGURE 18.2 Average CDF of the 27 benign (dotted red) and 26 malignant (solid blue) cases at different *b*-values: 100 (a); 200 (b); 300 (c); 400 (d); 500 (e); and 700 (f) s/mm².

It is worth noting that conventional classification methods directly employing the voxelwise ADCs of the entire prostate volume as discriminative features encounter at least two serious difficulties. Various input data sizes require unification by either data truncation for large prostate volumes, or zero padding for small ones. Both ways may decrease the accuracy of the classification. Techniques like bag-of-visual-words (BoVW) can be employed to overcome the difficulty of various input data sizes but the data has to be aligned and the accuracy of the BoVW technique is a function of the data resolution and the size of the bag. In addition, large ADC data volumes lead to considerable time expenditures for training and classification. In contrast, our SNCAE classifier exploits only the 100-component CDFs to describe the entire 3D ADC maps estimated at each *b*-value. This fixed data size helps overcome the above challenges and notably expedites the classification.

STACKED NONNEGATIVELY CONSTRAINED AUTOENCODERS (SNCAE)-BASED CLASSIFICATION

For the classification of prostates, our CAD system utilizes a deep neural network with a stack of autoencoders before the final softmax-regression-based classification layer that generalizes logistic regression to more than two categories. Two different structures of SNCAE were used to classify prostates into malignant or benign:

- *The first structure uses a single SNCAE*: Different combinations of *b*-values were examined to select the optimum *b*-value or values for the most accurate classification. SNCAE compresses the 100-component CDFs at some *b*-value inputted to it to capture the most noticeable variations and is built by linking the final hidden layer with a softmax classifier. SNCAE is first pre-trained one layer at a time using greedy unsupervised pre-training [63]. Then a supervised fine-tuning of all SNCAE layers is performed using error backpropagation to minimize the total loss for the given training data.
- *The second structure uses a two-phase structure of SNCAE*: In the first phase, seven SNCAE-based classifiers, one classifier for each of the seven *b*-values (100–700 s/mm²), are used to determine an initial classification probability of the prostate case. In the second phase, the resulting initial classification probabilities of the seven classifiers are then concatenated to form an initial classification probability vector that is fed into another SNCAE-based classifier to determine the final classification of the prostate case.

In the subsequent paragraphs, autoencoder (AE), the basic unsupervised feature learning algorithm is first introduced. Then, nonnegatively constrained autoencoders (NCAE), which imposes nonnegativity and sparsity constraints for learning robust feature representations is explained. Finally, SNCAE, the deep network architecture that is constructed by layer-wise stacking of multiple NCSAE is explained.

AE, the basic learning component of SNCAE, consists of three layers: input layer, hidden layer, and output layer. Each layer consists of a number of nodes. A node in a given layer is fully connected to all the nodes in the successive layer. The objective of AE is to learn a precise compressed representation of input data that could be used at a later stage to reconstruct the input data. In general, AE has two steps: encoding and decoding. The encoding layers hierarchically decrease the dimension of their inputs into codes to capture the most essential representations, while the decoding layers try to restore the original input from the codes in the hidden layers. Each AE compresses its input data to capture the most prominent variations and is built separately by greedy unsupervised pre-training [63]. The softmax output layer facilitates the subsequent supervised backpropagation-based fine-tuning of the entire classifier by minimizing the total loss (negative log-likelihood) for given training labeled data. Using the AEs with a nonnegativity constraint (NCAE) [64] yields both more reasonable data codes (features) during its unsupervised pre-training and better classification performance after the supervised refinement.

Let $\mathbf{W} = \{\mathbf{W}_j^e, \mathbf{W}_i^d : j = 1,\ldots,s; i = 1,\ldots n\}$ denote a set of column vectors of weights for encoding (e) and decoding (d) layers of a single AE in Figure 18.3a. Let T denote vector transposition. The AE converts an *n*-dimensional column vector $\mathbf{u} = [u_1, ..., u_n]^T$ of input signals into an *s*-dimensional column vector $\mathbf{h} = [h_1, ..., h_s]^T$ of hidden codes (features or activations), such that $s \ll n$, by uniform nonlinear transformation of *s* weighted linear combinations of signals:

$$h_j = \sigma\left(\mathbf{W}_{e:j}^T \mathbf{u}\right) \equiv \sigma\left(\sum_{i=1}^{n} w_{e:j:i} u_i\right)$$

where $\sigma(...)$ is a certain sigmoid, that is, a differentiable monotone scalar function with values in the range [0, 1]. Then, AE tries to reconstruct an approximation of the original input from the hidden feature representation. To learn a compressed representation, which helps discover the latent

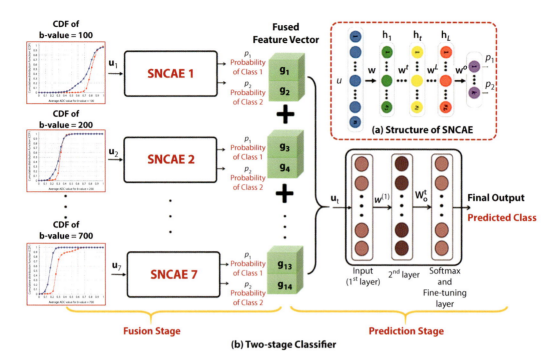

FIGURE 18.3   (a,b) Schematic overview of a DW-MRI-based CAD system for diagnosing prostate cancer.

structure of data in a high-dimensional space, and to avoid trivial solution of the minimization of the loss function of Equation 18.2 such as identity transformation, it is necessary that the hidden layer dimension be less than the input dimension, that is, $s \ll n$. Unsupervised pre-training of the AE minimizes total deviations between each given training input vector $\mathbf{u}_k$; $k = 1, ..., K$, and the same-dimensional vector, $\hat{\mathbf{u}}_{\mathbf{W}:k}$ reconstructed from its code, or activation vector, $\mathbf{h}_k$. The total reconstruction error of applying such AE to compress and decompress the K training input vectors integrates the ℓ_2-norms of the deviations:

$$J_{AE}(\mathbf{W}) = \frac{1}{2K} \sum_{k=1}^{K} \left\| \hat{\mathbf{u}}_{\mathbf{W}:k} - \mathbf{u}_k^2 \right\| \tag{18.2}$$

Here, the average sum-of-squared-differences represents the reconstruction error. The minimization of that reconstruction error indicates that the learned features preserve a significant amount of information about the input, which is a required criterion of precise representation of the original input. Inspired by nonnegative matrix factorization and by the proofs that neural activity in the human brain is sparse. NCSAE imposes two additional constraints on the basic AE, namely, nonnegativity constraint and sparsity constraint. The nonnegativity constraint enforces the autoencoder to learn additive part-based representation of the input data, while the sparsity constraint enforces the average activation of each hidden unit over the entire training dataset to be infinitesimal to improve the probability of linear separability. As suggested in Hosseini-Asl et al. [64], imposing the nonnegativity constraint on AE results in more precise data codes during the greedy unsupervised pre-training and improved classification accuracy after the supervised refinement. To reduce the number of negative weights and enforce sparsity of the NCAE, the reconstruction error of Equation 18.2 is appended, respectively, with quadratic negative weight penalties, $f(w_i) = (\min\{0, w_i\})^2$; $i = 1, ..., n$, and Kullback-Leibler (KL) divergence, $J_{KL}(\mathbf{h_{w_e}}; \gamma)$, of activations, $\mathbf{hw_e}$, obtained with the encoding weights $\mathbf{W}_e$ for the training data, from a fixed small positive average value, γ, near 0:

$$J_{NCAE}(\mathbf{W}) = J_{AE}(\mathbf{W}) + \alpha \sum_{j=1}^{s} \sum_{i=1}^{n} f\left(w_{j:i}\right) + \beta J_{KL}\left(\mathbf{h_{w_e}}; \gamma\right) \tag{18.3}$$

Here, the factors $\alpha \geq 0$ and $\beta \geq 0$ specify relative contributions of the nonnegativity and sparsity constraints to the overall loss, $J_{NCAE}(\mathbf{W})$, and

$$J_{KL}(\mathbf{h_{w_e}}, \gamma) = \sum_{j=1}^{s} h_{w_e:j} \log\left(\frac{h_{w_e:j}}{\gamma}\right) + \left(1 - h_{w_e:j}\right) \log\left(\frac{1 - h_{w_e:j}}{1 - \gamma}\right) \tag{18.4}$$

Recent studies have shown that a deep architecture is capable of learning complex and highly nonlinear features from data. In order to learn high-level features from data, NCSAE is used as a building block to construct a multilayer architecture of NCSAEs. In this architecture, the output vector from a low-level NCSAE is used as input to a high-level NCSAE and the output of the final NCSAE is used as input to a softmax-regression classifier. A good technique to train such deep architectures that does not have the limitations associated with full supervised training is to first pre-train the network one layer at a time using the unsupervised greedy algorithm.

The classifier is built by stacking the NCAE layers with an output softmax layer, as shown in Figure 18.3a. Each NCAE is pre-trained separately in the unsupervised mode, by using the activation vector of a lower layer as the input to the upper layer. In our case, the initial input data consisted of the 100-component CDFs, each of size 100. The bottom NCAE compresses the input vector to $s_1 = 50$ first-level activators, compressed by the next NCAE to $s_2 = 5$ second-level activators, which are reduced in turn by the output softmax layer to $s° = 2$ values.

Separate pre-training of the first and second layers by minimizing the loss of Equation 18.3 reduces the total reconstruction error, as well as increases sparsity of the extracted activations and numbers of the nonnegative weights. The activations of the second NCAE layer, $\mathbf{h}^{[2]} = \sigma(\mathbf{W}_{[2]}^{e}{}^{T}\mathbf{h}^{[1]})$, are inputs of the softmax classification layer, as sketched in Figure 18.3a to compute a plausibility of a decision in favor of each particular output class, $c = 1, 2$:

$$p\left(c; \mathbf{W}_{o:c}\right) = \frac{\exp\left(\mathbf{W}_{o:c}^{T}\mathbf{h}^{[2]}\right)}{\exp\left(\mathbf{W}_{o:1}^{T}\mathbf{h}^{[2]}\right) + \exp\left(\mathbf{W}_{o:2}^{T}\mathbf{h}^{[2]}\right)}; c = 1,2; \sum_{c=1}^{2} p\left(c; \mathbf{W}_{o:c}; \mathbf{h}^{[2]}\right) = 1$$

Its separate pre-training minimizes the total negative log-likelihood $J_o(\mathbf{W}_o)$ of the known training classes, appended with the negative weight penalties:

$$J_o\left(\mathbf{W}^o\right) = -\frac{1}{K} \sum_{k=1}^{K} \log p\left(c_k; \mathbf{W}_{o:c}\right) + \vartheta \sum_{c=1}^{2} \sum_{j=1}^{s_2} w_{o:c:j} \tag{18.5}$$

Finally, the entire stacked NCAE classifier (SNCAE) is fine-tuned on the labeled training data by the conventional error backpropagation through the network and penalizing only the negative weights of the softmax layer. In our experiments, $a = 0.03$, $b = 3$, and $\gamma = 0.1$.

In the first phase of the two-phase structure of SNCAE, the initial input data to each of the seven SNCAE is composed of the 100-component CDFs at some b-value (100–700 s/mm^2). The first NCSAE reduces the input vector dimension to $s_1 = 50$ first-level features (codes), which are reduced by the subsequent NCAE to $s_2 = 5$ second-level features (codes), which are finally decreased by the softmax layer to the goal $s° = 2$ values. In the second stage, each SNCAE's output probability is extracted and fused by concatenation, resulting in a vector of fused probability $\mathbf{u}_t = [\mathbf{g}_1, ..., \mathbf{g}_{14}]$ as shown in Figure 18.3b. To enhance the classification accuracy, this vector ($\mathbf{u}_t$) is fed into a new SNCAE to estimate the final classification as a class probability using the following equation:

$$p_t\left(c; \mathbf{W}_{o;c}^t\right) = \frac{\exp\left(\mathbf{W}_{o;c}^t{}^{\mathrm{T}} g_t\right)}{\sum_{c=1}^{C} \exp\left(\mathbf{W}_{o;c}^t{}^{\mathrm{T}} g_t\right)}; \quad c = 1, 2 \tag{18.6}$$

EXPERIMENTAL RESULTS

Experiments were conducted on 53 DW-MRI data sets (27 benign and 26 malignant) obtained using a body coil Signa Horizon GE scanner in axial plane with the following parameters: magnetic field strength: 1.5 T; TE: 84.6 ms; TR: 8000 ms; bandwidth: 142.86 kHz; FOV: 34 cm; slice thickness: 3 mm; inter-slice gap: 0 mm; acquisition sequence: conventional EPI; diffusion weighting directions: mono direction; the used range of b-values is from 0 to 700 s/mm^2. On average, 26 slices were obtained in 120 s to cover the prostate in each patient with voxel size of $1.25 \times 1.25 \times 3.00$ mm^3. The ground truths are performed on a slice-by-slice basis and obtained by manual segmentation using Slicer© (www.slicer.org). All annotations were verified by an expert. All the subjects were diagnosed using a biopsy and the Gleason scores for the malignant cases ranged from 6 to 8. The cases were evaluated as a whole and not per tumor. The experimental results of both the single SNCAE structure and the two-phase structure of SNCAE are explained in the sections titled "Diagnostic Results of the Single SNCAE Structure" and "Diagnostic Results of the Two-Phase Structure of SNCAE," respectively.

DIAGNOSTIC RESULTS OF THE SINGLE SNCAE STRUCTURE

To learn the statistical characteristics of both benign and malignant subjects, we trained our classifier by 53 DW-MRI datasets (27 benign and 26 malignant). The features involved for classification are the CDF of the normalized ADC maps for 7 different b-values of the segmented prostate tissue, as shown in Figure 18.2. To assess the accuracy of our system, we performed a leave-one-out cross-validation test with the whole 53 datasets. We tried many scenarios to choose the optimum b-value (or values) for the best classification results. After many trials and combinations, we reached the following result: among all available b-values, the b-value = 700 s/mm^2 is optimal. It outperforms all other available b-values. Moreover, it is better than using all b-values combined. In other words, training our classifier using only b-value = 700 s/mm^2 gives us a better classification result than taking the majority voting of all 7 b-values results. The overall diagnostic accuracy for different b-values are summarized in Figure 18.4. It is clear that b-value = 700 s/mm^2 has the highest accuracy results. And this is coincided with what we get in Figure 18.2f.

To highlight the merit of using SNCAE-based classifier, a comparison between our classifier and four other ready-to-use classifiers (K*, k-NN, random forest, and random tree classifiers implemented in Weka toolbox) [65] is summarized in Table 18.1. As demonstrated in this table and using b-value = 700 s/mm^2 only, our classifier achieves an overall accuracy of 100% for all testing datasets. Also, the proposed framework outperforms the other alternatives and holds promise of the proposed CAD system as a reliable noninvasive diagnostic tool.

Additionally, we plot the receiver operating characteristics (ROC) curve for the developed CAD system and other classifiers to test the performance of our diagnostic tool. The results are depicted in Figure 18.5.

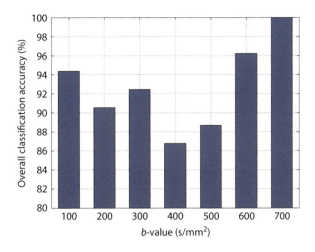

FIGURE 18.4   Classification accuracy of SNCAE classifier using DWI datasets with different *b*-values.

TABLE 18.1

Classification Accuracy, Sensitivity, and Specificity for Our CAD System and Different Classifiers from Weka Tool

Classifier	Accuracy	Sensitivity	Specificity
SNCAE (proposed)	100%	100%	100%
K* (K-star)	94.3%	94.3%	94.4%
k-NN-classifier (IBK)	88.67%	88.6%	88.7%
Random forest	86.7%	86.8%	86.8%
Random tree	84.9%	85.1%	84.9%

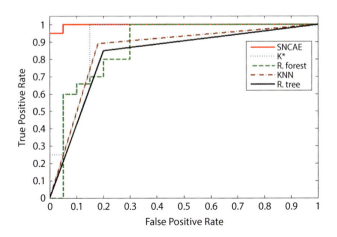

FIGURE 18.5   The ROC curve for different classifiers.

As shown in this figure, the area under the ROC curve of the proposed classifier is the maximum and approaches 1 in comparison to other alternative.

DIAGNOSTIC RESULTS OF THE TWO-PHASE STRUCTURE OF SNCAE

To learn the statistical characteristics of both benign and malignant subjects, we trained 7 different SNCAE, one for each b-value, by 53 DW-MRI datasets (27 benign and 26 malignant). All training was done inside leave-one-subject-out cross-validation framework. The features involved for classification are the CDF of the normalized ADC maps for 7 different b-values of the segmented prostate tissue. To assess the accuracy of our system, we perform a leave-one-subject-out cross-validation test for each AE with the whole 53 datasets. The overall diagnostic accuracy for different b-values are summarized in Table 18.2.

In the last stage of the classification, we concatenated the output probabilities from the 7 AEs. This vector of the fused probabilities is fed into the prediction stage SNCAE. Our classifier achieved an overall accuracy of 98.11% for all testing data sets, which is higher than all reported accuracies in Table 18.2.

To highlight the merit of using the proposed system, a comparison between our classifier and four other ready-to-use classifiers (K*, K-nearest neighbor, random forest, and random tree classifiers implemented in Weka toolbox) [65] is summarized in Table 18.3. The input features for each of those four classifiers are the 100-component CDFs. As demonstrated in Table 18.3, the proposed framework outperforms the other alternatives. The corresponding AUC of the receiver operating characteristics of those classifiers are shown in Figure 18.6. The AUC of the proposed classifier approaches 98.7%.

TABLE 18.2
Classification Accuracy of Our SNCAE Classifier at Different b-Values

Autoencoder	Correct Instance	Accuracy
SNCAE 1 (b-value = 100)	50 out of 53	94.34%
SNCAE 2 (b-value = 200)	48 out of 53	90.57%
SNCAE 3 (b-value = 300)	49 out of 53	92.45%
SNCAE 4 (b-value = 400)	47 out of 53	88.68%
SNCAE 5 (b-value = 500)	48 out of 53	90.57%
SNCAE 6 (b-value = 600)	49 out of 53	92.45%
SNCAE 7 (b-value = 700)	51 out of 53	96.23%

TABLE 18.3
Classification Accuracy, Sensitivity, Specificity, and AUC of Our SNCAE Classifier and Four Ready-to-Use Weka Classifiers

Classifier	Accuracy	Sensitivity	Specificity	AUC
SNCAE (proposed)	98.11%	96.15%	100%	98.7%
K* (K-star)	94.32%	94.33%	94.42%	92.6%
k-NN-classifier (IBK)	88.67%	88.63%	88.71%	88.7%
Random forest	88.64%	88.72%	88.60%	95.2%
Random tree	84.91%	85.13%	84.93%	85.1%

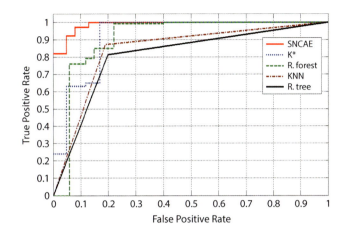

FIGURE 18.6 ROC curves for our SNCAE classifier and four ready-to-use Weka classifiers.

CONCLUSIONS AND FUTURE TRENDS

In this chapter, we presented an image-based CAD system for early diagnosis of prostate cancer from DW-MRI. The framework includes NMF-based segmentation, diffusion parameters estimation (CDFs of the ADC), and SNCAE-based classification. The proposed CAD system was tested on DW-MRI datasets from 53 subjects acquired at 7 different b-values (100–700 s/mm^2). Applications of the proposed approach yielded promising results that could, in the near future, replace the use of current technologies to diagnose prostate cancer.

This work could also be applied to various other applications in medical imaging, such as the kidney, the heart, the lung, and the retina.

One application is renal transplant functional assessment. Chronic kidney disease (CKD) affects about 26 million people in United States with 17,000 transplants being performed each year. In renal transplant patients, acute rejection is the leading cause of renal dysfunction. Given the limited number of donors, routine clinical post-transplantation evaluation is of immense importance to help clinicians initiate timely interventions with appropriate treatment and thus prevent graft loss. Accurate assessment of renal transplant function is critically important for graft survival. Although transplantation can improve a patient's well-being, there is a potential post-transplantation risk of kidney dysfunction that, if not treated in a timely manner, can lead to the loss of the entire graft, and even patient death. Thus, accurate assessment of renal transplant function is crucial for the identification of proper treatment. In recent years, an increased area of research has been dedicated to developing noninvasive image-based CAD systems for the assessment of renal transplant function utilizing different image modalities (e.g., ultrasound, CT, MRI, etc.). In particular, dynamic and diffusion MRI-based systems have been clinically used to assess transplanted kidneys with the advantage of providing information on each kidney separately. A variety of studies can be consulted for more details about renal transplant functional assessment [66–91].

The heart is also an important application for this work. The clinical assessment of myocardial perfusion plays a major role in the diagnosis, management, and prognosis of ischemic heart disease patients. Thus, there have been ongoing efforts to develop automated systems for accurate analysis of myocardial perfusion using first-pass images [92–108].

Another application for this work could be the detection of retinal abnormalities. The majority of ophthalmologists depend on visual interpretation for the identification of diseases types. However, inaccurate diagnosis will affect the treatment procedure which may lead to fatal results. Hence, there is a crucial need for computer automated diagnosis systems that yield highly accurate results. Optical coherence tomography (OCT) has become a powerful modality for noninvasive diagnosis of various retinal abnormalities such as glaucoma, diabetic macular edema, and macular degeneration. The problem with diabetic retinopathy (DR) is that the patient is not aware of the disease until the changes in the retina have progressed to a level at which treatment tends to be less effective. Therefore, automated early detection could limit the severity of the disease and assist ophthalmologists in investigating and treating it more efficiently [109,110].

Abnormalities of the lung could be another promising area of research and a related application for this work. Radiation-induced lung injury is the main side effect of radiation therapy for lung cancer patients. Although higher radiation doses increase the radiation therapy effectiveness for tumor control, this can lead to lung injury as a greater quantity of normal lung tissues is included in the treated area. Almost a third of patients who undergo radiation therapy develop lung injury following radiation treatment. The severity of radiation-induced lung injury ranges from ground-glass opacities and consolidation at the early phase to fibrosis and traction bronchiectasis in the late phase. Early detection of lung injury will thus help to improve treatment management [111–151].

This work can also be applied to other brain abnormalities, such as dyslexia and autism. Dyslexia is one of the most complicated developmental brain disorders that affect children's learning abilities. Dyslexia leads to the failure to develop age-appropriate reading skills in spite of a normal intelligence level and adequate reading instructions. Neuropathological studies have revealed an abnormal anatomy of some structures, such as the corpus callosum, in dyslexic brains. There has been a lot of work in the literature that aims at developing CAD systems for diagnosing this disorder, along with other brain disorders [152–174].

This work could also be applied for the extraction of blood vessels from phase contrast (PC) magnetic resonance angiography (MRA). Accurate cerebrovascular segmentation using noninvasive MRA is crucial for the early diagnosis and timely treatment of intracranial vascular diseases [157,158,175,176].

REFERENCES

1. Ferlay, J., Shin, H.R., Bray, F., Forman, D., Mathers, C., Parkin, D.M.: Estimates of worldwide burden of cancer in 2008: Globocan 2008. *International Journal of Cancer* **127**(12) (2010) 2893–2917.
2. Siegel, R.L., Miller, K.D., Jemal, A.: Cancer statistics, 2016. *CA: A Cancer Journal for Clinicians* **66**(1) (2016) 7–30.
3. Du, W., Liu, Y.P., Wang, S., Peng, Y., Oto, A.: Features extraction of prostate with graph spectral method for prostate cancer detection. In: *Software Engineering, Artificial Intelligence, Networking and Parallel/Distributed Computing (SNPD), 2016 17th IEEE/ACIS International Conference on*, IEEE (2016) pp. 663–668.
4. Cokkinides, V., Albano, J., Samuels, A., Ward, M., Thum, J.: American Cancer Society: Cancer facts and figures 2016. Atlanta, GA: American Cancer Society (2016).
5. Kalish, L.A., McDougal, W.S., McKinlay, J.B.: Family history and the risk of prostate cancer. *Urology* **56**(5) (2000) 803–806.
6. Steinberg, G.D., Carter, B.S., Beaty, T.H., Childs, B., Walsh, P.C.: Family history and the risk of prostate cancer. *The Prostate* **17**(4) (1990) 337–347.
7. Hoffman, R.M., Gilliland, F.D., Eley, J.W., Harlan, L.C., Stephenson, R.A., Stanford, J.L., Albertson, P.C., Hamilton, A.S., Hunt, W.C., Potosky, A.L.: Racial and ethnic differences in advanced-stage prostate cancer: the prostate cancer outcomes study. *Journal of the National Cancer Institute* **93**(5) (2001) 388–395.
8. Agalliu, I., Gern, R., Leanza, S., Burk, R.D.: Associations of high-grade prostate cancer with BRCA1 and BRCA2 founder mutations. *Clinical Cancer Research* **15**(3) (2009) 1112–1120.
9. Giovannucci, E., Liu, Y., Platz, E.A., Stampfer, M.J., Willett, W.C.: Risk factors for prostate cancer incidence and progression in the health professionals follow-up study. *International Journal of cancer* **121**(7) (2007) 1571–1578.

10. Rodriguez, C., Freedland, S.J., Deka, A., Jacobs, E.J., McCullough, M.L., Patel, A.V., Thun, M.J., Calle, E.E.: Body mass index, weight change, and risk of prostate cancer in the cancer prevention study ii nutrition cohort. *Cancer Epidemiology and Prevention Biomarkers* **16**(1) (2007) 63–69.

11. Ma, R.L., Chapman, K.: A systematic review of the effect of diet in prostate cancer prevention and treatment. *Journal of Human Nutrition and Dietetics* **22**(3) (2009) 187–199.

12. Mistry, K., Cable, G.: Meta-analysis of prostate-specific antigen and digital rectal examination as screening tests for prostate carcinoma. *The Journal of the American Board of Family Practice* **16**(2) (2003) 95–101.

13. Dijkstra, S., Mulders, P., Schalken, J.: Clinical use of novel urine and blood based prostate cancer biomarkers: a review. *Clinical Biochemistry* **47**(10) (2014) 889–896.

14. Davis, M., Sofer, M., Kim, S.S., Soloway, M.S.: The procedure of transrectal ultrasound guided biopsy of the prostate: a survey of patient preparation and biopsy technique. *The Journal of Urology* **167**(2) (2002) 566–570.

15. Gleason, D.F.: Classification of prostatic carcinomas. *Cancer Chemotherapy Reports.* Part 1 **50**(3) (1966) 125–128.

16. Gleason, D.F., Mellinger, G.T.: Prediction of prognosis for prostatic adenocarcinoma by combined histological grading and clinical staging. *The Journal of Urology* **111**(1) (1974) 58–64.

17. Montironi, R., Cheng, L., Lopez-Beltran, A., Scarpelli, M., Mazzucchelli, R., Mikuz, G., Kirkali, Z., Montorsi, F.: Original Gleason system versus 2005 ISUP modified Gleason system: the importance of indicating which system is used in the patient's pathology and clinical reports. *European Urology* **58**(3) (2010) 369–373.

18. Epstein, J.I., Allsbrook Jr, W.C., Amin, M.B., Egevad, L.L., Committee, I.G. et al.: The 2005 international society of urological pathology (ISUP) consensus conference on Gleason grading of prostatic carcinoma. *The American Journal of Surgical Pathology* **29**(9) (2005) 1228–1242.

19. DeMarzo, A.M., Nelson, W.G., Isaacs, W.B., Epstein, J.I.: Pathological and molecular aspects of prostate cancer. *The Lancet* **361**(9361) (2003) 955–964.

20. Schröder, F.H., Hugosson, J., Roobol, M.J., Tammela, T.L., Ciatto, S., Nelen, V., Kwiatkowski, M., Lujan, M., Lilja, H., Zappa, M. et al.: Screening and prostate-cancer mortality in a randomized european study. *New England Journal of Medicine* **360**(13) (2009) 1320–1328.

21. Schröder, F.H., Hugosson, J., Roobol, M.J., Tammela, T.L., Ciatto, S., Nelen, V., Kwiatkowski, M., Lujan, M., Lilja, H., Zappa, M. et al.: Prostate-cancer mortality at 11 years of follow-up. *New England Journal of Medicine* **366**(11) (2012) 981–990.

22. Hricak, H., Choyke, P.L., Eberhardt, S.C., Leibel, S.A., Scardino, P.T.: Imaging prostate cancer: A multidisciplinary perspective 1. *Radiology* **243**(1) (2007) 28–53.

23. Fichtinger, G., Krieger, A., Susil, R.C., Tanacs, A., Whitcomb, L.L., Atalar, E.: Transrectal prostate biopsy inside closed mri scanner with remote actuation, under real-time image guidance. In: *Medical Image Computing and Computer-Assisted InterventionMICCAI 2002.* Springer (2002) 91–98.

24. Applewhite, J.C., Matlaga, B., McCullough, D., Hall, M.: Transrectal ultrasound and biopsy in the early diagnosis of prostate cancer. *Cancer Control: Journal of the Moffitt Cancer Center* **8**(2) (2000) 141–150.

25. Fuchsjäger, M., Shukla-Dave, A., Akin, O., Barentsz, J., Hricak, H.: Prostate cancer imaging. *Acta Radiologica* **49**(1) (2008) 107–120.

26. Collins, D.J., Padhani, A.R.: Dynamic magnetic resonance imaging of tumor perfusion. *Engineering in Medicine and Biology Magazine, IEEE* **23**(5) (2004) 65–83.

27. Khalifa, F., Beache, G.M., Gimelfarb, G., El-Baz, A.: A novel cad system for analyzing cardiac firstpass MR images. In: *Pattern Recognition (ICPR), 2012 21st International Conference on, IEEE* (2012) 77–80.

28. El-Baz, A., Farag, A., Fahmi, R., Yuksela, S., El-Ghar, M., Eldiasty, T. et al.: Image analysis of renal DCE MRI for the detection of acute renal rejection. In: *Pattern Recognition, 2006. ICPR 2006. 18th International Conference on. Volume 3, IEEE* (2006) 822–825.

29. Farag, A., El-Baz, A., Yuksel, S.E., El-Ghar, M., Eldiasty, T. et al.: A framework for the detection of acute renal rejection with dynamic contrast enhanced magnetic resonance imaging. In: *Biomedical Imaging: Nano to Macro, 2006. 3rd IEEE International Symposium on, IEEE* (2006) 418–421.

30. El-Baz, A., Farag, A.A., Yuksel, S.E., El-Ghar, M.E., Eldiasty, T.A., Ghoneim, M.A.: Application of deformable models for the detection of acute renal rejection. In: *Deformable Models.* Springer (2007) 293–333.

31. El-Baz, A., Gimelfarb, G., El-Ghar, M.A.: New motion correction models for automatic identification of renal transplant rejection. In: *Medical Image Computing and Computer-Assisted Intervention–MICCAI 2007.* Springer (2007) 235–243.

32. El-Baz, A., Gimelfarb, G., El-Ghar, M. et al.: A novel image analysis approach for accurate identification of acute renal rejection. In: *Image Processing, 2008. ICIP 2008. 15th IEEE International Conference on, IEEE* (2008) 1812–1815.

33. El-Baz, A., Farb, G.G., El-Ghar, M. et al.: Image analysis approach for identification of renal transplant rejection. In: *Pattern Recognition, 2008. ICPR 2008. 19th International Conference on, IEEE* (2008) 1–4.

34. Khalifa, F., El-Baz, A., Gimelfarb, G., El-Ghar, M.A.: Non-invasive image-based approach for early detection of acute renal rejection. In: *Medical Image Computing and Computer-Assisted Intervention–MICCAI 2010.* Springer (2010) 10–18.

35. Firjani, A., Khalifa, F., Elnakib, A., Gimelfarb, G., El-Ghar, M.A., Elmaghraby, A., El-Baz, A.: A novel image-based approach for early detection of prostate cancer using DCE-MRI. In: *Computational Intelligence in Biomedical Imaging.* Springer (2014) 55–82.

36. Reda, I., Shalaby, A., Elmogy, M., Elfotouh, A.A., Khalifa, F., El-Ghar, M.A., Hosseini-Asl, E., Gimelfarb, G., Werghi, N., El-Baz, A.: A comprehensive non-invasive framework for diagnosing prostate cancer. *Computers in Biology and Medicine* **81** (2017) 148–158.

37. Reda, I., Shalaby, A., Elmogy, M., Aboulfotouh, A., Khalifa, F., El-Ghar, M.A., Gimelfarb, G., El-Baz, A.: Image-based computer-aided diagnostic system for early diagnosis of prostate cancer. In: *International Conference on Medical Image Computing and Computer-Assisted Intervention,* Springer (2016) 610–618.

38. Reda, I., Shalaby, A., El-Ghar, M.A., Khalifa, F., Elmogy, M., Aboulfotouh, A., Hosseini-Asl, E., El-Baz, A., Keynton, R.: A new nmf-autoencoder based cad system for early diagnosis of prostate cancer. In: *Biomedical Imaging (ISBI), 2016 IEEE 13th International Symposium on, IEEE* (2016) 1237–1240.

39. Reda, I., Shalaby, A., Khalifa, F., Elmogy, M., Aboulfotouh, A., El-Ghar, M.A., Hosseini-Asl, E., Werghi, N., Keynton, R., El-Baz, A.: Computer-aided diagnostic tool for early detection of prostate cancer. In: *Image Processing (ICIP), 2016 IEEE International Conference on, IEEE* (2016) 2668–2672.

40. Reda, I., Elmogy, M., Aboulfotouh, A., Ismail, M., El-Baz, A., Keynton, R.: Prostate segmentation using deformable model-based methods. *Biomedical Image Segmentation: Advances and Trends* (2016) 293–308.

41. Reda, I., Shalaby, A., Elmogy, M., Aboulfotouh, A., Werghi, N., Elmaghraby, A., El-Baz, A.: Prostate cancer diagnosis based on the fusion of imaging-markers with clinical-biomarkers. In: *Biomedical Engineering Society (BMES).* (2017).

42. Firjani, A., Elnakib, A., Khalifa, F., Gimelfarb, G., El-Ghar, M.A., Elmaghraby, A., El-Baz, A. et al.: A diffusion-weighted imaging based diagnostic system for early detection of prostate cancer. *Journal of Biomedical Science and Engineering* **6**(3) (2013) 346.

43. Sato, C., Naganawa, S., Nakamura, T., Kumada, H., Miura, S., Takizawa, O., Ishigaki, T.: Differentiation of noncancerous tissue and cancer lesions by apparent diffusion coefficient values in transition and peripheral zones of the prostate. *Journal of Magnetic Resonance Imaging* **21**(3) (2005) 258–262.

44. Bammer, R.: Basic principles of diffusion-weighted imaging. *European Journal of Radiology* **45**(3) (2003) 169–184.

45. Sundgren, P., Dong, Q., Gomez-Hassan, D., Mukherji, S., Maly, P., Welsh, R.: Diffusion tensor imaging of the brain: review of clinical applications. *Neuroradiology* **46**(5) (2004) 339–350.

46. Le Bihan, D., Mangin, J.F., Poupon, C., Clark, C.A., Pappata, S., Molko, N., Chabriat, H.: Diffusion tensor imaging: concepts and applications. *Journal of Magnetic Resonance Imaging* **13**(4) (2001) 534–546.

47. Wedeen, V.J., Wang, R., Schmahmann, J.D., Benner, T., Tseng, W., Dai, G., Pandya, D., Hagmann, P., D'Arceuil, H., de Crespigny, A.J.: Diffusion spectrum magnetic resonance imaging (DSI) tractography of crossing fibers. *Neuroimage* **41**(4) (2008) 1267–1277.

48. Hagmann, P., Jonasson, L., Maeder, P., Thiran, J.P., Wedeen, V.J., Meuli, R.: Understanding diffusion mr imaging techniques: From scalar diffusion-weighted imaging to diffusion tensor imaging and beyond 1. *Radiographics* **26**(suppl 1) (2006) S205–S223.

49. Liu, L., Tian, Z., Zhang, Z., Fei, B.: Computer-aided detection of prostate cancer with MRI: Technology and applications. *Academic Radiology* (2016) 1024–1046.

50. Ampeliotis, D., Antonakoudi, A., Berberidis, K., Psarakis, E., Kounoudes, A.: A computer-aided system for the detection of prostate cancer based on magnetic resonance image analysis. In: *Communications, Control and Signal Processing, 2008. ISCCSP 2008. 3rd International Symposium on,* IEEE (2008) 1372–1377.

51. Feleppa, E.J., Fair, W.R., Liu, T., Kalisz, A., Gnadt, W., Lizzi, F.L., Balaji, K., Porter, C.R., Tsai, H.: Two-dimensional and three-dimensional tissue-type imaging of the prostate based on ultrasonic spectrum analysis and neural network classification. In: *Medical Imaging 2000, International Society for Optics and Photonics* (2000) 152–160.

52. Duda, R.O., Hart, P.E., Stork, D.G.: *Pattern Classification*. Hoboken, NJ: John Wiley & Sons (2012).

53. Cortes, C., Vapnik, V.: Support-vector networks. *Machine Learning* **20**(3) (1995) 273–297.

54. Burges, C.J.: A tutorial on support vector machines for pattern recognition. *Data Mining and Knowledge Discovery* **2**(2) (1998) 121–167.

55. Ghose, S., Oliver, A., Marti, R., Lladó, X., Freixenet, J., Mitra, J., Vilanova, J.C., Meriaudeau, F.: A hybrid framework of multiple active appearance models and global registration for 3d prostate segmentation in mri. In: *SPIE Medical Imaging, International Society for Optics and Photonics* (2012) 83140S–83140S.

56. Niaf, E., Rouvière, O., Mège-Lechevallier, F., Bratan, F., Lartizien, C.: Computer-aided diagnosis of prostate cancer in the peripheral zone using multiparametric MRI. *Physics in Medicine and Biology* **57**(12) (2012) 3833.

57. Chan, I., Wells III, W., Mulkern, R.V., Haker, S., Zhang, J., Zou, K.H., Maier, S.E., Tempany, C.M.: Detection of prostate cancer by integration of line-scan diffusion, T2-mapping and T2-weighted magnetic resonance imaging; a multichannel statistical classifier. *Medical Physics* **30**(9) (2003) 2390–2398.

58. Litjens, G., Vos, P., Barentsz, J., Karssemeijer, N., Huisman, H.: Automatic computer aided detection of abnormalities in multi-parametric prostate MRI. In: *SPIE Medical Imaging, International Society for Optics and Photonics* (2011) 79630T–79630T.

59. Vos, P., Barentsz, J., Karssemeijer, N., Huisman, H.: Automatic computer-aided detection of prostate cancer based on multiparametric magnetic resonance image analysis. *Physics in Medicine and Biology* **57**(6) (2012) 1527.

60. McClure, P., Khalifa, F., Soliman, A., El-Ghar, M.A., Gimelfarb, G., Elmaghraby, A., El-Baz, A.: A novel nmf guided level-set for dwi prostate segmentation. *Journal of Computer Science and Systems Biology* **7** (2014) 209–216.

61. Le Bihan, D.: Apparent diffusion coefficient and beyond: what diffusion MR imaging can tell us about tissue structure. *Radiology* **268**(2) (2013) 318–322.

62. Litjens, G., Debats, O., Barentsz, J., Karssemeijer, N., Huisman, H.: Computer-aided detection of prostate cancer in MRI. *IEEE Transactions on Medical Imaging* **33**(5) (2014) 1083–1092.

63. Bengio, Y., Lamblin, P., Popovici, D., Larochelle, H.: Greedy layer-wise training of deep networks. *Advances in Neural Information Processing Systems* **19** (2007) 153–160.

64. Hosseini-Asl, E., Zurada, J., Nasraoui, O.: Deep learning of part-based representation of data using sparse autoencoders with nonnegativity constraints. *IEEE Transactions on Neural Networks and Learning Systems* **99** (2015) 1–13.

65. Hall, M., Frank, E., Holmes, G., Pfahringer, B., Reutemann, P., Witten, I.H.: The Weka data mining software: An update. *ACM SIGKDD Explorations* **11**(1) (2009) 10–18.

66. Ali, A.M., Farag, A.A., El-Baz, A.: Graph cuts framework for kidney segmentation with prior shape constraints. In: *Proceedings of International Conference on Medical Image Computing and Computer-Assisted Intervention, (MICCAI'07)*. Vol. 1, Brisbane, Australia, October 29–November 2 (2007) 384–392.

67. Chowdhury, A.S., Roy, R., Bose, S., Elnakib, F.K.A., El-Baz, A.: Non-rigid biomedical image registration using graph cuts with a novel data term. In: *Proceedings of IEEE International Symposium on Biomedical Imaging: From Nano to Macro, (ISBI'12)*, Barcelona, Spain, May 2–5 (2012) 446–449.

68. El-Baz, A., Farag, A.A., Yuksel, S.E., El-Ghar, M.E.A., Eldiasty, T.A., Ghoneim, M.A.: Application of deformable models for the detection of acute renal rejection. In Farag, A.A., Suri, J.S., eds.: *Deformable Models*. Vol. 1. (2007) 293–333.

69. El-Baz, A., Farag, A., Fahmi, R., Yuksel, S., El-Ghar, M.A., Eldiasty, T.: Image analysis of renal DCE MRI for the detection of acute renal rejection. In: *Proceedings of IAPR International Conference on Pattern Recognition (ICPR'06)*, Hong Kong, August 20–24 (2006) 822–825.

70. El-Baz, A., Farag, A., Fahmi, R., Yuksel, S., Miller, W., El-Ghar, M.A., El-Diasty, T., Ghoneim, M.: A new CAD system for the evaluation of kidney diseases using DCE-MRI. In: *Proceedings of International Conference on Medical Image Computing and Computer-Assisted Intervention, (MICCAI'08)*, Copenhagen, Denmark, October 1–6 (2006) 446–453.

71. El-Baz, A., Gimelfarb, G., El-Ghar, M.A.: A novel image analysis approach for accurate identification of acute renal rejection. In: *Proceedings of IEEE International Conference on Image Processing, (ICIP'08)*, San Diego, CA, October 12–15 (2008) 1812–1815.

72. El-Baz, A., Gimelfarb, G., El-Ghar, M.A.: Image analysis approach for identification of renal transplant rejection. In: *Proceedings of IAPR International Conference on Pattern Recognition, (ICPR'08)*, Tampa, FL, December 8–11 (2008) 1–4.

73. El-Baz, A., Gimelfarb, G., El-Ghar, M.A.: New motion correction models for automatic identification of renal transplant rejection. In: *Proceedings of International Conference on Medical Image Computing and Computer-Assisted Intervention, (MICCAI'07)*, Brisbane, Australia, October 29–November 2 (2007) 235–243.

74. Farag, A., El-Baz, A., Yuksel, S., El-Ghar, M.A., Eldiasty, T.: A framework for the detection of acute rejection with Dynamic Contrast Enhanced Magnetic Resonance Imaging. In: *Proceedings of IEEE International Symposium on Biomedical Imaging: From Nano to Macro, (ISBI'06)*, Arlington, VA, April 6–9 (2006) 418–421.

75. Khalifa, F., Beache, G.M., El-Ghar, M.A., El-Diasty, T., Gimelfarb, G., Kong, M., El-Baz, A.: Dynamic contrast-enhanced MRI-based early detection of acute renal transplant rejection. *IEEE Transactions on Medical Imaging* **32**(10) (2013) 1910–1927.

76. Khalifa, F., El-Baz, A., Gimelfarb, G., El-Ghar, M.A.: Non-invasive image-based approach for early detection of acute renal rejection. In: *Proceedings of International Conference Medical Image Computing and Computer-Assisted Intervention, (MICCAI'10)*, Beijing, China, September 20–24 (2010) 10–18.

77. Khalifa, F., El-Baz, A., Gimelfarb, G., Ouseph, R., El-Ghar, M.A.: Shape-appearance guided level-set deformable model for image segmentation. In: *Proceedings of IAPR International Conference on Pattern Recognition, (ICPR'10)*, Istanbul, Turkey, August 23–26 (2010) 4581–4584.

78. Khalifa, F., El-Ghar, M.A., Abdollahi, B., Frieboes, H., El-Diasty, T., El-Baz, A.: A comprehensive non-invasive framework for automated evaluation of acute renal transplant rejection using DCE-MRI. *NMR in Biomedicine* **26**(11) (2013) 1460–1470.

79. Khalifa, F., El-Ghar, M.A., Abdollahi, B., Frieboes, H.B., El-Diasty, T., El-Baz, A.: Dynamic contrast-enhanced MRI-based early detection of acute renal transplant rejection. In: *2014 Annual Scientific Meeting and Educational Course Brochure of the Society of Abdominal Radiology, (SAR'14)*, Boca Raton, FL, March 23–28 (2014) CID: 1855912.

80. Khalifa, F., Elnakib, A., Beache, G.M., Gimelfarb, G., El-Ghar, M.A., Sokhadze, G., Manning, S., McClure, P., El-Baz, A.: 3D kidney segmentation from CT images using a level set approach guided by a novel stochastic speed function. In: *Proceedings of International Conference Medical Image Computing and Computer-Assisted Intervention, (MICCAI'11)*, Toronto, Canada, September 18–22 (2011) 587–594.

81. Khalifa, F., Gimelfarb, G., El-Ghar, M.A., Sokhadze, G., Manning, S., McClure, P., Ouseph, R., El-Baz, A.: A new deformable model-based segmentation approach for accurate extraction of the kidney from abdominal CT images. In: *Proceedings of IEEE International Conference on Image Processing, (ICIP'11)*, Brussels, Belgium, September 11–14 (2011) 3393–3396.

82. Mostapha, M., Khalifa, F., Alansary, A., Soliman, A., Suri, J., El-Baz, A.: Computer-aided diagnosis systems for acute renal transplant rejection: Challenges and methodologies. In El-Baz, A., Saba J. Suri, L., eds.: *Abdomen and Thoracic Imaging*. Springer (2014) 1–35.

83. Shehata, M., Khalifa, F., Hollis, E., Soliman, A., Hosseini-Asl, E., El-Ghar, M.A., El-Baz, M., Dwyer, A.C., El-Baz, A., Keynton, R.: A new non-invasive approach for early classification of renal rejection types using diffusion-weighted mri. In: *IEEE International Conference on Image Processing (ICIP)*, 2016, IEEE (2016) 136–140.

84. Khalifa, F., Soliman, A., Takieldeen, A., Shehata, M., Mostapha, M., Shaffie, A., Ouseph, R., Elmaghraby, A., El-Baz, A.: Kidney segmentation from CT images using a 3D NMF-guided active contour model. In: *IEEE 13th International Symposium on Biomedical Imaging (ISBI)*, 2016, IEEE (2016) 432–435.

85. Shehata, M., Khalifa, F., Soliman, A., Takieldeen, A., El-Ghar, M.A., Shaffie, A., Dwyer, A.C., Ouseph, R., El-Baz, A., Keynton, R.: 3D diffusion MRI-based CAD system for early diagnosis of acute renal rejection. In: *Biomedical Imaging (ISBI), 2016 IEEE 13th International Symposium on*, IEEE (2016) 1177–1180.

86. Shehata, M., Khalifa, F., Soliman, A., Alrefai, R., El-Ghar, M.A., Dwyer, A.C., Ouseph, R., El-Baz, A.: A level set-based framework for 3D kidney segmentation from diffusion MR images. In: *IEEE International Conference on Image Processing (ICIP)*, 2015, IEEE (2015) 4441–4445.

87. Shehata, M., Khalifa, F., Soliman, A., El-Ghar, M.A., Dwyer, A.C., Gimelfarb, G., Keynton, R., El-Baz, A.: A promising non-invasive cad system for kidney function assessment. In: *International Conference on Medical Image Computing and Computer-Assisted Intervention*, Springer (2016) 613–621.

88. Khalifa, F., Soliman, A., Elmaghraby, A., Gimelfarb, G., El-Baz, A.: 3D kidney segmentation from abdominal images using spatial-appearance models. *Computational and Mathematical Methods in Medicine* **2017** (2017).

89. Hollis, E., Shehata, M., Khalifa, F., El-Ghar, M.A., El-Diasty, T., El-Baz, A.: Towards non-invasive diagnostic techniques for early detection of acute renal transplant rejection: A review. *The Egyptian Journal of Radiology and Nuclear Medicine* **48**(1) (2016) 257–269.

90. Shehata, M., Khalifa, F., Soliman, A., El-Ghar, M.A., Dwyer, A.C., El-Baz, A.: Assessment of renal transplant using image and clinical-based biomarkers. In: *Proceedings of 13th Annual Scientific Meeting of American Society for Diagnostics and Interventional Nephrology (ASDIN'17)*, New Orleans, LA, February 10–12, 2017. (2017).

91. Shehata, M., Khalifa, F., Soliman, A., El-Ghar, M.A., Dwyer, A.C., El-Baz, A.: Early assessment of acute renal rejection. In: *Proceedings of 12th Annual Scientific Meeting of American Society for Diagnostics and Interventional Nephrology (ASDIN'16)*, Pheonix, AZ, February 19–21, 2016. (2017).

92. Khalifa, F., Beache, G., El-Baz, A., Gimelfarb, G.: Deformable model guided by stochastic speed with application in cine images segmentation. In: *Proceedings of IEEE International Conference on Image Processing, (ICIP'10)*, Hong Kong, September 26–29 (2010) 1725–1728.

93. Khalifa, F., Beache, G.M., Elnakib, A., Sliman, H., Gimelfarb, G., Welch, K.C., El-Baz, A.: A new shape-based framework for the left ventricle wall segmentation from cardiac first-pass perfusion MRI. In: *Proceedings of IEEE International Symposium on Biomedical Imaging: From Nano to Macro, (ISBI'13)*, San Francisco, CA, April 7–11 (2013) 41–44.

94. Khalifa, F., Beache, G.M., Elnakib, A., Sliman, H., Gimelfarb, G., Welch, K.C., El-Baz, A.: A new non-rigid registration framework for improved visualization of transmural perfusion gradients on cardiac first–pass perfusion MRI. In: *Proceedings of IEEE International Symposium on Biomedical Imaging: From Nano to Macro, (ISBI'12)*, Barcelona, Spain, May 2–5 (2012) 828–831.

95. Khalifa, F., Beache, G.M., Firjani, A., Welch, K.C., Gimelfarb, G., El-Baz, A.: A new nonrigid registration approach for motion correction of cardiac first-pass perfusion MRI. In: *Proceedings of IEEE International Conference on Image Processing, (ICIP'12)*, Lake Buena Vista, FL, September 30–October 3 (2012) 1665–1668.

96. Khalifa, F., Beache, G.M., Gimelfarb, G., El-Baz, A.: A novel CAD system for analyzing cardiac first-pass MR images. In: *Proceedings of IAPR International Conference on Pattern Recognition (ICPR'12)*, Tsukuba Science City, Japan, November 11–15 (2012) 77–80.

97. Khalifa, F., Beache, G.M., Gimelfarb, G., El-Baz, A.: A novel approach for accurate estimation of left ventricle global indexes from short-axis cine MRI. In: *Proceedings of IEEE International Conference on Image Processing, (ICIP'11)*, Brussels, Belgium, September 11–14 (2011) 2645–2649.

98. Khalifa, F., Beache, G.M., Gimelfarb, G., Giridharan, G.A., El-Baz, A.: A new image-based framework for analyzing cine images. In El-Baz, A., Acharya, U.R., Mirmedhdi, M., Suri, J.S., eds.: *Handbook of Multi Modality State-of-the-Art Medical Image Segmentation and Registration Methodologies*. Vol. 2. Springer, New York (2011) 69–98.

99. Khalifa, F., Beache, G.M., Gimelfarb, G., Giridharan, G.A., El-Baz, A.: Accurate automatic analysis of cardiac cine images. *IEEE Transactions on Biomedical Engineering* **59**(2) (2012) 445–455.

100. Khalifa, F., Beache, G.M., Nitzken, M., Gimelfarb, G., Giridharan, G.A., El-Baz, A.: Automatic analysis of left ventricle wall thickness using short-axis cine CMR images. In: *Proceedings of IEEE International Symposium on Biomedical Imaging: From Nano to Macro, (ISBI'11)*, Chicago, IL, March 30–April 2 (2011) 1306–1309.

101. Nitzken, M., Beache, G., Elnakib, A., Khalifa, F., Gimelfarb, G., El-Baz, A.: Accurate modeling of tagged cmr 3D image appearance characteristics to improve cardiac cycle strain estimation. In: *Image Processing (ICIP), 2012 19th IEEE International Conference on*, Orlando, FL, IEEE (September 2012) 521–524.

102. Nitzken, M., Beache, G., Elnakib, A., Khalifa, F., Gimelfarb, G., El-Baz, A.: Improving full-cardiac cycle strain estimation from tagged cmr by accurate modeling of 3D image appearance characteristics. In: *Biomedical Imaging (ISBI), 2012 9th IEEE International Symposium on*, Barcelona, Spain, IEEE (May 2012) 462–465 (Selected for oral presentation).

103. Nitzken, M.J., El-Baz, A.S., Beache, G.M.: Markov-Gibbs random field model for improved full-cardiac cycle strain estimation from tagged CMR. *Journal of Cardiovascular Magnetic Resonance* **14**(1) (2012) 1–2.

104. Sliman, H., Elnakib, A., Beache, G., Elmaghraby, A., El-Baz, A.: Assessment of myocardial function from cine cardiac MRI using a novel 4D tracking approach. *Journal of Computer Science and Systems Biology* **7** (2014) 169–173.

105. Sliman, H., Elnakib, A., Beache, G.M., Soliman, A., Khalifa, F., Gimelfarb, G., Elmaghraby, A., El-Baz, A.: A novel 4D PDE-based approach for accurate assessment of myocardium function using cine cardiac magnetic resonance images. In: *Proceedings of IEEE International Conference on Image Processing (ICIP'14)*, Paris, France, October 27–30 (2014) 3537–3541.

106. Sliman, H., Khalifa, F., Elnakib, A., Beache, G.M., Elmaghraby, A., El-Baz, A.: A new segmentation-based tracking framework for extracting the left ventricle cavity from cine cardiac MRI. In: *Proceedings of IEEE International Conference on Image Processing, (ICIP'13)*, Melbourne, Australia, September 15–18 (2013) 685–689.

107. Sliman, H., Khalifa, F., Elnakib, A., Soliman, A., Beache, G.M., Elmaghraby, A., Gimelfarb, G., El-Baz, A.: Myocardial borders segmentation from cine MR images using bi-directional coupled parametric deformable models. *Medical Physics* **40**(9) (2013) 1–13.

108. Sliman, H., Khalifa, F., Elnakib, A., Soliman, A., Beache, G.M., Gimelfarb, G., Emam, A., Elmaghraby, A., El-Baz, A.: Accurate segmentation framework for the left ventricle wall from cardiac cine MRI. In: *Proceedings of International Symposium on Computational Models for Life Science, (CMLS'13)*. Vol. 1559, Sydney, Australia, November 27–29 (2013) 287–296.

109. Eladawi, N., Elmogy, M., Ghazal, M., Helmy, O., Aboelfetouh, A., Riad, A., Schaal, S., El-Baz, A.: Classification of retinal diseases based on oct images. *Frontiers in Bioscience Landmark Journal* **23** (2017) 247–264.

110. ElTanboly, A., Ismail, M., Shalaby, A., Switala, A., El-Baz, A., Schaal, S., Gimelfarb, G., El-Azab, M.: A computer aided diagnostic system for detecting diabetic retinopathy in optical coherence tomography images. *Medical Physics* **44** (2016) 914–923.

111. Abdollahi, B., Civelek, A.C., Li, X.F., Suri, J., El-Baz, A.: PET/CT nodule segmentation and diagnosis: A survey. In Saba, L., Suri, J.S., eds.: *Multi Detector CT Imaging*. Taylor & Francis Group (2014) 639–651.

112. Abdollahi, B., El-Baz, A., Amini, A.A.: A multi-scale non-linear vessel enhancement technique. In: *Engineering in Medicine and Biology Society, EMBC, 2011 Annual International Conference of the IEEE*, IEEE (2011) 3925–3929.

113. Abdollahi, B., Soliman, A., Civelek, A., Li, X.F., Gimelfarb, G., El-Baz, A.: A novel Gaussian scale space-based joint MGRF framework for precise lung segmentation. In: *Proceedings of IEEE International Conference on Image Processing, (ICIP'12)*, IEEE (2012) 2029–2032.

114. Abdollahi, B., Soliman, A., Civelek, A., Li, X.F., Gimelfarb, G., El-Baz, A.: A novel 3D joint MGRF framework for precise lung segmentation. In: *Machine Learning in Medical Imaging*. Springer (2012) 86–93.

115. Ali, A.M., El-Baz, A.S., Farag, A.A.: A novel framework for accurate lung segmentation using graph cuts. In: *Proceedings of IEEE International Symposium on Biomedical Imaging: From Nano to Macro, (ISBI'07)*, IEEE (2007) 908–911.

116. El-Baz, A., Beache, G.M., Gimelfarb, G., Suzuki, K., Okada, K.: Lung imaging data analysis. *International Journal of Biomedical Imaging* **2013** (2013).

117. El-Baz, A., Beache, G.M., Gimelfarb, G., Suzuki, K., Okada, K., Elnakib, A., Soliman, A., Abdollahi, B.: Computer-aided diagnosis systems for lung cancer: Challenges and methodologies. *International Journal of Biomedical Imaging* **2013** (2013).

118. El-Baz, A., Elnakib, A., Abou El-Ghar, M., Gimelfarb, G., Falk, R., Farag, A.: Automatic detection of 2D and 3D lung nodules in chest spiral CT scans. *International Journal of Biomedical Imaging* **2013** (2013).

119. El-Baz, A., Farag, A.A., Falk, R., La Rocca, R.: A unified approach for detection, visualization, and identification of lung abnormalities in chest spiral CT scans. In: *International Congress Series*. Vol. 1256, Elsevier (2003) 998–1004.

120. El-Baz, A., Farag, A.A., Falk, R., La Rocca, R.: Detection, visualization and identification of lung abnormalities in chest spiral CT scan: Phase-I. In: *Proceedings of International conference on Biomedical Engineering*, Cairo, Egypt. Vol. 12. (2002).

121. El-Baz, A., Farag, A., Gimelfarb, G., Falk, R., El-Ghar, M.A., Eldiasty, T.: A framework for automatic segmentation of lung nodules from low dose chest CT scans. In: *Proceedings of International Conference on Pattern Recognition, (ICPR'06)*. Vol. 3, IEEE (2006) 611–614.

122. El-Baz, A., Farag, A., Gimelfarb, G., Falk, R., El-Ghar, M.A.: A novel level set-based computer-aided detection system for automatic detection of lung nodules in low dose chest computed tomography scans. *Lung Imaging and Computer Aided Diagnosis* **10** (2011) 221–238.

123. El-Baz, A., Gimelfarb, G., Abou El-Ghar, M., Falk, R.: Appearance-based diagnostic system for early assessment of malignant lung nodules. In: *Proceedings of IEEE International Conference on Image Processing, (ICIP'12)*, IEEE (2012) 533–536.

124. El-Baz, A., Gimelfarb, G., Falk, R.: A novel 3D framework for automatic lung segmentation from low dose CT images. In El-Baz, A., Suri, J.S., eds.: *Lung Imaging and Computer Aided Diagnosis*. Taylor & Francis Group (2011) 1–16.

125. El-Baz, A., Gimelfarb, G., Falk, R., El-Ghar, M.: Appearance analysis for diagnosing malignant lung nodules. In: *Proceedings of IEEE International Symposium on Biomedical Imaging: From Nano to Macro (ISBI'10)*, IEEE (2010) 193–196.

126. El-Baz, A., Gimelfarb, G., Falk, R., El-Ghar, M.A.: A novel level set-based CAD system for automatic detection of lung nodules in low dose chest CT scans. In El-Baz, A., Suri, J.S., eds.: *Lung Imaging and Computer Aided Diagnosis*. Vol. 1. Taylor & Francis Group (2011) 221–238.

127. El-Baz, A., Gimelfarb, G., Falk, R., El-Ghar, M.A.: A new approach for automatic analysis of 3D low dose CT images for accurate monitoring the detected lung nodules. In: *Proceedings of International Conference on Pattern Recognition, (ICPR'08)*, IEEE (2008) 1–4.

128. El-Baz, A., Gimelfarb, G., Falk, R., El-Ghar, M.A.: A novel approach for automatic follow-up of detected lung nodules. In: *Proceedings of IEEE International Conference on Image Processing, (ICIP'07)*. Vol. 5, IEEE (2007) V–501.

129. El-Baz, A., Gimelfarb, G., Falk, R., El-Ghar, M.A.: A new CAD system for early diagnosis of detected lung nodules. In: *Image Processing, 2007. ICIP 2007. IEEE International Conference on*. Vol. 2, IEEE (2007) II–461.

130. El-Baz, A., Gimelfarb, G., Falk, R., El-Ghar, M.A., Refaie, H.: Promising results for early diagnosis of lung cancer. In: *Proceedings of IEEE International Symposium on Biomedical Imaging: From Nano to Macro, (ISBI'08)*, IEEE (2008) 1151–1154.

131. El-Baz, A., Gimelfarb, G.L., Falk, R., Abou El-Ghar, M., Holland, T., Shaffer, T.: A new stochastic framework for accurate lung segmentation. In: *Proceedings of Medical Image Computing and Computer-Assisted Intervention, (MICCAI'08)*. (2008) 322–330.

132. El-Baz, A., Gimelfarb, G.L., Falk, R., Heredis, D., Abou El-Ghar, M.: A novel approach for accurate estimation of the growth rate of the detected lung nodules. In: *Proceedings of International Workshop on Pulmonary Image Analysis*. (2008) 33–42.

133. El-Baz, A., Gimelfarb, G.L., Falk, R., Holland, T., Shaffer, T.: A framework for unsupervised segmentation of lung tissues from low dose computed tomography images. In: *Proceedings of British Machine Vision, (BMVC'08)*. (2008) 1–10.

134. El-Baz, A., Gimelfarb, G., Falk, R., El-Ghar, M.A.: 3D MGRF-based appearance modeling for robust segmentation of pulmonary nodules in 3D LDCT chest images. In: *Lung Imaging and Computer Aided Diagnosis*. chapter (2011) 51–63.

135. El-Baz, A., Gimelfarb, G., Falk, R., El-Ghar, M.A.: Automatic analysis of 3D low dose CT images for early diagnosis of lung cancer. *Pattern Recognition* **42**(6) (2009) 1041–1051.

136. El-Baz, A., Gimelfarb, G., Falk, R., El-Ghar, M.A., Rainey, S., Heredia, D., Shaffer, T.: Toward early diagnosis of lung cancer. In: *Proceedings of Medical Image Computing and Computer-Assisted Intervention, (MICCAI'09)*, Springer (2009) 682–689.

137. El-Baz, A., Gimelfarb, G., Falk, R., El-Ghar, M.A., Suri, J.: Appearance analysis for the early assessment of detected lung nodules. In: *Lung Imaging and Computer Aided Diagnosis*. (2011) 395–404.

138. El-Baz, A., Khalifa, F., Elnakib, A., Nitkzen, M., Soliman, A., McClure, P., Gimelfarb, G., El-Ghar, M.A.: A novel approach for global lung registration using 3D Markov Gibbs appearance model. In: *Proceedings of International Conference Medical Image Computing and Computer-Assisted Intervention, (MICCAI'12)*, Nice, France, October 1–5 (2012) 114–121.

139. El-Baz, A., Nitzken, M., Elnakib, A., Khalifa, F., Gimelfarb, G., Falk, R., El-Ghar, M.A.: 3D shape analysis for early diagnosis of malignant lung nodules. In: *Proceedings of International Conference Medical Image Computing and Computer-Assisted Intervention, (MICCAI'11)*, Toronto, Canada, September 18–22 (2011) 175–182.

140. El-Baz, A., Nitzken, M., Gimelfarb, G., Van Bogaert, E., Falk, R., El-Ghar, M.A., Suri, J.: Three-dimensional shape analysis using spherical harmonics for early assessment of detected lung nodules. In: *Lung Imaging and Computer Aided Diagnosis*. (2011) 421–438.

141. El-Baz, A., Nitzken, M., Khalifa, F., Elnakib, A., Gimelfarb, G., Falk, R., El-Ghar, M.A.: 3D shape analysis for early diagnosis of malignant lung nodules. In: *Proceedings of International Conference on Information Processing in Medical Imaging, (IPMI'11)*, Monastery Irsee, Germany, July 3–8 (2011) 772–783.

142. El-Baz, A., Nitzken, M., Vanbogaert, E., Gimelfarb, G., Falk, R., Abo El-Ghar, M.: A novel shape-based diagnostic approach for early diagnosis of lung nodules. In: *Biomedical Imaging: From Nano to Macro, 2011 IEEE International Symposium on*, IEEE (2011) 137–140.

143. El-Baz, A., Sethu, P., Gimelfarb, G., Khalifa, F., Elnakib, A., Falk, R., El-Ghar, M.A.: Elastic phantoms generated by microfluidics technology: Validation of an imaged-based approach for accurate measurement of the growth rate of lung nodules. *Biotechnology Journal* **6**(2) (2011) 195–203.

144. El-Baz, A., Sethu, P., Gimelfarb, G., Khalifa, F., Elnakib, A., Falk, R., El-Ghar, M.A.: A new validation approach for the growth rate measurement using elastic phantoms generated by state-of-the-art microfluidics technology. In: *Proceedings of IEEE International Conference on Image Processing, (ICIP'10)*, Hong Kong, September 26–29 (2010) 4381–4383.

145. El-Baz, A., Sethu, P., Gimelfarb, G., Khalifa, F., Elnakib, A., Falk, R., Suri, M.A.E.G.J.: Validation of a new imaged-based approach for the accurate estimating of the growth rate of detected lung nodules using real CT images and elastic phantoms generated by state-of-the-art microfluidics technology. In El-Baz, A., Suri, J.S., eds.: *Handbook of Lung Imaging and Computer Aided Diagnosis*. Vol. 1. Taylor & Francis Group, New York (2011) 405–420.

146. El-Baz, A., Soliman, A., McClure, P., Gimelfarb, G., El-Ghar, M.A., Falk, R.: Early assessment of malignant lung nodules based on the spatial analysis of detected lung nodules. In: *Proceedings of IEEE International Symposium on Biomedical Imaging: From Nano to Macro, (ISBI'12)*, IEEE (2012) 1463–1466.

147. El-Baz, A., Yuksel, S.E., Elshazly, S., Farag, A.A.: Non-rigid registration techniques for automatic follow-up of lung nodules. In: *Proceedings of Computer Assisted Radiology and Surgery, (CARS'05)*. Vol. 1281, Elsevier (2005) 1115–1120.

148. El-Baz, A.S., Suri, J.S.: Lung Imaging and Computer-Aided Diagnosis. CRC Press (2011)

149. Soliman, A., Khalifa, F., Shaffie, A., Liu, N., Dunlap, N., Wang, B., Elmaghraby, A., Gimelfarb, G., El-Baz, A.: Image-based CAD system for accurate identification of lung injury. In: *Proceedings of IEEE International Conference on Image Processing, (ICIP'16)*, IEEE (2016) 121–125.

150. Soliman, A., Khalifa, F., Dunlap, N., Wang, B., El-Ghar, M., El-Baz, A.: An iso-surfaces based local deformation handling framework of lung tissues. In: *Biomedical Imaging (ISBI), 2016 IEEE 13th International Symposium on*, IEEE (2016) 1253–1259.

151. Soliman, A., Khalifa, F., Shaffie, A., Dunlap, N., Wang, B., Elmaghraby, A., El-Baz, A.: Detection of lung injury using 4d-ct chest images. In: *Biomedical Imaging (ISBI), 2016 IEEE 13th International Symposium on*, IEEE (2016) 1274–1277.

152. Dombroski, B., Nitzken, M., Elnakib, A., Khalifa, F., El-Baz, A., Casanova, M.F.: Cortical surface complexity in a population-based normative sample. *Translational Neuroscience* **5**(1) (2014) 17–24.

153. El-Baz, A., Casanova, M., Gimelfarb, G., Mott, M., Switala, A.: An MRI-based diagnostic framework for early diagnosis of dyslexia. *International Journal of Computer Assisted Radiology and Surgery* **3**(3–4) (2008) 181–189.

154. El-Baz, A., Casanova, M., Gimelfarb, G., Mott, M., Switala, A., Vanbogaert, E., McCracken, R.: A new CAD system for early diagnosis of dyslexic brains. In: *Proceedings of International Conference on Image Processing (ICIP'2008)*, IEEE (2008) 1820–1823.

155. El-Baz, A., Casanova, M.F., Gimelfarb, G., Mott, M., Switwala, A.E.: A new image analysis approach for automatic classification of autistic brains. In: *Proceedings of IEEE International Symposium on Biomedical Imaging: From Nano to Macro (ISBI'2007)*, IEEE (2007) 352–355.

156. El-Baz, A., Elnakib, A., Khalifa, F., El-Ghar, M.A., McClure, P., Soliman, A., Gimelfarb, G.: Precise segmentation of 3-D magnetic resonance angiography. *IEEE Transactions on Biomedical Engineering* **59**(7) (2012) 2019–2029.

157. El-Baz, A., Farag, A.A., Gimelfarb, G.L., El-Ghar, M.A., Eldiasty, T.: Probabilistic modeling of blood vessels for segmenting mra images. In: *ICPR (3)*. (2006) 917–920.

158. El-Baz, A., Farag, A.A., Gimelfarb, G., El-Ghar, M.A., Eldiasty, T.: A new adaptive probabilistic model of blood vessels for segmenting MRA images. In: *Medical Image Computing and Computer-Assisted Intervention–MICCAI 2006*. Vol. 4191, Springer (2006) 799–806.

159. El-Baz, A., Farag, A.A., Gimelfarb, G., Hushek, S.G.: Automatic cerebrovascular segmentation by accurate probabilistic modeling of TOF-MRA images. In: *Medical Image Computing and Computer-Assisted Intervention–MICCAI 2005*. Springer (2005) 34–42.

160. El-Baz, A., Farag, A., Elnakib, A., Casanova, M.F., Gimelfarb, G., Switala, A.E., Jordan, D., Rainey, S.: Accurate automated detection of autism related corpus callosum abnormalities. *Journal of Medical Systems* **35**(5) (2011) 929–939.

161. El-Baz, A., Farag, A., Gimelfarb, G.: Cerebrovascular segmentation by accurate probabilistic modeling of TOF-MRA images. In: *Image Analysis*. Vol. 3540, Springer (2005) 1128–1137.

162. El-Baz, A., Gimelfarb, G., Falk, R., El-Ghar, M.A., Kumar, V., Heredia, D.: A novel 3D joint Markov-Gibbs model for extracting blood vessels from PC–MRA images. In: *Medical Image Computing and Computer-Assisted Intervention– MICCAI 2009*. Vol. 5762, Springer (2009) 943–950.

163. Elnakib, A., El-Baz, A., Casanova, M.F., Gimelfarb, G., Switala, A.E.: Image-based detection of corpus callosum variability for more accurate discrimination between dyslexic and normal brains. In: *Proceedings of IEEE International Symposium on Biomedical Imaging: From Nano to Macro (ISBI'2010)*, IEEE (2010) 109–112.

164. Elnakib, A., Casanova, M.F., Gimelfarb, G., Switala, A.E., El-Baz, A.: Autism diagnostics by center-line-based shape analysis of the corpus callosum. In: *Proceedings of IEEE International Symposium on Biomedical Imaging: From Nano to Macro (ISBI'2011)*, IEEE (2011) 1843–1846.

165. Elnakib, A., Nitzken, M., Casanova, M., Park, H., Gimelfarb, G., El-Baz, A.: Quantification of age-related brain cortex change using 3D shape analysis. In: *Pattern Recognition (ICPR), 2012 21ˢᵗ International Conference on*, IEEE (2012) 41–44.

166. Mostapha, M., Soliman, A., Khalifa, F., Elnakib, A., Alansary, A., Nitzken, M., Casanova, M.F., El-Baz, A.: A statistical framework for the classification of infant DT images. In: *Image Processing (ICIP), 2014 IEEE International Conference on*, IEEE (2014) 2222–2226.

167. Nitzken, M., Casanova, M., Gimelfarb, G., Elnakib, A., Khalifa, F., Switala, A., El-Baz, A.: 3D shape analysis of the brain cortex with application to dyslexia. In: *Image Processing (ICIP), 2011 18th IEEE International Conference on*, Brussels, Belgium, IEEE (September 2011) 2657–2660 (Selected for oral presentation. Oral acceptance rate is 10 percent and the overall acceptance rate is 35 percent).

168. El-Gamal, F.E.Z.A., Elmogy, M., Ghazal, M., Atwan, A., Barnes, G., Casanova, M., Keynton, R., El-Baz, A.: A novel CAD system for local and global early diagnosis of Alzheimer's disease based on PIB-PET scans. In: *Image Processing (ICIP), 2017 IEEE International Conference on*, Beijing, China, IEEE (2017).

169. Ismail, M., Soliman, A., Ghazal, M., Switala, A.E., Gimelfarb, G., Barnes, G.N., Khalil, A. and El-Baz, A.: A fast stochastic framework for automatic MR brain images segmentation. *PloS one* **12** (2017) e0187391.

170. Ismail, M.M., Keynton, R.S., Mostapha, M.M., ElTanboly, A.H., Casanova, M.F., Gimelfarb, G.L., El-Baz, A.: Studying autism spectrum disorder with structural and diffusion magnetic resonance imaging: A survey. *Frontiers in Human Neuroscience* **10** (2016)

171. Alansary, A., Ismail, M., Soliman, A., Khalifa, F., Nitzken, M., Elnakib, A., Mostapha, M., Black, A., Stinebruner, K., Casanova, M.F. et al.: Infant brain extraction in T1-weighted MR images using bet and refinement using LCDG and MRGF models. *IEEE Journal of Biomedical and Health Informatics* **20**(3) (2016) 925–935

172. Ismail, M., Barnes, G., Nitzken, M., Switala, A., Shalaby, A., Hosseini-Asl, E., Casanova, M., Keynton, R., Khalil, A. and El-Baz, A.: A new deep-learning approach for early detection of shape variations in autism using structural MRI. In Image Processing (ICIP), *2017 IEEE International Conference on*, IEEE (2017) 1057–1061.

173. Ismail, M., Soliman, A., ElTanboly, A., Switala, A., Mahmoud, M., Khalifa, F., Gimelfarb, G., Casanova, M.F., Keynton, R., El-Baz, A.: Detection of white matter abnormalities in mr brain images for diagnosis of autism in children. In: *Biomedical Imaging (ISBI), 2016 IEEE 13th International Symposium on*, IEEE (2016) 6–9.

174. Ismail, M., Mostapha, M., Soliman, A., Nitzken, M., Khalifa, F., Elnakib, A., Gimelfarb, G., Casanova, M., El-Baz, A.: Segmentation of infant brain MR images based on adaptive shape prior and higher-order MRGF. In: *Image Processing (ICIP), 2015 IEEE International Conference on*, IEEE (2015) 4327–4331.

175. Shalaby, A., Taher, F., El-Baz, M., Ghazal, v., Abou El-Ghar, M., Takieldeen, A., El-Baz, A.: Probabilistic modeling of blood vessels for segmenting magnetic resonance angiography images. In: *Medical Research Archive-MRA*. KEI (2017) 34–42.

176. Chowdhury, A.S., Rudra, A.K., Sen, M., Elnakib, A., El-Baz, A.: Cerebral white matter segmentation from MRI using probabilistic graph cuts and geometric shape priors. In: *ICIP*. (2010) 3649–3652.

19 MRI Imaging of Seminal Vesicle Invasion (SVI) in Prostate Adenocarcinoma

Samuel A. Gold, Graham R. Hale, Kareem N. Rayn, Vladimir Valera, Jonathan B. Bloom, and Peter A. Pinto

CONTENTS

INTRODUCTION

Prostate cancer (PCa) is an adenocarcinoma of prostate glandular tissue that is most often localized to the prostate. Rather than a solitary primary tumor focus, PCa is typically multifocal; it is estimated that nearly 80% of PCa cases have more than one tumor located within the prostate [1,2]. Generally, the prostate contains a dominant lesion demonstrating high oncologic activity as is evidenced by its increased size and higher grade. This lesion is termed the "index lesion" and according to contemporary thinking, represents the oncologic engine driving malignant growth [3,4]. The other lesions comprising the multifocal character of this cancer are termed "satellite lesions." They are often smaller, less active tumors located discontinuously throughout the prostate, which makes detection of satellite lesions especially challenging both preoperatively on imaging and biopsy, and postoperatively on final pathologic investigation [5]. Therefore, it is possible that rates of multifocal prostate adenocarcinoma are even higher than currently reported.

Given the tendency of PCa to produce multiple tumors within the prostate, spread of malignant cells beyond the prostate is of great concern. Fortunately, rates of invasive or metastatic PCa are low relative to localized PCa [6]. In recent years, the increase in public awareness about the need for PCa screening and the widespread adoption of prostate-specific antigen (PSA) as an effective, yet controversial screening method has dramatically improved the early detection and treatment of PCa to reduce rates of invasive or metastatic PCa [7].

The prostate gland is surrounded by the prostatic capsule, which is not a true capsule, but instead a fibromuscular layer on the exterior of the prostate. It is made up of an outer collagen band with an inner smooth muscle component that together cannot be separated from the prostatic tissue. The prostatic capsule covers the entire prostate with the key exceptions of the prostatic apex and the points of insertion for the ejaculatory ducts near the seminal vesicles [8]. Surrounding the prostate and the prostatic capsule is periprostatic adipose tissue. Furthermore, posterior to the prostate is the rectoprosatic fascia, also named Denonvilliers' fascia. It functions as a physical barrier between the prostate and the muscular rectum beneath.

If the capsule is breached and cancer is detected beyond its margins, then extraprostatic extension (EPE) is diagnosed. In staging, this is classified as T3 (or greater) cancer. Pathologic T3a (pT3a) cancer is defined as extension (either unilateral or bilateral) beyond the prostatic capsule and pT3b cancer is defined as invasion of one or both seminal vesicles (pT3b); pT4 cancer involves invasion of the bladder or rectum (Table 19.1) [9]. PCa staging also includes any potential involvement of regional lymph nodes or distant metastatic disease for TNM classification (Figure 19.1).

TABLE 19.1

Clinical Staging of Prostate Cancer

Clinical Staging of Prostate Cancer:

- T1 = undetectable on clinical exam
- T2 = palpable nodule without extraprostatic extension
- T3 = extends beyond prostate
  - T3a = extension beyond prostatic capsule
  - T3b = invasion of seminal vesicles
- T4 = extends to adjacent structures (other than seminal vesicles)
  - T4a = invasion of bladder neck, external sphincter, or rectum
  - T4b = invasion of floor or wall of the pelvis

Source: Partin, A.W. et al., *JAMA*, 277, 1445–1451, 1997.

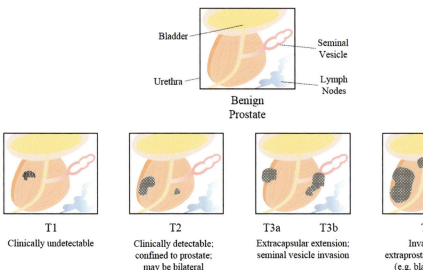

FIGURE 19.1   Stages of prostate cancer progression.

Cancer contained within the prostate is most often treated with radical prostatectomy (RP). In this procedure, the prostate (retained within the capsule) is excised along with the seminal vesicles and portions of the vas deferens. This has shown to be a very successful procedure because cancer localized within the prostatic capsule is completely removed and rates of PCa-specific survival following 10 years are very high [10]. However, if the cancer has invaded beyond the capsule (T3 disease), the risks of pathologic complications and poor outcomes are significantly higher. Extraprostatic extension is shown to increase the rates of surgical margins positive for cancerous tissue (absolute risk increase [ARI] 20%) and biochemical recurrence (ARI 10% over 15 years), and decrease cancer-specific survival (absolute risk reduction [ARR] 9% over 15 years) [11].

Due to these potential complications, extraprostatic extension is a dreaded finding for urologists. Its presence alters preoperative surgical planning, administration of neoadjuvant or adjuvant therapies, postoperative monitoring, and overall patient prognosis. It is therefore clear that accurate detection of pT3 disease is vital for oncologic management. This chapter will review the preoperative diagnosis of extraprostatic extension—specifically seminal vesical invasion—in primary prostate adenocarcinoma.

SEMINAL VESICLE INVASION

The seminal vesicles are extraprostatic structures located posteriolaterally to the prostate near the base of the prostate. They are glandular structures each comprised of a singular tube repeatedly folded on itself. The seminal vesicles have a thick muscular layer surrounding the luminal mucosa that is utilized for production and excretion of seminal fluid. During ejaculation, seminal fluid is pushed through the seminal vesicle lumen where it meets the ipsilateral vas deferens to form the ejaculatory ducts at the prostate. The seminal fluid moves through the ejaculatory duct as it passes through the prostate, mixes with prostatic fluid, and enters the prostatic urethra at the verumontanum where it is ultimately ejaculated as semen.

Questions remain about if the seminal vesicles are completely extraprostatic structures. There is evidence suggesting that the most proximal segments of the seminal vesicle do not abruptly transition to ejaculatory duct at the margin of the prostate, but instead invaginate into the prostatic base. This finding is termed invaginated extraprostatic space (IES) [12]. As mentioned above, the openings of the ejaculatory ducts are not covered by the prostatic capsule. They are directly connected to prostatic stroma, providing a convenient method of cancerous extension beyond the prostate to the seminal vesicles.

SVI is reported in 3.1%–26% of radical prostatectomy specimens [13–17]. The mechanism of PCa invasion into the seminal vesicles is not uniform. Currently, SVI is categorized into three modes of cancerous invasion. Type I SVI describes spread via the IES/ejaculatory ducts into the seminal vesicles [15]. The precise route of spread is not totally understood. According to the 2009 International Society of Urological Pathology conference, SVI should only be diagnosed with cancerous invasion of the muscular wall of the extraprostatic part of the seminal vesicle, rather than possible extension into the seminal vesicle epithelium of IES, which is difficult to discern from ejaculatory duct epithelium [12,15,18–20]. Furthermore, seminal vesicle epithelium has also been shown to resemble prostatic intraepithelial neoplasia, atypical acinar proliferations, and prostatic adenocarcinoma [21]. Type II SVI describes invasion through the prostatic capsule and into the seminal vesicles. This is further subdivided into type IIa, which signifies invasion through the base of the prostate directly into the seminal vesicle, and type IIb, which signifies retrograde invasion into the seminal vesicles via involvement of the periprostatic nerves [15,19,20]. Type III SVI describes discontinuous or meta-static lesions in the seminal vesicles [15] (Table 19.2) (Figure 19.2).

Numerous studies have evaluated the prognostic importance of seminal vesicle invasion. Most importantly, SVI decreases long-term survival in radical prostatectomy patients. An early study on the natural history of pT3b disease without nodal involvement or metastases (T3bN0M0) demon-strated that SVI decreased 7-year survival rate from 67% to 32% [22]. Looking at PCa progression, multiple studies demonstrated varying rates of 5-year biochemical recurrence-free survival. Rates ranged from 5% to 60% with a median value of 36% [23–30].

SVI is often found in cases of PCa characterized by other features independently associated with more aggressive cancer and worse prognosis. For example, incidence of SVI is associated with increasing tumor volume and increasing tumor grade as measured by Gleason score [15]. These features signify increased risks of extraprostatic extension, metastatic disease, biochemical recur-rence, and PCa-related mortality [9]. However, the presence of SVI is associated with additional risk of extraprostatic extension and lymph node metastasis [15,31].

It is very important to note that the presence of SVI does not automatically portend a con-sistently poor outcome. For example, the type of cancerous invasion is significantly correlated with prognosis. Type I spread is the most common form of SVI while type III is the least com-mon, but type I SVI is associated with worse outcomes than type III [15,30,32]. In fact, type III SVI cancers had rates of 5-year progression-free survival similar to cancers with extrapros-tatic extension but without SVI [15]. In addition, type II cancer invading directly through the

---

TABLE 19.2

Patterns of Seminal Vesicle Invasion

Patterns of Seminal Vesicle Invasion:
- Type I—via IES/ejaculatory ducts
- Type IIa—via direct invasion through prostatic base
- Type IIb—via retrograde invasion of periprostatic nerves
- Type III—discontinuous/metastatic

Source: Ohori, M. et al., *Am. J. Surg. Pathol.*, 17, 1252–1261, 1993.

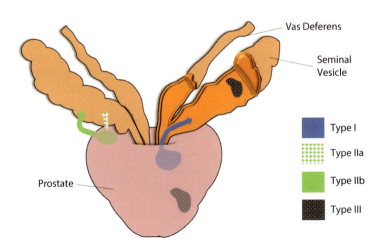

FIGURE 19.2 Types of seminal vesicle invasion.

prostatic capsule was found to have higher rates of lymph node involvement than type I, which suggests that the route of type II invasion through periprostatic soft tissue near the base of the prostate increases the likelihood of lymphatic involvement as compared to type I invasion through the ejaculatory ducts [15].

In addition, there is a difference in outcomes between intraprostatic invasion of the seminal vesicles (occurring at sites of invaginated extraprostatic space) and extraprostatic invasion of the seminal vesicles. In one study, patients with invasion limited to the intraprostatic seminal vesicle had a 5-year biochemical progression-free likelihood of 74%, which was similar to biochemical progression-free likelihood in patients without seminal vesicle invasion [19]. This was significantly higher than the less than 20% likelihood of 5-year biochemical progression-free survival for patients with extraprostatic invasion of the seminal vesicles [19].

The classification of T3b disease does not distinguish between bilateral and unilateral SVI, but research suggests that this distinction is also quite important for patient prognosis. In a study by Lee et al. [33], bilateral SVI was associated with markedly worse 5-year biochemical recurrence-free survival (4.3%) than unilateral SVI (19.8%).

CLINICAL DETECTION AND CLINICAL IMPLICATIONS OF SVI

Given the negative association of SVI with patient outcomes, clinical practice patterns for management of PCa are greatly influenced by discovery of SVI. Many surgeons consider the clinical diagnosis of SVI enough to justify excluding a patient from surgical candidacy. The argument is that rates of recurrence for cases with SVI are too high to justify exposing patients to the morbidity of radical prostatectomy. A similar argument is made for patients with very high-risk (Gleason 9 or 10) disease that may harbor subclinical metastases. Other considerations for the presence of T3 disease include the use of neoadjuvant or adjuvant androgen deprivation therapy, chemotherapy, or radiation; in addition to more careful postoperative monitoring for biochemical recurrence or local recurrence of PCa.

While SVI is a very significant feature for PCa staging, its detection poses a serious challenge. Historically, the gold standard for confirming SVI was either perioperative or postoperative pathologic analysis, but at this point the patient had already been exposed to the increased morbidity of an intensive surgical procedure. An early, accurate assessment of SVI for PCa staging is hugely beneficial to effectively and safely manage patients with PCa.

There is no one test to specifically identify SVI and traditional methods for diagnosing PCa are not ideal in this circumstance. Classically, even before the advent of PSA testing, the digital rectal examination was the standard-of-care screening method for PCa. In fact, the digital rectal examination is still a hallmark of PCa screening now used in conjunction with an elevated PSA value (generally considered to be >4.0 ng/mL) [34]. However, the digital rectal examination is limited in many ways. Primarily, a positive finding can only be detected in men with PCa of clinical stage cT2 or higher, which describes the presence of a palpable nodule suspicious for malignancy on the prostatic capsule (cT2 disease) or palpation of malignant extension to adjacent structures (cT3–4 disease) [9]. Any nonpalpable cancer (cT1 disease) will evade detection on digital rectal exam. Even cancers causing capsular bulges or extension may go undetected due to the inherent challenges presented by the prostatic anatomy relative to the rectum. A digital rectal examination preferentially samples the posterior aspects of the prostate while undersampling the apex, base, and anterior aspects [35]. If extraprostatic extension were to occur outside the region sampled by digital rectal examination, existing T3 disease may be mistakenly understaged as T1 disease. Given the location of the seminal vesicles in relation to the area commonly sampled by digital rectal examination, potentially palpable lesions of the seminal vesicles may often go undiagnosed with this screening method [36].

ULTRASOUND IMAGING AND BIOPSY FOR SVI DETECTION

The most widespread and tested method for PCa diagnosis is the transrectal ultrasound (TRUS)-guided systematic biopsy (Figure 19.3). Using real-time ultrasound imaging, the prostate is visualized and a biopsy needle is passed repeatedly through the wall of the rectum and into the prostate via the posterior aspect of the gland. Common practice is to divide the prostate into six regions and sample each region twice, medially and laterally, to obtain 12 biopsy specimens. The systematic biopsy, also termed sextant biopsy, is effectively random. The biopsy cores do not target suspicious areas of the prostate preferentially, but instead sample the same six regions regardless of differences in pre-procedure screening or imaging.

TRUS imaging alone does have some utility in preoperative PCa staging. A study by Eisenberg et al. [37] compared the accuracy of PCa staging utilizing TRUS as compared to digital rectal examination. The authors found that of the 157 patients with evidence of extraprostatic extension on final pathologic analysis, only 2 were detected on digital rectal examination. Furthermore, 50 patients (22%) without palpable disease on digital rectal examination were found to have confirmed extraprostatic extension on final pathology. These patients would be staged as cT1c (organ-confined disease) without ultrasound imaging. Regarding TRUS, an increase in suspicion for findings of extraprostatic extension correlated directly with likelihood of pathologic confirmation of pT3 disease. Of patients with no evidence of extraprostatic extension on ultrasound, 15.3% were found to have pT3 disease on final pathology as compared to 63.3% of patients with strong suspicion of extraprostatic extension on ultrasound [37]. Overall, the authors found that using TRUS to detect extraprostatic extension in nonpalpable tumors demonstrated an area under the receiver operator curve (AUC) of 0.88. Looking at long-term follow-up, the study also demonstrated a significantly improved 5-year biochemical failure-free rate for patients without evidence of extraprostatic extension on ultrasound (87%) as compared to those patients with any ultrasound evidence of extraprostatic extension (64%) [37]. For TRUS detection of SVI specifically, the authors recorded findings of 4% sensitivity, 99.8% specificity, 67% positive predictive value, 93% negative predictive value, and an AUC of 0.76 [37].

In recent years, inherent inadequacies of the TRUS-guided systematic biopsy have come to light. Much of its shortcomings resemble those of the digital rectal examination because they share a rectal approach to detect prostate pathology. Again, the apex, base, and anterior regions of the prostate

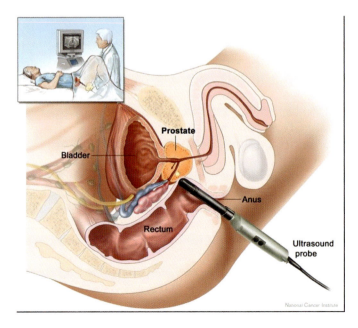

FIGURE 19.3 Transrectal ultrasound (TRUS) of the prostate.

are more difficult to sample via this biopsy approach. Additionally, TRUS-guided biopsies do not routinely sample areas outside the prostate, which includes the seminal vesicles.

However, research has demonstrated that certain preoperative characteristics indicate need for TRUS-guided biopsy of the seminal vesicles. For example, presence of bilateral samples of the prostate base positive for cancer on systematic biopsy was most significantly correlated with malignant extension into the seminal vesicles. In a study conducted by Guillonneau et al., 73.33% of patients with bilateral positive basal prostatic biopsies had extraprostatic SVI confirmed on final pathology. In comparison, 10.25% of patients with unilateral positive basal prostatic biopsies and 0% of patients with negative basal prostatic biopsies had confirmed SVI [28]. Of note, this study did not find a significant association between PSA values and SVI [28]. In a separate study, Panache-Navarrete et al. [38] suggest performing biopsy of seminal vesicles when the following are present: direct visualization during TRUS biopsy, PSA > 19.6 ng/mL, suspicious digital rectal exam findings, and small prostate volumes (<41 mL). To date, however, there is no consensus on when to biopsy seminal vesicles.

Ideally, a seminal vesicle lesion suspicious for malignancy would be visualized on TRUS imaging. A study by Wymenga et al. [39] detailed a model for targeting suspicious seminal vesicle lesions with TRUS-guided biopsy. On ultrasound, suspicious lesions are generally hypoechoic relative to the echogenicity of the peripheral zone of the prostate [39]. Once identified, the surgeon can direct the transrectal biopsy needle toward the proximal extraprostatic section of the seminal vesicle taking care to avoid sampling of the prostatic base and the distal seminal vesicle (Figure 19.4). As mentioned above, SVI can present bilaterally, which indicates a worse prognosis than unilateral SVI [33]. Therefore, it is prudent to biopsy both seminal vesicles when a suspicious lesion is identified. In this study, the surgeons successfully acquired seminal vesicle tissue in biopsies at a rate of 91%, but limited final pathology specimens were available for confirmation of seminal vesicle biopsies positive or negative for malignancy [39].

Taken together with the study conducted by Eisenberg et al. [37], this study demonstrates that use of TRUS imaging and biopsy is feasible for identification and sampling of lesions suspicious for SVI. However, the extremely low sensitivity value reported by Eisenberg et al. raises the question as to whether TRUS dramatically under-visualizes possible SVI. Lending support to this question, Enlund et al. [40] reported that 60% of pT3 prostate tumors are missed with direct ultrasound visualization.

Without improved modalities to visualize and sample seminal vesicle lesions, final pathologic analysis is the only true determination of proof for SVI. If ultrasound and systematic biopsies routinely fail to identify possible SVI, patients may be inappropriately staged and allowed to defer definitive surgical treatment in favor of active surveillance, for example. Even in cases when

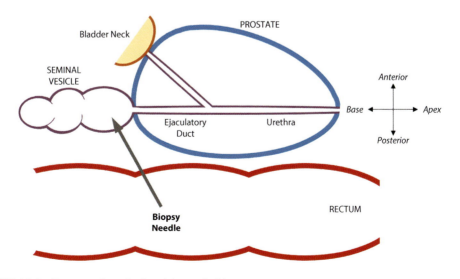

FIGURE 19.4 Transrectal seminal vesicle needle biopsy.

ultrasound does effectively diagnose T3b disease, there is little evidence suggesting it can effectively characterize the degree or type of SVI. As detailed above, the type of SVI has strong prognostic implications for disease-free survival and presence of lymph node metastasis. One can imagine how failure to detect SVI with a high degree of precision may have rippling clinical consequences. There is a clear need for more sensitive detection of SVI.

MRI FOR DETECTION OF PCa AND EXTRAPROSTATIC EXTENSION

Despite the virtually universal adoption of ultrasound imaging and guidance for prostate biopsies, magnetic resonance imaging (MRI) has gained ground as a highly effective modality for detecting and characterizing prostate lesions. More specifically, multiparametric MRI (mpMRI) has garnered attention for this purpose [41].

In present clinical practice, mpMRI incorporates T2-weighted images, diffusion-weighted images (DWI), and dynamic contrast-enhanced (DCE) MR perfusion to best assess for suspicious lesions in the prostate. T2-weighted imaging provides the highest spatial resolution and the clearest anatomy of the prostate and can identify lesions that are hypointense relative to the benign high-intensity signal tissue. Additionally, higher-grade PCa shows lower signal intensity on T2 imaging [41,42]. DWI measures the random movement of water molecules in tissue and can detect intraprostatic lesions as hyperintense due to the increased density of tumor tissue [42,43]. DWI can be used to calculate the apparent diffusion coefficient (ADC), which acts as a proxy to represent the capillary perfusion and diffusion characteristics. The numerical value gives the radiologist insight into the macroscopic architecture of the lesion [41]. DCE measures the movement of contrast agent through vasculature in rapid sequences; aberrant hypervascularity in prostate tumors results in early and pronounced enhancement distinct from benign prostatic tissue [44]. Gadolinium contrast alone is insufficient to differentiate PCa from benign tissue due to the highly vascular nature of the gland [41]. T1-weighted images are often utilized to detect the prostate contour, possible hemorrhage, or regional nodal disease (Table 19.3) [45].

Multiparametric MRI has improved detection of clinically significant PCa (Gleason score ≥7) well beyond the bounds of ultrasound imaging. It better estimates the tumor location, size, and grade; and multiple clinical studies have demonstrated high sensitivities (44%–87%) and very high negative predictive values (92%–94%) [46–50]. To aid in standardizing the correlation between mpMRI features and likelihood of clinically significant PCa, the Prostate Imaging Reporting and Data System, version 2 (PI-RADS v2) was created [51]. This is based on integration of information from each parameter of mpMRI to generate an overall risk assessment on a per-lesion basis.

In addition, mpMRI has also proven to be a successful modality for detection of extraprostatic extension via capsule invasion. In a study conducted by Raskolnikov et al. [52] on mpMRI detection of extraprostatic extension, specificity was 73.9% with a negative predictive value of 82.8%. Sensitivity for imaging identification of extraprostatic extension remains an opportunity for additional improvement [52]. However, additional research on mpMRI for pathologically confirmed extraprostatic extension reported sensitivity, specificity, positive predictive value, and negative

TABLE 19.3
mpMRI Modalities and Associated PCa Findings

MRI Modality	Imaging Function	PCa Lesion Trait
T2-weighted	Displays anatomy in high resolution	Hypointense focus
DWI	Detects tissue density	Hyperintense focus
DCE	Measures vascularity	Early enhancement
MRS	Detects metabolite resonance in 3D	Elevated choline-plus-creatine-to-citrate ratio
T1-weighted	Detects hemorrhage and nodal disease	Not used for lesion assessment

Source: Hoeks, C.M. et al., *Radiology*, 261, 46–66, 2011.

predictive value as 70.7%, 90.6%, 57.1%, and 95.1%, respectively [53]. PI-RADS v2 has also proven effective over the prior criteria (PI-RADS v1) in detecting extraprostatic extension by demonstrating increased negative predictive value (96.3%–97.1% for PI-RADS v2 versus 84.9%–89.1% for PI-RADS v1) [54]. Therefore, mpMRI continues to reduce the risk of preoperative understaging.

Research by Radtke et al. [55] retrospectively investigated how integration of mpMRI technology would change the detection of extraprostatic extension and clinical management according to well-established National Comprehensive Cancer Network (NCCN) criteria. The authors determined that mpMRI in moderate- and high-risk cohorts yielded a positive predictive value of 90.0% and 88.9%, respectively. Furthermore, the authors found that use of an mpMRI-based prognostic measure would have altered the initial surgical plan in 31.1% of cases [55]. There is also research evaluating imaging features such as distance to prostatic capsule and length of tumor contact with prostatic capsule to better predict pathologic extraprostatic extension [56,57].

MRI FOR DETECTION OF SVI

Due to the high resolution and functional capabilities of mpMRI, detection of SVI is an active area of research. The principles that make mpMRI such an attractive imaging option for visualization of prostatic lesions hold true for imaging of seminal vesicle lesions, as well. On MRI, the seminal vesicle lumen, septations, and seminal fluid are all visualized. The tissue composition appears similar to that of the prostate (benign tissue has high signal intensity on T2-weighted imaging) with the addition of high-signal intensity seminal fluid on T2-weighted MRI [58]. The similarities between benign prostate and benign seminal vesicle tissue aid in identifying malignant extension of prostate tissue.

For SVI, a set of diagnostic criteria guide detection of this pathologic feature (Table 19.4). Loss of normal seminal vesicle architecture and presence of a seminal vesicle enlargement or mass with hypointensity on T2 MRI are key in diagnosis of SVI [59,60]. Loss of seminal vesicle architecture is the most specific feature for SVI on MRI and hypointense focus on T2 MRI is the most sensitive (Figure 19.1). Predictive utility of mpMRI increases when evidence of capsular invasion is observed at the prostatic base [59]. Loss of visualization of the angle between the prostate and the seminal vesicles is also suggestive of SVI [59,61].

Magnetic resonance spectroscopy (MRS) has also been investigated for the detection of SVI. MRS images are derived from the unique resonance frequencies of protons in metabolites of selected tissue. In malignant cells, cellular metabolism is altered, which in prostate tumor tissue manifests as decreased production of citrate by epithelial cells. In addition, increased cell turnover results in increased choline-containing molecules that are involved in cell membrane maintenance. In total, the primary biomarker visualized on MRS for PCa detection is choline-plus-creatine-to-citrate ratio [41]. While MRS is able to visualize PCa in three-dimensions and may characterize tumor grade, its application is significantly limited for seminal vesical imaging [41,62]. This is because seminal vesicles have naturally elevated levels of choline and decreased levels of citrate thereby mimicking the pattern abnormality of intraprostatic lesions [63]. Furthermore, MRS demands a high level of expertise and significant time investment by patients and practitioners, which together limits its clinical practicality [41] (Table 19.5).

TABLE 19.4

mpMRI Criteria for Identification of SVI

- Loss of normal seminal vesicle architecture
- Hypointense focus on T2-weighted MRI
- Loss of visualization of angle between prostatic capsule and seminal vesicles

Source: Sala, E. et al., *Radiology*, 238, 929–937, 2006; Claus, F.G. et al., *Radiographics*, 24, S167–S180, 2004; Tyloch, J.F. et al., *J. Ultrason.*, 17, 43–58, 2017.

TABLE 19.5

Summary of Clinical Studies Evaluating MRI Detection of SVI

Author, Year	Lee et al. (2017)	Kim et al. (2010)	Ghafoori et al. (2015)	Morlacco et al. (2016)	Soylu et al. (2013)
Journal	*Can Urol Assoc J*	*Can Urol Urol J*	*Iran J Radiology*	*J Eur Uro*	*Radiology*
Data collection, enrollment years	Single-center retrospective review, 2009–2013	Single-center retrospective review, 2003–2006	Single-center retrospective, 2011–2013	Single-center retrospective, 2003–2013	Single-center retrospective, 2007–2010
n	48	32	238	501	131
Inclusion criteria	Preoperative MRI, adverse path features (PSA > 10, F/T < 0.1, PSAD > 0.15, cT3, GS > 4 or 5, or high volume disease	All intermediate- and high-risk RP patients, preoperative mpMRI	All patients with biopsy proven cancer, MRI, radical prostatectomy	All RP patients who underwent MRI with endorectal coil	Endorectal mpMRI with subsequent RP
Imaging modality/ parameters	3T MRI	1.5T MRI	1.5T MRI	1.5T MRI	1.5T MRI
	Pelvic phased array (PPA), multiparametric	PPA surface coil	Endorectal coil, PPA, T2, and contrast enhancement	Multiple, NR	mpMRI, phase array surface coil, endorectal coil
Radiologist experience	1 radiologist, >10 years	1 radiologist, NR	1 radiologist, >8 years	Multiple, NR	2 radiologists, 9 yrs, 2 yrs
Reporting	EPE and SVI	EPE SVI	Accuracy of MRI in prostate staging	Prediction of clinical variables before and after addition of MRI	Sensitivity, specificity, NPV, PPV of 3 imaging modalities (T2, DW, DCE) and agreement between radiologists
Sensitivity, specificity	EPE: 39%, 56% / SVI: 33%, 95%	EPE: 82.4%, 87.2% / SVI: 83.3%, 92.3%	SVI: 97%, 98%	NR	61%–78%, 96.6%
NPV, PPV	EPE: 45%, 50% / SVI: 50%, 91%	EPE: 93.2%, 70% / SVI: 96%, 71.4%	SVI: 99%, 94%	NR	92.2%–95.4%, 98.3%
Gold Standard comparison	Radical prostatectomy (RP) specimen	RP specimen	RP specimen	RP specimen	RP specimen
Imaging utility in prediction	Questionable	Surface coil seems to be good alternative to endorectal coil	Highly accurate	MRI adds additional predictive value to clinical models	
Notes	Prevalence of SVI 12.5%, GS 7–9 patients revealed sensitivity = 33.3% and specificity 94.9% for predicting SVI; no endorectal coil used; authors noted lower than expected results	Surface coil, small sample size	Endorectal coil significantly higher PSA and GS in patient with SVI		Between experienced and inexperienced radiologist, NPV improved significantly with T2 and DW together

Source: Soylu, F.N. et al., *Radiology*, 267, 797–806, 2013; Ghafoori, M. et al., *Iran J. Radiol.*, 12, e14556, 2015; Kim, B. et al., *Can. Urol. Assoc. J.*, 4, 257–262, 2010; Lee, T. et al., *Can. Urol. Assoc. J.*, 11, E174–E178, 2017; Morlacco, A. et al., *Eur. Urol.*, 71, 701–704, 2017.

The measured dimensions of the seminal vesicles can show rather significant variability. In a series of 82 patients who underwent radical prostatectomy, the average length was 31 ± 10.3 mm. However, the measured lengths were not associated with age, body mass index (BMI), prostate size, presence of prostatic adenoma, or sexual or urinary functional metrics (e.g., sexual health inventory for men (SHIM) and international prostate symptoms score (IPSS) scores) [64]. Therefore, the inherent anatomical variability makes seminal vesicle size an unreliable method for detection of abnormal growth or invasion. On the contrary, the manner in which the composition of the components of the seminal vesicles is displayed on mpMRI (e.g., septations, seminal fluid) is relatively consistent. For example, in a study conducted by Maeda et al. [65], abnormal signal hyperintensity on T1-weighted MRI in the seminal vesicles was observed in only 1.7% of the screening population and no associated clinical significance was found. Examinations of signal intensity or architecture on mpMRI are therefore better indicators of seminal vesicle malignancy.

LITERATURE REVIEW FOR MRI DETECTION OF SVI

A number of clinical studies have attempted to measure the diagnostic impact of mpMRI in prostate cancer staging (Table 19.6). Those that specifically address SVI are reviewed here.

In a single-center retrospective review, Soylu et al. [66] used an experienced radiologist (9 years) and an inexperienced radiologist (2 years) to read mpMRIs of the seminal vesicles in 131 patients. They compared accuracy of the reads using T2-weighted alone, T2+DWI, T2+DWI+DCE, and agreement between readers. They found that T2-weighted, when combined with DWI imaging, improved sensitivity and positive predictive value in both radiologists (sensitivity 65%–78% and 56.5%–61%, PPV 60%–82%, 52–82) [66]. Adding DCE imaging to the combined T2-weighted and DWI MR images showed no improvement in detection of SVI with either radiologist [66]. Lastly, they note that the major limitation to diagnosing SVI on MRI is that the criteria for diagnosis relies heavily on luminal extension of the tumor. Microscopic invasion of the seminal vesicle wall or microscopic foci are nearly impossible to detect without a luminal component [66]. This potentially limits the radiologist's ability to diagnose SVI in addition to creating areas for discordant reads among different practitioners.

There are several additional equipment, physician, and patient considerations to note when looking at the role of MRI in predicting SVI. As mentioned above, mpMRI is the most accurate modality with which to visualize the prostate and diagnose SVI [41].

Second, radiologist experience and expertise should be considered. In a single-center analysis of 56 patients, Allen et al. reported that an expert radiologist can increase reporting accuracy when compared to radical prostatectomy specimen (sensitivity of EPE detection increased from 50% to 72%; specificity remained the same) [67].

TABLE 19.6
Pathologies Mimicking SVI on mpMRI

SVI Mimic	Cause	mpMRI Features Similar to SVI	mpMRI Features Different from SVI
Hemorrhage	Localized trauma	T2 hypointensity	T1 hyperintensity indicative of bleeding
Amyloidosis	Aging, chronic inflammation	Narrowed/thickened seminal vesicles, T2 hypointensity	Absence of restricted diffusion on DWI
Calculi	Unknown	Focal T2 hypointensity	Low-signal DCE-MRI
Seminal vesiculitis	Prostatitis	Diffuse, focal wall thickening	Diffuse wall enhancement
Seminal vesicle atrophy	Post-radiation therapy	Fibrotic seminal vesicle wall thickening	Usually bilateral and symmetric

Source: Reddy, M.N. and Verma, S., *J. Clin. Imaging Sci.*, 4, 61, 2014.

Third, the use of endorectal coils versus surface coils has been discussed with the consensus being that endorectal coils are more accurate but that surface coils can be an acceptable alternative [68–70]. The use of endorectal coils was first detailed by Schnall et al. in 1989 to better visualize conditions in the prostate, periprostatic tissues, and seminal vesicles. In a series of 15 patients they reported increased spatial and contrast resolution, which showed promise in a more accurate assessment of tumor volume and extracapsular extension [68]. MRI technology has improved significantly since the 1980s and the practice of employing of endorectal coils to provide better resolution persists.

In a single-center retrospective analysis of 238 patients, Ghafoori et al. reported the sensitivity, specificity, negative predictive value, and positive predictive values of endorectal coils to be 97%, 98%, 99%, and 94%, respectively [69].

In a separate single-center retrospective review, Kim et al. reported that in 31 patients with elevated risk of extracapsular extension, the use of a surface coil attained a sensitivity, specificity, negative predictive value, and positive predictive value of 83.3%, 92.3%, 96%, and 71.4%, respectively. The authors surmised that while this is less accurate that endorectal coils, it is an acceptable alternative in centers without access to endorectal coils [70].

Lastly, the effects of fluid volume in the seminal vesicle must be considered when evaluating the seminal vesicles on imaging. Diagnosis of SVI requires the luminal component of the tumor to be visible [66]. When the lumen is collapsed, it may not be possible to view tumor extension into the lumen or to adequately access the seminal vesicle walls. In a single-center prospective study of 15 healthy male patients, the effects of ejaculatory abstinence were studied. Volunteers underwent 3T MRI at baseline, 1, 2, and 3 days post-ejaculation. The authors reported that seminal vesicle volume was significantly reduced 24 hours post-ejaculation and remained lower than baseline at day 2, but the volumes significantly increased over the next 2 days post-ejaculation. The authors also note that the average seminal vesicle volume was 12.47 cm³ and that ADC values reduced as volume reduced. They concluded that a period of abstinence of 3 days should be recommended for a complete exam. They also noted that standardization of pre-mpMRI procedures may reduce variability of ADC values and improve the quality and analysis of mpMRI imaging [71].

In a retrospective study of 238 patients, Kabakus et al. sought to explore the effects of abstinence on seminal vesicle volume and diagnosis of seminal vesical invasion in a clinical setting [72]. Patients were divided into groups of ejaculatory abstinence (ejaculation >3 days prior, $n = 196$) and non-abstinent (most recent ejaculation within 3 days of MRI, $n = 42$). They found that abstinent patients had statistically significantly larger seminal vesical volumes than non-abstinent (6.0 mL vs. 8.8 mL, $p = 0.011$). Additionally, they reported that in men over 60 years old who did not abstain from ejaculation starting 3 days before imaging, there was a higher risk in having a non-diagnostic study. They concluded that in men over 60, abstinence from ejaculation starting 3 days before mpMRI resulted in larger seminal vesicle volumes and decreased rates of non-diagnostic studies [72].

The study and review of seminal vesicle invasion in the clinical setting is highly important, but does not come without challenges. SVI is usually reported as a smaller component in a broader study, rather than the primary focus of studies. Studies that do focus or report on SVI typically have low numbers of enrolled patients when compared to the relatively large numbers of other prostate cancer studies. There also exist wide ranges of reported NPV (50%–90%), PPV (74%–98.3%), sensitivity (33%–97%), and specificity (92.3%–98%) in the detection of SVI with MRI [66,69,70,73,74].

There are several equipment, physician, and patient components that offer sources of variability that may complicate reporting on SVI consistently. Although consensus was reached that mpMRI is the best imaging modality for the seminal vesicles in 2011, there was a wide variety of techniques being used before then [41]. There are differences in magnetic field strength (1.5T vs. 3T) between the machines used, as well. Experience of the radiologist also plays a role as more experienced radiologists can increase the accuracy of reporting on conditions inside the seminal vesicles [67]. Components of the MRI (endorectal and surface coils) also offer variability in the detection of SVI. Although endorectal coils are considered more accurate, surface coils are used as an alternative in centers for a variety of reasons [68–70].

In addition, patient factors play a role in the rate of non-diagnostic evaluations of the seminal vesicles. The amount of fluid in the seminal vesicles, which is impacted by recent ejaculation, leads to a smaller volume of fluid in the seminal vesicles and higher rates of non-diagnostic examinations [72]. Overall, the technology and practices for evaluating conditions within the seminal vesicles are continuing to improve, but greater standardization of methodologies is needed before larger conclusions can be drawn.

DIFFERENTIAL DIAGNOSIS FOR ABNORMAL SEMINAL VESICLE MRI FINDINGS

The loss of seminal vesicle architecture or the presence of a hypointense lesion are suggestive of SVI, but can be found in association with other benign conditions (Table 19.7).

Hemorrhage into the seminal vesicles can create a localized hypointensity on T2-weighted MRI that resembles a malignant invasion [75]. Specifically, low signal intensity on T2 imaging likely represents fresh bleeding, whereas high signal intensity is more strongly correlated with old bleeding [76]. It is common to see hemorrhage in patients being worked up for PCa due to the local trauma caused by prostate needle biopsy. Most urologists defer post-biopsy MRI for at least 4 weeks to reduce the incidence of hemorrhage, but prostate hemorrhage can persist up to 4 months [75,77]. T1-weighted MR images will reveal this lesion as hemorrhage as opposed to malignancy due to the marked high-signal intensity from methemoglobin that is not normally seen in the seminal vesicles or SVI (Figure 19.2) [65,75,78].

Amyloidosis of the seminal vesicles can also resemble SVI and is relatively common in elderly men. Amyloidosis in the seminal vesicles is generally asymptomatic, but on mpMRI shows narrowed and thickened seminal vesicles lumens, and hypointensity on T2 MRI—features shared by SVI [79]. However, seminal vesicle amyloidosis will not show the restricted diffusion on DWI that is characteristic of prostate malignancy [75].

Although rare, seminal vesicle calculi can also mimic SVI with focal hypointensity [75]. They are usually symptomatic causing hematospermia and dysorgasmia [80]. Unlike SVI, seminal vesicle calculi display a low signal on DCE-MRI (Figure 19.3).

Additional pathologies that may resemble SVI include seminal vasculitis and seminal vesicle atrophy [81]. Fortunately, the multiple modalities of mpMRI and the consistent features of SVI help distinguish evidence of T3b PCa from less significant pathologies.

TABLE 19.7

Key Take Away Points of PCa Recurrence in Seminal Vesicles

- mpMRI is a very reliable imaging tool to detect local PCa recurrence in patients with BCR after primary treatment
- mpMRI after RP is indicated to diagnose small local cancer recurrence
- mpMRI can be used to more effectively target the recurrent PCa nodule with salvage RT, while minimizing complications
- Preoperative PSA and Gleason score are likely to be predictive of progression in patients with isolated SVI while positive surgical margins and capsular invasion may not necessarily be associated with progression in these patients

MRI-TRUS FUSION-GUIDED BIOPSY OF THE SEMINAL VESICLES

Although mpMRI has vastly improved the visualization of seminal vesicle lesions, the addition of tissue sampling provides more substantial evidence of SVI. TRUS biopsy of the seminal vesicles is severely limited by the low sensitivity of detecting suspicious seminal vesicle lesions on ultrasound. Instead, an MRI-based biopsy approach makes use of improved detection and characterization of intra- and extraprostatic lesions. This advantage has spurred the development of targeted biopsies.

In brief, an mpMRI-TRUS fusion-guided biopsy combines the high spatial resolution provided by mpMRI with the real-time imaging of the ultrasound during biopsy. While some practitioners are able to visualize the mpMR and ultrasound images separately to guide biopsy target location (termed "cognitive fusion"), this technique is heavily influenced by practitioner experience and does not make use of the full breadth of information provided by mpMRI [82]. Another approach, in-gantry MRI for transperineal prostate biopsies, was developed to utilize real-time MRI findings, but it is a resource- and time-intensive procedure. Instead, multiple software-device platforms digitally combine the mpMRI with the real-time ultrasound (termed "fusion biopsy") to aid in overcoming potential learning curves and more precisely sample lesions [48,82]. Targeted biopsies more accurately sample clinically significant PCa lesions and decrease the risk of cancer upgrading on final pathology to better inform therapeutic approaches [46,83,84].

As discussed earlier, systematic biopsies rely on a sextant strategy that may undersample lesions in the anterior, apical, or basal prostate in addition to the seminal vesicles. Fusion biopsies allow for histologic confirmation of those patients who require investigation of the seminal vesicles.

A study by Raskolnikov et al. [63] set forth a model for seminal vesical biopsy via a fusion platform. Between 2007 and 2013, 25 out of 822 scanned patients were found to have lesions suspicious for SVI based on mpMRI. In this protocol, mpMRI of the prostate was performed on a 3 T MRI machine with use of an endorectal coil. Sequences included tri-planar T2-weighted, DCE, DWI, and MRS. Patients then underwent a TRUS-guided systematic biopsy in addition to targeted biopsies of each lesion visible on MRI in the same biopsy session. When clinically indicated, patients underwent robotic-assisted radical prostatectomy and specimens were analyzed by a single genitourinary pathologist. Thirty-one lesions suspicious for SVI were identified within the 25 selected patients; 20/31 (65%) lesions had targeted biopsy findings positive for SVI, 6 sampled benign tissue, and 5 contained only fibroadipose tissue. Although only four patients underwent both targeted seminal vesical biopsy and radical prostatectomy, all four of these patients had agreement of SVI on biopsy and final pathology [63].

In a case study presented by Somwaru et al. [85], fusion biopsy was able to successfully detect a focus of malignant ectopic prostate tissue in one seminal vesicle. Repeat 12-core sextant biopsies yielded benign prostatic tissue (including at the prostatic base), but with use of mpMRI-TRUS fusion-guided biopsy, a suspicious lesion was visualized in the left seminal vesicle and sampled to confirm Gleason 7 (4 + 3) primary PCa arising in the seminal vesicle without glandular or transcapsular involvement. This was staged as T3b disease and the patient was treated with external beam radiation plus androgen deprivation therapy [85]. The repeated benign systematic biopsies may have merely indicated follow-up PSA testing without intervention.

By extending the established principles of mpMRI-TRUS fusion-guided prostate biopsy to include lesions of the seminal vesicles, SVI can potentially be detected with greater accuracy and confidence than with systematic biopsies or mpMRI alone.

PREDICTIVE NOMOGRAMS FOR SVI RISK ESTIMATION

Predictive nomograms have been developed in order to assign risk of SVI (and other pathologic features) to a patient through consideration of various sources of information including demographic, clinical, and pathologic data. Prior to adoption of mpMRI in PCa staging, clinicians sought to bridge the gap in predicting extraprostatic extension and associated clinical outcomes with nomograms. Widely used nomograms for prediction of SVI prior to radical prostatectomy include the 2007 update of Partin tables, the European Society for Urologic Oncology (ESUO), the Gallina nomogram, the Kattan staging nomogram, and the Cancer of the Prostate Risk Assessment (CAPRA) score [74,86–89]. Together these models utilize preoperative PSA, age, clinical staging, and systematic biopsy data such as Gleason score and percentage of positive cores. In comparing the relative value in predicting SVI between the 2007 Partin, ESUO, and Gallina nomograms, the AUC for each was found to be 0.805, 0.792, and 0.692, respectively. All of the nomograms demonstrated high sensitivities, but low specificities and extremely low positive predictive values [90].

Of note, none of the three nomograms above utilize imaging data as part of their predictive modeling. Wang et al. [89] studied the potential effect of imaging on predictive capability by including MRI with the Kattan staging nomogram. Using a 1.5T endorectal MRI, the authors established that the AUC for MRI plus Kattan nomogram (0.87) was significantly improved over either the Kattan nomogram (0.80) or MRI (0.76) alone [89].

In a separate study, Morlacco et al. [74] evaluated the predictive effect of adding preoperative 1.5T endorectal MRI to the Partin and CAPRA nomograms. They identified that the AUC for predicting SVI with was markedly improved when using the Partin table with MRI (0.82 vs. 0.75) and the CAPRA score with MRI (0.83 vs. 0.75) versus the nomograms alone [74]. Based on these findings, there is clear opportunity for improvement in predictive capabilities of nomograms by formally incorporating MRI information and even seminal vesicle targeted biopsy data.

USE OF MRI FOR DETECTION OF PCa RECURRENCE IN THE SEMINAL VESICLES

The role of mpMRI is not only limited to detection, localization, and staging of prostate cancer but also extends to cases of active surveillance, patients refusing biopsy, targeted biopsy, and diagnosis of recurrence after treatment [91]. The definition of biochemical failure (BCR) differs between radical prostatectomy (RP), defined as two consecutive PSA values > 0.2 ng/mL, and radiation therapy (RT), defined as a PSA increase >2 ng/mL higher than the initial PSA nadir value [92,93]. However, it is important to note that BCR detected through a persistently elevated PSA does not necessarily imply local recurrence but can also be due to distant metastases or residual glandular healthy tissue in the post-prostatectomy bed. Therefore, an imaging procedure is often carried out in patients with BCR after primary treatment to distinguish between local PCa recurrence and distant spread of disease [94]. Compared to other imaging modalities such as PET/CT, which has a poor detection rate of small lesions, mpMRI possesses superior contrast and spatial resolution and is emerging as a promising modality for evaluation of recurrent PCa [95].

Salvage RT is generally performed when post-RP local recurrence is recognized. The accurate identification of local recurrence with mpMRI represents an emerging modality for evaluation of the prostatic fossa after RP, potentially improving the effectiveness of salvage RT by allowing for a targeted increase in radiation dose in areas of known disease recurrence [96]. Local recurrence in the seminal vesicles appears similar to SVI on mpMRI (Table 19.4). This is apparent with cases of failed focal therapy or brachytherapy for which the prostate is not excised (Figure 19.4). Following RP with removal of the prostate and seminal vesicles, however, a recurrent PCa can be recognized as an area of slightly increased T2 signal intensity relative to adjacent musculature in a soft tissue mass in the surgical bed, with rapid wash-in and washout, as well as restricted diffusion on DCE [97].

Common sites of local recurrence are retrovesical, at the vesicourethral anastomosis around the urinary bladder or membranous urethra, at the resection site of the vas deferens and at the anterior or lateral surgical margins of the prostatectomy bed. After RP, fibrosis and atrophic remnants of seminal vesicles are observed in approximately 20% of patients and must be distinguished from local relapse. Fibrotic remnants of seminal vesicles demonstrate very low signal intensity. In cases where a seminal vesicle shows an area of focally increased T2 signal intensity, it may be mimicking a local recurrence. However, retained seminal vesicles would not demonstrate diffusion restriction or rapid contrast wash-in and washout on DCE as a recurrent PCa would [98].

Local salvage therapy should be undertaken early in patients with local recurrence after RT, as the median time to development of distant metastases is approximately 3 years [99]. Salvage therapies in patients with local recurrence after RT include additional irradiation of the prostate, RP, cryosurgery, transrectal high-intensity focused ultrasound (HIFU), and laser ablation [100]. In order to perform focal salvage therapies more effectively, there is an increased need for imaging techniques to be able to identify and localize recurrent PCa.

Currently, mpMRI is considered to be the gold standard imaging technique in localizing recurrent PCa in patients with BCR after RT. Compared to recurrent PCa after RP, which shows a lightly high signal intensity in T2-weighted images, recurrent PCa after radiotherapy shows a low signal intensity on T2 MRI. However, the findings on DWI and DCE are the same for both recurrent PCa after RT and recurrent PCa after RP with restricted diffusion on DWI and rapid wash-in and wash-out on DCE.

In addition to the finding of decreased signal intensity on T2-weighted images, the entire prostate and the seminal vesicles are decreased in size after RT and the peripheral, central, and transition zones appear less distinct from each other [98,101]. RT induces glandular atrophy and fibrosis that may result in changes in PCa such as decreased size, reduced capsular bulging, capsular irregularity, or decreased extracapsular extension as well as changes in the appearance of adjacent anatomic structures including increased bladder or rectal wall thickness, thickening of the perirectal fascia, and increased signal intensity of the pelvic side wall musculature. Because both the recurrent tumor and the normal surrounding parenchyma appear hypointense on T2 MRI, T2 MRI alone is limited in its ability to detect recurrent PCa after RT [102]. It is hypothesized that detecting PCa recurrence after RT may still be possible on T2 MRI alone if the PCa recurrence produces an additional focal reduction in signal intensity [103,104]. However, it may be easier to identify a recurrent disease using DCE than with T2 MRI because of the different patterns between recurrence and post-radiation fibrosis on DCE. Recurrent tissue presents as a hypervascular early enhancing homogenous nodule after RT, whereas the surrounding prostatic tissue has homogenous, slow and low enhancement [94]. Due to an increase in perfusion and blood volume as a result of inflammation after RT, DCE should be performed at least 3 months after RT.

Using TRUS-guided biopsy as the standard of reference, Roy et al. [105] evaluated the sensitivity in the detection of post-RT local PCa recurrence of the three types of functional MRI. Thirty-two patients with local recurrence after external beam radiation therapy (EBRT) were enrolled in this study. The sensitivity was highest for T2+DWI+DCE (100%) followed by, in decreasing order: T2+DWI, DCE alone, and DWI alone (94%); T2+DCE (91%); T2+DWI+DCE+MRS (76%); T2WI and MRSI alone (74%); and lastly T2+MRSI (44%).

RISK FACTORS FOR PROGRESSION AFTER RP WITH SVI

There have been several studies attempting to evaluate the risk factors for progression after RP in patients with SVI. Epstein et al. [106] demonstrated that in a group of 45 patients with SVI, Gleason score of the RP specimen, capsular invasion, as well as surgical margin status were independent risk factors for progression. However, when the analysis was restricted to tumors with seminal vesicle invasion without lymph node involvement, the surgical margin and the Gleason score were not statistically significant predictors. Tefilli et al. [29] demonstrated in a study of 93 patients with isolated SVI that positive surgical margins, Gleason score greater than 7, and preoperative PSA level greater than 10 ng/mL were independent predictive factors for progression. In another study of 137 patients with isolated seminal vesicle invasion without lymph node involvement, Salomon et al. [107] found that preoperative PSA and Gleason score of the RP specimen were independent factors for progression. Neither capsular invasion nor positive surgical margins predicted progression.

In addition to Salomon et al. [107] and Epstein et al. [106], Debras et al. [108], Ohori et al. [30], and Sofer et al. [109] also found that positive surgical margins are not an independent risk factor for progression in patients with isolated SVI without lymph node involvement. In their study of

52 patients, Debras et al. [108] distinguished between proximal invasion of the seminal vesicles from invasion of the free part of the seminal vesicle. On multivariate analysis, they found that invasion of the free, distal part of the seminal vesicle as well as the Gleason score of the RP specimen were the only independent factors predictive of progression. According to this model, the tumor volume, extracapsular extension, and surgical margin status were not significant predictive factors of progression [108].

If positive surgical margins are not predictive of progression in patients with isolated SVI after RP, it may be because SVI is per se a poor prognostic factor [107]. Despite SVI being associated with a poor prognosis, it is not equivalent to having metastatic disease; for example, 34% of patients in the study by Salomon et al. [107] were free of biochemical progression at 5 years, 65% of the patients with SVI and negative surgical margins were progression free 5 years after RP in the study by Tefilli et al. [29], and 53% of the patients were progression free after approximately 4 years in the study by Sofer et al. [109].

CONCLUSIONS

As the urologic oncology community moves further into an era of MR imaging for PCa assessment, the ability of MRI to stage PCa for extraprostatic extension will have great utility. Based on the success of mpMRI and fusion-guided targeted biopsy to improve diagnosis of PCa, MRI-based detection of extraprostatic pathologic features shows significant potential. At present, formalization of this clinical practice is still in a relatively nascent stage, while MRI technology is advancing at a rapid pace.

Current literature presents a wide range of results regarding the effectiveness of MRI for SVI detection, which makes determination of the best imaging parameters challenging. Previous studies have established that mpMRI detection of SVI is feasible and displays many advantages over traditional imaging modalities. One example of this is the potential utilization of fusion-guided targeted biopsies to obtain seminal vesicle samples for presurgical histopathologic confirmation. However, while the management implications of incorrectly staging PCa are apparent and significant, additional studies capturing a greater number of patients are needed to better understand how MRI will truly impact clinical decisions and outcomes.

Greater adoption of MRI is consistently hampered by the resource and financial demands of this technology. PCa is a common malignancy that is being treated in various healthcare settings, not solely in large academic medical centers, so access to MRI is not consistent. As more clinical studies measure the accuracy of SVI detection via MRI, future work should aim to identify the financial and quality-of-life implications of this PCa staging approach. Given the wide-ranging impact of initial clinical decisions, which may be based on incorrect staging, and the dramatic consequences of extraprostatic extension on long-term prognosis, there is great potential for MRI staging to reduce these painful (and potentially avoidable) outcomes.

As is true with other urologic malignancies, MRI for SVI detection shows promise. With continued development, MRI may be able to diagnose extraprostatic extension with the same degree of sophistication as is seen for diagnosis of intraprostatic lesions.

REFERENCES

1. A. Villers, J. E. McNeal, F. S. Freiha, and T. A. Stamey, Multiple cancers in the prostate: Morphologic features of clinically recognized versus incidental tumors, *Cancer*, 70, 2313–18, 1992.
2. A. M. Wise, T. A. Stamey, J. E. McNeal, and J. L. Clayton, Morphologic and clinical significance of multifocal prostate cancers in radical prostatectomy specimens, *Urology*, 60, 264–9, 2002.
3. S. R. Bott, H. U. Ahmed, R. G. Hindley, A. Abdul-Rahman, A. Freeman, and M. Emberton, The index lesion and focal therapy: An analysis of the pathological characteristics of prostate cancer, *BJU Int*, 106, 1607–11, 2010.
4. W. Liu, S. Laitinen, S. Khan, M. Vihinen, J. Kowalski, G. Yu, et al., Copy number analysis indicates monoclonal origin of lethal metastatic prostate cancer, *Nat Med*, 15, 559–65, 2009.

5. M. Noguchi, T. A. Stamey, J. E. McNeal, and R. Nolley, Prognostic factors for multifocal prostate cancer in radical prostatectomy specimens: Lack of significance of secondary cancers, *J Urol*, 170, 459–63, 2003.

6. J. Li, J. A. Djenaba, A. Soman, S. H. Rim, and V. A. Master, Recent trends in prostate cancer incidence by age, cancer stage, and grade, the United States, 2001–2007, *Prostate Cancer*, 2012, 691380, 2012.

7. C. Buzzoni, A. Auvinen, M. J. Roobol, S. Carlsson, S. M. Moss, D. Puliti, et al., Metastatic prostate cancer incidence and prostate-specific antigen testing: New insights from the European randomized study of screening for prostate cancer, *Eur Urol*, 68, 885–90, 2015.

8. C. H. Lee, O. Akin-Olugbade, and A. Kirschenbaum, Overview of prostate anatomy, histology, and pathology, *Endocrinol Metab Clin North Am*, 40, 565–75, viii–ix, 2011.

9. A. W. Partin, M. W. Kattan, E. N. Subong, P. C. Walsh, K. J. Wojno, J. E. Oesterling, et al., Combination of prostate-specific antigen, clinical stage, and Gleason score to predict pathological stage of localized prostate cancer: A multi-institutional update, *JAMA*, 277, 1445–51, 1997.

10. M. Peacock, J. Quirt, W. James Morris, A. So, C. K. Sing, T. Pickles, et al., Population-based 10-year event-free survival after radical prostatectomy for patients with prostate cancer in British Columbia, *Can Urol Assoc J*, 9, 409–13, 2015.

11. J. Mikel Hubanks, S. A. Boorjian, I. Frank, M. T. Gettman, R. Houston Thompson, L. J. Rangel, et al., The presence of extracapsular extension is associated with an increased risk of death from prostate cancer after radical prostatectomy for patients with seminal vesicle invasion and negative lymph nodes, *Urol Oncol*, 32, 26 e1–7, 2014.

12. K. Miyai, A. Kristiansen, L. Egevad, S. Pina-Oviedo, M. K. Divatia, S. S. Shen, et al., Seminal vesicle intraepithelial involvement by prostate cancer: Putative mechanism and clinicopathological significance, *Hum Pathol*, 45, 1805–12, 2014.

13. Y. Huang, S. Isharwal, A. Haese, F. K. Chun, D. V. Makarov, Z. Feng, et al., Prediction of patient-specific risk and percentile cohort risk of pathological stage outcome using continuous prostate-specific antigen measurement, clinical stage and biopsy Gleason score, *BJU Int*, 107, 1562–9, 2011.

14. T. A. Masterson, J. A. Pettus, R. G. Middleton, and R. A. Stephenson, Isolated seminal vesicle invasion imparts better outcomes after radical retropubic prostatectomy for clinically localized prostate cancer: Prognostic stratification of pt3b disease by nodal and margin status, *Urology*, 66, 152–5, 2005.

15. M. Ohori, P. T. Scardino, S. L. Lapin, C. Seale-Hawkins, J. Link, and T. M. Wheeler, The mechanisms and prognostic significance of seminal vesicle involvement by prostate cancer, *Am J Surg Pathol*, 17, 1252–61, 1993.

16. A. A. Villers, J. E. McNeal, E. A. Redwine, F. S. Freiha, and T. A. Stamey, Pathogenesis and biological significance of seminal vesicle invasion in prostatic adenocarcinoma, *J Urol*, 143, 1183–7, 1990.

17. E. Mukamel, J. B. deKernion, J. Hannah, R. B. Smith, D. G. Skinner, and W. E. Goodwin, The incidence and significance of seminal vesicle invasion in patients with adenocarcinoma of the prostate, *Cancer*, 59, 1535–8, 1987.

18. D. M. Berney, T. M. Wheeler, D. J. Grignon, J. I. Epstein, D. F. Griffiths, P. A. Humphrey, et al., International Society of Urological Pathology (ISUP) Consensus Conference on Handling and Staging of Radical Prostatectomy Specimens. Working group 4: Seminal vesicles and lymph nodes, *Mod Pathol*, 24, 39–47, 2011.

19. S. R. Potter, J. I. Epstein, and A. W. Partin, Seminal vesicle invasion by prostate cancer: Prognostic significance and therapeutic implications, *Rev Urol*, 2, 190–5, 2000.

20. M. Ohori, M. W. Kattan, C. Yu, K. Matsumoto, T. Satoh, J. Ishii, et al., Nomogram to predict seminal vesicle invasion using the status of cancer at the base of the prostate on systematic biopsy, *Int J Urol*, 17, 534–40, 2010.

21. J. Arista-Nasr, A. Trolle-Silva, E. Aguilar-Ayala, and B. Martinez-Benitez, Seminal epithelium in prostate biopsy can mimic malignant and premalignant prostatic lesions, *Actas Urol Esp*, 40, 17–22, 2016.

22. D. P. Byar and F. K. Mostofi, Carcinoma of the prostate: Prognostic evaluation of certain pathologic features in 208 radical prostatectomies: Examined by the step-section technique, *Cancer*, 30, 5–13, 1972.

23. A. V. D'Amico, R. Whittington, S. B. Malkowicz, D. Schultz, M. Schnall, J. E. Tomaszewski, et al., A multivariate analysis of clinical and pathological factors that predict for prostate specific antigen failure after radical prostatectomy for prostate cancer, *J Urol*, 154, 131–8, 1995.

24. D. van den Ouden, W. C. Hop, R. Kranse, and F. H. Schroder, Tumour control according to pathological variables in patients treated by radical prostatectomy for clinically localized carcinoma of the prostate, *Br J Urol*, 79, 203–11, 1997.

25. W. J. Catalona and D. S. Smith, 5-year tumor recurrence rates after anatomical radical retropubic prostatectomy for prostate cancer, *J Urol*, 152, 1837–42, 1994.

26. J. G. Trapasso, J. B. deKernion, R. B. Smith, and F. Dorey, The incidence and significance of detectable levels of serum prostate specific antigen after radical prostatectomy, *J Urol*, 152, 1821–5, 1994.
27. J. I. Epstein, A. W. Partin, J. Sauvageot, and P. C. Walsh, Prediction of progression following radical prostatectomy: A multivariate analysis of 721 men with long-term follow-up, *Am J Surg Pathol*, 20, 286–92, 1996.
28. B. Guillonneau, B. Debras, B. Veillon, J. Bougaran, E. Chambon, and G. Vallancien, Indications for preoperative seminal vesicle biopsies in staging of clinically localized prostatic cancer, *Eur Urol*, 32, 160–5, 1997.
29. M. V. Tefilli, E. L. Gheiler, R. Tiguert, M. Banerjee, W. Sakr, D. J. Grignon, et al., Prognostic indicators in patients with seminal vesicle involvement following radical prostatectomy for clinically localized prostate cancer, *J Urol*, 160, 802–6, 1998.
30. M. Ohori, T. M. Wheeler, M. W. Kattan, Y. Goto, and P. T. Scardino, Prognostic significance of positive surgical margins in radical prostatectomy specimens, *J Urol*, 154, 1818–24, 1995.
31. N. N. Stone, R. G. Stock, D. Parikh, P. Yeghiayan, and P. Unger, Perineural invasion and seminal vesicle involvement predict pelvic lymph node metastasis in men with localized carcinoma of the prostate, *J Urol*, 160, 1722–6, 1998.
32. A. Kristiansen, F. Wiklund, P. Wiklund, and L. Egevad, Prognostic significance of patterns of seminal vesicle invasion in prostate cancer, *Histopathology*, 62, 1049–56, 2013.
33. H. J. Lee, J. H. Han, D. H. Lee, J. K. Nam, T. N. Kim, M. K. Chung, et al., Does bilateral seminal vesicle invasion at radical prostatectomy predict worse prognosis than unilateral invasion among patients with pT3b prostate cancers? *Int J Urol*, 23, 758–63, 2016.
34. J. Philip, S. Dutta Roy, M. Ballal, C. S. Foster, and P. Javle, Is a digital rectal examination necessary in the diagnosis and clinical staging of early prostate cancer? *BJU Int*, 95, 969–71, 2005.
35. C. Bolenz, M. Gierth, R. Grobholz, T. Kopke, A. Semjonow, C. Weiss, et al., Clinical staging error in prostate cancer: Localization and relevance of undetected tumour areas, *BJU Int*, 103, 1184–9, 2009.
36. W. J. Catalona, J. P. Richie, F. R. Ahmann, M. A. Hudson, P. T. Scardino, R. C. Flanigan, et al., Comparison of digital rectal examination and serum prostate specific antigen in the early detection of prostate cancer: Results of a multicenter clinical trial of 6,630 men, *J Urol*, 197, S200–S207, 2017.
37. M. L. Eisenberg, J. E. Cowan, B. J. Davies, P. R. Carroll, and K. Shinohara, The importance of tumor palpability and transrectal ultrasonographic appearance in the contemporary clinical staging of prostate cancer, *Urol Oncol*, 29, 171–6, 2011.
38. J. Panach-Navarrete, F. Garcia-Morata, J. A. Hernandez-Medina, and J. M. Martinez-Jabaloyas, When to biopsy seminal vesicles, *Actas Urol Esp*, 39, 203–209, 2015.
39. L. F. Wymenga, F. J. Duisterwinkel, K. Groenier, and H. J. Mensink, Ultrasound-guided seminal vesicle biopsies in prostate cancer, *Prostate Cancer Prostatic Dis*, 3, 100–106, 2000.
40. A. Enlund, K. Pedersen, B. Boeryd, and E. Varenhorst, Transrectal ultrasonography compared to histo-pathological assessment for local staging of prostatic carcinoma, *Acta Radiol*, 31, 597–600, 1990.
41. C. M. Hoeks, J. O. Barentsz, T. Hambrock, D. Yakar, D. M. Somford, S. W. Heijmink, et al., Prostate cancer: Multiparametric MR imaging for detection, localization, and staging, *Radiology*, 261, 46–66, 2011.
42. H. Hricak, P. L. Choyke, S. C. Eberhardt, S. A. Leibel, and P. T. Scardino, Imaging prostate cancer: A multidisciplinary perspective, *Radiology*, 243, 28–53, 2007.
43. A. Qayyum, Diffusion-weighted imaging in the abdomen and pelvis: Concepts and applications, *Radiographics*, 29, 1797–810, 2009.
44. S. Verma, B. Turkbey, N. Muradyan, A. Rajesh, F. Cornud, M. A. Haider, et al., Overview of dynamic contrast-enhanced MRI in prostate cancer diagnosis and management, *AJR Am J Roentgenol*, 198, 1277–88, 2012.
45. D. Bonekamp, M. A. Jacobs, R. El-Khouli, D. Stoianovici, and K. J. Macura, Advancements in MR imaging of the prostate: From diagnosis to interventions, *Radiographics*, 31, 677–703, 2011.
46. M. M. Siddiqui, S. Rais-Bahrami, B. Turkbey, A. K. George, J. Rothwax, N. Shakir, et al., Comparison of MR/ultrasound fusion-guided biopsy with ultrasound-guided biopsy for the diagnosis of prostate cancer, *JAMA*, 313, 390–7, 2015.
47. A. R. Rastinehad, B. Turkbey, S. S. Salami, O. Yaskiv, A. K. George, M. Fakhoury, et al., Improving detection of clinically significant prostate cancer: Magnetic resonance imaging/transrectal ultrasound fusion guided prostate biopsy, *J Urol*, 191, 1749–54, 2014.
48. J. S. Wysock, A. B. Rosenkrantz, W. C. Huang, M. D. Stifelman, H. Lepor, F. M. Deng, et al., A prospective, blinded comparison of magnetic resonance (MR) imaging-ultrasound fusion and visual estimation in the performance of MR-targeted prostate biopsy: The PROFUS trial, *Eur Urol*, 66, 343–51, 2014.

49. B. Calio, A. Sidana, D. Sugano, S. Gaur, A. Jain, M. Maruf, et al., Changes in prostate cancer detection rate of MRI-TRUS fusion vs systematic biopsy over time: Evidence of a learning curve, *Prostate Cancer Prostatic Dis*, 2017.

50. J. J. Futterer, A. Briganti, P. De Visschere, M. Emberton, G. Giannarini, A. Kirkham, et al., Can clinically significant prostate cancer be detected with multiparametric magnetic resonance imaging? A systematic review of the literature, *Eur Urol*, 68, 1045–53, 2015.

51. H. A. Vargas, A. M. Hotker, D. A. Goldman, C. S. Moskowitz, T. Gondo, K. Matsumoto, et al., Updated prostate imaging reporting and data system (PIRADS v2) recommendations for the detection of clinically significant prostate cancer using multiparametric MRI: Critical evaluation using whole-mount pathology as standard of reference, *Eur Radiol*, 26, 1606–12, 2016.

52. D. Raskolnikov, A. K. George, S. Rais-Bahrami, B. Turkbey, M. M. Siddiqui, N. A. Shakir, et al., The role of magnetic resonance image guided prostate biopsy in stratifying men for risk of extracapsular extension at radical prostatectomy, *J Urol*, 194, 105–11, 2015.

53. T. S. Feng, A. R. Sharif-Afshar, S. C. Smith, J. Miller, C. Nguyen, Q. Li, et al., Multiparametric magnetic resonance imaging localizes established extracapsular extension of prostate cancer, *Urol Oncol*, 33, 109 e15–22, 2015.

54. Y. Matsuoka, J. Ishioka, H. Tanaka, T. Kimura, S. Yoshida, K. Saito, et al., Impact of the prostate imaging reporting and data system, Version 2, on MRI diagnosis for extracapsular extension of prostate cancer, *AJR Am J Roentgenol*, 209, W76–84, 2017.

55. J. P. Radtke, S. Boxler, T. H. Kuru, M. B. Wolf, C. D. Alt, I. V. Popeneciu, et al., Improved detection of anterior fibromuscular stroma and transition zone prostate cancer using biparametric and multiparametric MRI with MRI-targeted biopsy and MRI-US fusion guidance, *Prostate Cancer Prostatic Dis*, 18, 288–96, 2015.

56. E. Baco, E. Rud, L. Vlatkovic, A. Svindland, H. B. Eggesbo, A. J. Hung, et al., Predictive value of magnetic resonance imaging determined tumor contact length for extracapsular extension of prostate cancer, *J Urol*, 193, 466–72, 2015.

57. R. Gupta, R. O'Connell, A. M. Haynes, P. D. Stricker, W. Barrett, J. J. Turner, et al., Extraprostatic extension (EPE) of prostatic carcinoma: Is its proximity to the surgical margin or Gleason score important?, *BJU Int*, 116, 343–50, 2015.

58. B. Kim, A. Kawashima, J. A. Ryu, N. Takahashi, R. P. Hartman, and B. F. King, Jr., Imaging of the seminal vesicle and vas deferens, *Radiographics*, 29, 1105–21, 2009.

59. E. Sala, O. Akin, C. S. Moskowitz, H. F. Eisenberg, K. Kuroiwa, N. M. Ishill, et al., Endorectal MR imaging in the evaluation of seminal vesicle invasion: Diagnostic accuracy and multivariate feature analysis, *Radiology*, 238, 929–37, 2006.

60. F. G. Claus, H. Hricak, and R. R. Hattery, Pretreatment evaluation of prostate cancer: Role of MR imaging and 1H MR spectroscopy, *Radiographics*, 24 Suppl 1, S167–80, 2004.

61. J. F. Tyloch and A. P. Wieczorek, The standards of an ultrasound examination of the prostate gland. Part 2, *J Ultrason*, 17, 43–58, 2017.

62. T. Kobus, T. Hambrock, C. A. Hulsbergen-van de Kaa, A. J. Wright, J. O. Barentsz, A. Heerschap, et al., In vivo assessment of prostate cancer aggressiveness using magnetic resonance spectroscopic imaging at 3 T with an endorectal coil, *Eur Urol*, 60, 1074–80, 2011.

63. D. Raskolnikov, A. K. George, S. Rais-Bahrami, B. Turkbey, N. A. Shakir, C. Okoro, et al., Multiparametric magnetic resonance imaging and image-guided biopsy to detect seminal vesicle invasion by prostate cancer, *J Endourol*, 28, 1283–9, 2014.

64. O. N. Gofrit, K. C. Zorn, J. B. Taxy, G. P. Zagaja, G. D. Steinberg, and A. L. Shalhav, The dimensions and symmetry of the seminal vesicles, *J Robot Surg*, 3, 29–33, 2009.

65. E. Maeda, M. Katsura, W. Gonoi, T. Yoshikawa, N. Hayashi, H. Ohtsu, et al., Abnormal signal intensities of the seminal vesicles in a screening population, *J Magn Reson Imaging*, 39, 1426–30, 2014.

66. F. N. Soylu, Y. Peng, Y. Jiang, S. Wang, C. Schmid-Tannwald, I. Sethi, et al., Seminal vesicle invasion in prostate cancer: Evaluation by using multiparametric endorectal MR imaging, *Radiology*, 267, 797–806, 2013.

67. D. J. Allen, R. Hindley, S. Clovis, P. O'Donnell, D. Cahill, G. Rottenberg, et al., Does body-coil magnetic-resonance imaging have a role in the preoperative staging of patients with clinically localized prostate cancer?, *BJU Int*, 94, 534–8, 2004.

68. M. D. Schnall, R. E. Lenkinski, H. M. Pollack, Y. Imai, and H. Y. Kressel, Prostate: MR imaging with an endorectal surface coil, *Radiology*, 172, 570–4, 1989.

69. M. Ghafoori, M. Alavi, M. Shakiba, and K. Hoseini, The value of prostate MRI with endorectal coil in detecting seminal vesicle involvement in patients with prostate cancer, *Iran J Radiol*, 12, e14556, 2015.

70. B. Kim, R. H. Breau, D. Papadatos, D. Fergusson, S. Doucette, I. Cagiannos, et al., Diagnostic accuracy of surface coil magnetic resonance imaging at 1.5 T for local staging of elevated risk prostate cancer, *Can Urol Assoc J*, 4, 257–62, 2010.

71. T. Barrett, J. Tanner, A. B. Gill, R. A. Slough, J. Wason, and F. A. Gallagher, The longitudinal effect of ejaculation on seminal vesicle fluid volume and whole-prostate ADC as measured on prostate MRI, *Eur Radiol*, 27, 12, 5236–5243, 2017.

72. I. M. Kabakus, S. Borofsky, F. V. Mertan, M. Greer, D. Daar, B. J. Wood, et al., Does abstinence from ejaculation before prostate MRI improve evaluation of the seminal vesicles? *AJR Am J Roentgenol*, 207, 1205–1209, 2016.

73. T. Lee, J. Hoogenes, I. Wright, E. D. Matsumoto, and B. Shayegan, Utility of preoperative 3 Tesla pelvic phased-array multiparametric magnetic resonance imaging in prediction of extracapsular extension and seminal vesicle invasion of prostate cancer and its impact on surgical margin status: Experience at a Canadian academic tertiary care centre, *Can Urol Assoc J*, 11, E174–8, 2017.

74. A. Morlacco, V. Sharma, B. R. Viers, L. J. Rangel, R. E. Carlson, A. T. Froemming, et al., The incremental role of magnetic resonance imaging for prostate cancer staging before radical prostatectomy, *Eur Urol*, 71, 701–704, 2017.

75. M. N. Reddy and S. Verma, Lesions of the seminal vesicles and their MRI characteristics, *J Clin Imaging Sci*, 4, 61, 2014.

76. S. Furuya, R. Furuya, N. Masumori, T. Tsukamoto, and M. Nagaoka, Magnetic resonance imaging is accurate to detect bleeding in the seminal vesicles in patients with hemospermia, *Urology*, 72, 838–42, 2008.

77. S. White, H. Hricak, R. Forstner, J. Kurhanewicz, D. B. Vigneron, C. J. Zaloudek, et al., Prostate cancer: Effect of postbiopsy hemorrhage on interpretation of MR images, *Radiology*, 195, 385–90, 1995.

78. S. A. Mirowitz, Seminal vesicles: Biopsy-related hemorrhage simulating tumor invasion at endorectal MR imaging, *Radiology*, 185, 373–6, 1992.

79. Y. Kaji, K. Sugimura, S. Nagaoka, and T. Ishida, Amyloid deposition in seminal vesicles mimicking tumor invasion from bladder cancer: MR findings, *J Comput Assist Tomogr*, 16, 989–91, 1992.

80. A. Parnham, Rare cause of painful ejaculation, *J Sex Med*, 13, S201–S202, 2016.

81. G. Dagur, K. Warren, Y. Suh, N. Singh, and S. A. Khan, Detecting diseases of neglected seminal vesicles using imaging modalities: A review of current literature, *Int J Reprod Biomed (Yazd)*, 14, 293–302, 2016.

82. G. A. Sonn, D. J. Margolis, and L. S. Marks, Target detection: Magnetic resonance imaging-ultrasound fusion-guided prostate biopsy, *Urol Oncol*, 32, 903–11, 2014.

83. M. M. Siddiqui, A. K. George, R. Rubin, S. Rais-Bahrami, H. L. Parnes, M. J. Merino, et al., Efficiency of prostate cancer diagnosis by MR/ultrasound fusion-guided biopsy vs standard extended-sextant biopsy for MR-visible lesions, *J Natl Cancer Inst*, 108, 2016.

84. M. M. Siddiqui, S. Rais-Bahrami, H. Truong, L. Stamatakis, S. Vourganti, J. Nix, et al., Magnetic resonance imaging/ultrasound-fusion biopsy significantly upgrades prostate cancer versus systematic 12-core transrectal ultrasound biopsy, *Eur Urol*, 64, 713–19, 2013.

85. A. S. Somwaru, D. Alex, and A. K. Zaheer, Prostate cancer arising in ectopic prostatic tissue within the left seminal vesicle: A rare case diagnosed with multi-parametric magnetic resonance imaging and magnetic resonance imaging-transrectal ultrasound fusion biopsy, *BMC Med Imaging*, 16, 16, 2016.

86. D. V. Makarov, B. J. Trock, E. B. Humphreys, L. A. Mangold, P. C. Walsh, J. I. Epstein, et al., Updated nomogram to predict pathologic stage of prostate cancer given prostate-specific antigen level, clinical stage, and biopsy Gleason score (Partin tables) based on cases from 2000 to 2005, *Urology*, 69, 1095–101, 2007.

87. A. R. Zlotta, T. Roumeguere, V. Ravery, P. Hoffmann, F. Montorsi, L. Turkeri, et al., Is seminal vesicle ablation mandatory for all patients undergoing radical prostatectomy? A multivariate analysis on 1283 patients, *Eur Urol*, 46, 42–9, 2004.

88. A. Gallina, F. K. Chun, A. Briganti, S. F. Shariat, F. Montorsi, A. Salonia, et al., Development and split-sample validation of a nomogram predicting the probability of seminal vesicle invasion at radical prostatectomy, *Eur Urol*, 52, 98–105, 2007.

89. L. Wang, H. Hricak, M. W. Kattan, H. N. Chen, K. Kuroiwa, H. F. Eisenberg, et al., Prediction of seminal vesicle invasion in prostate cancer: Incremental value of adding endorectal MR imaging to the Kattan nomogram, *Radiology*, 242, 182–8, 2007.

90. G. Lughezzani, K. C. Zorn, L. Budaus, M. Sun, D. I. Lee, A. L. Shalhav, et al., Comparison of three different tools for prediction of seminal vesicle invasion at radical prostatectomy, *Eur Urol*, 62, 590–6, 2012.

91. J. O. Barentsz, J. Richenberg, R. Clements, P. Choyke, S. Verma, G. Villeirs, et al., ESUR prostate MR guidelines 2012, *Eur Radiol*, 22, 746–57, 2012.

92. M. Roach, 3rd, G. Hanks, H. Thames, Jr., P. Schellhammer, W. U. Shipley, G. H. Sokol, et al., Defining biochemical failure following radiotherapy with or without hormonal therapy in men with clinically localized prostate cancer: Recommendations of the RTOG-ASTRO Phoenix Consensus Conference, *Int J Radiat Oncol Biol Phys*, 65, 965–74, 2006.

93. S. A. Boorjian, R. H. Thompson, M. K. Tollefson, L. J. Rangel, E. J. Bergstralh, M. L. Blute, et al., Long-term risk of clinical progression after biochemical recurrence following radical prostatectomy: The impact of time from surgery to recurrence, *Eur Urol*, 59, 893–9, 2011.

94. O. Rouviere, T. Vitry, and D. Lyonnet, Imaging of prostate cancer local recurrences: Why and how? *Eur Radiol*, 20, 1254–66, 2010.

95. F. Barchetti and V. Panebianco, Multiparametric MRI for recurrent prostate cancer post radical prostatectomy and postradiation therapy, *Biomed Res Int*, 2014, 316272, 2014.

96. C. R. King and M. T. Spiotto, Improved outcomes with higher doses for salvage radiotherapy after prostatectomy, *Int J Radiat Oncol Biol Phys*, 71, 23–7, 2008.

97. A. Heidenreich, J. Bellmunt, M. Bolla, S. Joniau, M. Mason, V. Matveev, et al., EAU guidelines on prostate cancer. Part 1: Screening, diagnosis, and treatment of clinically localised disease, *Eur Urol*, 59, 61–71, 2011.

98. V. Panebianco, F. Barchetti, M. D. Grompone, A. Colarieti, V. Salvo, G. Cardone, et al., Magnetic resonance imaging for localization of prostate cancer in the setting of biochemical recurrence, *Urol Oncol*, 34, 303–10, 2016.

99. F. J. Bianco, Jr., P. T. Scardino, A. J. Stephenson, C. J. Diblasio, P. A. Fearn, and J. A. Eastham, Long-term oncologic results of salvage radical prostatectomy for locally recurrent prostate cancer after radiotherapy, *Int J Radiat Oncol Biol Phys*, 62, 448–53, 2005.

100. G. L. Gravina, V. Tombolini, M. Di Staso, P. Franzese, P. Bonfili, A. Gennarelli, et al., Advances in imaging and in non-surgical salvage treatments after radiorecurrence in prostate cancer: What does the oncologist, radiotherapist and radiologist need to know?, *Eur Radiol*, 22, 2848–58, 2012.

101. F. V. Coakley, H. Hricak, A. E. Wefer, J. L. Speight, J. Kurhanewicz, and M. Roach, Brachytherapy for prostate cancer: Endorectal MR imaging of local treatment-related changes, *Radiology*, 219, 817–21, 2001.

102. A. C. Westphalen, G. D. Reed, P. P. Vinh, C. Sotto, D. B. Vigneron, and J. Kurhanewicz, Multiparametric 3T endorectal MRI after external beam radiation therapy for prostate cancer, *J Magn Reson Imaging*, 36, 430–7, 2012.

103. D. M. Nudell, A. E. Wefer, H. Hricak, and P. R. Carroll, Imaging for recurrent prostate cancer, *Radiol Clin North Am*, 38, 213–29, 2000.

104. D. Yakar, T. Hambrock, H. Huisman, C. A. Hulsbergen-van de Kaa, E. van Lin, H. Vergunst, et al., Feasibility of 3T dynamic contrast-enhanced magnetic resonance-guided biopsy in localizing local recurrence of prostate cancer after external beam radiation therapy, *Invest Radiol*, 45, 121–5, 2010.

105. C. Roy, F. Foudi, J. Charton, M. Jung, H. Lang, C. Saussine, et al., Comparative sensitivities of functional MRI sequences in detection of local recurrence of prostate carcinoma after radical prostatectomy or external-beam radiotherapy, *AJR Am J Roentgenol*, 200, W361–8, 2013.

106. J. I. Epstein, M. Carmichael, and P. C. Walsh, Adenocarcinoma of the prostate invading the seminal vesicle: Definition and relation of tumor volume, grade and margins of resection to prognosis, *J Urol*, 149, 1040–5, 1993.

107. L. Salomon, A. G. Anastasiadis, C. W. Johnson, J. M. McKiernan, E. T. Goluboff, C. C. Abbou, et al., Seminal vesicle involvement after radical prostatectomy: Predicting risk factors for progression, *Urology*, 62, 304–309, 2003.

108. B. Debras, B. Guillonneau, J. Bougaran, E. Chambon, and G. Vallancien, Prognostic significance of seminal vesicle invasion on the radical prostatectomy specimen: Rationale for seminal vesicle biopsies, *Eur Urol*, 33, 271–7, 1998.

109. M. Sofer, M. Savoie, S. S. Kim, F. Civantos, and M. S. Soloway, Biochemical and pathological predictors of the recurrence of prostatic adenocarcinoma with seminal vesicle invasion, *J Urol*, 169, 153–6, 2003.

Index

Note: Page numbers in italic and bold refer to figures and tables respectively.